MW01533464

Association.

2020
AMERICAN HEART ASSOCIATION
GUIDELINES
FOR CPR AND ECC

Supplement to ***Circulation*** • Volume 142 • Number 16 • Supplement 2 • October 20, 2020

ISBN 978-1-61669-767-9
Printed in the United States of America

First American Heart Association Printing November 2020
5 4 3 2 1

Circulation

SUPPLEMENT

2020 AMERICAN HEART ASSOCIATION GUIDELINES FOR CARDIOPULMONARY RESUSCITATION AND EMERGENCY CARDIOVASCULAR CARE

70th ANNIVERSARY

American Heart Association.

ISSN 0009-7322
Volume 142. Number 16. Suppl 2. October 20, 2020
www.ahajournals.org/journal/circ

Supplement to Circulation

2020 American Heart Association Guidelines for Cardiopulmonary Resuscitation and Emergency Cardiovascular Care

On behalf of the American Heart Association Emergency Cardiovascular Care Committee

Editors

Eric J. Lavonas, MD, MS (Coeditor)
David J. Magid, MD, MPH (Coeditor)

Associate Editors

Eric J. Lavonas, MD, MS (Coeditor)
David J. Magid, MD, MPH (Coeditor)
Khalid Aziz, MBBS, MA, MEd(IT) (Neonatal Writing Group Chair)
Katherine M. Berg, MD (Adult Writing Group Vice Chair)
Adam Cheng, MD (EIT Writing Group Chair)
Aaron Donoghue, MD, MSCE (EIT Writing Group Vice Chair)
Henry C. Lee, MD (Neonatal Writing Group Vice Chair)
Raina M. Merchant, MD, MSHP (ECC Chair)
Ashish R. Panchal, MD, PhD (Adult Writing Group Chair)
Tia T. Raymond, MD (Pediatric Writing Group Vice Chair)
Alexis A. Topjian, MD, MSCE (Pediatric Writing Group Chair)

Acknowledgments

We acknowledge the considerable contributions made by Amber Hoover, Melissa Mahgoub, Amber Rodriguez, and Veronica Zamora, as well as Paula Blackwell, Jenna Joiner, Michelle Reneau, Kara Robinson, Dava Walker, Joe Loftin, Jody Hundley, Julie Scroggins, Sarah Johnson, and Gabrielle Hayes.

American Heart Association.

Circulation

Part 1: Executive Summary

2020 American Heart Association Guidelines for Cardiopulmonary Resuscitation and Emergency Cardiovascular Care

Raina M. Merchant, MD, MSHP
Alexis A. Topjian, MD, MSCE
Ashish R. Panchal, MD, PhD
Adam Cheng, MD
Khalid Aziz, MBBS, MA, MEd(IT)
Katherine M. Berg, MD
Eric J. Lavonas, MD, MS
David J. Magid, MD, MPH
On behalf of the Adult Basic and Advanced Life Support, Pediatric Basic and Advanced Life Support, Neonatal Life Support, Resuscitation Education Science, and Systems of Care Writing Groups

INTRODUCTION

The *2020 American Heart Association* (AHA) *Guidelines for Cardiopulmonary Resuscitation* (CPR) *and Emergency Cardiovascular Care* provides a comprehensive review of evidence-based recommendations for resuscitation and emergency cardiovascular care. The initial guidelines for CPR were published in 1966 by an ad hoc CPR Committee of the Division of Medical Sciences, National Academy of Sciences—National Research Council.[1] This occurred in response to requests from several organizations and agencies about the need for standards and guidelines regarding training and response.

Since then, CPR guidelines have been reviewed, updated, and published periodically by the AHA.[2–9] In 2015, the process of 5-year updates was transitioned to an online format that uses a continuous evidence evaluation process rather than periodic reviews. This allowed for significant changes in science to be reviewed in an expedited manner and then incorporated directly into the guidelines if deemed appropriate. The intent was that this would increase the potential for more immediate transitions from guidelines to bedside. The approach for this 2020 guidelines document reflects alignment with the International Liaison Committee on Resuscitation (ILCOR) and associated member councils and includes varying levels of evidence reviews specific to the scientific questions considered of greatest clinical significance and new evidence.

Over a half-century after the initial guidelines were published, cardiac arrest remains a leading cause of mortality and morbidity in the United States and other countries worldwide. As reported in the AHA "Heart Disease and Stroke Statistics—2020 Update," emergency medical services respond to more than 347 000 adults and more than 7000 children (less than 18 years of age) with out-of-hospital cardiac arrest (OHCA) each year in the United States.[10] In-hospital cardiac arrest (IHCA) is estimated to occur in 9.7 per 1000 adult cardiac arrests (approximately 292 000 events annually) and 2.7 pediatric events per 1000 hospitalizations.[11] In addition, approximately 1% of newly born infants in the United States need intensive resuscitative measures to restore cardiorespiratory function.[12,13]

Overall, although both adult and pediatric IHCA outcomes have improved steadily since 2004, similar gains are not being seen in OHCA.[10] The proportion of adult patients with return of spontaneous circulation (ROSC) following OHCA that is attended by emergency medical services has remained essentially unchanged since 2012.[10]

Much of the variation in survival rates is thought to be due to the strength of the Chain of Survival (Figure 1), the critical actions that must occur in rapid succession to maximize the chance of survival from cardiac arrest.[14] A sixth link, recovery, has been added to each Chain with this version of the guidelines to emphasize the importance of recovery and survivorship for resuscitation outcomes. Analogous Chains of Survival have also been developed for pediatric OHCA and for both adult and pediatric IHCA. Similarly, successful neonatal resuscitation depends on a continuum of integrated lifesaving steps that begins with careful assessment and

Key Words: AHA Scientific Statements ■ apnea ■ automated external defibrillator ■ capnography ■ cardiopulmonary resuscitation ■ defibrillators ■ delivery of health care ■ echocardiography ■ electric countershock ■ epinephrine ■ extracorporeal membrane oxygenation ■ heart arrest ■ infusions, intraosseous ■ intubation, intratracheal ■ life support care ■ respiration, artificial ■ shock, cardiogenic ■ shock, septic

https://www.ahajournals.org/journal/circ

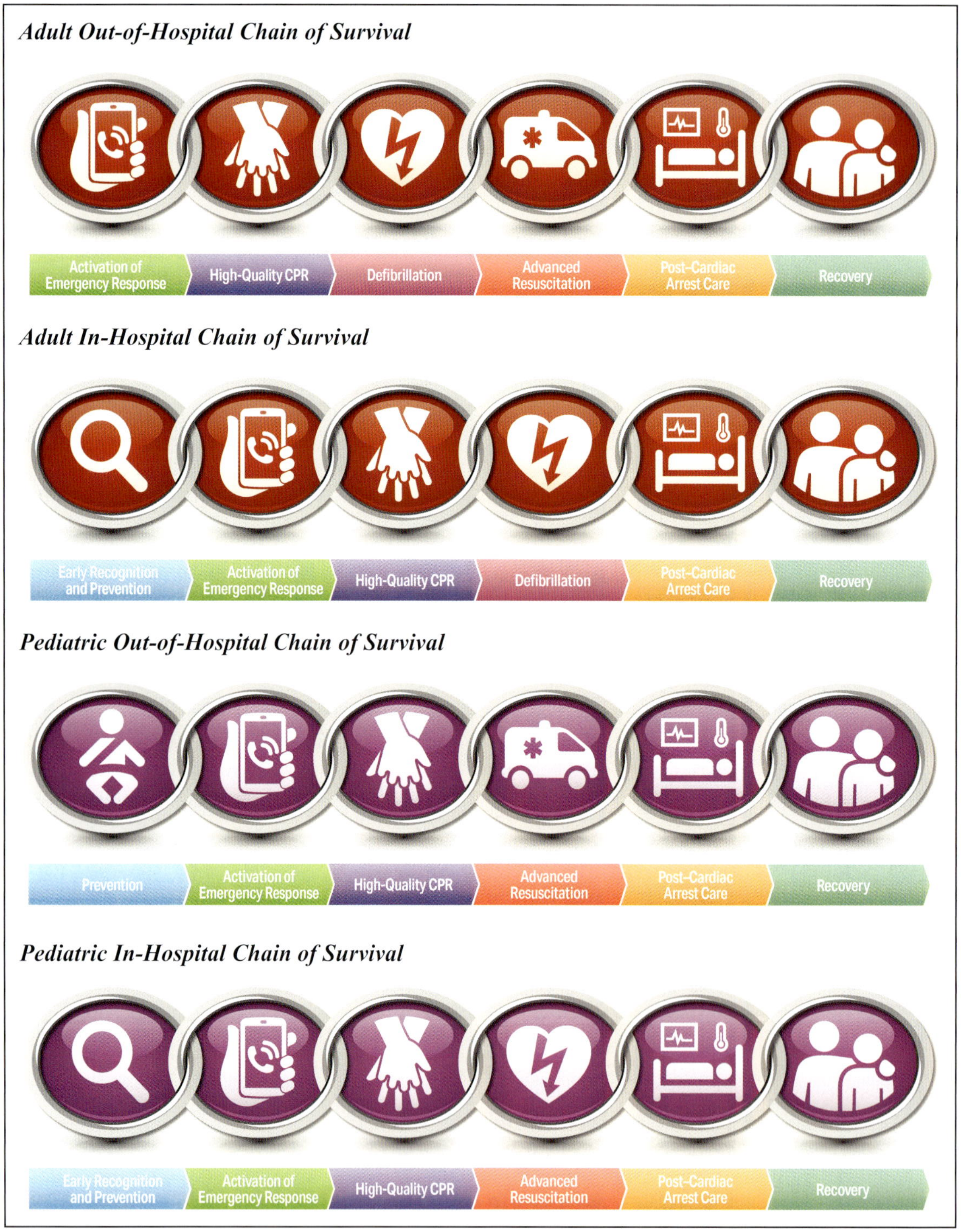

Figure 1. The American Heart Association Chains of Survival.
CPR indicates cardiopulmonary resuscitation.

preparation in advance of birth as well as resuscitation and stabilization at the time of birth and through the first 28 days after birth.[15]

This executive summary provides an overview of and orientation to the 2020 AHA Guidelines, which are organized around the Utstein Formula for Survival (Figure 2).[16]

Each section in this summary describes the scope of each guideline Part, along with a list of the most significant and impactful new or updated recommendations for that Part. Each section also includes a list of critical knowledge gaps that highlights important research questions and significant opportunities for enhancing the Chain of Survival. This executive summary does not contain extensive external reference citations; the reader is referred to Parts 2 through 7 for more detailed reviews of the scientific evidence and corresponding recommendations.[15,17–21]

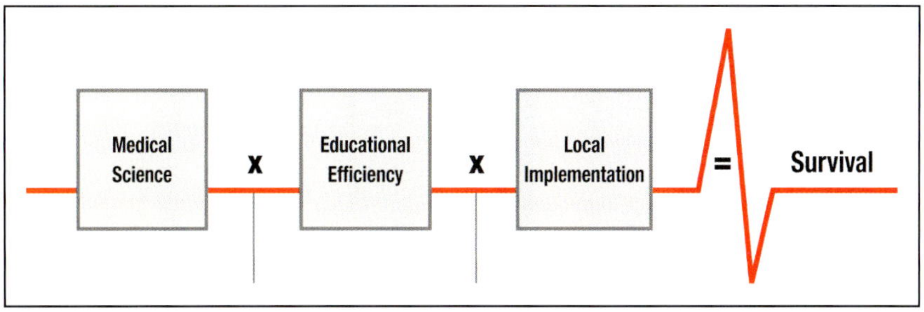

Figure 2. The Utstein Formula for Survival, emphasizing the 3 components essential to improving survival.[16]

Coronavirus Disease 2019 (COVID-19) Guidance

Together with other professional societies, the AHA has provided interim guidance for basic life support (BLS) and advanced life support (ALS) in adults, children, and neonates with suspected or confirmed COVID-19 infection. Because the evidence and guidance are evolving with the COVID-19 situation, that information is maintained separately from the ECC guidelines. Readers are directed to the AHA website[22] for the most recent guidance.

EVIDENCE EVALUATION AND GUIDELINES DEVELOPMENT[19]

The 2020 Guidelines are based on the extensive evidence evaluation performed in conjunction with ILCOR and the affiliated ILCOR member councils. Three different types of evidence reviews (systematic reviews, scoping reviews, and evidence updates) were used in the 2020 process. Each of these resulted in a description of the literature that facilitated guideline development.[23–28] The ILCOR evidence reviews used Grading of Recommendations Assessment, Development, and Evaluation methodology and terminology.[29] These AHA treatment recommendations followed standard AHA processes and nomenclature, which are described fully in "Part 2: Evidence Evaluation and Guidelines Development."[19]

Each AHA writing group reviewed all relevant and current AHA guidelines for CPR and emergency cardiovascular care,[30–41] pertinent *2020 International Consensus on CPR and Emergency Cardiovascular Care Science With Treatment Recommendations* evidence evaluations and recommendations,[42–48] and all relevant evidence update worksheets to determine whether current guidelines should be reaffirmed, updated, or retired or if new recommendations were needed. The writing groups then drafted, reviewed, and approved recommendations, assigning to each a Class of Recommendation (COR; ie, strength) and Level of Evidence (LOE; ie, quality) (as outlined in Table 3 in Part 2 of this supplement).[19]

The 2020 Guidelines contain 491 recommendations (Table). Despite recent improvements in support for resuscitation research, 51% of these recommendations are based on limited data and 17% on expert opinion. This highlights the persistent knowledge gaps in resuscitation science that need to be addressed through expanded research initiatives and funding opportunities. With reference to these gaps, we acknowledge the importance of addressing the values and preferences of our key stakeholders: the patients, families, and teams who are involved in the process of resuscitation.

The 2020 Guidelines are organized into knowledge chunks, grouped into discrete modules of information on specific topics or management issues.[49] Each modular knowledge chunk includes a table of recommendations, a brief introduction or synopsis, recommendation-specific supportive text, hyperlinked references, and, when relevant, figures, flow diagrams of algorithms, and additional tables.

Abbreviations

Abbreviation	Meaning/Phrase
ACLS	advanced cardiovascular life support
AED	automated external defibrillator
AHA	American Heart Association
ALS	advanced life support
BLS	basic life support
COR	Class of Recommendation
CPR	cardiopulmonary resuscitation
IHCA	in-hospital cardiac arrest
ILCOR	International Liaison Committee on Resuscitation
LOE	Level of Evidence
OHCA	out-of-hospital cardiac arrest
PPV	positive-pressure ventilation
ROSC	return of spontaneous circulation

ADULT BASIC AND ADVANCED LIFE SUPPORT[20]

"Part 3: Adult Basic and Advanced Life Support" includes a comprehensive set of recommendations for the care of adult victims of OHCA and IHCA. We reaffirm the critical steps in the Chain of Survival, expand on the postresuscitative care section with the addition of an updated algorithm, and introduce a new link in the Chain of Survival, for recovery and survivorship. The main focus in managing adult cardiac arrest includes

Table. Recommendations in the 2020 Guidelines

Classification	Adult Basic and Advanced Life Support	Pediatric Basic and Advanced Life Support	Neonatal Resuscitation	Resuscitation Education Science	Systems of Care	Total	Percent
Class (Strength) of Recommendation							
1 (strong)	78	53	16	5	9	161	33%
2a (moderate)	57	42	14	13	10	135	27%
2b (weak)	89	30	21	11	6	158	32%
3: No benefit (moderate)	15	1	3	0	0	19	4%
3: Harm (strong)	11	4	3	0	0	18	4%
Level (Quality) of Evidence							
A	2	1	2	1	0	6	1%
B-R	37	3	8	7	1	55	11%
B-NR	57	19	8	5	8	97	20%
C-LD	123	70	24	15	15	248	51%
C-EO	31	37	15	1	1	85	17%
Total	250	130	57	29	25	491	

EO indicates expert opinion; LD, limited data; NR, nonrandomized; and R, randomized.

rapid recognition, prompt provision of CPR, and defibrillation of ventricular fibrillation and pulseless ventricular tachycardia. Since 2010, the AHA has directed efforts at minimizing the time to provision of chest compressions by focusing the universal sequence of responses on compressions followed by airway and breathing. The 2020 Guidelines continue to highlight the critical importance of chest compressions and leverage current relevant evidence to optimize care and improve survival. Additional recommendations relevant to adult resuscitation appear in "Part 7: Systems of Care."[18]

Adult Basic and Advanced Life Support: Significant New, Updated, and Reaffirmed Recommendations

- *CPR reaffirmed:* Provision of CPR has long been the hallmark of cardiac arrest management. Updated evidence from an analysis of over 12 500 patients[50] reaffirms the importance of chest compression quality as well as the following:
  - During manual CPR, rescuers should perform chest compressions to a depth of at least 2 inches, or 5 cm, for an average adult while avoiding excessive chest compression depths (greater than 2.4 inches, or 6 cm)(Class 1, LOE B-NR).[51–54]
  - It is reasonable for rescuers to perform chest compressions at a rate of 100 to 120/min (Class 2a, LOE B-NR).[50,55]

Furthermore, from a new systematic review,[44] we recommend that lay rescuers initiate CPR for presumed cardiac arrest because the risk of harm to patients is low if they are not in cardiac arrest (Class 1, LOE C-LD).[56–59]

- *Double sequential defibrillation:* Along with CPR, early defibrillation is critical to survival when sudden cardiac arrest is caused by ventricular fibrillation or pulseless ventricular tachycardia. However, rescuers may encounter victims who are refractory to defibrillation attempts. Double sequential defibrillation—shock delivery by 2 defibrillators nearly simultaneously—has emerged as a new technological approach to manage these patients.[60–64] At this time, a systematic review reveals that the usefulness of double sequential defibrillation for refractory shockable rhythm has not been established (Class 2b, LOE C-LD).[48]
- *Intravenous (IV) before intraosseous (IO):* The peripheral IV route has been the traditional approach for giving emergency pharmacotherapy, although the IO route has grown in popularity and is increasingly implemented as a first-line approach for vascular access. New evidence suggests some uncertainty about the efficacy of the IO route compared with the IV route.[65–69] Therefore, it is reasonable for providers to first attempt establishing IV access for drug administration in cardiac arrest (Class 2a, LOE B-NR). IO access may be considered if attempts at IV access are unsuccessful or not feasible (Class 2b, LOE B-NR).
- *Early epinephrine administration reaffirmed:* In 2 randomized clinical trials,[70,71] administration of epinephrine increased ROSC and survival, leading to a recommendation that epinephrine be administered for patients in cardiac arrest (Class 1, LOE B-R).[40,72] Uncertainty about the effect of epinephrine on neurological outcome, in addition to the variation in outcomes based on timing and initial rhythm, supported the following new concepts:
  - With respect to timing, for cardiac arrest with a nonshockable rhythm, it is reasonable to administer epinephrine as soon as feasible (Class 2a, C-LD).

Circulation. 2020;142(suppl 2):S337–S357. DOI: 10.1161/CIR.0000000000000918

- With respect to timing, for cardiac arrest with a shockable rhythm, it may be reasonable to administer epinephrine after initial defibrillation attempts have failed (Class 2b, C-LD).

The Adult Cardiac Arrest Algorithm has been updated to emphasize the early administration of epinephrine for patients with nonshockable rhythms.

- *Individualized management of resuscitation:* Not all cardiac arrest events are identical, and specialized management may be critical for optimal patient outcome, such as when the primary etiology of arrest is respiratory, a gravid uterus impedes venous return, or resuscitation involves a viable fetus. In the Special Circumstances of Resuscitation section, we highlight 2 such areas (opioid overdose and cardiac arrest in pregnancy):
  - *Opioid overdose:* The opioid epidemic has resulted in an increase in respiratory and cardiac arrests due to opioid overdose.[73] To address this public health crisis, we present 2 new algorithms for the management of opioid-associated emergencies, highlighting that lay rescuers and trained responders should not delay activating emergency response systems while awaiting the patient's response to naloxone or other interventions (Class 1, LOE E-O). Additionally, for patients known or suspected to be in cardiac arrest, in the absence of a proven benefit from the use of naloxone, standard resuscitative measures should take priority over naloxone administration, with a focus on high-quality CPR (compressions plus ventilation) (Class 1, LOE E-O).[73]
  - *Cardiac arrest in pregnancy:* We present updated recommendations and a new algorithm highlighting the concept that the best outcomes for both mother and fetus are through successful maternal resuscitation.[74] Team planning for cardiac arrest in pregnancy should be done in collaboration with the obstetric, neonatal, emergency, anesthesiology, intensive care, and cardiac arrest services (Class 1, LOE C-LD). Priorities for treating the pregnant woman in cardiac arrest should include provision of high-quality CPR and relief of aortocaval compression through left lateral uterine displacement (Class 1, LOE C-LD). If the pregnant woman with a fundus height at or above the umbilicus has not obtained ROSC with usual resuscitation measures plus manual left lateral uterine displacement, it is advisable to prepare to evacuate the uterus while resuscitation continues (Class 1, LOE C-LD).[75–79] To accomplish delivery early, ideally within 5 minutes after the time of arrest, it is reasonable to immediately prepare for perimortem cesarean delivery while initial BLS and advanced cardiovascular life support (ACLS) interventions are being performed (Class 2a, LOE C-EO), although provider skill set and available personnel and resources may also logically influence this timing.[74]
- *Point-of-care ultrasound for prognostication:* Many have attempted to leverage the use of new technologies like portable ultrasound machines to provide guidance in making decisions on futility and termination of resuscitation. However, on the basis of a synthesis of the evidence,[48] we suggest against the use of point-of-care ultrasound for prognostication during CPR (Class 3: No benefit, LOE C-LD). This recommendation does not preclude the use of ultrasound to identify potentially reversible causes of cardiac arrest or detect ROSC.
- *Postresuscitative care:* Post–cardiac arrest care, a critical component of the Chain of Survival, demands a comprehensive, structured, multidisciplinary system of care that should be implemented in a consistent manner for the treatment of post–cardiac arrest patients (Class 1, LOE B-NR).[40,80] We present a new algorithm that describes the initial stabilization phase and additional emergency activities after ROSC. Key considerations include blood pressure management, monitoring for and treatment of seizures, and targeted temperature management.
- *Improving neuroprognostication*: Accurate neurological prognostication in cardiac arrest survivors who do not regain consciousness with ROSC is critically important to ensure that patients with significant potential for recovery are not destined for certain poor outcomes due to care withdrawal.[81] With updated systematic reviews on multiple aspects of neuroprognostication,[48] in patients who remain comatose after cardiac arrest, we recommend that neuroprognostication involve a multimodal approach and not be based on any single finding (Class 1, LOE B-NR).[48,81] To assist in this process, we have developed evidence-based guidance to facilitate multimodal prognostication. This includes the following:
  - In patients who remain comatose after cardiac arrest, we recommend that neuroprognostication be delayed until adequate time has passed to ensure avoidance of confounding by medication effect or a transiently poor examination in the early postinjury period (Class 1, LOE B-NR).[82]
  - In patients who remain comatose after cardiac arrest, it is reasonable to perform multimodal neuroprognostication at a minimum of 72 hours after the return to normothermia, though individual prognostic tests may be obtained earlier than this (Class 2a, LOE B-NR).[48]

Further, we provide specific guidance on the use of clinical examination, serum biomarkers, electrophysiological tests, and neuroimaging for neuroprognostication.

- *Recovery and survivorship:* Finally, we have added an additional link in the Chain of Survival: recovery from cardiac arrest. Recovery expectations and survivorship plans that address treatment, surveillance, and rehabilitation need to be provided to cardiac arrest survivors and their caregivers at hospital discharge to address the sequelae of cardiac arrest and optimize transitions of care to independent physical, social, emotional, and role function.[83] Recommendations that are critically important to this concept include the following:
  - We recommend structured assessment for anxiety, depression, posttraumatic stress, and fatigue for cardiac arrest survivors and their caregivers (Class 1, LOE B-NR)[83–87]
  - We recommend that cardiac arrest survivors have multimodal rehabilitation assessment and treatment for physical, neurological, cardiopulmonary, and cognitive impairments before discharge from the hospital (Class 1, LOE C-LD).[83,88–90]
  - We recommend that cardiac arrest survivors and their caregivers receive comprehensive, multidisciplinary discharge planning, to include medical and rehabilitative treatment recommendations and return to activity/work expectations (Class 1, LOE C-LD).[83]

Knowledge Gaps

Some of the most pertinent gaps in adult resuscitation research include the following:

- What are optimal strategies to enhance lay rescuer performance of CPR?
- For patients with an arterial line in place, does targeting CPR to a particular blood pressure improve outcomes?
- Can artifact-filtering algorithms for analysis of ECG rhythms during CPR in a real-time clinical setting decrease pauses in chest compressions and improve outcomes?
- Does preshock waveform analysis lead to improved outcome?
- Does double sequential defibrillation and/or alternative defibrillator pad positioning affect outcome in cardiac arrest with shockable rhythm?
- Is the IO route of drug administration safe and efficacious in cardiac arrest, and does efficacy vary by IO site?
- Does epinephrine, when administered early after cardiac arrest, improve survival with favorable neurological outcome?
- Does the use of point-of-care cardiac ultrasound during cardiac arrest improve outcomes?
- Is targeting a specific partial pressure of end-tidal carbon dioxide ($ETCO_2$) value during CPR beneficial, and what degree of rise in $ETCO_2$ indicates ROSC?
- Which populations are most likely to benefit from extracorporeal CPR?
- Does the treatment of nonconvulsive seizures, which are common in postarrest patients, improve patient outcomes?
- Do neuroprotective agents improve favorable neurological outcome after cardiac arrest?
- What is the most efficacious management approach for postarrest cardiogenic shock, including pharmacological, catheter intervention, or implantable device?
- Does targeted temperature management, compared with strict normothermia, improve outcomes?
- What is the optimal duration for targeted temperature management before rewarming?
- What is the best approach to rewarming postarrest patients after treatment with targeted temperature management?
- Are glial fibrillary acidic protein, serum tau protein, and neurofilament light chain measurements valuable for neuroprognostication?
- Do more uniform definitions for status epilepticus, malignant electroencephalogram patterns, and other electroencephalogram patterns enable better comparisons of their prognostic values across studies?
- Is there a consistent threshold value for prognostication for gray-white ratio or apparent diffusion coefficient?
- What do survivor-derived outcome measures of the impact of cardiac arrest survival look like, and how do they differ from current generic or clinician-derived measures?
- Does hospital-based protocolized discharge planning for cardiac arrest survivors improve access to/referral to rehabilitation services or patient outcomes?
- Is there benefit to naloxone administration in patients with opioid-associated cardiac arrest who are receiving CPR with ventilation?
- What is the ideal initial dose of naloxone in a setting where fentanyl and fentanyl analogues are responsible for a large proportion of opioid overdose?
- In cases of suspected opioid overdose managed by a non–healthcare provider who is not capable of reliably checking a pulse, is initiation of CPR beneficial?

- What is the ideal timing of perimortem cesarean delivery for a pregnant woman in cardiac arrest?
- Which patients with cardiac arrest due to "suspected" pulmonary embolism benefit from emergency thrombolysis during resuscitation?

PEDIATRIC BASIC AND ADVANCED LIFE SUPPORT[21]

Part 4 of the 2020 Guidelines, "Pediatric Basic and Advanced Life Support," includes recommendations for the treatment of pediatric OHCA and IHCA, including postresuscitation care and survivorship. The causes, treatment, and outcomes of cardiac arrest in children differ from cardiac arrest in adults. For example, pediatric cardiac arrests are more often due to respiratory causes. These guidelines contain recommendations for pediatric BLS and ALS, excluding the newborn period, and are based on the best available resuscitation science. Expansions to pediatric ALS recommendations include care of the child with pulmonary hypertension, congenital heart disease, and post–cardiac arrest recovery. This summary highlights the new and updated recommendations in pediatric BLS and ALS since 2015 that we believe will have a significant impact on process and on patient-related outcomes from cardiac arrest. Additional recommendations related to pediatric resuscitation can be found in "Part 7: Systems of Care."

Significant New and Updated Recommendations

- *Respiratory rate:* Respiratory rates during pediatric CPR have previously been extrapolated from adult data, because of lack of pediatric studies. New data about respiratory rates during CPR in children are now available. Although limited, these data support a higher respiratory rate for children with an advanced airway than was previously recommended.[91] When performing CPR in infants and children with an advanced airway, it may be reasonable to target a respiratory rate range of 1 breath every 2 to 3 seconds (20–30 breaths/min), accounting for age and clinical condition. Rates exceeding these recommendations may compromise hemodynamics (Class 2b, LOE C-LD).[91] For infants and children with a pulse but absent or inadequate respiratory effort, it is reasonable to give 1 breath every 2 to 3 seconds (20–30 breaths/min) (Class 2a, LOE C-EO).[91]
- *Cuffed endotracheal tubes:* Intubation with a cuffed endotracheal tube can improve capnography and ventilation in patients with poor pulmonary compliance and decrease the need for endotracheal tube changes. It is reasonable to choose cuffed endotracheal tubes over uncuffed endotracheal tubes for intubating infants and children (Class 2a, LOE C-LD).[92–98]
- *Cricoid pressure:* Although cricoid pressure may be useful in certain circumstances, routine use can impede visualization during laryngoscopy and chest rise with bag-mask ventilation. Clinical studies show that routine use of cricoid pressure reduces the rate of first-attempt intubation success. Routine use of cricoid pressure is not recommended during endotracheal intubation of pediatric patients (Class 3: No benefit, LOE C-LD),[99,100] and if cricoid pressure is used, discontinue if it interferes with ventilation or the speed or ease of intubation (Class 3: Harm, LOE C-LD).[99,100]
- *Early epinephrine:* The goal of epinephrine administration during CPR is to optimize coronary perfusion pressure and maintain cerebral perfusion pressure. Earlier administration of epinephrine during CPR may increase survival-to-discharge rates. For pediatric patients in any setting, it is reasonable to administer the initial dose of epinephrine within 5 minutes from the start of chest compressions (Class 2a, LOE C-LD).[101–104]
- *Diastolic blood pressure to guide CPR:* For patients with continuous invasive arterial blood pressure monitoring in place at the time of cardiac arrest, it is reasonable for providers to use diastolic blood pressure to assess CPR quality (Class 2a, LOE C-LD).[105] Although ideal blood pressure targets during CPR are not known, diastolic blood pressure is the main driver of coronary blood flow and may be used to guide interventions if an arterial line is in place.
- *Seizures after cardiac arrest:* Post–cardiac arrest seizures are common. Many are nonconvulsive, which can be detected only with electroencephalography monitoring. When resources are available, continuous electroencephalography monitoring is recommended for the detection of seizures after cardiac arrest in patients with persistent encephalopathy (Class 1, LOE C-LD).[106–109] It is recommended to treat clinical seizures that follow cardiac arrest (Class 1, LOE C-LD).[110,111] It is reasonable to treat nonconvulsive status epilepticus that follows cardiac arrest, in consultation with experts (Class 2a, LOE C-EO).[110,111]
- *Recovery and survivorship:* New neurological morbidity after cardiac arrest is common and should be addressed with ongoing assessment and intervention to support patients after hospital discharge. It is recommended that pediatric cardiac arrest survivors be evaluated for rehabilitation services (Class 1, LOE C-LD).[112–117] It is reasonable to refer pediatric cardiac arrest survivors for ongoing neurological

evaluation for at least the first year after cardiac arrest (Class 2a, LOE C-LD).[81,83,115,117–122]

- *Septic shock:* Previous AHA guidelines for the management of septic shock included aggressive (20 mL/kg) fluid boluses and lacked additional guidance. In these 2020 Guidelines, a more tailored approach to fluid administration is suggested, and vasopressor recommendations are provided.
  - In patients with septic shock, it is reasonable to administer fluid in 10-mL/kg or 20-mL/kg aliquots with frequent reassessment (Class 2a, LOE C-LD).[123] Providers should reassess the patient after every fluid bolus to assess for fluid responsiveness and for signs of volume overload (Class 1, LOE C-LD).[123–125]
  - Either isotonic crystalloids or colloids can be effective as the initial fluid choice for resuscitation (Class 2a, LOE B-R).[126] Either balanced or unbalanced solutions can be effective as the fluid choice for resuscitation (Class 2a, LOE B-NR).[127–129]
  - In infants and children with fluid-refractory septic shock, it is reasonable to use either epinephrine or norepinephrine as an initial vasoactive infusion (Class 2a, LOE C-LD).[130–135]
- *Opioid overdose:* Although most victims of opioid overdose are adults, young children suffer opioid overdose from exploratory behavior, and adolescents through opioid abuse or self-harm exposure. Opioid overdose causes respiratory depression, which can progress to respiratory arrest and then cardiac arrest. Pediatric opioid overdose management is the same as for adults. For a patient with suspected opioid overdose who has a definite pulse but no normal breathing or only gasping (ie, a respiratory arrest), in addition to providing standard pediatric BLS or ALS care, it is reasonable for responders to administer intramuscular or intranasal naloxone (Class 2a, LOE B-NR).[136–149] Empirical administration of intramuscular or intranasal naloxone to all unresponsive opioid-associated life-threatening emergency patients may be reasonable as an adjunct to standard first aid and non–healthcare provider BLS protocols (Class 2b, LOE C-EO).[137–145,147–150] New opioid-associated emergency algorithms for lay rescuers and healthcare professionals are provided.

Knowledge Gaps

Some of the most pertinent gaps in pediatric resuscitation research include the following:

- What is the optimal route of medication delivery during CPR: IV or IO?
- In what time frame should the first dose of epinephrine be administered during pulseless cardiac arrest?
- With what frequency should subsequent doses of epinephrine be administered?
- With what frequency should the rhythm be checked during CPR?
- What are the optimal chest compression rate and ventilation rate during CPR? Are they age dependent? Do they differ when an advanced airway is in place?
- Are there specific situations in which advanced airway placement is either beneficial or harmful in OHCA or IHCA? Do they differ based on the etiology of cardiac arrest?
- Can echocardiography improve CPR quality or outcomes from cardiac arrest?
- What is the role of extracorporeal CPR for infants and children with OHCA and IHCA due to noncardiac causes?
- What is the optimal timing and dosing of defibrillation for ventricular fibrillation and pulseless ventricular tachycardia?
- What clinical tools can be used to help in the decision to terminate pediatric IHCA and OHCA resuscitation?
- What is the optimal blood pressure target during the post–cardiac arrest period?
- What are the reliable methods for postarrest prognostication?
- What rehabilitation therapies and follow-up should be provided to improve outcomes after cardiac arrest?
- What are the most effective and safe medications for adenosine-refractory supraventricular tachycardia?

NEONATAL LIFE SUPPORT[15]

Part 5 of the AHA 2020 Guidelines, "Neonatal Life Support,"[15] includes recommendations on how to follow the algorithm that include anticipation and preparation, umbilical cord management at delivery, initial actions, heart rate monitoring, respiratory support, chest compressions, intravascular access and therapies, withholding and discontinuation of resuscitation, postresuscitation care, and human factors and performance. Consistent with the Utstein Formula for Survival, the 2020 Guidelines provide a comprehensive review of recommendations for neonatal resuscitation, including new and updated recommendations that are based on the latest evidence from studies published in the medical literature and reviews completed by ILCOR.

Significant New and Updated Recommendations

- *Skin-to-skin contact:* Placing healthy newborn infants who do not require resuscitation skin-to-skin after birth can be effective in improving breastfeeding, temperature control, and blood glucose stability (Class 2a, LOE B-R). A Cochrane systematic review found that healthy infants receiving skin-to-skin contact were more likely to be breastfed at 1 to 4 months of age. In addition, blood glucose after birth was meaningfully higher and cardiorespiratory stability was also improved with skin-to-skin contact.[151]
- *Intubation for meconium:* For nonvigorous newborns (presenting with apnea or ineffective breathing effort) delivered through meconium-stained amniotic fluid, routine laryngoscopy, with or without tracheal suctioning, is not recommended (Class 3: No benefit, LOE C-LD). For nonvigorous newborns delivered through meconium-stained amniotic fluid who have evidence of airway obstruction during positive-pressure ventilation (PPV), intubation and tracheal suction can be beneficial (Class 2a, LOE C-EO). Endotracheal suctioning is indicated only if airway obstruction is suspected after providing PPV.[46]
- *Vascular access*: For babies requiring vascular access at the time of delivery, the umbilical vein is the recommended route (Class 1, LOE C-EO). If IV access is not feasible, it may be reasonable to use the IO route (Class 2b, LOE C-EO). Babies who have failed to respond to PPV and chest compressions require vascular access to infuse epinephrine and/or volume expanders. Umbilical venous catheterization is the preferred technique in the delivery room.[46,152] IO access is an alternative if umbilical venous access is not feasible or care is being provided outside of the delivery room.[46]
- *Termination of resuscitation:* In newly born babies receiving resuscitation, if there is no heart rate and all the steps of resuscitation have been performed, cessation of resuscitation efforts should be discussed with the healthcare team and the family. A reasonable time frame for this change in goals of care is around 20 minutes after birth (Class 1, LOE C-LD). Newly born babies who have failed to respond to resuscitative efforts by approximately 20 minutes of age have a low likelihood of survival. For this reason, a time frame for decisions relating to discontinuation of resuscitation efforts is suggested, emphasizing engagement of parents and the resuscitation team before redirecting care.[46,153]

Knowledge Gaps

Some of the most pertinent gaps in neonatal resuscitation research include the following:

- What is the optimal management of the umbilical cord at delivery, especially in the baby who appears to need respiratory support?
- What is the optimal oxygen management at all stages of resuscitation, including when initiating PPV, when providing chest compressions, and after resuscitation?
- What are the optimal dosing, timing, and route of administration for epinephrine?
- What is the optimal management for the detection and treatment of hypovolemia?
- How should neonatal resuscitation be modified in non–delivery room settings?
- What strategies are most effective for optimizing provider and team performance, including training methods, the frequency of retraining intervals, and the approach to briefing, debriefing, and feedback?

RESUSCITATION EDUCATION SCIENCE[17]

Part 6 of the 2020 Guidelines, "Resuscitation Education Science," includes recommendations about various instructional design features in resuscitation training, including deliberate practice, spaced learning, booster training, teamwork and leadership training, in situ education, manikin fidelity, CPR feedback devices, virtual reality and gamified learning, and precourse preparation.[17] We also discuss educational strategies to support lay rescuer training and efforts to address the opioid epidemic. The second section of Part 6 describes how specific provider considerations may influence the impact of educational interventions. We offer recommendations to address disparities in education and in willingness to provide CPR, and we outline how practitioner experience and participation in ACLS courses influence patient outcomes from cardiac arrest. Additional recommendations related to resuscitation education science can be found in "Part 7: Systems of Care."[18]

Significant New and Updated Recommendations

- *Booster training:* It is recommended to implement booster sessions when using a massed learning approach for resuscitation training (Class 1, LOE B-R). Most current resuscitation courses use a massed learning approach: a single training event lasting hours or days coupled with retraining every 1 to 2 years.[154] The addition of booster training sessions (ie, brief, frequent sessions focused on repetition of prior content) to resuscitation courses is associated with improved CPR skill retention over 12 months.[155–161] The frequency of booster sessions should be balanced against learner attrition (ie, higher attrition rates with more frequent sessions[155]) and the availability of resources to support implementation of booster training.

- *Spaced learning:* It is reasonable to use a spaced learning approach in place of a massed learning approach for resuscitation training (Class 2a, LOE B-R).[162–164] In contrast to the traditional or massed learning approach involving a 1- or 2-day course, a spaced learning approach separates training into multiple sessions over time, with intervals of weeks to months between sessions. Each spaced session involves the presentation of new content and may include repetition of content from prior sessions.[162–164] Two randomized clinical trials in pediatric resuscitation training report that a spaced learning approach results in improved clinical performance and technical skills (IO insertion, bag-mask ventilation) in comparison to a traditional 1- or 2-day course.[162,164] Because new content and/or skills are presented at each session, learner attendance across all sessions is required to ensure course completion.
- *Deliberate practice and mastery learning:* Incorporating a deliberate practice and mastery learning model into BLS or ALS courses may be considered for improving skill acquisition and performance (Class 2b, LOE B-NR). *Deliberate practice* is a training approach where learners are given (1) a discrete goal to achieve, (2) immediate feedback on their performance, and (3) ample time for repetition to improve performance.[165] *Mastery learning* is the use of deliberate-practice training along with testing that uses a set of criteria to define a minimum passing standard that implies mastery of the tasks being learned.[166] Studies incorporating a deliberate-practice and mastery-learning model into training demonstrated improved learner performance in resuscitation skills.[167–174] Coupling repetition with feedback and allowing sufficient time to achieve competency are key elements associated with improved outcomes.
- *In situ simulation training:* It is reasonable to conduct in situ simulation-based resuscitation training in addition to traditional training (Class 2a, LOE C-LD). In situ simulation is a form of simulation training activities that occurs in actual patient-care areas.[175] One advantage of in situ training is that it provides learners with a more realistic training environment. In situ training can be focused on the development of individual provider technical skills or team-based skills, including communication, leadership, role allocation, and situational awareness.[176,177] When added to other educational strategies, in situ training has a positive impact on learning and on performance outcomes.[161,164,178–182] The advantages of in situ training should be weighed against the risks of training in clinical spaces.
- *Lay rescuer training:* A combination of self-instruction and instructor-led teaching with hands-on training is recommended as an alternative to instructor-led courses for lay rescuers. If instructor-led training is not available, self-directed training is recommended for lay rescuers (Class 1, LOE C-LD).[183–186] The primary goal of resuscitation training for lay rescuers (ie, non–healthcare professionals) is to increase immediate bystander CPR rates, automated external defibrillator (AED) use, and timely emergency response system activation during an OHCA. Studies comparing self-instruction or video-based instruction with instructor-led training demonstrate no significant differences in performance outcomes.[183–186] A shift to more self-directed training may lead to a higher proportion of trained lay rescuers, thus increasing the chances that a trained lay rescuer will be available during OHCA.
- *Training school-age children:* It is recommended to train middle school– and high school–age children in how to perform high-quality CPR (Class 1, LOE C-LD).[187–195] Training school-age children to perform CPR instills confidence and a positive attitude toward responding to an OHCA event.[187–195] Targeting this population with CPR training helps to build the future cadre of community-based, trained lay rescuers.
- *Disparities in CPR training:* Eliminating disparities in CPR training could improve bystander CPR rates and outcomes from cardiac arrest in populations with historically low rates of bystander CPR. Communities with predominantly black and Hispanic populations and those with lower socioeconomic status have lower rates of bystander CPR and CPR training.[196–206] It is recommended to target and tailor lay rescuer CPR training to specific racial and ethnic populations and neighborhoods in the United States (Class 1, LOE B-NR).[196–200,207–211] It is recommended to target low–socioeconomic status populations and neighborhoods for layperson CPR training and awareness efforts (Class 1, LOE B-NR).[201–206,212–215] Targeting training efforts should consider barriers such as language, financial considerations, and poor access to information.
- *Barriers to bystander CPR for women:* Women are often less likely to receive bystander CPR because rescuers often fear accusations of inappropriate touching, sexual assault, or injuring the victim.[216,217] It is reasonable to address barriers to

bystander CPR for female victims through educational training and public awareness efforts (Class 2a, LOE C-LD).[216–219] Targeted training may help to overcome these barriers and improve bystander CPR rates for female victims.

- *Advanced Cardiovascular Life Support course participation:* It is reasonable for healthcare professionals to take an adult ACLS course or equivalent training (Class 2a, LOE C-LD).[220–228] For more than 3 decades, the ACLS course has been recognized as an essential component of resuscitation training for frontline, acute-care providers. A recent systematic review found that having resuscitation teams with 1 or more team members trained in ACLS results in improved patient outcomes.[228] This recommendation supports the use of the ACLS course as foundational training for acute-care providers.

Knowledge Gaps

Some of the most pertinent gaps in resuscitation education research include the following:

- Which educational interventions most impact real-world performance and clinical outcomes, as opposed to educational outcomes or performance in training?
- How can instructional design features be combined or blended to optimize outcomes? Future studies should evaluate the synergistic effects of instructional design features when used in a blended manner (eg, in situ simulation training delivered as booster sessions).
- What are the most effective ways to train and develop resuscitation instructors? Future research should evaluate the impact of various faculty-development strategies on instructor skills and learner outcomes.

SYSTEMS OF CARE[18]

Part 7 of the 2020 Guidelines focuses on systems of care, with an emphasis on elements that are relevant to a broad range of resuscitation situations and to persons of all ages. The systems of care guidelines are organized around the Chain of Survival, beginning with prevention and early identification of cardiac arrest and proceeding through resuscitation to post–cardiac arrest care and survivorship. Recommendations focused on OHCA include community initiatives to promote cardiac arrest recognition, CPR, public access defibrillation, the use of mobile phone technologies to summon first responders, and an enhanced role for emergency telecommunicators. Relevant to IHCA are recommendations about the recognition and stabilization of hospital patients at risk for developing cardiac arrest. Additional recommendations address clinical debriefing, transport to specialized cardiac arrest centers, organ donation, and performance measurement.

Significant New and Updated Recommendations

- *Summoning willing bystanders:* Emergency dispatch systems should alert willing bystanders to nearby events that may require CPR or AED use through mobile phone technology (Class 1, LOE B-NR). Despite the recognized role of lay rescuers in improving OHCA outcomes, most communities experience low rates of bystander CPR and AED use.[229,230] Mobile phone technology, such as text messages and mobile phone apps, is available to summon trained members of the general public to nearby events to assist in CPR and to direct those responders to the nearest AED.[231] Notification of lay rescuers via a mobile phone app results in improved bystander response times, higher bystander CPR rates, shorter time to defibrillation, and higher rates of survival to hospital discharge.[47] As this technology becomes more ubiquitous, studies exploring the impact of these alerts on cardiac arrest outcomes for diverse patient, community, and geographic contexts are needed.
- *Cognitive aids and checklists:* It may be reasonable to use cognitive aids to improve team performance of healthcare providers during CPR (Class 2b, LOE C-LD). Cognitive aids are prompts designed to help individuals and teams to recall information, complete tasks, and adhere to guideline recommendations.[232] Examples include pocket cards, posters, checklists, mobile apps, and mnemonics. Although the use of cognitive aids in trauma resuscitation improves adherence to resuscitation guidelines, reduces errors, and improves survival,[233–236] there are no studies evaluating their use by healthcare teams in cardiac arrest.[47]
- *Data for continuous improvement:* Continuous improvement starts with disciplined collection and evaluation of data on resuscitation performance and outcomes. It is reasonable for organizations that treat cardiac arrest patients to collect processes-of-care data and outcomes (Class 2a, LOE C-LD). Clinical registries collect information on the processes of care (CPR performance, defibrillation times) and outcomes of care (ROSC, survival) associated with real-world management of cardiac arrest. Registries provide information that can be used to identify opportunities to improve the quality of care. A recent systematic review found improvement in cardiac arrest survival in organizations and communities that implemented cardiac arrest registries.[47]

Knowledge Gaps

Some of the most pertinent gaps in systems of care research include the following:

- Which interventions improve the willingness of the general public to perform CPR and use AEDs, especially for populations and communities with low bystander response rates?
- Does just-in-time AED delivery, including drone delivery of AEDs, increase the number of patients receiving timely defibrillation and improve resuscitation outcomes?
- Which clinical criteria accurately identify patients at increased risk for IHCA?
- What are the ideal components of a hospital rapid response system and rapid response team? How can these factors be integrated into a realistic and effective response model for the prevention of IHCA?
- What is the best structure for individual, team, and system feedback to achieve performance improvement?
- In what settings are community CPR and AED programs cost-effective?

IMPLEMENTING THE GUIDELINES

In this executive summary, we presented an overview of the guidelines process, recommendations, and knowledge gaps that can be translated into practice. Future efforts can focus on evaluating the feasibility and acceptability of recommendations, their cost-effectiveness, and their impact on equity, although such evaluations are outside the scope of this document.

SUMMARY

Cardiac arrest remains a condition with considerable morbidity and mortality that broadly affects individuals across age, gender, race, geography, and socioeconomic status. Although there have been modest improvements in survival, there is still considerable work to be done to address the significant burden of this disease. This executive summary provides an overview of new or updated recommendations that are based on rigorous evidence evaluations and included in the 2020 Guidelines.

To continue to make progress toward addressing this condition over the next decade will require further strengthening the Chain of Survival and enhancing coordinated systems of care. Knowledge gaps identified in the 2020 Guidelines point to critically important research questions that should be addressed and that represent opportunities for funding the future trajectory of resuscitation science. Developing guidelines is an important initial step that can advance efforts that will ultimately result in improved outcomes for patients.

ARTICLE INFORMATION

The American Heart Association requests that this document be cited as follows: Merchant RM, Topjian AA, Panchal AR, Cheng A, Aziz K, Berg KM, Lavonas EJ, Magid DJ; on behalf of the Adult Basic and Advanced Life Support, Pediatric Basic and Advanced Life Support, Neonatal Life Support, Resuscitation Education Science, and Systems of Care Writing Groups. Part 1: executive summary: 2020 American Heart Association Guidelines for Cardiopulmonary Resuscitation and Emergency Cardiovascular Care. *Circulation*. 2020;142(suppl 2):S337–S357. doi: 10.1161/CIR.0000000000000918

Acknowledgments

The writing group acknowledges the members of the Adult Basic and Advanced Life Support, Pediatric Basic and Advanced Life Support, Neonatal Life Support, Resuscitation Education Science, and Systems of Care Writing Groups.

Disclosures

Writing Group Disclosures

Writing Group Member	Employment	Research Grant	Other Research Support	Speakers' Bureau/ Honoraria	Expert Witness	Ownership Interest	Consultant/ Advisory Board	Other
Raina M. Merchant	University of Pennsylvania	NIH (R01 PI not specific to cardiac arrest: "Digital Phenotyping and Cardiovascular Health")*	None	None	None	None	None	None
Khalid Aziz	University of Alberta (Canada)	None	None	None	None	None	None	None
Katherine M. Berg	Beth Israel Deaconess Medical Center	NHLBI Grant K23 HL128814†	None	None	None	None	None	None
Adam Cheng	Alberta Children's Hospital (Canada)	None	None	None	None	None	None	None

(Continued)

Writing Group Disclosures Continued

Writing Group Member	Employment	Research Grant	Other Research Support	Speakers' Bureau/ Honoraria	Expert Witness	Ownership Interest	Consultant/ Advisory Board	Other
Eric J. Lavonas	Denver Health Emergency Medicine	BTG Pharmaceuticals (Denver Health (Dr Lavonas' employer) has research, call center, consulting, and teaching agreements with BTG Pharmaceuticals. BTG manufactures the digoxin antidote, DigiFab. Dr Lavonas does not receive bonus or incentive compensation, and these agreements involve an unrelated product. When these guidelines were developed, Dr Lavonas recused from discussions related to digoxin poisoning.)†	None	None	None	None	None	American Heart Association (Senior Science Editor)†
David J. Magid	University of Colorado	NIH†; NHLBI†; CMS†; AHA†	None	None	None	None	None	American Heart Association (Senior Science Editor)†
Ashish R. Panchal	The Ohio State University	None	None	None	None	None	None	None
Alexis A. Topjian	The Children's Hospital of Philadelphia, University of Pennsylvania	NIH*	None	None	None	None	None	None

This table represents the relationships of writing group members that may be perceived as actual or reasonably perceived conflicts of interest as reported on the Disclosure Questionnaire, which all members of the writing group are required to complete and submit. A relationship is considered to be "significant" if (a) the person receives $10 000 or more during any 12-month period, or 5% or more of the person's gross income; or (b) the person owns 5% or more of the voting stock or share of the entity, or owns $10 000 or more of the fair market value of the entity. A relationship is considered to be "modest" if it is less than "significant" under the preceding definition.

*Modest.

†Significant.

Reviewer Disclosures

Reviewer	Employment	Research Grant	Other Research Support	Speakers' Bureau/ Honoraria	Expert Witness	Ownership Interest	Consultant/ Advisory Board	Other
Aarti Bavare	Baylor College of Medicine	None	None	None	None	None	None	None
Raúl J. Gazmuri	Rosalind Franklin University of Medicine and Science	Zoll Foundation (received–Myocardial Effects of Shock Burden During Defibrillation Attempts. Work conducted in a swine model)†; Zoll Foundation (received–Amplitude Spectral Area to Assess Hemodynamic and Metabolic Interventions during Cardiac Arrest. Work conducted in a swine model)†; Zoll Foundation (Does Erythropoietin Reduce Adverse Post-Resuscitation Myocardial and Cerebral Effects of Epinephrine Resulting in Improved Survival with Good Neurological Function? Work in a swine model)†	None	None	None	None	None	None
Julia Indik	University of Arizona	None	None	None	None	None	None	None
Steven L. Kronick	University of Michigan	NIH (Enhancing Pre-Hospital Outcomes for Cardiac Arrest [EPOC])*	None	None	None	None	None	None

(Continued)

Reviewer Disclosures Continued

Reviewer	Employment	Research Grant	Other Research Support	Speakers' Bureau/ Honoraria	Expert Witness	Ownership Interest	Consultant/ Advisory Board	Other
Eddy Lang	University of Calgary (Canada)	None	None	None	None	None	None	None
Alexandra Marquez	Children's Hospital of Philadelphia	Labatt Innovation Fund (seed fund grant (≈25K) for device development project to create a "rapid access" ECLS cannulation deployment system)†	None	None	None	None	None	None
Mary Ann McNeil	University of Minnesota	None	None	None	None	None	None	None
Robert D. Nelson	Wake Forest University Health Sciences	None	None	None	None	None	None	None
Donald H. Shaffner	Johns Hopkins Hospital	None	None	None	None	None	None	None

This table represents the relationships of reviewers that may be perceived as actual or reasonably perceived conflicts of interest as reported on the Disclosure Questionnaire, which all reviewers are required to complete and submit. A relationship is considered to be "significant" if (a) the person receives $10 000 or more during any 12-month period, or 5% or more of the person's gross income; or (b) the person owns 5% or more of the voting stock or share of the entity, or owns $10 000 or more of the fair market value of the entity. A relationship is considered to be "modest" if it is less than "significant" under the preceding definition.

*Modest.

†Significant.

REFERENCES

1. National Academy of Sciences. Cardiopulmonary resuscitation. *JAMA*. 1966;198:372–379.
2. Standards for cardiopulmonary resuscitation (CPR) and emergency cardiac care (ECC), 3: advanced life support. *JAMA*. 1974;227(suppl):852–860.
3. Standards and guidelines for cardiopulmonary resuscitation (CPR) and emergency cardiac care (ECC). *JAMA*. 1980;244:453–509.
4. Standards and guidelines for cardiopulmonary resuscitation (CPR) and emergency cardiac care (ECC): National Academy of Sciences—National Research Council. *JAMA*. 1986;255:2905–2989.
5. Guidelines for cardiopulmonary resuscitation and emergency cardiac care: Emergency Cardiac Care Committee and Subcommittees, American Heart Association, Part I: introduction. *JAMA*. 1992;268:2171–2183.
6. The American Heart Association in collaboration with the International Liaison Committee on Resuscitation. Guidelines 2000 for Cardiopulmonary Resuscitation and Emergency Cardiovascular Care: Part 6: advanced cardiovascular life support: 7D: the tachycardia algorithms. *Circulation*. 2000;102(suppl):I158–I165.
7. ECC Committee, Subcommittees, Task Forces of the American Heart Association. 2005 American Heart Association Guidelines for Cardiopulmonary Resuscitation and Emergency Cardiovascular Care. *Circulation*. 2005;112(suppl):IV1–IV203. doi: 10.1161/CIRCULATIONAHA.105.166550
8. Field JM, Hazinski MF, Sayre MR, Chameides L, Schexnayder SM, Hemphill R, Samson RA, Kattwinkel J, Berg RA, Bhanji F, et al. Part 1: executive summary: 2010 American Heart Association Guidelines for Cardiopulmonary Resuscitation and Emergency Cardiovascular Care. *Circulation*. 2010;122(suppl 3):S640–S656. doi: 10.1161/CIRCULATIONAHA.110.970889
9. Neumar RW, Shuster M, Callaway CW, Gent LM, Atkins DL, Bhanji F, Brooks SC, de Caen AR, Donnino MW, Ferrer JM, et al. Part 1: executive summary: 2015 American Heart Association Guidelines Update for Cardiopulmonary Resuscitation and Emergency Cardiovascular Care. *Circulation*. 2015;132(suppl 2):S315–S367. doi: 10.1161/CIR.0000000000000252
10. Virani SS, Alonso A, Benjamin EJ, Bittencourt MS, Callaway CW, Carson AP, Chamberlain AM, Chang AR, Cheng S, Delling FN, et al: on behalf of the American Heart Association Council on Epidemiology and Prevention Statistics Committee and Stroke Statistics Subcommittee. Heart disease and stroke statistics—2020 update: a report from the American Heart Association. *Circulation*. 2020;141:e139–e596. doi: 10.1161/CIR.0000000000000757
11. Holmberg MJ, Ross CE, Fitzmaurice GM, Chan PS, Duval-Arnould J, Grossestreuer AV, Yankama T, Donnino MW, Andersen LW; American Heart Association's Get With The Guidelines–Resuscitation Investigators. Annual Incidence of Adult and Pediatric In-Hospital Cardiac Arrest in the United States. *Circ Cardiovasc Qual Outcomes*. 2019;12:e005580. doi: 10.1161/CIRCOUTCOMES.119.005580
12. Perlman JM, Risser R. Cardiopulmonary resuscitation in the delivery room: associated clinical events. *Arch Pediatr Adolesc Med*. 1995;149:20–25. doi: 10.1001/archpedi.1995.02170130022005
13. Barber CA, Wyckoff MH. Use and efficacy of endotracheal versus intravenous epinephrine during neonatal cardiopulmonary resuscitation in the delivery room. *Pediatrics*. 2006;118:1028–1034. doi: 10.1542/peds.2006-0416
14. Cummins RO, Ornato JP, Thies WH, Pepe PE. Improving survival from sudden cardiac arrest: the "chain of survival" concept. A statement for health professionals from the Advanced Cardiac Life Support Subcommittee and the Emergency Cardiac Care Committee, American Heart Association. *Circulation*. 1991;83:1832–1847. doi: 10.1161/01.cir.83.5.1832
15. Aziz K, Lee HC, Escobedo MB, Hoover AV, Kamath-Rayne BD, Kapadia VS, Magid DJ, Niermeyer S, Schmölzer GM, Szyld E, et al. Part 5: neonatal resuscitation: 2020 American Heart Association Guidelines for Cardiopulmonary Resuscitation and Emergency Cardiovascular Care. *Circulation*. 2020;142(suppl 2):S524–S550. doi: 10.1161/CIR.0000000000000902
16. Søreide E, Morrison L, Hillman K, Monsieurs K, Sunde K, Zideman D, Eisenberg M, Sterz F, Nadkarni VM, Soar J, Nolan JP; Utstein Formula for Survival Collaborators. The formula for survival in resuscitation. *Resuscitation*. 2013;84:1487–1493. doi: 10.1016/j.resuscitation.2013.07.020
17. Cheng A, Magid DJ, Auerbach M, Bhanji F, Bigham BL, Blewer AL, Dainty KN, Diederich E, Lin Y, Leary M, et al. Part 6: resuscitation education science: 2020 American Heart Association Guidelines for Cardiopulmonary Resuscitation and Emergency Cardiovascular Care. *Circulation*. 2020;142(suppl 2):S551–S579. doi: 10.1161/CIR.0000000000000903
18. Berg KM, Cheng A, Panchal AR, Topjian AA, Aziz K, Bhanji F, Bigham BL, Hirsch KG, Hoover AV, Kurz MC, et al; on behalf of the Adult Basic and Advanced Life Support, Pediatric Basic and Advanced Life Support, Neonatal Life Support, and Resuscitation Education Science Writing Groups. Part 7: systems of care: 2020 American Heart Association Guidelines for Cardiopulmonary Resuscitation and Emergency Cardiovascular Care. *Circulation*. 2020;142(suppl 2):S580–S604. doi: 10.1161/CIR.0000000000000899
19. Magid DJ, Aziz K, Cheng A, Hazinski MF, Hoover AV, Mahgoub M, Panchal AR, Sasson C, Topjian AA, Rodriguez AJ, et al. Part 2: evidence evaluation and guidelines development: 2020 American Heart Association Guidelines for Cardiopulmonary Resuscitation and Emergency Cardiovascular Care. *Circulation*. 2020;142(suppl 2):S358–S365. doi: 10.1161/CIR.0000000000000898
20. Panchal AR, Bartos JA, Cabañas JG, Donnino MW, Drennan IR, Hirsch KG, Kudenchuk PJ, Kurz MC, Lavonas EJ, Morley PT, et al; on behalf of the Adult Basic and Advanced Life Support Writing Group. Part 3: adult basic and advanced life support: 2020 American Heart Association Guidelines for Cardiopulmonary Resuscitation and Emergency

Cardiovascular Care. *Circulation*. 2020;142(suppl 2):S366–S468. doi: 10.1161/CIR.0000000000000916
21. Topjian AA, Raymond TT, Atkins D, Chan M, Duff JP, Joyner BL Jr, Lasa JJ, Lavonas EJ, Levy A, Mahgoub M, et al; on behalf of the Pediatric Basic and Advanced Life Support Collaborators. Part 4: pediatric basic and advanced life support: 2020 American Heart Association Guidelines for Cardiopulmonary Resuscitation and Emergency Cardiovascular Care. *Circulation*. 2020;142(suppl 2):S469–S523. doi: 10.1161/CIR.0000000000000901
22. American Heart Association. Coronavirus (COVID-19) resources for CPR training & resuscitation. https://cpr.heart.org/en/resources/coronavirus-covid19-resources-for-cpr-training. Accessed June 24, 2020.
23. International Liaison Committee on Resuscitation. Continuous evidence evaluation guidance and templates. https://www.ilcor.org/documents/continuous-evidence-evaluation-guidance-and-templates. Accessed December 31, 2019.
24. Institute of Medicine (US) Committee of Standards for Systematic Reviews of Comparative Effectiveness Research. *Finding What Works in Health Care: Standards for Systematic Reviews*. Washington, DC: The National Academies Press; 2011.
25. Tricco AC, Lillie E, Zarin W, O'Brien KK, Colquhoun H, Levac D, Moher D, Peters MDJ, Horsley T, Weeks L, Hempel S, Akl EA, Chang C, McGowan J, Stewart L, Hartling L, Aldcroft A, Wilson MG, Garritty C, Lewin S, Godfrey CM, Macdonald MT, Langlois EV, Soares-Weiser K, Moriarty J, Clifford T, Tunçalp Ö, Straus SE. PRISMA Extension for Scoping Reviews (PRISMA-ScR): Checklist and Explanation. *Ann Intern Med*. 2018;169:467–473. doi: 10.7326/M18-0850
26. PRISMA. PRISMA for scoping reviews. http://www.prisma-statement.org/Extensions/ScopingReviews. Accessed December 31, 2019.
27. International Liaison Committee on Resuscitation (ILCOR). Continuous evidence evaluation guidance and templates: 2020 evidence update worksheet final. https://www.ilcor.org/documents/continuous-evidence-evaluation-guidance-and-templates#Templates. Accessed December 31, 2019.
28. International Liaison Committee on Resuscitation (ILCOR). Continuous evidence evaluation guidance and templates: 2020 evidence update process final. https://www.ilcor.org/documents/continuous-evidence-evaluation-guidance-and-templates. Accessed December 31, 2019.
29. Guyatt GH, Oxman AD, Vist GE, Kunz R, Falck-Ytter Y, Alonso-Coello P, Schünemann HJ; GRADE Working Group. GRADE: an emerging consensus on rating quality of evidence and strength of recommendations. *BMJ*. 2008;336:924–926. doi: 10.1136/bmj.39489.470347.AD
30. 2010 American Heart Association Guidelines for Cardiopulmonary Resuscitation and Emergency Cardiovascular Care Science. *Circulation*. 2010;122(suppl 3):S640–S946.
31. 2015 American Heart Association Guidelines Update for Cardiopulmonary Resuscitation and Emergency Cardiovascular Care. *Circulation*. 2015;132(suppl 2):S315–S589.
32. Atkins DL, de Caen AR, Berger S, Samson RA, Schexnayder SM, Joyner BL Jr, Bigham BL, Niles DE, Duff JP, Hunt EA, Meaney PA. 2017 American Heart Association Focused Update on Pediatric Basic Life Support and Cardiopulmonary Resuscitation Quality: An Update to the American Heart Association Guidelines for Cardiopulmonary Resuscitation and Emergency Cardiovascular Care. *Circulation*. 2018;137:e1–e6. doi: 10.1161/CIR.0000000000000540
33. Charlton NP, Pellegrino JL, Kule A, Slater TM, Epstein JL, Flores GE, Goolsby CA, Orkin AM, Singletary EM, Swain JM. 2019 American Heart Association and American Red Cross Focused Update for First Aid: Presyncope: An Update to the American Heart Association and American Red Cross Guidelines for First Aid. *Circulation*. 2019;140:e931–e938. doi: 10.1161/CIR.0000000000000730
34. Duff JP, Topjian A, Berg MD, Chan M, Haskell SE, Joyner BL Jr, Lasa JJ, Ley SJ, Raymond TT, Sutton RM, Hazinski MF, Atkins DL. 2018 American Heart Association Focused Update on Pediatric Advanced Life Support: An Update to the American Heart Association Guidelines for Cardiopulmonary Resuscitation and Emergency Cardiovascular Care. *Circulation*. 2018;138:e731–e739. doi: 10.1161/CIR.0000000000000612
35. Duff JP, Topjian AA, Berg MD, Chan M, Haskell SE, Joyner BL Jr, Lasa JJ, Ley SJ, Raymond TT, Sutton RM, Hazinski MF, Atkins DL. 2019 American Heart Association Focused Update on Pediatric Advanced Life Support: An Update to the American Heart Association Guidelines for Cardiopulmonary Resuscitation and Emergency Cardiovascular Care. *Circulation*. 2019;140:e904–e914. doi: 10.1161/CIR.0000000000000731
36. Duff JP, Topjian AA, Berg MD, Chan M, Haskell SE, Joyner BL Jr, Lasa JJ, Ley SJ, Raymond TT, Sutton RM, et al. 2019 American Heart Association focused update on pediatric basic life support: an update to the American Heart Association guidelines for cardiopulmonary resuscitation and emergency cardiovascular care. *Circulation*. 2019;140:e915–e921. doi: 10.1161/CIR.0000000000000736
37. Escobedo MB, Aziz K, Kapadia VS, Lee HC, Niermeyer S, Schmölzer GM, Szyld E, Weiner GM, Wyckoff MH, Yamada NK, Zaichkin JG. 2019 American Heart Association Focused Update on Neonatal Resuscitation: An Update to the American Heart Association Guidelines for Cardiopulmonary Resuscitation and Emergency Cardiovascular Care. *Circulation*. 2019;140:e922–e930. doi: 10.1161/CIR.0000000000000729
38. Kleinman ME, Goldberger ZD, Rea T, Swor RA, Bobrow BJ, Brennan EE, Terry M, Hemphill R, Gazmuri RJ, Hazinski MF, Travers AH. 2017 American Heart Association Focused Update on Adult Basic Life Support and Cardiopulmonary Resuscitation Quality: An Update to the American Heart Association Guidelines for Cardiopulmonary Resuscitation and Emergency Cardiovascular Care. *Circulation*. 2018;137:e7–e13. doi: 10.1161/CIR.0000000000000539
39. Panchal AR, Berg KM, Cabañas JG, Kurz MC, Link MS, Del Rios M, Hirsch KG, Chan PS, Hazinski MF, Morley PT, Donnino MW, Kudenchuk PJ. 2019 American Heart Association Focused Update on Systems of Care: Dispatcher-Assisted Cardiopulmonary Resuscitation and Cardiac Arrest Centers: An Update to the American Heart Association Guidelines for Cardiopulmonary Resuscitation and Emergency Cardiovascular Care. *Circulation*. 2019;140:e895–e903. doi: 10.1161/CIR.0000000000000733
40. Panchal AR, Berg KM, Hirsch KG, Kudenchuk PJ, Del Rios M, Cabañas JG, Link MS, Kurz MC, Chan PS, Morley PT, et al. 2019 American Heart Association focused update on advanced cardiovascular life support: use of advanced airways, vasopressors, and extracorporeal cardiopulmonary resuscitation during cardiac arrest: an update to the American Heart Association guidelines for cardiopulmonary resuscitation and emergency cardiovascular care. *Circulation*. 2019;140:e881–e894. doi: 10.1161/CIR.0000000000000732
41. Panchal AR, Berg KM, Kudenchuk PJ, Del Rios M, Hirsch KG, Link MS, Kurz MC, Chan PS, Cabañas JG, Morley PT, Hazinski MF, Donnino MW. 2018 American Heart Association Focused Update on Advanced Cardiovascular Life Support Use of Antiarrhythmic Drugs During and Immediately After Cardiac Arrest: An Update to the American Heart Association Guidelines for Cardiopulmonary Resuscitation and Emergency Cardiovascular Care. *Circulation*. 2018;138:e740–e749. doi: 10.1161/CIR.0000000000000613
42. Nolan JP, Maconochie I, Soar J, Olasveengen TM, Greif R, Wyckoff MH, Singletary EM, Aickin R, Berg KM, Mancini ME, et al. Executive summary: 2020 International Consensus on Cardiopulmonary Resuscitation and Emergency Cardiovascular Care Science With Treatment Recommendations. *Circulation*. 2020;142(suppl 1):S2–S27. doi: 10.1161/CIR.0000000000000890
43. Morley PT, Atkins DL, Finn JC, Maconochie I, Nolan JP, Rabi Y, Singletary EM, Wang TL, Welsford M, Olasveengen TM, et al. Evidence evaluation process and management of potential conflicts of interest: 2020 International Consensus on Cardiopulmonary Resuscitation and Emergency Cardiovascular Care Science With Treatment Recommendations. *Circulation*. 2020;142(suppl 1):S28–S40. doi: 10.1161/CIR.0000000000000891
44. Olasveengen TM, Mancini ME, Perkins GD, Avis S, Brooks S, Castrén M, Chung SP, Considine J, Couper K, Escalante R, et al; on behalf of the Adult Basic Life Support Collaborators. Adult basic life support: 2020 International Consensus on Cardiopulmonary Resuscitation and Emergency Cardiovascular Care Science With Treatment Recommendations. *Circulation*. 2020;142(suppl 1):S41–S91. doi: 10.1161/CIR.0000000000000892
45. Maconochie IK, Aickin R, Hazinski MF, Atkins DL, Bingham R, Couto TB, Guerguerian A-M, Nadkarni VM, Ng K-C, Nuthall GA, et al; on behalf of the Pediatric Life Support Collaborators. Pediatric life support: 2020 International Consensus on Cardiopulmonary Resuscitation and Emergency Cardiovascular Care Science With Treatment Recommendations. *Circulation*. 2020;142(suppl 1):S140–S184. doi: 10.1161/CIR.0000000000000894
46. Wyckoff MH, Wyllie J, Aziz K, de Almeida MF, Fabres J, Fawke J, Guinsburg R, Hosono S, Isayama T, Kapadia VS, et al; on behalf of the Neonatal Life Support Collaborators. Neonatal life support: International Consensus on Cardiopulmonary Resuscitation and Emergency Cardiovascular Care Science With Treatment Recommendations. *Circulation*. 2020;142(suppl 1):S185–S221. doi: 10.1161/CIR.0000000000000895
47. Greif R, Bhanji F, Bigham BL, Bray J, Breckwoldt J, Cheng A, Duff JP, Gilfoyle E, Hsieh M-J, Iwami T, et al; on behalf of the Education, Implementation, and Teams Collaborators. Education, implementation, and teams: 2020 International Consensus on Cardiopulmonary Resuscitation and Emergency Cardiovascular Care Science With Treatment

Recommendations. *Circulation.* 2020;142(suppl 1):S222–S283. doi: 10.1161/CIR.0000000000000896
48. Berg KM, Soar J, Andersen LW, Böttiger BW, Cacciola S, Callaway CW, Couper K, Cronberg T, D'Arrigo S, Deakin CD, et al; on behalf of the Adult Advanced Life Support Collaborators. Adult advanced life support: 2020 International Consensus on Cardiopulmonary Resuscitation and Emergency Cardiovascular Care Science With Treatment Recommendations. *Circulation.* 2020;142(suppl 1):S92–S139. doi: 10.1161/CIR.0000000000000893
49. Levine GN, O'Gara PT, Beckman JA, Al-Khatib SM, Birtcher KK, Cigarroa JE, de Las Fuentes L, Deswal A, Fleisher LA, Gentile F, Goldberger ZD, Hlatky MA, Joglar JA, Piano MR, Wijeysundera DN. Recent Innovations, Modifications, and Evolution of ACC/AHA Clinical Practice Guidelines: An Update for Our Constituencies: A Report of the American College of Cardiology/American Heart Association Task Force on Clinical Practice Guidelines. *Circulation.* 2019;139:e879–e886. doi: 10.1161/CIR.0000000000000651
50. Considine J, Gazmuri RJ, Perkins GD, Kudenchuk PJ, Olasveengen TM, Vaillancourt C, Nishiyama C, Hatanaka T, Mancini ME, Chung SP, Escalante-Kanashiro R, Morley P. Chest compression components (rate, depth, chest wall recoil and leaning): A scoping review. *Resuscitation.* 2020;146:188–202. doi: 10.1016/j.resuscitation.2019.08.042
51. Stiell IG, Brown SP, Nichol G, Cheskes S, Vaillancourt C, Callaway CW, Morrison LJ, Christenson J, Aufderheide TP, Davis DP, Free C, Hostler D, Stouffer JA, Idris AH; Resuscitation Outcomes Consortium Investigators. What is the optimal chest compression depth during out-of-hospital cardiac arrest resuscitation of adult patients? *Circulation.* 2014;130:1962–1970. doi: 10.1161/CIRCULATIONAHA.114.008671
52. Stiell IG, Brown SP, Christenson J, Cheskes S, Nichol G, Powell J, Bigham B, Morrison LJ, Larsen J, Hess E, Vaillancourt C, Davis DP, Callaway CW; Resuscitation Outcomes Consortium (ROC) Investigators. What is the role of chest compression depth during out-of-hospital cardiac arrest resuscitation? *Crit Care Med.* 2012;40:1192–1198. doi: 10.1097/CCM.0b013e31823bc8bb
53. Edelson DP, Abella BS, Kramer-Johansen J, Wik L, Myklebust H, Barry AM, Merchant RM, Hoek TL, Steen PA, Becker LB. Effects of compression depth and pre-shock pauses predict defibrillation failure during cardiac arrest. *Resuscitation.* 2006;71:137–145. doi: 10.1016/j.resuscitation.2006.04.008
54. Babbs CF, Kemeny AE, Quan W, Freeman G. A new paradigm for human resuscitation research using intelligent devices. *Resuscitation.* 2008;77:306–315. doi: 10.1016/j.resuscitation.2007.12.018
55. Hwang SO, Cha KC, Kim K, Jo YH, Chung SP, You JS, Shin J, Lee HJ, Park YS, Kim S, et al. A randomized controlled trial of compression rates during cardiopulmonary resuscitation. *J Korean Med Sci.* 2016;31:1491–1498. doi: 10.3346/jkms.2016.31.9.1491
56. White L, Rogers J, Bloomingdale M, Fahrenbruch C, Culley L, Subido C, Eisenberg M, Rea T. Dispatcher-assisted cardiopulmonary resuscitation: risks for patients not in cardiac arrest. *Circulation.* 2010;121:91–97. doi: 10.1161/CIRCULATIONAHA.109.872366
57. Haley KB, Lerner EB, Pirrallo RG, Croft H, Johnson A, Uihlein M. The frequency and consequences of cardiopulmonary resuscitation performed by bystanders on patients who are not in cardiac arrest. *Prehosp Emerg Care.* 2011;15:282–287. doi: 10.3109/10903127.2010.541981
58. Moriwaki Y, Sugiyama M, Tahara Y, Iwashita M, Kosuge T, Harunari N, Arata S, Suzuki N. Complications of bystander cardiopulmonary resuscitation for unconscious patients without cardiopulmonary arrest. *J Emerg Trauma Shock.* 2012;5:3–6. doi: 10.4103/0974-2700.93094
59. Tanaka Y, Nishi T, Takase K, Yoshita Y, Wato Y, Taniguchi J, Hamada Y, Inaba H. Survey of a protocol to increase appropriate implementation of dispatcher-assisted cardiopulmonary resuscitation for out-of-hospital cardiac arrest. *Circulation.* 2014;129:1751–1760. doi: 10.1161/CIRCULATIONAHA.113.004409
60. Beck LR, Ostermayer DG, Ponce JN, Srinivasan S, Wang HE. Effectiveness of Prehospital Dual Sequential Defibrillation for Refractory Ventricular Fibrillation and Ventricular Tachycardia Cardiac Arrest. *Prehosp Emerg Care.* 2019;23:597–602. doi: 10.1080/10903127.2019.1584256
61. Mapp JG, Hans AJ, Darrington AM, Ross EM, Ho CC, Miramontes DA, Harper SA, Wampler DA; Prehospital Research and Innovation in Military and Expeditionary Environments (PRIME) Research Group. Prehospital Double Sequential Defibrillation: A Matched Case-Control Study. *Acad Emerg Med.* 2019;26:994–1001. doi: 10.1111/acem.13672
62. Ross EM, Redman TT, Harper SA, Mapp JG, Wampler DA, Miramontes DA. Dual defibrillation in out-of-hospital cardiac arrest: A retrospective cohort analysis. *Resuscitation.* 2016;106:14–17. doi: 10.1016/j.resuscitation.2016.06.011
63. Emmerson AC, Whitbread M, Fothergill RT. Double sequential defibrillation therapy for out-of-hospital cardiac arrests: The London experience. *Resuscitation.* 2017;117:97–101. doi: 10.1016/j.resuscitation.2017.06.011
64. Cheskes S, Dorian P, Feldman M, McLeod S, Scales DC, Pinto R, Turner L, Morrison LJ, Drennan IR, Verbeek PR. Double sequential external defibrillation for refractory ventricular fibrillation: the DOSE VF pilot randomized controlled trial. *Resuscitation.* 2020;150:178–184. doi: 10.1016/j.resuscitation.2020.02.010
65. Granfeldt A, Avis SR, Lind PC, Holmberg MJ, Kleinman M, Maconochie I, Hsu CH, Fernanda de Almeida M, Wang TL, Neumar RW, Andersen LW. Intravenous vs. intraosseous administration of drugs during cardiac arrest: A systematic review. *Resuscitation.* 2020;149:150–157. doi: 10.1016/j.resuscitation.2020.02.025
66. Feinstein BA, Stubbs BA, Rea T, Kudenchuk PJ. Intraosseous compared to intravenous drug resuscitation in out-of-hospital cardiac arrest. *Resuscitation.* 2017;117:91–96. doi: 10.1016/j.resuscitation.2017.06.014
67. Kawano T, Grunau B, Scheuermeyer FX, Gibo K, Fordyce CB, Lin S, Stenstrom R, Schlamp R, Jenneson S, Christenson J. Intraosseous Vascular Access Is Associated With Lower Survival and Neurologic Recovery Among Patients With Out-of-Hospital Cardiac Arrest. *Ann Emerg Med.* 2018;71:588–596. doi: 10.1016/j.annemergmed.2017.11.015
68. Clemency B, Tanaka K, May P, Innes J, Zagroba S, Blaszak J, Hostler D, Cooney D, McGee K, Lindstrom H. Intravenous vs. intraosseous access and return of spontaneous circulation during out of hospital cardiac arrest. *Am J Emerg Med.* 2017;35:222–226. doi: 10.1016/j.ajem.2016.10.052
69. Nguyen L, Suarez S, Daniels J, Sanchez C, Landry K, Redfield C. Effect of Intravenous Versus Intraosseous Access in Prehospital Cardiac Arrest. *Air Med J.* 2019;38:147–149. doi: 10.1016/j.amj.2019.02.005
70. Jacobs IG, Finn JC, Jelinek GA, Oxer HF, Thompson PL. Effect of adrenaline on survival in out-of-hospital cardiac arrest: a randomised double-blind placebo-controlled trial. *Resuscitation.* 2011;82:1138–1143. doi: 10.1016/j.resuscitation.2011.06.029
71. Perkins GD, Ji C, Deakin CD, Quinn T, Nolan JP, Scomparin C, Regan S, Long J, Slowther A, Pocock H, Black JJM, Moore F, Fothergill RT, Rees N, O'Shea L, Docherty M, Gunson I, Han K, Charlton K, Finn J, Petrou S, Stallard N, Gates S, Lall R; PARAMEDIC2 Collaborators. A Randomized Trial of Epinephrine in Out-of-Hospital Cardiac Arrest. *N Engl J Med.* 2018;379:711–721. doi: 10.1056/NEJMoa1806842
72. Holmberg MJ, Issa MS, Moskowitz A, Morley P, Welsford M, Neumar RW, Paiva EF, Coker A, Hansen CK, Andersen LW, Donnino MW, Berg KM; International Liaison Committee on Resuscitation Advanced Life Support Task Force Collaborators. Vasopressors during adult cardiac arrest: A systematic review and meta-analysis. *Resuscitation.* 2019;139:106–121. doi: 10.1016/j.resuscitation.2019.04.008
73. Dezfulian C, Orkin AM, Maron BA, Elmer J, Girota S, Gladwin MT, Merchant RM, Panchal AR, Perman SM, Starks M, et al; on behalf of the American Heart Association Council on Cardiopulmonary, Critical Care, Perioperative and Resuscitation; Council on Arteriosclerosis, Thrombosis and Vascular Biology; Council on Cardiovascular and Stroke Nursing; and Council on Clinical Cardiology. Opioid-associated out-of-hospital cardiac arrest: distinctive clinical features and implications for healthcare and public responses: a scientific statement from the American Heart Association. *Circulation.* In press.
74. Jeejeebhoy FM, Zelop CM, Lipman S, Carvalho B, Joglar J, Mhyre JM, Katz VL, Lapinsky SE, Einav S, Warnes CA, Page RL, Griffin RE, Jain A, Dainty KN, Arafeh J, Windrim R, Koren G, Callaway CW; American Heart Association Emergency Cardiovascular Care Committee, Council on Cardiopulmonary, Critical Care, Perioperative and Resuscitation, Council on Cardiovascular Diseases in the Young, and Council on Clinical Cardiology. Cardiac Arrest in Pregnancy: A Scientific Statement From the American Heart Association. *Circulation.* 2015;132:1747–1773. doi: 10.1161/CIR.0000000000000300
75. Dijkman A, Huisman CM, Smit M, Schutte JM, Zwart JJ, van Roosmalen JJ, Oepkes D. Cardiac arrest in pregnancy: increasing use of perimortem caesarean section due to emergency skills training? *BJOG.* 2010;117:282–287. doi: 10.1111/j.1471-0528.2009.02461.x
76. Page-Rodriguez A, Gonzalez-Sanchez JA. Perimortem cesarean section of twin pregnancy: case report and review of the literature. *Acad Emerg Med.* 1999;6:1072–1074. doi: 10.1111/j.1553-2712.1999.tb01199.x
77. Cardosi RJ, Porter KB. Cesarean delivery of twins during maternal cardiopulmonary arrest. *Obstet Gynecol.* 1998;92(4 Pt 2):695–697. doi: 10.1016/s0029-7844(98)00127-6
78. Rees SG, Thurlow JA, Gardner IC, Scrutton MJ, Kinsella SM. Maternal cardiovascular consequences of positioning after spinal anaesthesia for

Caesarean section: left 15 degree table tilt vs. left lateral. *Anaesthesia.* 2002;57:15–20. doi: 10.1046/j.1365-2044.2002.02325.x
79. Mendonca C, Griffiths J, Ateleanu B, Collis RE. Hypotension following combined spinal-epidural anaesthesia for Caesarean section. Left lateral position vs. tilted supine position. *Anaesthesia.* 2003;58:428–431. doi: 10.1046/j.1365-2044.2003.03090.x
80. Callaway CW, Donnino MW, Fink EL, Geocadin RG, Golan E, Kern KB, Leary M, Meurer WJ, Peberdy MA, Thompson TM, et al. Part 8: post–cardiac arrest care: 2015 American Heart Association Guidelines Update for Cardiopulmonary Resuscitation and Emergency Cardiovascular Care. *Circulation.* 2015;132(suppl 2):S465–482. doi: 10.1161/cir.0000000000000262
81. Geocadin RG, Callaway CW, Fink EL, Golan E, Greer DM, Ko NU, Lang E, Licht DJ, Marino BS, McNair ND, Peberdy MA, Perman SM, Sims DB, Soar J, Sandroni C; American Heart Association Emergency Cardiovascular Care Committee. Standards for Studies of Neurological Prognostication in Comatose Survivors of Cardiac Arrest: A Scientific Statement From the American Heart Association. *Circulation.* 2019;140:e517–e542. doi: 10.1161/CIR.0000000000000702
82. Samaniego EA, Mlynash M, Caulfield AF, Eyngorn I, Wijman CA. Sedation confounds outcome prediction in cardiac arrest survivors treated with hypothermia. *Neurocritical care.* 2011;15:113–119. doi: 10.1007/s12028-010-9412-8
83. Sawyer KN, Camp-Rogers TR, Kotini-Shah P, Del Rios M, Gossip MR, Moitra VK, Haywood KL, Dougherty CM, Lubitz SA, Rabinstein AA, Rittenberger JC, Callaway CW, Abella BS, Geocadin RG, Kurz MC; American Heart Association Emergency Cardiovascular Care Committee; Council on Cardiovascular and Stroke Nursing; Council on Genomic and Precision Medicine; Council on Quality of Care and Outcomes Research; and Stroke Council. Sudden Cardiac Arrest Survivorship: A Scientific Statement From the American Heart Association. *Circulation.* 2020;141:e654–e685. doi: 10.1161/CIR.0000000000000747
84. Wilder Schaaf KP, Artman LK, Peberdy MA, Walker WC, Ornato JP, Gossip MR, Kreutzer JS; Virginia Commonwealth University ARCTIC Investigators. Anxiety, depression, and PTSD following cardiac arrest: a systematic review of the literature. *Resuscitation.* 2013;84:873–877. doi: 10.1016/j.resuscitation.2012.11.021
85. Presciutti A, Verma J, Pavol M, Anbarasan D, Falo C, Brodie D, Rabbani LE, Roh DJ, Park S, Claassen J, Agarwal S. Posttraumatic stress and depressive symptoms characterize cardiac arrest survivors' perceived recovery at hospital discharge. *Gen Hosp Psychiatry.* 2018;53:108–113. doi: 10.1016/j.genhosppsych.2018.02.006
86. Presciutti A, Sobczak E, Sumner JA, Roh DJ, Park S, Claassen J, Kronish I, Agarwal S. The impact of psychological distress on long-term recovery perceptions in survivors of cardiac arrest. *J Crit Care.* 2019;50:227–233. doi: 10.1016/j.jcrc.2018.12.011
87. Lilja G, Nilsson G, Nielsen N, Friberg H, Hassager C, Koopmans M, Kuiper M, Martini A, Mellinghoff J, Pelosi P, Wanscher M, Wise MP, Östman I, Cronberg T. Anxiety and depression among out-of-hospital cardiac arrest survivors. *Resuscitation.* 2015;97:68–75. doi: 10.1016/j.resuscitation.2015.09.389
88. Nolan JP, Soar J, Cariou A, Cronberg T, Moulaert VR, Deakin CD, Bottiger BW, Friberg H, Sunde K, Sandroni C. European Resuscitation Council and European Society of Intensive Care Medicine 2015 guidelines for post-resuscitation care. *Intensive Care Med.* 2015;41:2039–2056. doi: 10.1007/s00134-015-4051-3
89. Moulaert VR, Verbunt JA, Bakx WG, Gorgels AP, de Krom MC, Heuts PH, Wade DT, van Heugten CM. 'Stand still., and move on', a new early intervention service for cardiac arrest survivors and their caregivers: rationale and description of the intervention. *Clin Rehabil.* 2011;25:867–879. doi: 10.1177/0269215511399937
90. Cowan MJ, Pike KC, Budzynski HK. Psychosocial nursing therapy following sudden cardiac arrest: impact on two-year survival. *Nurs Res.* 2001;50:68–76. doi: 10.1097/00006199-200103000-00002
91. Sutton RM, Reeder RW, Landis WP, Meert KL, Yates AR, Morgan RW, Berger JT, Newth CJ, Carcillo JA, McQuillen PS, Harrison RE, Moler FW, Pollack MM, Carpenter TC, Notterman DA, Holubkov R, Dean JM, Nadkarni VM, Berg RA; Eunice Kennedy Shriver National Institute of Child Health and Human Development Collaborative Pediatric Critical Care Research Network (CPCCRN). Ventilation Rates and Pediatric In-Hospital Cardiac Arrest Survival Outcomes. *Crit Care Med.* 2019;47:1627–1636. doi: 10.1097/CCM.0000000000003898
92. Chen L, Zhang J, Pan G, Li X, Shi T, He W. Cuffed versus uncuffed endotracheal tubes in pediatrics: a meta-analysis. *Open Med (Wars).* 2018;13:366–373. doi: 10.1515/med-2018-0055
93. Shi F, Xiao Y, Xiong W, Zhou Q, Huang X. Cuffed versus uncuffed endotracheal tubes in children: a meta-analysis. *J Anesth.* 2016;30:3–11. doi: 10.1007/s00540-015-2062-4
94. De Orange FA, Andrade RG, Lemos A, Borges PS, Figueiroa JN, Kovatsis PG. Cuffed versus uncuffed endotracheal tubes for general anaesthesia in children aged eight years and under. *Cochrane Database Syst Rev.* 2017;11:CD011954. doi: 10.1002/14651858.CD011954.pub2
95. Chambers NA, Ramgolam A, Sommerfield D, Zhang G, Ledowski T, Thurm M, Lethbridge M, Hegarty M, von Ungern-Sternberg BS. Cuffed vs. uncuffed tracheal tubes in children: a randomised controlled trial comparing leak, tidal volume and complications. *Anaesthesia.* 2018;73:160–168. doi: 10.1111/anae.14113
96. de Wit M, Peelen LM, van Wolfswinkel L, de Graaff JC. The incidence of postoperative respiratory complications: A retrospective analysis of cuffed vs uncuffed tracheal tubes in children 0-7 years of age. *Paediatr Anaesth.* 2018;28:210–217. doi: 10.1111/pan.13340
97. Schweiger C, Marostica PJ, Smith MM, Manica D, Carvalho PR, Kuhl G. Incidence of post-intubation subglottic stenosis in children: prospective study. *J Laryngol Otol.* 2013;127:399–403. doi: 10.1017/S002221511300025X
98. Dorsey DP, Bowman SM, Klein MB, Archer D, Sharar SR. Perioperative use of cuffed endotracheal tubes is advantageous in young pediatric burn patients. *Burns.* 2010;36:856–860. doi: 10.1016/j.burns.2009.11.011
99. Kojima T, Laverriere EK, Owen EB, Harwayne-Gidansky I, Shenoi AN, Napolitano N, Rehder KJ, Adu-Darko MA, Nett ST, Spear D, et al; and the National Emergency Airway Registry for Children (NEAR4KIDS) Collaborators and Pediatric Acute Lung Injury and Sepsis Investigators (PALISI). Clinical impact of external laryngeal manipulation during laryngoscopy on tracheal intubation success in critically ill children. *Pediatr Crit Care Med.* 2018;19:106–114. doi: 10.1097/PCC.0000000000001373
100. Kojima T, Harwayne-Gidansky I, Shenoi AN, Owen EB, Napolitano N, Rehder KJ, Adu-Darko MA, Nett ST, Spear D, Meyer K, Giuliano JS Jr, Tarquinio KM, Sanders RC Jr, Lee JH, Simon DW, Vanderford PA, Lee AY, Brown CA III, Skippen PW, Breuer RK, Toedt-Pingel I, Parsons SJ, Gradidge EA, Glater LB, Culver K, Nadkarni VM, Nishisaki A; National Emergency Airway Registry for Children (NEAR4KIDS) and Pediatric Acute Lung Injury and Sepsis Investigators (PALISI). Cricoid Pressure During Induction for Tracheal Intubation in Critically Ill Children: A Report From National Emergency Airway Registry for Children. *Pediatr Crit Care Med.* 2018;19:528–537. doi: 10.1097/PCC.0000000000001531
101. Andersen LW, Berg KM, Saindon BZ, Massaro JM, Raymond TT, Berg RA, Nadkarni VM, Donnino MW; American Heart Association Get With the Guidelines–Resuscitation Investigators. Time to Epinephrine and Survival After Pediatric In-Hospital Cardiac Arrest. *JAMA.* 2015;314:802–810. doi: 10.1001/jama.2015.9678
102. Lin YR, Wu MH, Chen TY, Syue YJ, Yang MC, Lee TH, Lin CM, Chou CC, Chang CF, Li CJ. Time to epinephrine treatment is associated with the risk of mortality in children who achieve sustained ROSC after traumatic out-of-hospital cardiac arrest. *Crit Care.* 2019;23:101. doi: 10.1186/s13054-019-2391-z
103. Lin YR, Li CJ, Huang CC, Lee TH, Chen TY, Yang MC, Chou CC, Chang CF, Huang HW, Hsu HY, Chen WL. Early Epinephrine Improves the Stabilization of Initial Post-resuscitation Hemodynamics in Children With Non-shockable Out-of-Hospital Cardiac Arrest. *Front Pediatr.* 2019;7:220. doi: 10.3389/fped.2019.00220
104. Fukuda T, Kondo Y, Hayashida K, Sekiguchi H, Kukita I. Time to epinephrine and survival after paediatric out-of-hospital cardiac arrest. *Eur Heart J Cardiovasc Pharmacother.* 2018;4:144–151. doi: 10.1093/ehjcvp/pvx023
105. Berg RA, Sutton RM, Reeder RW, Berger JT, Newth CJ, Carcillo JA, McQuillen PS, Meert KL, Yates AR, Harrison RE, Moler FW, Pollack MM, Carpenter TC, Wessel DL, Jenkins TL, Notterman DA, Holubkov R, Tamburro RF, Dean JM, Nadkarni VM; Eunice Kennedy Shriver National Institute of Child Health and Human Development Collaborative Pediatric Critical Care Research Network (CPCCRN) PICqCPR (Pediatric Intensive Care Quality of Cardio-Pulmonary Resuscitation) Investigators. Association Between Diastolic Blood Pressure During Pediatric In-Hospital Cardiopulmonary Resuscitation and Survival. *Circulation.* 2018;137:1784–1795. doi: 10.1161/CIRCULATIONAHA.117.032270
106. Herman ST, Abend NS, Bleck TP, Chapman KE, Drislane FW, Emerson RG, Gerard EE, Hahn CD, Husain AM, Kaplan PW, LaRoche SM, Nuwer MR, Quigg M, Riviello JJ, Schmitt SE, Simmons LA, Tsuchida TN, Hirsch LJ; Critical Care Continuous EEG Task Force of the American Clinical Neurophysiology Society. Consensus statement on continuous EEG in critically ill adults and children, part I: indications. *J Clin Neurophysiol.* 2015;32:87–95. doi: 10.1097/WNP.0000000000000166

107. Abend NS, Topjian A, Ichord R, Herman ST, Helfaer M, Donnelly M, Nadkarni V, Dlugos DJ, Clancy RR. Electroencephalographic monitoring during hypothermia after pediatric cardiac arrest. *Neurology.* 2009;72:1931–1940. doi: 10.1212/WNL.0b013e3181a82687
108. Topjian AA, Gutierrez-Colina AM, Sanchez SM, Berg RA, Friess SH, Dlugos DJ, Abend NS. Electrographic status epilepticus is associated with mortality and worse short-term outcome in critically ill children. *Crit Care Med.* 2013;41:215–223. doi: 10.1097/CCM.0b013e3182668035
109. Ostendorf AP, Hartman ME, Friess SH. Early Electroencephalographic Findings Correlate With Neurologic Outcome in Children Following Cardiac Arrest. *Pediatr Crit Care Med.* 2016;17:667–676. doi: 10.1097/PCC.0000000000000791
110. Brophy GM, Bell R, Claassen J, Alldredge B, Bleck TP, Glauser T, Laroche SM, Riviello JJ Jr, Shutter L, Sperling MR, Treiman DM, Vespa PM; Neurocritical Care Society Status Epilepticus Guideline Writing Committee. Guidelines for the evaluation and management of status epilepticus. *Neurocrit Care.* 2012;17:3–23. doi: 10.1007/s12028-012-9695-z
111. Topjian AA, Sánchez SM, Shults J, Berg RA, Dlugos DJ, Abend NS. Early Electroencephalographic Background Features Predict Outcomes in Children Resuscitated From Cardiac Arrest. *Pediatr Crit Care Med.* 2016;17:547–557. doi: 10.1097/PCC.0000000000000740
112. Moler FW, Silverstein FS, Holubkov R, Slomine BS, Christensen JR, Nadkarni VM, Meert KL, Clark AE, Browning B, Pemberton VL, Page K, Shankaran S, Hutchison JS, Newth CJ, Bennett KS, Berger JT, Topjian A, Pineda JA, Koch JD, Schleien CL, Dalton HJ, Ofori-Amanfo G, Goodman DM, Fink EL, McQuillen P, Zimmerman JJ, Thomas NJ, van der Jagt EW, Porter MB, Meyer MT, Harrison R, Pham N, Schwarz AJ, Nowak JE, Alten J, Wheeler DS, Bhalala US, Lidsky K, Lloyd E, Mathur M, Shah S, Wu T, Theodorou AA, Sanders RC Jr, Dean JM; THAPCA Trial Investigators. Therapeutic hypothermia after out-of-hospital cardiac arrest in children. *N Engl J Med.* 2015;372:1898–1908. doi: 10.1056/NEJMoa1411480
113. Moler FW, Silverstein FS, Holubkov R, Slomine BS, Christensen JR, Nadkarni VM, Meert KL, Browning B, Pemberton VL, Page K, et al; on behalf of the THAPCA Trial Investigators. Therapeutic hypothermia after in-hospital cardiac arrest in children. *N Engl J Med.* 2017;376:318–329. doi: 10.1056/NEJMoa1610493
114. Slomine BS, Silverstein FS, Page K, Holubkov R, Christensen JR, Dean JM, Moler FW; Therapeutic Hypothermia after Pediatric Cardiac Arrest (THAPCA) Trial Investigators. Relationships between three and twelve month outcomes in children enrolled in the therapeutic hypothermia after pediatric cardiac arrest trials. *Resuscitation.* 2019;139:329–336. doi: 10.1016/j.resuscitation.2019.03.020
115. Slomine BS, Silverstein FS, Christensen JR, Holubkov R, Telford R, Dean JM, Moler FW; Therapeutic Hypothermia after Paediatric Cardiac Arrest (THAPCA) Trial Investigators. Neurobehavioural outcomes in children after In-Hospital cardiac arrest. *Resuscitation.* 2018;124:80–89. doi: 10.1016/j.resuscitation.2018.01.002
116. Slomine BS, Silverstein FS, Christensen JR, Page K, Holubkov R, Dean JM, Moler FW. Neuropsychological Outcomes of Children 1 Year After Pediatric Cardiac Arrest: Secondary Analysis of 2 Randomized Clinical Trials. *JAMA Neurol.* 2018;75:1502–1510. doi: 10.1001/jamaneurol.2018.2628
117. Slomine BS, Silverstein FS, Christensen JR, Holubkov R, Page K, Dean JM, Moler FW; on behalf of the THAPCA Trial Group. Neurobehavioral outcomes in children after out-of-hospital cardiac arrest. *Pediatrics.* 2016;137:e20153412. doi: 10.1542/peds.2015–3412
118. van Zellem L, Buysse C, Madderom M, Legerstee JS, Aarsen F, Tibboel D, Utens EM. Long-term neuropsychological outcomes in children and adolescents after cardiac arrest. *Intensive Care Med.* 2015;41:1057–1066. doi: 10.1007/s00134-015-3789-y
119. van Zellem L, Utens EM, Legerstee JS, Cransberg K, Hulst JM, Tibboel D, Buysse C. Cardiac Arrest in Children: Long-Term Health Status and Health-Related Quality of Life. *Pediatr Crit Care Med.* 2015;16:693–702. doi: 10.1097/PCC.0000000000000452
120. van Zellem L, Utens EM, Madderom M, Legerstee JS, Aarsen F, Tibboel D, Buysse C. Cardiac arrest in infants, children, and adolescents: long-term emotional and behavioral functioning. *Eur J Pediatr.* 2016;175:977–986. doi: 10.1007/s00431-016-2728-4
121. Topjian AA, Scholefield BR, Pinto NP, Fink EL, Buysse CMP, Haywood K, Maconochie I, Nadkarni VM, de Caen A, Escalante-Kanashiro R, Ng K-C, et al. P-COSCA (Pediatric Core Outcome Set for Cardiac Arrest) in children: an advisory statement from the International Liaison Committee on Resuscitation. *Circulation.* 2020;142:e000-e000. doi: 10.1161/CIR.0000000000000911
122. Topjian AA, de Caen A, Wainwright MS, Abella BS, Abend NS, Atkins DL, Bembea MM, Fink EL, Guerguerian AM, Haskell SE, Kilgannon JH, Lasa JJ, Hazinski MF. Pediatric Post-Cardiac Arrest Care: A Scientific Statement From the American Heart Association. *Circulation.* 2019;140:e194–e233. doi: 10.1161/CIR.0000000000000697
123. Inwald DP, Canter R, Woolfall K, Mouncey P, Zenasni Z, O'Hara C, Carter A, Jones N, Lyttle MD, Nadel S, et al; on behalf of PERUKI (Paediatric Emergency Research in the UK and Ireland) and PICS SG (Paediatric Intensive Care Society Study Group). Restricted fluid bolus volume in early septic shock: results of the Fluids in Shock pilot trial. *Archives of disease in childhood.* 2019;104:426–431. doi: 10.1136/archdischild-2018–314924
124. van Paridon BM, Sheppard C, Garcia Guerra G, Joffe AR; on behalf of the Alberta Sepsis Network. Timing of antibiotics, volume, and vasoactive infusions in children with sepsis admitted to intensive care. *Crit Care.* 2015;19:293. doi: 10.1186/s13054-015-1010-x
125. Sankar J, Ismail J, Sankar MJ, C P S, Meena RS. Fluid Bolus Over 15-20 Versus 5-10 Minutes Each in the First Hour of Resuscitation in Children With Septic Shock: A Randomized Controlled Trial. *Pediatr Crit Care Med.* 2017;18:e435–e445. doi: 10.1097/PCC.0000000000001269
126. Medeiros DN, Ferranti JF, Delgado AF, de Carvalho WB. Colloids for the Initial Management of Severe Sepsis and Septic Shock in Pediatric Patients: A Systematic Review. *Pediatr Emerg Care.* 2015;31:e11–e16. doi: 10.1097/PEC.0000000000000601
127. Balamuth F, Kittick M, McBride P, Woodford AL, Vestal N, Casper TC, Metheney M, Smith K, Atkin NJ, Baren JM, Dean JM, Kuppermann N, Weiss SL. Pragmatic Pediatric Trial of Balanced Versus Normal Saline Fluid in Sepsis: The PRoMPT BOLUS Randomized Controlled Trial Pilot Feasibility Study. *Acad Emerg Med.* 2019;26:1346–1356. doi: 10.1111/acem.13815
128. Weiss SL, Keele L, Balamuth F, Vendetti N, Ross R, Fitzgerald JC, Gerber JS. Crystalloid Fluid Choice and Clinical Outcomes in Pediatric Sepsis: A Matched Retrospective Cohort Study. *J Pediatr.* 2017;182:304–310.e10. doi: 10.1016/j.jpeds.2016.11.075
129. Emrath ET, Fortenberry JD, Travers C, McCracken CE, Hebbar KB. Resuscitation With Balanced Fluids Is Associated With Improved Survival in Pediatric Severe Sepsis. *Crit Care Med.* 2017;45:1177–1183. doi: 10.1097/CCM.0000000000002365
130. Ventura AM, Shieh HH, Bousso A, Góes PF, de Cássia F O Fernandes I, de Souza DC, Paulo RL, Chagas F, Gilio AE. Double-Blind Prospective Randomized Controlled Trial of Dopamine Versus Epinephrine as First-Line Vasoactive Drugs in Pediatric Septic Shock. *Crit Care Med.* 2015;43:2292–2302. doi: 10.1097/CCM.0000000000001260
131. Ramaswamy KN, Singhi S, Jayashree M, Bansal A, Nallasamy K. Double-Blind Randomized Clinical Trial Comparing Dopamine and Epinephrine in Pediatric Fluid-Refractory Hypotensive Septic Shock. *Pediatr Crit Care Med.* 2016;17:e502–e512. doi: 10.1097/PCC.0000000000000954
132. Davis AL, Carcillo JA, Aneja RK, Deymann AJ, Lin JC, Nguyen TC, Okhuysen-Cawley RS, Relvas MS, Rozenfeld RA, Skippen PW, Stojadinovic BJ, Williams EA, Yeh TS, Balamuth F, Brierley J, de Caen AR, Cheifetz IM, Choong K, Conway E Jr, Cornell T, Doctor A, Dugas MA, Feldman JD, Fitzgerald JC, Flori HR, Fortenberry JD, Graciano AL, Greenwald BM, Hall MW, Han YY, Hernan LJ, Irazuzta JE, Iselin E, van der Jagt EW, Jeffries HE, Kache S, Katyal C, Kissoon N, Kon AA, Kutko MC, MacLaren G, Maul T, Mehta R, Odetola F, Parbuoni K, Paul R, Peters MJ, Ranjit S, Reuter-Rice KE, Schnitzler EJ, Scott HF, Torres A Jr, Weingarten-Arams J, Weiss SL, Zimmerman JJ, Zuckerberg AL. American College of Critical Care Medicine Clinical Practice Parameters for Hemodynamic Support of Pediatric and Neonatal Septic Shock. *Crit Care Med.* 2017;45:1061–1093. doi: 10.1097/CCM.0000000000002425
133. Lampin ME, Rousseaux J, Botte A, Sadik A, Cremer R, Leclerc F. Noradrenaline use for septic shock in children: doses, routes of administration and complications. *Acta Paediatr.* 2012;101:e426–e430. doi: 10.1111/j.1651-2227.2012.02725.x
134. Deep A, Goonasekera CD, Wang Y, Brierley J. Evolution of haemodynamics and outcome of fluid-refractory septic shock in children. *Intensive Care Med.* 2013;39:1602–1609. doi: 10.1007/s00134-013-3003-z
135. Weiss SL, Peters MJ, Alhazzani W, Agus MSD, Flori HR, Inwald DP, Nadel S, Schlapbach LJ, Tasker RC, Argent AC, Brierley J, Carcillo J, Carrol ED, Carroll CL, Cheifetz IM, Choong K, Cies JJ, Cruz AT, De Luca D, Deep A, Faust SN, De Oliveira CF, Hall MW, Ishimine P, Javouhey E, Joosten KFM, Joshi P, Karam O, Kneyber MCJ, Lemson J, MacLaren G, Mehta NM, Møller MH, Newth CJL, Nguyen TC, Nishisaki A, Nunnally ME, Parker MM, Paul RM, Randolph AG, Ranjit S, Romer LH, Scott HF, Tume LN, Verger JT, Williams EA, Wolf J, Wong HR, Zimmerman JJ, Kissoon N, Tissieres P. Surviving Sepsis Campaign International Guidelines for the Management of Septic Shock and Sepsis-Associated Organ

Dysfunction in Children. *Pediatr Crit Care Med.* 2020;21:e52–e106. doi: 10.1097/PCC.0000000000002198
136. Kelly LK, Porta NF, Goodman DM, Carroll CL, Steinhorn RH. Inhaled prostacyclin for term infants with persistent pulmonary hypertension refractory to inhaled nitric oxide. *J Pediatr.* 2002;141:830–832. doi: 10.1067/mpd.2002.129849
137. Kerr D, Kelly AM, Dietze P, Jolley D, Barger B. Randomized controlled trial comparing the effectiveness and safety of intranasal and intramuscular naloxone for the treatment of suspected heroin overdose. *Addiction.* 2009;104:2067–2074. doi: 10.1111/j.1360-0443.2009.02724.x
138. Wanger K, Brough L, Macmillan I, Goulding J, MacPhail I, Christenson JM. Intravenous vs subcutaneous naloxone for out-of-hospital management of presumed opioid overdose. *Acad Emerg Med.* 1998;5:293–299. doi: 10.1111/j.1553-2712.1998.tb02707.x
139. Barton ED, Colwell CB, Wolfe T, Fosnocht D, Gravitz C, Bryan T, Dunn W, Benson J, Bailey J. Efficacy of intranasal naloxone as a needleless alternative for treatment of opioid overdose in the prehospital setting. *J Emerg Med.* 2005;29:265–271. doi: 10.1016/j.jemermed.2005.03.007
140. Robertson TM, Hendey GW, Stroh G, Shalit M. Intranasal naloxone is a viable alternative to intravenous naloxone for prehospital narcotic overdose. *Prehosp Emerg Care.* 2009;13:512–515. doi: 10.1080/10903120903144866
141. Cetrullo C, Di Nino GF, Melloni C, Pieri C, Zanoni A. [Naloxone antagonism toward opiate analgesic drugs. Clinical experimental study]. *Minerva Anestesiol.* 1983;49:199–204.
142. Osterwalder JJ. Naloxone–for intoxications with intravenous heroin and heroin mixtures–harmless or hazardous? A prospective clinical study. *J Toxicol Clin Toxicol.* 1996;34:409–416. doi: 10.3109/15563659609013811
143. Sporer KA, Firestone J, Isaacs SM. Out-of-hospital treatment of opioid overdoses in an urban setting. *Acad Emerg Med.* 1996;3:660–667. doi: 10.1111/j.1553-2712.1996.tb03487.x
144. Stokland O, Hansen TB, Nilsen JE. [Prehospital treatment of heroin intoxication in Oslo in 1996]. *Tidsskr Nor Laegeforen.* 1998;118:3144–3146.
145. Buajordet I, Naess AC, Jacobsen D, Brørs O. Adverse events after naloxone treatment of episodes of suspected acute opioid overdose. *Eur J Emerg Med.* 2004;11:19–23. doi: 10.1097/00063110-200402000-00004
146. Cantwell K, Dietze P, Flander L. The relationship between naloxone dose and key patient variables in the treatment of non-fatal heroin overdose in the prehospital setting. *Resuscitation.* 2005;65:315–319. doi: 10.1016/j.resuscitation.2004.12.012
147. Boyd JJ, Kuisma MJ, Alaspää AO, Vuori E, Repo JV, Randell TT. Recurrent opioid toxicity after pre-hospital care of presumed heroin overdose patients. *Acta Anaesthesiol Scand.* 2006;50:1266–1270. doi: 10.1111/j.1399-6576.2006.01172.x
148. Nielsen K, Nielsen SL, Siersma V, Rasmussen LS. Treatment of opioid overdose in a physician-based prehospital EMS: frequency and long-term prognosis. *Resuscitation.* 2011;82:1410–1413. doi: 10.1016/j.resuscitation.2011.05.027
149. Wampler DA, Molina DK, McManus J, Laws P, Manifold CA. No deaths associated with patient refusal of transport after naloxone-reversed opioid overdose. *Prehosp Emerg Care.* 2011;15:320–324. doi: 10.3109/10903127.2011.569854
150. Kelly AM, Kerr D, Dietze P, Patrick I, Walker T, Koutsogiannis Z. Randomised trial of intranasal versus intramuscular naloxone in prehospital treatment for suspected opioid overdose. *Med J Aust.* 2005;182:24–27.
151. Moore ER, Bergman N, Anderson GC, Medley N. Early skin-to-skin contact for mothers and their healthy newborn infants. *Cochrane Database Syst Rev.* 2016;11:CD003519. doi: 10.1002/14651858.CD003519.pub4
152. de Almeida MF, Guinsburg R, Velaphi S, Aziz K, Perlman JM, Szyld E, Kim HS, Hosono S, Liley HG, Mildenhall L, et al. Intravenous vs. intraosseus administration of drugs during cardiac arrest: International Liaison Committee on Resuscitation (ILCOR) Neonatal Life Support Task Force. 2019. https://costr.ilcor.org/document/intravenous-vs-intraosseous-administration-of-drugs-during-cardiac-arrest-nls-task-force-systematic-review-costr. Updated February 20, 2020. Accessed March 2, 2020.
153. Foglia EE, Weiner G, de Almeida MF, Liley HG, Aziz K, Fabres J, Fawke J, Hosono S, Isayama T, Kapadia VS, et al. Impact of duration of intensive resuscitation (NLS #895): systematic review: International Liaison Committee on Resuscitation (ILCOR) Neonatal Life Support Task Force. 2020. https://costr.ilcor.org/document/impact-of-duration-of-intensive-resuscitation-nls-896-systematic-review. Updated February 19, 2020. Accessed March 1, 2020.
154. Cheng A, Nadkarni VM, Mancini MB, Hunt EA, Sinz EH, Merchant RM, Donoghue A, Duff JP, Eppich W, Auerbach M, Bigham BL, Blewer AL, Chan PS, Bhanji F; American Heart Association Education Science Investigators; and on behalf of the American Heart Association Education Science and Programs Committee, Council on Cardiopulmonary, Critical Care, Perioperative and Resuscitation; Council on Cardiovascular and Stroke Nursing; and Council on Quality of Care and Outcomes Research. Resuscitation Education Science: Educational Strategies to Improve Outcomes From Cardiac Arrest: A Scientific Statement From the American Heart Association. *Circulation.* 2018;138:e82–e122. doi: 10.1161/CIR.0000000000000583
155. Anderson R, Sebaldt A, Lin Y, Cheng A. Optimal training frequency for acquisition and retention of high-quality CPR skills: A randomized trial. *Resuscitation.* 2019;135:153–161. doi: 10.1016/j.resuscitation.2018.10.033
156. Lin Y, Cheng A, Grant VJ, Currie GR, Hecker KG. Improving CPR quality with distributed practice and real-time feedback in pediatric healthcare providers - A randomized controlled trial. *Resuscitation.* 2018;130:6–12. doi: 10.1016/j.resuscitation.2018.06.025
157. O'Donnell CM, Skinner AC. An evaluation of a short course in resuscitation training in a district general hospital. *Resuscitation.* 1993;26:193–201. doi: 10.1016/0300-9572(93)90179-t
158. Oermann MH, Kardong-Edgren SE, Odom-Maryon T. Effects of monthly practice on nursing students' CPR psychomotor skill performance. *Resuscitation.* 2011;82:447–453. doi: 10.1016/j.resuscitation.2010.11.022
159. Kardong-Edgren S, Oermann MH, Odom-Maryon T. Findings from a nursing student CPR study: implications for staff development educators. *J Nurses Staff Dev.* 2012;28:9–15. doi: 10.1097/NND.0b013e318240a6ad
160. Nishiyama C, Iwami T, Murakami Y, Kitamura T, Okamoto Y, Marukawa S, Sakamoto T, Kawamura T. Effectiveness of simplified 15-min refresher BLS training program: a randomized controlled trial. *Resuscitation.* 2015;90:56–60. doi: 10.1016/j.resuscitation.2015.02.015
161. Sullivan NJ, Duval-Arnould J, Twilley M, Smith SP, Aksamit D, Boone-Guercio P, Jeffries PR, Hunt EA. Simulation exercise to improve retention of cardiopulmonary resuscitation priorities for in-hospital cardiac arrests: A randomized controlled trial. *Resuscitation.* 2015;86:6–13. doi: 10.1016/j.resuscitation.2014.10.021
162. Patocka C, Cheng A, Sibbald M, Duff JP, Lai A, Lee-Nobbee P, Levin H, Varshney T, Weber B, Bhanji F. A randomized education trial of spaced versus massed instruction to improve acquisition and retention of paediatric resuscitation skills in emergency medical service (EMS) providers. *Resuscitation.* 2019;141:73–80. doi: 10.1016/j.resuscitation.2019.06.010
163. Patocka C, Khan F, Dubrovsky AS, Brody D, Bank I, Bhanji F. Pediatric resuscitation training-instruction all at once or spaced over time? *Resuscitation.* 2015;88:6–11. doi: 10.1016/j.resuscitation.2014.12.003
164. Kurosawa H, Ikeyama T, Achuff P, Perkel M, Watson C, Monachino A, Remy D, Deutsch E, Buchanan N, Anderson J, Berg RA, Nadkarni VM, Nishisaki A. A randomized, controlled trial of in situ pediatric advanced life support recertification ("pediatric advanced life support reconstructed") compared with standard pediatric advanced life support recertification for ICU frontline providers*. *Crit Care Med.* 2014;42:610–618. doi: 10.1097/CCM.0000000000000024
165. Ericsson KA. Deliberate practice and the acquisition and maintenance of expert performance in medicine and related domains. *Acad Med.* 2004;79(suppl):S70–81. doi: 10.1097/00001888-200410001-00022
166. McGaghie WC. When I say … mastery learning. *Med Educ.* 2015;49:558–559. doi: 10.1111/medu.12679
167. Magee MJ, Farkouh-Karoleski C, Rosen TS. Improvement of Immediate Performance in Neonatal Resuscitation Through Rapid Cycle Deliberate Practice Training. *J Grad Med Educ.* 2018;10:192–197. doi: 10.4300/JGME-D-17-00467.1
168. Diederich E, Lineberry M, Blomquist M, Schott V, Reilly C, Murray M, Nazaran P, Rourk M, Werner R, Broski J. Balancing Deliberate Practice and Reflection: A Randomized Comparison Trial of Instructional Designs for Simulation-Based Training in Cardiopulmonary Resuscitation Skills. *Simul Healthc.* 2019;14:175–181. doi: 10.1097/SIH.0000000000000375
169. Braun L, Sawyer T, Smith K, Hsu A, Behrens M, Chan D, Hutchinson J, Lu D, Singh R, Reyes J, Lopreiato J. Retention of pediatric resuscitation performance after a simulation-based mastery learning session: a multicenter randomized trial. *Pediatr Crit Care Med.* 2015;16:131–138. doi: 10.1097/PCC.0000000000000315
170. Cordero L, Hart BJ, Hardin R, Mahan JD, Nankervis CA. Deliberate practice improves pediatric residents' skills and team behaviors during simulated neonatal resuscitation. *Clin Pediatr (Phila).* 2013;52:747–752. doi: 10.1177/0009922813488646
171. Hunt EA, Duval-Arnould JM, Chime NO, Jones K, Rosen M, Hollingsworth M, Aksamit D, Twilley M, Camacho C, Nogee DP, Jung J, Nelson-McMillan K, Shilkofski N, Perretta JS. Integration of in-hospital cardiac arrest contextual curriculum into a basic life support course: a

randomized, controlled simulation study. *Resuscitation.* 2017;114:127–132. doi: 10.1016/j.resuscitation.2017.03.014
172. Hunt EA, Duval-Arnould JM, Nelson-McMillan KL, Bradshaw JH, Diener-West M, Perretta JS, Shilkofski NA. Pediatric resident resuscitation skills improve after "rapid cycle deliberate practice" training. *Resuscitation.* 2014;85:945–951. doi: 10.1016/j.resuscitation.2014.02.025
173. Jeffers J, Eppich W, Trainor J, Mobley B, Adler M. Development and Evaluation of a Learning Intervention Targeting First-Year Resident Defibrillation Skills. *Pediatr Emerg Care.* 2016;32:210–216. doi: 10.1097/PEC.0000000000000765
174. Reed T, Pirotte M, McHugh M, Oh L, Lovett S, Hoyt AE, Quinones D, Adams W, Gruener G, McGaghie WC. Simulation-Based Mastery Learning Improves Medical Student Performance and Retention of Core Clinical Skills. *Simul Healthc.* 2016;11:173–180. doi: 10.1097/SIH.0000000000000154
175. Kurup V, Matei V, Ray J. Role of in-situ simulation for training in healthcare: opportunities and challenges. *Curr Opin Anaesthesiol.* 2017;30:755–760. doi: 10.1097/ACO.0000000000000514
176. Goldshtein D, Krensky C, Doshi S, Perelman VS. In situ simulation and its effects on patient outcomes: a systematic review. *BMJ Simulation and Technology Enhanced Learning.* 2020;6:3–9. doi: 10.1136/bmjstel-2018-000387
177. Rosen MA, Hunt EA, Pronovost PJ, Federowicz MA, Weaver SJ. In situ simulation in continuing education for the health care professions: a systematic review. *J Contin Educ Health Prof.* 2012;32:243–254. doi: 10.1002/chp.21152
178. Steinemann S, Berg B, Skinner A, DiTulio A, Anzelon K, Terada K, Oliver C, Ho HC, Speck C. In situ, multidisciplinary, simulation-based teamwork training improves early trauma care. *J Surg Educ.* 2011;68:472–477. doi: 10.1016/j.jsurg.2011.05.009
179. Clarke SO, Julie IM, Yao AP, Bang H, Barton JD, Alsomali SM, Kiefer MV, Al Khulaif AH, Aljahany M, Venugopal S, Bair AE. Longitudinal exploration of in situ mock code events and the performance of cardiac arrest skills. *BMJ Simul Technol Enhanc Learn.* 2019;5:29–33. doi: 10.1136/bmjstel-2017-000255
180. Rubio-Gurung S, Putet G, Touzet S, Gauthier-Moulinier H, Jordan I, Beissel A, Labaune JM, Blanc S, Amamra N, Balandras C, Rudigoz RC, Colin C, Picaud JC. In situ simulation training for neonatal resuscitation: an RCT. *Pediatrics.* 2014;134:e790–e797. doi: 10.1542/peds.2013-3988
181. Saqe-Rockoff A, Ciardiello AV, Schubert FD. Low-Fidelity, In-Situ Pediatric Resuscitation Simulation Improves RN Competence and Self-Efficacy. *J Emerg Nurs.* 2019;45:538–544.e1. doi: 10.1016/j.jen.2019.02.003
182. Katznelson JH, Wang J, Stevens MW, Mills WA. Improving Pediatric Preparedness in Critical Access Hospital Emergency Departments: Impact of a Longitudinal In Situ Simulation Program. *Pediatr Emerg Care.* 2018;34:17–20. doi: 10.1097/PEC.0000000000001366
183. Reder S, Cummings P, Quan L. Comparison of three instructional methods for teaching cardiopulmonary resuscitation and use of an automatic external defibrillator to high school students. *Resuscitation.* 2006;69:443–453. doi: 10.1016/j.resuscitation.2005.08.020
184. Roppolo LP, Pepe PE, Campbell L, Ohman K, Kulkarni H, Miller R, Idris A, Bean L, Bettes TN, Idris AH. Prospective, randomized trial of the effectiveness and retention of 30-min layperson training for cardiopulmonary resuscitation and automated external defibrillators: The American Airlines Study. *Resuscitation.* 2007;74:276–285. doi: 10.1016/j.resuscitation.2006.12.017
185. de Vries W, Turner NM, Monsieurs KG, Bierens JJ, Koster RW. Comparison of instructor-led automated external defibrillation training and three alternative DVD-based training methods. *Resuscitation.* 2010;81:1004–1009. doi: 10.1016/j.resuscitation.2010.04.006
186. Saraç L, Ok A. The effects of different instructional methods on students' acquisition and retention of cardiopulmonary resuscitation skills. *Resuscitation.* 2010;81:555–561. doi: 10.1016/j.resuscitation.2009.08.030
187. Zeleke BG, Biswas ES, Biswas M. Teaching Cardiopulmonary Resuscitation to Young Children (<12 Years Old). *Am J Cardiol.* 2019;123:1626–1627. doi: 10.1016/j.amjcard.2019.02.011
188. Schmid KM, García RQ, Fernandez MM, Mould-Millman NK, Lowenstein SR. Teaching Hands-Only CPR in Schools: A Program Evaluation in San José, Costa Rica. *Ann Glob Health.* 2018;84:612–617. doi: 10.9204/aogh.2367
189. Li H, Shen X, Xu X, Wang Y, Chu L, Zhao J, Wang Y, Wang H, Xie G, Cheng B, et al. Bystander cardiopulmonary resuscitation training in primary and secondary school children in China and the impact of neighborhood socioeconomic status: A prospective controlled trial. *Medicine (Baltimore).* 2018;97:e12673. doi: 10.1097/MD.0000000000012673
190. Paglino M, Contri E, Baggiani M, Tonani M, Costantini G, Bonomo MC, Baldi E. A video-based training to effectively teach CPR with long-term retention: the ScuolaSalvaVita.it ("SchoolSavesLives.it") project. *Intern Emerg Med.* 2019;14:275–279. doi: 10.1007/s11739-018-1946-3
191. Magid KH, Heard D, Sasson C. Addressing Gaps in Cardiopulmonary Resuscitation Education: Training Middle School Students in Hands-Only Cardiopulmonary Resuscitation. *J Sch Health.* 2018;88:524–530. doi: 10.1111/josh.12634
192. Andrews T, Price L, Mills B, Holmes L. Young adults' perception of mandatory CPR training in Australian high schools: a qualitative investigation. *Austr J Paramedicine.* 2018;15. doi: 10.33151/ajp.15.2.577
193. Aloush S, Tubaishat A, ALBashtawy M, Suliman M, Alrimawi I, Al Sabah A, Banikhaled Y. Effectiveness of Basic Life Support Training for Middle School Students. *J Sch Nurs.* 2019;35:262–267. doi: 10.1177/1059840517753879
194. Gabriel IO, Aluko JO. Theoretical knowledge and psychomotor skill acquisition of basic life support training programme among secondary school students. *World J Emerg Med.* 2019;10:81–87. doi: 10.5847/wjem.j.1920-8642.2019.02.003
195. Brown LE, Carroll T, Lynes C, Tripathi A, Halperin H, Dillon WC. CPR skill retention in 795 high school students following a 45-minute course with psychomotor practice. *Am J Emerg Med.* 2018;36:1110–1112. doi: 10.1016/j.ajem.2017.10.026
196. Brookoff D, Kellermann AL, Hackman BB, Somes G, Dobyns P. Do blacks get bystander cardiopulmonary resuscitation as often as whites? *Ann Emerg Med.* 1994;24:1147–1150. doi: 10.1016/s0196-0644(94)70246-2
197. Vadeboncoeur TF, Richman PB, Darkoh M, Chikani V, Clark L, Bobrow BJ. Bystander cardiopulmonary resuscitation for out-of-hospital cardiac arrest in the Hispanic vs the non-Hispanic populations. *Am J Emerg Med.* 2008;26:655–660. doi: 10.1016/j.ajem.2007.10.002
198. Anderson ML, Cox M, Al-Khatib SM, Nichol G, Thomas KL, Chan PS, Saha-Chaudhuri P, Fosbol EL, Eigel B, Clendenen B, Peterson ED. Rates of cardiopulmonary resuscitation training in the United States. *JAMA Intern Med.* 2014;174:194–201. doi: 10.1001/jamainternmed.2013.11320
199. Fosbøl EL, Dupre ME, Strauss B, Swanson DR, Myers B, McNally BF, Anderson ML, Bagai A, Monk L, Garvey JL, Bitner M, Jollis JG, Granger CB. Association of neighborhood characteristics with incidence of out-of-hospital cardiac arrest and rates of bystander-initiated CPR: implications for community-based education intervention. *Resuscitation.* 2014;85:1512–1517. doi: 10.1016/j.resuscitation.2014.08.013
200. Blewer AL, Schmicker RH, Morrison LJ, Aufderheide TP, Daya M, Starks MA, May S, Idris AH, Callaway CW, Kudenchuk PJ, Vilke GM, Abella BS; Resuscitation Outcomes Consortium Investigators. Variation in Bystander Cardiopulmonary Resuscitation Delivery and Subsequent Survival From Out-of-Hospital Cardiac Arrest Based on Neighborhood-Level Ethnic Characteristics. *Circulation.* 2020;141:34–41. doi: 10.1161/CIRCULATIONAHA.119.041541
201. Mitchell MJ, Stubbs BA, Eisenberg MS. Socioeconomic status is associated with provision of bystander cardiopulmonary resuscitation. *Prehosp Emerg Care.* 2009;13:478–486. doi: 10.1080/10903120903144833
202. Vaillancourt C, Lui A, De Maio VJ, Wells GA, Stiell IG. Socioeconomic status influences bystander CPR and survival rates for out-of-hospital cardiac arrest victims. *Resuscitation.* 2008;79:417–423. doi: 10.1016/j.resuscitation.2008.07.012
203. Chiang WC, Ko PC, Chang AM, Chen WT, Liu SS, Huang YS, Chen SY, Lin CH, Cheng MT, Chong KM, Wang HC, Yang CW, Liao MW, Wang CH, Chien YC, Lin CH, Liu YP, Lee BC, Chien KL, Lai MS, Ma MH. Bystander-initiated CPR in an Asian metropolitan: does the socioeconomic status matter? *Resuscitation.* 2014;85:53–58. doi: 10.1016/j.resuscitation.2013.07.033
204. Moncur L, Ainsborough N, Ghose R, Kendal SP, Salvatori M, Wright J. Does the level of socioeconomic deprivation at the location of cardiac arrest in an English region influence the likelihood of receiving bystander-initiated cardiopulmonary resuscitation? *Emerg Med J.* 2016;33:105–108. doi: 10.1136/emermed-2015-204643
205. Dahan B, Jabre P, Karam N, Misslin R, Tafflet M, Bougouin W, Jost D, Beganton F, Marijon E, Jouven X. Impact of neighbourhood socio-economic status on bystander cardiopulmonary resuscitation in Paris. *Resuscitation.* 2017;110:107–113. doi: 10.1016/j.resuscitation.2016.10.028
206. Brown TP, Booth S, Hawkes CA, Soar J, Mark J, Mapstone J, Fothergill RT, Black S, Pocock H, Bichmann A, Gunson I, Perkins GD. Characteristics of neighbourhoods with high incidence of out-of-hospital cardiac arrest and low bystander cardiopulmonary resuscitation rates in England. *Eur Heart J Qual Care Clin Outcomes.* 2019;5:51–62. doi: 10.1093/ehjqcco/qcy026
207. Liu KY, Haukoos JS, Sasson C. Availability and quality of cardiopulmonary resuscitation information for Spanish-speaking

population on the Internet. *Resuscitation.* 2014;85:131–137. doi: 10.1016/j.resuscitation.2013.08.274
208. Yip MP, Ong B, Tu SP, Chavez D, Ike B, Painter I, Lam I, Bradley SM, Coronado GD, Meischke HW. Diffusion of cardiopulmonary resuscitation training to chinese immigrants with limited english proficiency. *Emerg Med Int.* 2011;2011:685249. doi: 10.1155/2011/685249
209. Meischke H, Taylor V, Calhoun R, Liu Q, Sos C, Tu SP, Yip MP, Eisenberg D. Preparedness for cardiac emergencies among Cambodians with limited English proficiency. *J Community Health.* 2012;37:176–180. doi: 10.1007/s10900-011-9433-z
210. Sasson C, Haukoos JS, Bond C, Rabe M, Colbert SH, King R, Sayre M, Heisler M. Barriers and facilitators to learning and performing cardiopulmonary resuscitation in neighborhoods with low bystander cardiopulmonary resuscitation prevalence and high rates of cardiac arrest in Columbus, OH. *Circ Cardiovasc Qual Outcomes.* 2013;6:550–558. doi: 10.1161/CIRCOUTCOMES.111.000097
211. Sasson C, Haukoos JS, Ben-Youssef L, Ramirez L, Bull S, Eigel B, Magid DJ, Padilla R. Barriers to calling 911 and learning and performing cardiopulmonary resuscitation for residents of primarily Latino, high-risk neighborhoods in Denver, Colorado. *Ann Emerg Med.* 2015;65:545–552.e2. doi: 10.1016/j.annemergmed.2014.10.028
212. Blewer AL, Ibrahim SA, Leary M, Dutwin D, McNally B, Anderson ML, Morrison LJ, Aufderheide TP, Daya M, Idris AH, et al. Cardiopulmonary resuscitation training disparities in the United States *J Am Heart Assoc.* 2017;6:e006124. doi: 10.1161/JAHA.117.006124
213. Abdulhay NM, Totolos K, McGovern S, Hewitt N, Bhardwaj A, Buckler DG, Leary M, Abella BS. Socioeconomic disparities in layperson CPR training within a large U.S. city. *Resuscitation.* 2019;141:13–18. doi: 10.1016/j.resuscitation.2019.05.038
214. Sasson C, Keirns CC, Smith DM, Sayre MR, Macy ML, Meurer WJ, McNally BF, Kellermann AL, Iwashyna TJ. Examining the contextual effects of neighborhood on out-of-hospital cardiac arrest and the provision of bystander cardiopulmonary resuscitation. *Resuscitation.* 2011;82:674–679. doi: 10.1016/j.resuscitation.2011.02.002
215. Root ED, Gonzales L, Persse DE, Hinchey PR, McNally B, Sasson C. A tale of two cities: the role of neighborhood socioeconomic status in spatial clustering of bystander CPR in Austin and Houston. *Resuscitation.* 2013;84:752–759. doi: 10.1016/j.resuscitation.2013.01.007
216. Becker TK, Gul SS, Cohen SA, Maciel CB, Baron-Lee J, Murphy TW, Youn TS, Tyndall JA, Gibbons C, Hart L, Alviar CL; Florida Cardiac Arrest Resource Team. Public perception towards bystander cardiopulmonary resuscitation. *Emerg Med J.* 2019;36:660–665. doi: 10.1136/emermed-2018-208234
217. Perman SM, Shelton SK, Knoepke C, Rappaport K, Matlock DD, Adelgais K, Havranek EP, Daugherty SL. Public Perceptions on Why Women Receive Less Bystander Cardiopulmonary Resuscitation Than Men in Out-of-Hospital Cardiac Arrest. *Circulation.* 2019;139:1060–1068. doi: 10.1161/CIRCULATIONAHA.118.037692
218. Blewer AL, McGovern SK, Schmicker RH, May S, Morrison LJ, Aufderheide TP, Daya M, Idris AH, Callaway CW, Kudenchuk PJ, Vilke GM, Abella BS; Resuscitation Outcomes Consortium (ROC) Investigators. Gender Disparities Among Adult Recipients of Bystander Cardiopulmonary Resuscitation in the Public. *Circ Cardiovasc Qual Outcomes.* 2018;11:e004710. doi: 10.1161/CIRCOUTCOMES.118.004710
219. Kramer CE, Wilkins MS, Davies JM, Caird JK, Hallihan GM. Does the sex of a simulated patient affect CPR? *Resuscitation.* 2015;86:82–87. doi: 10.1016/j.resuscitation.2014.10.016
220. Camp BN, Parish DC, Andrews RH. Effect of advanced cardiac life support training on resuscitation efforts and survival in a rural hospital. *Ann Emerg Med.* 1997;29:529–533. doi: 10.1016/s0196-0644(97)70228-2
221. Dane FC, Russell-Lindgren KS, Parish DC, Durham MD, Brown TD. In-hospital resuscitation: association between ACLS training and survival to discharge. *Resuscitation.* 2000;47:83–87. doi: 10.1016/s0300-9572(00)00210-0
222. Lowenstein SR, Sabyan EM, Lassen CF, Kern DC. Benefits of training physicians in advanced cardiac life support. *Chest.* 1986;89:512–516. doi: 10.1378/chest.89.4.512
223. Makker R, Gray-Siracusa K, Evers M. Evaluation of advanced cardiac life support in a community teaching hospital by use of actual cardiac arrests. *Heart Lung.* 1995;24:116–120. doi: 10.1016/s0147-9563(05)80005-6
224. Moretti MA, Cesar LA, Nusbacher A, Kern KB, Timerman S, Ramires JA. Advanced cardiac life support training improves long-term survival from in-hospital cardiac arrest. *Resuscitation.* 2007;72:458–465. doi: 10.1016/j.resuscitation.2006.06.039
225. Pottle A, Brant S. Does resuscitation training affect outcome from cardiac arrest? *Accid Emerg Nurs.* 2000;8:46–51. doi: 10.1054/aaen.1999.0089
226. Sanders AB, Berg RA, Burress M, Genova RT, Kern KB, Ewy GA. The efficacy of an ACLS training program for resuscitation from cardiac arrest in a rural community. *Ann Emerg Med.* 1994;23:56–59. doi: 10.1016/s0196-0644(94)70009-5
227. Sodhi K, Singla MK, Shrivastava A. Impact of advanced cardiac life support training program on the outcome of cardiopulmonary resuscitation in a tertiary care hospital. *Indian J Crit Care Med.* 2011;15:209–212. doi: 10.4103/0972-5229.92070
228. Lockey A, Lin Y, Cheng A. Impact of adult advanced cardiac life support course participation on patient outcomes-A systematic review and meta-analysis. *Resuscitation.* 2018;129:48–54. doi: 10.1016/j.resuscitation.2018.05.034
229. Girotra S, van Diepen S, Nallamothu BK, Carrel M, Vellano K, Anderson ML, McNally B, Abella BS, Sasson C, Chan PS; CARES Surveillance Group and the HeartRescue Project. Regional Variation in Out-of-Hospital Cardiac Arrest Survival in the United States. *Circulation.* 2016;133:2159–2168. doi: 10.1161/CIRCULATIONAHA.115.018175
230. Zijlstra JA, Stieglis R, Riedijk F, Smeekes M, van der Worp WE, Koster RW. Local lay rescuers with AEDs, alerted by text messages, contribute to early defibrillation in a Dutch out-of-hospital cardiac arrest dispatch system. *Resuscitation.* 2014;85:1444–1449. doi: 10.1016/j.resuscitation.2014.07.020
231. Berglund E, Claesson A, Nordberg P, Djärv T, Lundgren P, Folke F, Forsberg S, Riva G, Ringh M. A smartphone application for dispatch of lay responders to out-of-hospital cardiac arrests. *Resuscitation.* 2018;126:160–165. doi: 10.1016/j.resuscitation.2018.01.039
232. Fletcher KA, Bedwell WL. Cognitive aids: design suggestions for the medical field. *Proc Int Symp Human Factors Ergonomics Health Care.* 2014;3:148–152. doi: 10.1177/2327857914031024
233. Fitzgerald M, Cameron P, Mackenzie C, Farrow N, Scicluna P, Gocentas R, Bystrzycki A, Lee G, O'Reilly G, Andrianopoulos N, Dziukas L, Cooper DJ, Silvers A, Mori A, Murray A, Smith S, Xiao Y, Stub D, McDermott FT, Rosenfeld JV. Trauma resuscitation errors and computer-assisted decision support. *Arch Surg.* 2011;146:218–225. doi: 10.1001/archsurg.2010.333
234. Bernhard M, Becker TK, Nowe T, Mohorovicic M, Sikinger M, Brenner T, Richter GM, Radeleff B, Meeder PJ, Büchler MW, Böttiger BW, Martin E, Gries A. Introduction of a treatment algorithm can improve the early management of emergency patients in the resuscitation room. *Resuscitation.* 2007;73:362–373. doi: 10.1016/j.resuscitation.2006.09.014
235. Kelleher DC, Carter EA, Waterhouse LJ, Parsons SE, Fritzeen JL, Burd RS. Effect of a checklist on advanced trauma life support task performance during pediatric trauma resuscitation. *Acad Emerg Med.* 2014;21:1129–1134. doi: 10.1111/acem.12487
236. Lashoher A, Schneider EB, Juillard C, Stevens K, Colantuoni E, Berry WR, Bloem C, Chadbunchachai W, Dharap S, Dy SM, Dziekan G, Gruen RL, Henry JA, Huwer C, Joshipura M, Kelley E, Krug E, Kumar V, Kyamanywa P, Mefire AC, Musafir M, Nathens AB, Ngendahayo E, Nguyen TS, Roy N, Pronovost PJ, Khan IQ, Razzak JA, Rubiano AM, Turner JA, Varghese M, Zakirova R, Mock C. Implementation of the World Health Organization Trauma Care Checklist Program in 11 Centers Across Multiple Economic Strata: Effect on Care Process Measures. *World J Surg.* 2017;41:954–962. doi: 10.1007/s00268-016-3759-8

Circulation

Part 2: Evidence Evaluation and Guidelines Development

2020 American Heart Association Guidelines for Cardiopulmonary Resuscitation and Emergency Cardiovascular Care

ABSTRACT: The *2020 American Heart Association* (AHA) *Guidelines for Cardiopulmonary Resuscitation and Emergency Cardiovascular Care* is based on the extensive evidence evaluation performed in conjunction with the International Liaison Committee on Resuscitation. The Adult Basic and Advanced Life Support, Pediatric Basic and Advanced Life Support, Neonatal Life Support, Resuscitation Education Science, and Systems of Care Writing Groups drafted, reviewed, and approved recommendations, assigning to each recommendation a Class of Recommendation (ie, strength) and Level of Evidence (ie, quality). The 2020 Guidelines are organized in knowledge chunks that are grouped into discrete modules of information on specific topics or management issues. The 2020 Guidelines underwent blinded peer review by subject matter experts and were also reviewed and approved for publication by the AHA Science Advisory and Coordinating Committee and the AHA Executive Committee. The AHA has rigorous conflict-of-interest policies and procedures to minimize the risk of bias or improper influence during development of the guidelines. Anyone involved in any part of the guideline development process disclosed all commercial relationships and other potential conflicts of interest.

David J. Magid, MD, MPH
Khalid Aziz, MBBS, MA, MEd(IT)
Adam Cheng, MD
Mary Fran Hazinski, RN, MSN
Amber V. Hoover, RN, MSN
Melissa Mahgoub, PhD
Ashish R. Panchal, MD, PhD
Comilla Sasson, MD, PhD
Alexis A. Topjian, MD, MSCE
Amber J. Rodriguez, PhD
Aaron Donoghue, MD, MSCE
Katherine M. Berg, MD
Henry C. Lee, MD
Tia T. Raymond, MD
Eric J. Lavonas, MD, MS

INTRODUCTION

This Part describes the process of creating the *2020 American Heart Association* (AHA) *Guidelines for Cardiopulmonary Resuscitation* (CPR) *and Emergency Cardiovascular Care* (ECC). The process of evidence evaluation, the format of the guideline document; the formation of the AHA writing groups; the guideline development, review, and approval process; and the management of potential conflicts of interest are described.

METHODOLOGY AND EVIDENCE REVIEW

The 2020 Guidelines are designed to present a comprehensive yet succinct compilation of guidance for CPR and ECC. These adult basic and advanced life support, pediatric basic and advanced life support, neonatal life support, resuscitation education science, and systems of care guidelines are based on the extensive evidence evaluation performed in conjunction with the International Liaison Committee on Resuscitation (ILCOR), as detailed in the *2020 International Consensus on CPR and ECC Science With Treatment Recommendations* (CoSTR).[1–7]

Key Words: AHA Scientific Statements ■ cardiac arrest ■ evidence evaluation ■ resuscitation

https://www.ahajournals.org/journal/circ

Table 1. GRADE Terminology for Strength of Recommendation and Criteria for Evidence Certainty Assessment[34]

Strength of Recommendation			
Strong Recommendation = We Recommend		Weak Recommendation = We Suggest	
Assessment Criteria for Certainty of Effect			
Study Design	**Certainty of Effect Begins at This Level**	**Lower if**	**Higher if**
Randomized trial	High or moderate	Risk of bias Inconsistency Indirectness Imprecision Publication bias	Large effect Dose response All plausible confounding would reduce demonstrated effect or would suggest a spurious effect when results show no effect
Observational trial	Low or very low		

GRADE indicates Grading of Recommendations, Assessment, Development, and Evaluation.

The AHA partnered with the ILCOR task forces, as well as with other ILCOR member councils, in the evidence review process. The ILCOR Scientific Advisory Committee, consisting of methodological experts, created a methodological governance process for evidence evaluation. Although the *2015 AHA Guidelines Update for CPR and ECC* relied primarily on systematic reviews, the 2020 Guidelines used 3 types of evidence reviews (systematic reviews, scoping reviews, and evidence updates), each of which resulted in a description of the published evidence that facilitated guideline development.[4,8]

Systematic Review

The first type of evidence review is the systematic review, conducted according to the recommendations of the National Academy of Medicine,[9] by using the methodological approach proposed by the Grading of Recommendations, Assessment, Development, and Evaluation (GRADE) Working Group.[10] Each ILCOR task force identified and prioritized questions to be addressed by using the PICOST (population, intervention, comparator, outcome, study design, time frame) format[11] and determined the important outcomes to be reported. A detailed search for relevant publications was performed on MEDLINE, Embase, and Cochrane Library databases, with identified publications screened for further evaluation.

Two systematic reviewers conducted a risk-of-bias assessment for each relevant study by using Cochrane and GRADE criteria for randomized controlled trials (RCTs),[12] Quality Assessment of Diagnostic Accuracy Studies (QUADAS)-2 for studies of diagnostic accuracy,[13] and GRADE criteria for observational and interventional studies informing therapy or prognosis questions.[10] In addition to assessing scientific bias, the Cochrane risk-of-bias tool also considers both the source of funding and potential conflicts of interest of authors of the study. The reviewers created evidence profile tables containing information on all study outcomes.[14] The quality of the evidence (ie, confidence in the estimate of the effect) was categorized as high, moderate, low, or very low[15] on the basis of the study methodologies and the GRADE domains of bias, inconsistency, indirectness, imprecision, and publication bias[10] (Tables 1 and 2). Any unresolved disparity between reviewer assessments was resolved through discussions and consensus with the task force representative of the Scientific Advisory Committee and, if disagreement remained, by the larger ILCOR task force.

The ILCOR task forces reviewed, discussed, and debated the studies and systematic review analyses, drafting a consensus on science statement and a written summary of identified evidence and evidence quality for each outcome. When there was consensus, the task force developed consensus treatment recommendations, labeled as strong or weak and either for or against a therapy, prognostic tool, or diagnostic test, noting the certainty of the evidence. In addition, each topic summary included the PICOST question and a justification and evidence-to-decision framework section, capturing the values and preferences considered by the task force as well as a list of knowledge gaps. Public input was sought at multiple stages, including PICOST development and draft CoSTR statements.[4] The task forces considered all public comments when finalizing the CoSTR statements. All 2020 CoSTR statements underwent peer review by at least 5 subject matter experts and were endorsed by the ILCOR board before publication.

Scoping Review

The second type of evidence review is the scoping review. The purpose of a scoping review is to provide an overview of the available research evidence related to a specific topic and to determine if sufficient evidence is identified to recommend performance of a systematic review. One difference between scoping reviews and systematic reviews is that scoping reviews have broader inclusion criteria, whereas traditional systematic reviews address a narrow, clearly defined question. Unlike the treatment recommendations that can arise from a systematic review, scoping reviews cannot result in a new ILCOR treatment recommendation or modification of an existing ILCOR treatment recommendation.

The methodology for the scoping review was based on the Preferred Reporting Items for Systematic Reviews

Table 2. GRADE Terminology[34]

Risk of bias	Study limitations in randomized trials include lack of allocation concealment, lack of blinding, incomplete accounting of patients and outcome events, selective outcome reporting bias, and stopping early for benefit. Study limitations in observational studies include failure to apply appropriate eligibility criteria, flawed measurement of exposure and outcome, failure to adequately control confounding, and incomplete follow-up.
Inconsistency	Criteria for inconsistency in results include the following: Point estimates vary widely across studies; CIs show minimal or no overlap; statistical test for heterogeneity shows a low *P* value; and the I^2 is large (a measure of variation in point estimates resulting from among-study differences).
Indirectness	Sources of indirectness include data from studies with differences in population (eg, OHCA instead of IHCA, adults instead of children), differences in the intervention (eg, different compression-ventilation ratios), differences in outcome, and indirect comparisons.
Imprecision	Low event rates or small sample sizes will generally result in wide CIs and therefore imprecision.
Publication bias	Several sources of publication bias include tendency not to publish negative studies and the influence of industry-sponsored studies. An asymmetrical funnel plot increases suspicion of publication bias.
Good practice statements	Guideline panels often consider it necessary to issue guidance on specific topics that do not lend themselves to a formal review of research evidence. The reason might be that research into the topic is unlikely to be located or would be considered unethical or infeasible. Criteria for issuing a nongraded good practice statement include the following: There is overwhelming certainty that the benefits of the recommended guidance will outweigh harms, and a specific rationale is provided; the statements should be clear and actionable to a specific target population; the guidance is deemed necessary and might be overlooked by some providers if not specifically communicated; and the recommendations should be readily implementable by the specific target audience to which the guidance is directed.

GRADE indicates Grading of Recommendations, Assessment, Development, and Evaluation; IHCA, in-hospital cardiac arrest; and OHCA, out-of-hospital cardiac arrest.

and Meta-analyses (PRISMA) Extension for Scoping Reviews.[8,16,17] Each task force identified questions to be reviewed, presented in the PICOST format. The MEDLINE, Embase, and Cochrane databases were then searched to identify relevant publications. Those performing the scoping reviews extracted data to create summary tables. The task force then reviewed the studies and the evidence tables, developing a consensus narrative summary of the evidence and an overview of the task force insights. Each topic narrative summary and overview of task force insights as well as the complete scoping review were posted on the ILCOR website for public review and input,[4] with final versions included in the appendix and summarized in the body of the relevant task force CoSTR publication.

Evidence Update

The evidence update is the third type of review supporting the 2020 CoSTR and the 2020 Guidelines. This review is used for questions not undergoing a systematic or scoping review. Evidence updates were performed by AHA writing group members, AHA volunteers, or other ILCOR member council volunteers. The evidence update reviewers used PubMed to conduct searches of English language publications indexed in the MEDLINE database. When the search strategies from previous reviews were available, these were repeated. Searching beyond the MEDLINE database was optional, at the discretion of the reviewer. Reviewers identified relevant new studies, guidelines, and systematic reviews, and completed an evidence update worksheet,[8] which included the research question, the search strategy, and a table summarizing any new evidence. After review by the ILCOR Science Advisory Committee Chair, the evidence update worksheet was included in the relevant 2020 CoSTR task force publication appendix and cited within the body of the manuscript.

GUIDELINE FORMAT

In contrast to prior ECC Guidelines, the 2020 Guidelines are organized in knowledge chunks, grouped into discrete modules of information on specific topics or management issues.[18] Each modular knowledge chunk includes a table of recommendations, a brief introduction or synopsis, recommendation-specific supportive text, and, when appropriate, figures, flow diagrams of algorithms, and additional tables. Hyperlinked references are provided to facilitate quick access and review.

FORMATION OF THE AHA GUIDELINE WRITING GROUPS

The AHA strives to ensure that each guideline writing group includes requisite expertise and diversity, representative of the broader medical community by selecting experts from a wide array of backgrounds, geographic regions of North America, sexes, races, ethnicities, intellectual perspectives, and scopes of clinical practice. Volunteers with an interest and recognized expertise in resuscitation are nominated by the writing group chair, selected by the AHA ECC Committee and approved by the AHA Manuscript Oversight Committee. The Adult Basic and Advanced Life Support Writing Group included experts in emergency medicine, critical care, cardiology, toxicology, neurology, emergency medical services, education, research, and public health. The Pediatric Basic

Table 3. Applying Class of Recommendation and Level of Evidence to Clinical Strategies, Interventions, Treatments, or Diagnostic Testing in Patient Care (Updated May 2019)*

CLASS (STRENGTH) OF RECOMMENDATION

CLASS 1 (STRONG) — **Benefit >>> Risk**

Suggested phrases for writing recommendations:
- Is recommended
- Is indicated/useful/effective/beneficial
- Should be performed/administered/other
- Comparative-Effectiveness Phrases†:
  - Treatment/strategy A is recommended/indicated in preference to treatment B
  - Treatment A should be chosen over treatment B

CLASS 2a (MODERATE) — **Benefit >> Risk**

Suggested phrases for writing recommendations:
- Is reasonable
- Can be useful/effective/beneficial
- Comparative-Effectiveness Phrases†:
  - Treatment/strategy A is probably recommended/indicated in preference to treatment B
  - It is reasonable to choose treatment A over treatment B

CLASS 2b (WEAK) — **Benefit ≥ Risk**

Suggested phrases for writing recommendations:
- May/might be reasonable
- May/might be considered
- Usefulness/effectiveness is unknown/unclear/uncertain or not well-established

CLASS 3: No Benefit (MODERATE) — **Benefit = Risk**
(Generally, LOE A or B use only)

Suggested phrases for writing recommendations:
- Is not recommended
- Is not indicated/useful/effective/beneficial
- Should not be performed/administered/other

Class 3: Harm (STRONG) — **Risk > Benefit**

Suggested phrases for writing recommendations:
- Potentially harmful
- Causes harm
- Associated with excess morbidity/mortality
- Should not be performed/administered/other

LEVEL (QUALITY) OF EVIDENCE‡

LEVEL A
- High-quality evidence‡ from more than 1 RCT
- Meta-analyses of high-quality RCTs
- One or more RCTs corroborated by high-quality registry studies

LEVEL B-R — **(Randomized)**
- Moderate-quality evidence‡ from 1 or more RCTs
- Meta-analyses of moderate-quality RCTs

LEVEL B-NR — **(Nonrandomized)**
- Moderate-quality evidence‡ from 1 or more well-designed, well-executed nonrandomized studies, observational studies, or registry studies
- Meta-analyses of such studies

LEVEL C-LD — **(Limited Data)**
- Randomized or nonrandomized observational or registry studies with limitations of design or execution
- Meta-analyses of such studies
- Physiological or mechanistic studies in human subjects

LEVEL C-EO — **(Expert Opinion)**
- Consensus of expert opinion based on clinical experience

COR and LOE are determined independently (any COR may be paired with any LOE).

A recommendation with LOE C does not imply that the recommendation is weak. Many important clinical questions addressed in guidelines do not lend themselves to clinical trials. Although RCTs are unavailable, there may be a very clear clinical consensus that a particular test or therapy is useful or effective.

* The outcome or result of the intervention should be specified (an improved clinical outcome or increased diagnostic accuracy or incremental prognostic information).

† For comparative-effectiveness recommendations (COR 1 and 2a; LOE A and B only), studies that support the use of comparator verbs should involve direct comparisons of the treatments or strategies being evaluated.

‡ The method of assessing quality is evolving, including the application of standardized, widely-used, and preferably validated evidence grading tools; and for systematic reviews, the incorporation of an Evidence Review Committee.

COR indicates Class of Recommendation; EO, expert opinion; LD, limited data; LOE, Level of Evidence; NR, nonrandomized; R, randomized; and RCT, randomized controlled trial.

This tool has been used in all AHA ECC Guidelines and focused updates since its initial publication in the 2015 Guidelines Update.[35]

and Advanced Life Support Writing Group consisted of pediatric clinicians including intensivists, cardiac intensivists, cardiologists, and emergency physicians and emergency medicine nurses. The Neonatal Life Support Writing Group included neonatal physicians and nurses with backgrounds in clinical medicine, education, research, and public health. The Resuscitation Education Science Writing Group consisted of experts in resuscitation education, clinical medicine (ie, pediatrics, intensive care, emergency medicine), nursing, prehospital care, and health services and education research. The Systems of Care Writing Group included experts in clinical medicine, education, research, and public health. Before appointment, writing group members completed a disclosure of relevant relationships with industry. Writing group members also adhered to all AHA requirements for management of any potential conflicts of interest.

GUIDELINES DEVELOPMENT, REVIEW, AND APPROVAL

Each AHA writing group reviewed all relevant and current AHA guidelines for CPR and ECC,[19–30] pertinent 2020 CoSTR evidence and recommendations,[1–3,6,7] and all relevant evidence update worksheets to determine if current guidelines should be reaffirmed, revised, or retired, or if new recommendations were needed. The writing groups then drafted, reviewed, and approved recommendations, assigning to each recommendation a Class of Recommendation (COR) (ie, strength) and Level of Evidence (LOE) (ie, quality) (Table 3). Each of the 2020 Guidelines articles was submitted for blinded peer review to 5 subject matter experts nominated by the AHA. Before appointment, all peer reviewers were required to disclose relationships with industry and any other potential conflicts of interest, and all disclosures were reviewed by AHA staff. Peer reviewer feedback was provided for guidelines in draft format and again in final format. All guidelines were reviewed and approved for publication by the AHA Science Advisory and Coordinating Committee and AHA Executive Committee.

MANAGEMENT OF POTENTIAL CONFLICTS OF INTEREST

The AHA and ILCOR have rigorous conflict-of-interest policies and procedures to minimize the risk of bias or improper influence during development of the CoSTRs and the AHA guidelines. Both organizations followed these policies[31–33] throughout the 2020 evidence evaluation and document preparation process, and anyone involved in any part of this process was required to disclose all commercial relationships and other potential conflicts (including intellectual) both before joining the writing group and during writing group activities. These disclosures were reviewed before assignment of task force chairs and members, writing group chairs and members, consultants, and peer reviewers. In keeping with the AHA conflict of interest policy, the chair and most members of each ILCOR and AHA writing group had to be free of relevant conflicts. Writing group members do not draft text or vote on any recommendation for which they had a relevant conflict. Appendix 1 lists writing group members' disclosure information. Peer reviewers were also required to disclose relationships with industry and any other potential conflicts of interest; these disclosures appear in Appendix 2.

ARTICLE INFORMATION

The American Heart Association requests that this document be cited as follows: Magid DJ, Aziz K, Cheng A, Hazinski MF, Hoover AV, Mahgoub M, Panchal AR, Sasson C, Topjian AA, Rodriguez AJ, Donoghue A, Berg KM, Lee HC, Raymond T, Lavonas EJ. Part 2: evidence evaluation and guidelines development: 2020 American Heart Association Guidelines for Cardiopulmonary Resuscitation and Emergency Cardiovascular Care. *Circulation*. 2020;142(suppl 2):S358–S365. doi: 10.1161/CIR.0000000000000898

Disclosures

Appendix 1. Writing Group Disclosures

Writing Group Member	Employment	Research Grant	Other Research Support	Speakers' Bureau/ Honoraria	Expert Witness	Ownership Interest	Consultant/ Advisory Board	Other
David J. Magid	University of Colorado	NIH†; NHLBI†; CMS†; AHA†	None	None	None	None	None	American Heart Association (Senior Science Editor)†
Khalid Aziz	University of Alberta Pediatrics	None	None	None	None	None	None	Salary: University of Alberta†
Katherine M. Berg	Beth Israel Deaconess Medical Center Pulmonary and Critical Care	NHLBI Grant K23 HL128814†	None	None	None	None	None	None
Adam Cheng	Alberta Children's Hospital	None	None	None	None	None	None	None
Aaron Donoghue	The Children's Hospital of Philadelphia, University of Pennsylvania School of Medicine	None	None	None	Atkinson, Haskins, Nellis, Brittingham, Gladd & Fiasco*	None	None	None
Mary Fran Hazinski	Vanderbilt University School of Nursing	None	None	None	None	None	American Heart Association†	None
Amber V. Hoover	American Heart Association	None	None	None	None	None	None	None

(*Continued*)

Appendix 1. Continued

Writing Group Member	Employment	Research Grant	Other Research Support	Speakers' Bureau/ Honoraria	Expert Witness	Ownership Interest	Consultant/ Advisory Board	Other
Eric J. Lavonas	Denver Health Emergency Medicine	BTG Pharmaceuticals (Denver Health (Dr Lavonas' employer) has research, call center, consulting, and teaching agreements with BTG Pharmaceuticals. BTG manufactures the digoxin antidote, DigiFab. Dr Lavonas does not receive bonus or incentive compensation, and these agreements involve an unrelated product. When these guidelines were developed, Dr Lavonas recused from discussions related to digoxin poisoning.)†	None	None	None	None	None	American Heart Association (Senior Science Editor)†
Henry C. Lee	Stanford University	NICHD (PI of R01 grant examining intensive care for infants born at extremely early gestational age)*	None	None	None	None	None	None
Melissa Mahgoub	American Heart Association	None	None	None	None	None	None	None
Ashish R. Panchal	The Ohio State University Wexner Medical Center Emergency Medicine	None	None	None	None	None	None	None
Tia T. Raymond	Medical City Children's Hospital Congenital Heart Surgery Unit	None	None	None	None	None	None	None
Amber J. Rodriguez	American Heart Association National Center Emergency Cardiovascular Care	None	None	None	None	None	None	None
Comilla Sasson	American Heart Association	None	None	None	None	None	None	None
Alexis A. Topjian	The Children's Hospital of Philadelphia, University of Pennsylvania School of Medicine Anesthesia and Critical Care	None	None	None	None	None	None	None

This table represents the relationships of writing group members that may be perceived as actual or reasonably perceived conflicts of interest as reported on the Disclosure Questionnaire, which all members of the writing group are required to complete and submit. A relationship is considered to be "significant" if (a) the person receives $10 000 or more during any 12-month period, or 5% or more of the person's gross income; or (b) the person owns 5% or more of the voting stock or share of the entity, or owns $10 000 or more of the fair market value of the entity. A relationship is considered to be "modest" if it is less than "significant" under the preceding definition.

*Modest.

†Significant.

Appendix 2. Reviewer Disclosures

Reviewer	Employment	Research Grant	Other Research Support	Speakers' Bureau/ Honoraria	Expert Witness	Ownership Interest	Consultant/Advisory Board	Other
Fredrik Folke	Gentofte University Hospital (Denmark)	None	None	None	None	None	None	None
Joel Lexchin	University Health Network, Toronto (Canada)	None	None	None	None	None	None	None
Robert T. Mallet	University North Texas Health Science Center	None	None	None	None	None	AHA (service on study sections reviewing grant applications to support resuscitation research)*	None
Mary Ann McNeil	University of Minnesota	None	None	None	None	None	None	None
Taylor Sawyer	Seattle Children's Hospital/ University of Washington	None	None	None	None	None	None	None
Will Smith	Wilderness and Emergency Medicine Consulting (WEMC)	None	None	None	None	None	None	None
Lorrel E. B. Toft	University of Nevada Reno	None	None	None	None	None	None	None

This table represents the relationships of reviewers that may be perceived as actual or reasonably perceived conflicts of interest as reported on the Disclosure Questionnaire, which all reviewers are required to complete and submit. A relationship is considered to be "significant" if (a) the person receives $10 000 or more during any 12-month period, or 5% or more of the person's gross income; or (b) the person owns 5% or more of the voting stock or share of the entity, or owns $10 000 or more of the fair market value of the entity. A relationship is considered to be "modest" if it is less than "significant" under the preceding definition.

*Modest.

REFERENCES

1. Berg KM, Soar J, Andersen LW, Böttiger BW, Cacciola S, Callaway CW, Couper K, Cronberg T, D'Arrigo S, Deakin CD, et al; on behalf of the Adult Advanced Life Support Collaborators. Adult advanced life support: 2020 International Consensus on Cardiopulmonary Resuscitation and Emergency Cardiovascular Care Science With Treatment Recommendations. *Circulation*. 2020;142(suppl 1):S92–S139. doi: 10.1161/CIR.0000000000000893
2. Greif R, Bhanji F, Bigham BL, Bray J, Breckwoldt J, Cheng A, Duff JP, Gilfoyle E, Hsieh M-J, Iwami T, et al; on behalf of the Education, Implementation, and Teams Collaborators. Education, implementation, and teams: 2020 International Consensus on Cardiopulmonary Resuscitation and Emergency Cardiovascular Care Science With Treatment Recommendations. *Circulation*. 2020;142(suppl 1):S222–S283. doi: 10.1161/CIR.0000000000000896
3. Maconochie IK, Aickin R, Hazinski MF, Atkins DL, Bingham R, Couto TB, Guerguerian A-M, Nadkarni VM, Ng K-C, Nuthall GA, et al; on behalf of the Pediatric Life Support Collaborators. Pediatric life support: 2020 International Consensus on Cardiopulmonary Resuscitation and Emergency Cardiovascular Care Science With Treatment Recommendations *Circulation*. 2020;142(suppl 1):S140–S184. doi: 10.1161/CIR.0000000000000894
4. Morley PT, Atkins DL, Finn JC, Maconochie I, Nolan JP, Rabi Y, Singletary EM, Wang TL, Welsford M, Olasveengen TM, et al. Evidence evaluation process and management of potential conflicts of interest: 2020 International Consensus on Cardiopulmonary Resuscitation and Emergency Cardiovascular Care Science With Treatment Recommendations. *Circulation*. 2020;142(suppl 1):S28–S40. doi: 10.1161/CIR.0000000000000891
5. Nolan JP, Maconochie I, Soar J, Olasveengen TM, Greif R, Wyckoff MH, Singletary EM, Aickin R, Berg KM, Mancini ME, et al. Executive summary: 2020 International Consensus on Cardiopulmonary Resuscitation and Emergency Cardiovascular Care Science With Treatment Recommendations. *Circulation*. 2020;142(suppl 1):S2–S27. doi: 10.1161/CIR.0000000000000890
6. Olasveengen TM, Mancini ME, Perkins GD, Avis S, Brooks S, Castrén M, Chung SP, Considine J, Couper K, Escalante R, et al; on behalf of the Adult Basic Life Support Collaborators. Adult basic life support: 2020 International Consensus on Cardiopulmonary Resuscitation and Emergency Cardiovascular Care Science With Treatment Recommendations. *Circulation*. 2020;142(suppl 1):S41–S91. doi: 10.1161/CIR.0000000000000892
7. Wyckoff MH, Wyllie J, Aziz K, de Almeida MF, Fabres J, Fawke J, Guinsburg R, Hosono S, Isayama T, Kapadia VS, et al; on behalf of the Neonatal Life Support Collaborators. Neonatal life support: 2020 International Consensus on Cardiopulmonary Resuscitation and Emergency Cardiovascular Care Science With Treatment Recommendations. *Circulation*. 2020;142(suppl 1):S185–S221. doi: 10.1161/CIR.0000000000000895
8. International Liaison Committee on Resuscitation. Continuous evidence evaluation guidance and templates. https://www.ilcor.org/documents/continuous-evidence-evaluation-guidance-and-templates. Accessed December 31, 2019.
9. Institute of Medicine (US) Committee of Standards for Systematic Reviews of Comparative Effectiveness Research. *Finding What Works in Health Care: Standards for Systematic Reviews*. Washington, DC: The National Academies Press; 2011.
10. GRADE Working Group. 5.2.1. Study limitations (risk of bias). In: Schünemann HJ, Brożek J, Guyatt G, Oxman A., eds. *GRADE Handbook*. 2013. https://gdt.gradepro.org/app/handbook/handbook.html. Accessed December 31, 2019.
11. Cochrane Training. Chapter 5: defining the review questions and developing criteria for including studies. In: O'Connor D, Higgins J, Green S, eds. *Cochrane Handbook for Systematic Reviews of Interventions*. Version 5.1.0. 2011. https://handbook-5-1.cochrane.org/chapter_5/5_defining_the_review_question_and_developing_criteria_for.htm. Accessed December 31, 2019.
12. Cochrane Training. Chapter 8: assessing risk of bias in included studies. In: Higgins JPT, Altman DG, Sterne J, eds. *Cochrane Handbook for Systematic Reviews of Interventions*. Version 5.1.0. 2011. https://handbook-5-1.cochrane.org/chapter_8/8_assessing_risk_of_bias_in_included_studies.htm. Accessed December 31, 2019.
13. Whiting PF, Rutjes AW, Westwood ME, Mallett S, Deeks JJ, Reitsma JB, Leeflang MM, Sterne JA, Bossuyt PM; QUADAS-2 Group. QUADAS-2: a revised tool for the quality assessment of diagnostic accuracy studies. *Ann Intern Med*. 2011;155:529–536. doi: 10.7326/0003-4819-155-8-201110180-00009
14. Evidence Prime. GRADEpro GDT—an introduction to the system. https://gdt.gradepro.org/app/help/user_guide/index.html. Accessed December 31, 2019.
15. Schünemann HJ, Oxman AD, Brozek J, Glasziou P, Jaeschke R, Vist GE, Williams JW Jr, Kunz R, Craig J, Montori VM, Bossuyt P, Guyatt GH; GRADE Working Group. Grading quality of evidence and strength of recommendations for diagnostic tests and strategies. *BMJ*. 2008;336:1106–1110. doi: 10.1136/bmj.39500.677199.AE
16. Tricco AC, Lillie E, Zarin W, O'Brien KK, Colquhoun H, Levac D, Moher D, Peters MDJ, Horsley T, Weeks L, Hempel S, Akl EA, Chang C, McGowan J, Stewart L, Hartling L, Aldcroft A, Wilson MG, Garritty C, Lewin S, Godfrey CM, Macdonald MT, Langlois EV, Soares-Weiser K, Moriarty J, Clifford T,

Tunçalp Ö, Straus SE. PRISMA extension for scoping reviews (PRISMA-ScR): checklist and explanation. *Ann Intern Med.* 2018;169:467–473. doi: 10.7326/M18-0850
17. PRISMA. PRISMA for scoping reviews. http://www.prisma-statement.org/Extensions/ScopingReviews. Accessed December 31, 2019.
18. Levine GN, O'Gara PT, Beckman JA, Al-Khatib SM, Birtcher KK, Cigarroa JE, de Las Fuentes L, Deswal A, Fleisher LA, Gentile F, Goldberger ZD, Hlatky MA, Joglar JA, Piano MR, Wijeysundera DN. Recent innovations, modifications, and evolution of ACC/AHA clinical practice guidelines: an update for our constituencies: a report of the American College of Cardiology/American Heart Association Task Force on Clinical Practice Guidelines. *Circulation.* 2019;139:e879–e886. doi: 10.1161/CIR.0000000000000651
19. Field JM, Hazinski MF, Sayre MR, Chameides L, Schexnayder SM, Hemphill R, Samson RA, Kattwinkel J, Berg RA, Bhanji F, et al. Part 1: executive summary: 2010 American Heart Association Guidelines for Cardiopulmonary Resuscitation and Emergency Cardiovascular Care. *Circulation.* 2010;122(suppl 3):S640–S656. doi: 10.1161/CIRCULATIONAHA.110.970889
20. Neumar RW, Shuster M, Callaway CW, Gent LM, Atkins DL, Bhanji F, Brooks SC, de Caen AR, Donnino MW, Ferrer JM, et al. Part 1: executive summary: 2015 American Heart Association Guidelines Update for Cardiopulmonary Resuscitation and Emergency Cardiovascular Care. *Circulation.* 2015;132(suppl 2):S315–S367. doi: 10.1161/CIR.0000000000000252
21. Kleinman ME, Goldberger ZD, Rea T, Swor RA, Bobrow BJ, Brennan EE, Terry M, Hemphill R, Gazmuri RJ, Hazinski MF, Travers AH. 2017 American Heart Association focused update on adult basic life support and cardiopulmonary resuscitation quality: an update to the American Heart Association Guidelines for Cardiopulmonary Resuscitation and Emergency Cardiovascular Care. *Circulation.* 2018;137:e7–e13. doi: 10.1161/CIR.0000000000000539
22. Escobedo MB, Aziz K, Kapadia VS, Lee HC, Niermeyer S, Schmölzer GM, Szyld E, Weiner GM, Wyckoff MH, Yamada NK, Zaichkin JG. 2019 American Heart Association focused update on neonatal resuscitation: an update to the American Heart Association Guidelines for Cardiopulmonary Resuscitation and Emergency Cardiovascular Care. *Circulation.* 2019;140:e922–e930. doi: 10.1161/CIR.0000000000000729
23. Panchal AR, Berg KM, Cabañas JG, Kurz MC, Link MS, Del Rios M, Hirsch KG, Chan PS, Hazinski MF, Morley PT, Donnino MW, Kudenchuk PJ. 2019 American Heart Association focused update on systems of care: dispatcher-assisted cardiopulmonary resuscitation and cardiac arrest centers: an update to the American Heart Association Guidelines for Cardiopulmonary Resuscitation and Emergency Cardiovascular Care. *Circulation.* 2019;140:e895–e903. doi: 10.1161/CIR.0000000000000733
24. Panchal AR, Berg KM, Hirsch KG, Kudenchuk PJ, Del Rios M, Cabañas JG, Link MS, Kurz MC, Chan PS, Morley PT, et al. 2019 American Heart Association focused update on advanced cardiovascular life support: use of advanced airways, vasopressors, and extracorporeal cardiopulmonary resuscitation during cardiac arrest: an update to the American Heart Association guidelines for cardiopulmonary resuscitation and emergency cardiovascular care. *Circulation.* 2019;140:e881–e894. doi: 10.1161/CIR.0000000000000732
25. Panchal AR, Berg KM, Kudenchuk PJ, Del Rios M, Hirsch KG, Link MS, Kurz MC, Chan PS, Cabañas JG, Morley PT, Hazinski MF, Donnino MW. 2018 American Heart Association focused update on advanced cardiovascular life support use of antiarrhythmic drugs during and immediately after cardiac arrest: an update to the American Heart Association Guidelines for Cardiopulmonary Resuscitation and Emergency Cardiovascular Care. *Circulation.* 2018;138:e740–e749. doi: 10.1161/CIR.0000000000000613
26. Atkins DL, de Caen AR, Berger S, Samson RA, Schexnayder SM, Joyner BL Jr, Bigham BL, Niles DE, Duff JP, Hunt EA, Meaney PA. 2017 American Heart Association focused update on pediatric basic life support and cardiopulmonary resuscitation quality: an update to the American Heart Association Guidelines for Cardiopulmonary Resuscitation and Emergency Cardiovascular Care. *Circulation.* 2018;137:e1–e6. doi: 10.1161/CIR.0000000000000540
27. Charlton NP, Pellegrino JL, Kule A, Slater TM, Epstein JL, Flores GE, Goolsby CA, Orkin AM, Singletary EM, Swain JM. 2019 American Heart Association and American Red Cross focused update for first aid: presyncope: an update to the American Heart Association and American Red Cross Guidelines for First Aid. *Circulation.* 2019;140:e931–e938. doi: 10.1161/CIR.0000000000000730
28. Duff JP, Topjian A, Berg MD, Chan M, Haskell SE, Joyner BL Jr, Lasa JJ, Ley SJ, Raymond TT, Sutton RM, Hazinski MF, Atkins DL. 2018 American Heart Association focused update on pediatric advanced life support: an update to the American Heart Association Guidelines for Cardiopulmonary Resuscitation and Emergency Cardiovascular Care. *Circulation.* 2018;138:e731–e739. doi: 10.1161/CIR.0000000000000612
29. Duff JP, Topjian AA, Berg MD, Chan M, Haskell SE, Joyner BL Jr, Lasa JJ, Ley SJ, Raymond TT, Sutton RM, Hazinski MF, Atkins DL. 2019 American Heart Association focused update on pediatric advanced life support: an update to the American Heart Association Guidelines for Cardiopulmonary Resuscitation and Emergency Cardiovascular Care. *Circulation.* 2019;140:e904–e914. doi: 10.1161/CIR.0000000000000731
30. Duff JP, Topjian AA, Berg MD, Chan M, Haskell SE, Joyner BL Jr, Lasa JJ, Ley SJ, Raymond TT, Sutton RM, et al. 2019 American Heart Association focused update on pediatric basic life support: an update to the American Heart Association guidelines for cardiopulmonary resuscitation and emergency cardiovascular care. *Circulation.* 2019;140:e915–e921. doi: 10.1161/CIR.0000000000000736
31. American Heart Association. Conflict of interest policy. https://www.heart.org/en/about-us/statements-and-policies/conflict-of-interest-policy. Accessed December 31, 2019.
32. American Heart Association. MOC policies and procedures regarding relationships with industry for writing group members. https://professional.heart.org/idc/groups/ahamah-public/@wcm/@sop/@spub/documents/downloadable/ucm_495614.pdf. Accessed April 30, 2020.
33. American College of Cardiology Foundation, American Heart Association. Methodology manual and policies from the ACCF/AHA task force on practice guidelines. 2010. https://professional.heart.org/idc/groups/ahamah-public/@wcm/@sop/documents/downloadable/ucm_319826.pdf. Accessed April 30, 2020.
34. Soar J, Maconochie I, Wyckoff MH, Olasveengen TM, Singletary EM, Greif R, Aickin R, Bhanji F, Donnino MW, Mancini ME, Wyllie JP, Zideman D, Andersen LW, Atkins DL, Aziz K, Bendall J, Berg KM, Berry DC, Bigham BL, Bingham R, Couto TB, Böttiger BW, Borra V, Bray JE, Breckwoldt J, Brooks SC, Buick J, Callaway CW, Carlson JN, Cassan P, Castrén M, Chang WT, Charlton NP, Cheng A, Chung SP, Considine J, Couper K, Dainty KN, Dawson JA, de Almeida MF, de Caen AR, Deakin CD, Drennan IR, Duff JP, Epstein JL, Escalante R, Gazmuri RJ, Gilfoyle E, Granfeldt A, Guerguerian AM, Guinsburg R, Hatanaka T, Holmberg MJ, Hood N, Hosono S, Hsieh MJ, Isayama T, Iwami T, Jensen JL, Kapadia V, Kim HS, Kleinman ME, Kudenchuk PJ, Lang E, Lavonas E, Liley H, Lim SH, Lockey A, Lofgren B, Ma MH, Markenson D, Meaney PA, Meyran D, Mildenhall L, Monsieurs KG, Montgomery W, Morley PT, Morrison LJ, Nadkarni VM, Nation K, Neumar RW, Ng KC, Nicholson T, Nikolaou N, Nishiyama C, Nuthall G, Ohshimo S, Okamoto D, O'Neil B, Yong-Kwang Ong G, Paiva EF, Parr M, Pellegrino JL, Perkins GD, Perlman J, Rabi Y, Reis A, Reynolds JC, Ristagno G, Roehr CC, Sakamoto T, Sandroni C, Schexnayder SM, Scholefield BR, Shimizu N, Skrifvars MB, Smyth MA, Stanton D, Swain J, Szyld E, Tijssen J, Travers A, Trevisanuto D, Vaillancourt C, Van de Voorde P, Velaphi S, Wang TL, Weiner G, Welsford M, Woodin JA, Yeung J, Nolan JP, Hazinski MF. 2019 International Consensus on Cardiopulmonary Resuscitation and Emergency Cardiovascular Care Science With Treatment Recommendations: summary from the Basic Life Support; Advanced Life Support; Pediatric Life Support; Neonatal Life Support; Education, Implementation, and Teams; and First Aid Task Forces. *Circulation.* 2019; 140:e826–e880. doi: 10.1161/CIR.0000000000000734
35. Morrison LJ, Gent LM, Lang E, Nunnally ME, Parker MJ, Callaway CW, Nadkarni VM, Fernandez AR, Billi JE, Egan JR, et al. Part 2: evidence evaluation and management of conflicts of interest: 2015 American Heart Association Guidelines Update for Cardiopulmonary Resuscitation and Emergency Cardiovascular Care. *Circulation.* 2015;132(suppl 2):S368–S382. doi: 10.1161/CIR.0000000000000253

Circulation

Part 3: Adult Basic and Advanced Life Support

2020 American Heart Association Guidelines for Cardiopulmonary Resuscitation and Emergency Cardiovascular Care

Ashish R. Panchal, MD, PhD, Chair
Jason A. Bartos, MD, PhD
José G. Cabañas, MD, MPH
Michael W. Donnino, MD
Ian R. Drennan, ACP, PhD(C)
Karen G. Hirsch, MD
Peter J. Kudenchuk, MD
Michael C. Kurz, MD, MS
Eric J. Lavonas, MD, MS
Peter T. Morley, MBBS
Brian J. O'Neil, MD
Mary Ann Peberdy, MD
Jon C. Rittenberger, MD, MS
Amber J. Rodriguez, PhD
Kelly N. Sawyer, MD, MS
Katherine M. Berg, MD, Vice Chair
On behalf of the Adult Basic and Advanced Life Support Writing Group

TOP 10 TAKE-HOME MESSAGES FOR ADULT CARDIOVASCULAR LIFE SUPPORT

1. On recognition of a cardiac arrest event, a layperson should simultaneously and promptly activate the emergency response system and initiate cardiopulmonary resuscitation (CPR).
2. Performance of high-quality CPR includes adequate compression depth and rate while minimizing pauses in compressions,
3. Early defibrillation with concurrent high-quality CPR is critical to survival when sudden cardiac arrest is caused by ventricular fibrillation or pulseless ventricular tachycardia.
4. Administration of epinephrine with concurrent high-quality CPR improves survival, particularly in patients with nonshockable rhythms.
5. Recognition that all cardiac arrest events are not identical is critical for optimal patient outcome, and specialized management is necessary for many conditions (eg, electrolyte abnormalities, pregnancy, after cardiac surgery).
6. The opioid epidemic has resulted in an increase in opioid-associated out-of-hospital cardiac arrest, with the mainstay of care remaining the activation of the emergency response systems and performance of high-quality CPR.
7. Post–cardiac arrest care is a critical component of the Chain of Survival and demands a comprehensive, structured, multidisciplinary system that requires consistent implementation for optimal patient outcomes.
8. Prompt initiation of targeted temperature management is necessary for all patients who do not follow commands after return of spontaneous circulation to ensure optimal functional and neurological outcome.
9. Accurate neurological prognostication in brain-injured cardiac arrest survivors is critically important to ensure that patients with significant potential for recovery are not destined for certain poor outcomes due to care withdrawal.
10. Recovery expectations and survivorship plans that address treatment, surveillance, and rehabilitation need to be provided to cardiac arrest survivors and their caregivers at hospital discharge to optimize transitions of care to home and to the outpatient setting.

PREAMBLE

In 2015, approximately 350 000 adults in the United States experienced nontraumatic out-of-hospital cardiac arrest (OHCA) attended by emergency medical services (EMS) personnel.[1] Approximately 10.4% of patients with OHCA survive their initial hospitalization, and 8.2% survive with good functional status. The key drivers of successful resuscitation from OHCA are lay rescuer cardiopulmonary

Key Words: AHA Scientific Statements ■ apnea ■ cardiopulmonary resuscitation ■ defibrillators ■ delivery of health care ■ electric countershock ■ heart arrest ■ life support care

https://www.ahajournals.org/journal/circ

resuscitation (CPR) and public use of an automated external defibrillator (AED). Despite recent gains, only 39.2% of adults receive layperson-initiated CPR, and the general public applied an AED in only 11.9% of cases.[1] Survival rates from OHCA vary dramatically between US regions and EMS agencies.[2,3] After significant improvements, survival from OHCA has plateaued since 2012.

Approximately 1.2% of adults admitted to US hospitals suffer in-hospital cardiac arrest (IHCA).[1] Of these patients, 25.8% were discharged from the hospital alive, and 82% of survivors have good functional status at the time of discharge. Despite steady improvement in the rate of survival from IHCA, much opportunity remains.

The International Liaison Committee on Resuscitation (ILCOR) Formula for Survival emphasizes 3 essential components for good resuscitation outcomes: guidelines based on sound resuscitation science, effective education of the lay public and resuscitation providers, and implementation of a well-functioning Chain of Survival.[4]

These guidelines contain recommendations for basic life support (BLS) and advanced life support (ALS) for adult patients and are based on the best available resuscitation science. The Chain of Survival, introduced in Major Concepts, is now expanded to emphasize the important component of survivorship during recovery from cardiac arrest, requires coordinated efforts from medical professionals in a variety of disciplines and, in the case of OHCA, from lay rescuers, emergency dispatchers, and first responders. In addition, specific recommendations about the training of resuscitation providers are provided in "Part 6: Resuscitation Education Science," and recommendations about systems of care are provided in "Part 7: Systems of Care."

INTRODUCTION

Scope of the Guidelines

These guidelines are designed primarily for North American healthcare providers who are looking for an up-to-date summary for BLS and ALS for adults as well as for those who are seeking more in-depth information on resuscitation science and gaps in current knowledge. The BLS care of adolescents follows adult guidelines. This Part of the *2020 American Heart Association* (AHA) *Guidelines for CPR and Emergency Cardiovascular Care* includes recommendations for clinical care of adults with cardiac arrest, including those with life-threatening conditions in whom cardiac arrest is imminent, and after successful resuscitation from cardiac arrest.

Some recommendations are directly relevant to lay rescuers who may or may not have received CPR training and who have little or no access to resuscitation equipment. Other recommendations are relevant to persons with more advanced resuscitation training, functioning either with or without access to resuscitation drugs and devices, working either within or outside of a hospital. Some treatment recommendations involve medical care and decision-making after return of spontaneous circulation (ROSC) or when resuscitation has been unsuccessful. Importantly, recommendations are provided related to team debriefing and systematic feedback to increase future resuscitation success.

Organization of the Writing Group

The Adult Cardiovascular Life Support Writing Group included a diverse group of experts with backgrounds in emergency medicine, critical care, cardiology, toxicology, neurology, EMS, education, research, and public health, along with content experts, AHA staff, and the AHA senior science editors. Each recommendation was developed and formally approved by the writing group.

The AHA has rigorous conflict of interest policies and procedures to minimize the risk of bias or improper influence during the development of guidelines. Before appointment, writing group members disclosed all commercial relationships and other potential (including intellectual) conflicts. These procedures are described more fully in "Part 2: Evidence Evaluation and Guidelines Development." Disclosure information for writing group members is listed in Appendix 1.

Methodology and Evidence Review

These guidelines are based on the extensive evidence evaluation performed in conjunction with the ILCOR and affiliated ILCOR member councils. Three different types of evidence reviews (systematic reviews, scoping reviews, and evidence updates) were used in the 2020 process. Each of these resulted in a description of the literature that facilitated guideline development. A more comprehensive description of these methods is provided in "Part 2: Evidence Evaluation and Guidelines Development."

Class of Recommendation and Level of Evidence

As with all AHA guidelines, each 2020 recommendation is assigned a Class of Recommendation (COR) based on the strength and consistency of the evidence, alternative treatment options, and the impact on patients and society (Table 1). The Level of Evidence (LOE) is based on the quality, quantity, relevance, and consistency of the available evidence. For each recommendation, the writing group discussed and approved specific recommendation wording and the COR and LOE assignments. In determining the COR, the writing group considered the LOE and other factors, including systems issues,

Table 1. Applying Class of Recommendation and Level of Evidence to Clinical Strategies, Interventions, Treatments, or Diagnostic Testing in Patient Care (Updated May 2019)*

CLASS (STRENGTH) OF RECOMMENDATION	
CLASS 1 (STRONG)	**Benefit >>> Risk**
Suggested phrases for writing recommendations: • Is recommended • Is indicated/useful/effective/beneficial • Should be performed/administered/other • Comparative-Effectiveness Phrases†: – Treatment/strategy A is recommended/indicated in preference to treatment B – Treatment A should be chosen over treatment B	
CLASS 2a (MODERATE)	**Benefit >> Risk**
Suggested phrases for writing recommendations: • Is reasonable • Can be useful/effective/beneficial • Comparative-Effectiveness Phrases†: – Treatment/strategy A is probably recommended/indicated in preference to treatment B – It is reasonable to choose treatment A over treatment B	
CLASS 2b (WEAK)	**Benefit ≥ Risk**
Suggested phrases for writing recommendations: • May/might be reasonable • May/might be considered • Usefulness/effectiveness is unknown/unclear/uncertain or not well-established	
CLASS 3: No Benefit (MODERATE) **(Generally, LOE A or B use only)**	**Benefit = Risk**
Suggested phrases for writing recommendations: • Is not recommended • Is not indicated/useful/effective/beneficial • Should not be performed/administered/other	
Class 3: Harm (STRONG)	**Risk > Benefit**
Suggested phrases for writing recommendations: • Potentially harmful • Causes harm • Associated with excess morbidity/mortality • Should not be performed/administered/other	

LEVEL (QUALITY) OF EVIDENCE‡	
LEVEL A	
• High-quality evidence‡ from more than 1 RCT • Meta-analyses of high-quality RCTs • One or more RCTs corroborated by high-quality registry studies	
LEVEL B-R	**(Randomized)**
• Moderate-quality evidence‡ from 1 or more RCTs • Meta-analyses of moderate-quality RCTs	
LEVEL B-NR	**(Nonrandomized)**
• Moderate-quality evidence‡ from 1 or more well-designed, well-executed nonrandomized studies, observational studies, or registry studies • Meta-analyses of such studies	
LEVEL C-LD	**(Limited Data)**
• Randomized or nonrandomized observational or registry studies with limitations of design or execution • Meta-analyses of such studies • Physiological or mechanistic studies in human subjects	
LEVEL C-EO	**(Expert Opinion)**
• Consensus of expert opinion based on clinical experience	

COR and LOE are determined independently (any COR may be paired with any LOE).

A recommendation with LOE C does not imply that the recommendation is weak. Many important clinical questions addressed in guidelines do not lend themselves to clinical trials. Although RCTs are unavailable, there may be a very clear clinical consensus that a particular test or therapy is useful or effective.

* The outcome or result of the intervention should be specified (an improved clinical outcome or increased diagnostic accuracy or incremental prognostic information).

† For comparative-effectiveness recommendations (COR 1 and 2a; LOE A and B only), studies that support the use of comparator verbs should involve direct comparisons of the treatments or strategies being evaluated.

‡ The method of assessing quality is evolving, including the application of standardized, widely-used, and preferably validated evidence grading tools; and for systematic reviews, the incorporation of an Evidence Review Committee.

COR indicates Class of Recommendation; EO, expert opinion; LD, limited data; LOE, Level of Evidence; NR, nonrandomized; R, randomized; and RCT, randomized controlled trial.

economic factors, and ethical factors such as equity, acceptability, and feasibility. These evidence-review methods, including specific criteria used to determine COR and LOE, are described more fully in "Part 2: Evidence Evaluation and Guidelines Development." The Adult Basic and Advanced Life Support Writing Group members had final authority over and formally approved these recommendations.

Unfortunately, despite improvements in the design and funding support for resuscitation research, the overall certainty of the evidence base for resuscitation science is low. Of the 250 recommendations in these guidelines, only 2 recommendations are supported by Level A evidence (high-quality evidence from more than 1 randomized controlled trial [RCT], or 1 or more RCT corroborated by high-quality registry studies.) Thirty-seven recommendations are supported by Level B-Randomized Evidence (moderate evidence from 1 or more RCTs) and 57 by Level B-Nonrandomized evidence. The majority of recommendations are based on Level C evidence, including those based on limited data (123 recommendations) and expert opinion (31 recommendations). Accordingly, the strength of recommendations is weaker than optimal: 78 Class 1 (strong) recommendations, 57 Class 2a (moderate) recommendations, and 89 Class 2b (weak) recommendations are included in these guidelines. In addition, 15 recommendations are designated Class 3: No Benefit, and 11 recommendations are Class 3: Harm. Clinical trials in resuscitation are sorely needed.

Guideline Structure

The 2020 Guidelines are organized into knowledge chunks, grouped into discrete modules of information on specific topics or management issues.[5] Each modular knowledge chunk includes a table of recommendations that uses standard AHA nomenclature of COR and LOE. A brief introduction or short synopsis is provided to put the recommendations into context with important background information and overarching management or treatment concepts. Recommendation-specific text clarifies the rationale and key study data supporting the recommendations. When appropriate, flow diagrams or additional tables are included. Hyperlinked references are provided to facilitate quick access and review.

Document Review and Approval

Each of the 2020 Guidelines documents was submitted for blinded peer review to 5 subject-matter experts nominated by the AHA. Before appointment, all peer reviewers were required to disclose relationships with industry and any other conflicts of interest, and all disclosures were reviewed by AHA staff. Peer reviewer feedback was provided for guidelines in draft format and again in final format. All guidelines were reviewed and approved for publication by the AHA Science Advisory and Coordinating Committee and the AHA Executive Committee. Disclosure information for peer reviewers is listed in Appendix 2.

REFERENCES

1. Virani SS, Alonso A, Benjamin EJ, Bittencourt MS, Callaway CW, Carson AP, Chamberlain AM, Chang AR, Cheng S, Delling FN, et al: on behalf of the American Heart Association Council on Epidemiology and Prevention Statistics Committee and Stroke Statistics Subcommittee. Heart disease and stroke statistics—2020 update: a report from the American Heart Association. *Circulation*. 2020;141:e139–e596. doi: 10.1161/CIR.0000000000000757
2. Okubo M, Schmicker RH, Wallace DJ, Idris AH, Nichol G, Austin MA, Grunau B, Wittwer LK, Richmond N, Morrison LJ, Kurz MC, Cheskes S, Kudenchuk PJ, Zive DM, Aufderheide TP, Wang HE, Herren H, Vaillancourt C, Davis DP, Vilke GM, Scheuermeyer FX, Weisfeldt ML, Elmer J, Colella R, Callaway CW; Resuscitation Outcomes Consortium Investigators. Variation in Survival After Out-of-Hospital Cardiac Arrest Between Emergency Medical Services Agencies. *JAMA Cardiol.* 2018;3:989–999. doi: 10.1001/jamacardio.2018.3037
3. Zive DM, Schmicker R, Daya M, Kudenchuk P, Nichol G, Rittenberger JC, Aufderheide T, Vilke GM, Christenson J, Buick JE, Kaila K, May S, Rea T, Morrison LJ; ROC Investigators. Survival and variability over time from out of hospital cardiac arrest across large geographically diverse communities participating in the Resuscitation Outcomes Consortium. *Resuscitation*. 2018;131:74–82. doi: 10.1016/j.resuscitation.2018.07.023
4. Søreide E, Morrison L, Hillman K, Monsieurs K, Sunde K, Zideman D, Eisenberg M, Sterz F, Nadkarni VM, Soar J, Nolan JP; Utstein Formula for Survival Collaborators. The formula for survival in resuscitation. *Resuscitation*. 2013;84:1487–1493. doi: 10.1016/j.resuscitation.2013.07.020
5. Levine GN, O'Gara PT, Beckman JA, Al-Khatib SM, Birtcher KK, Cigarroa JE, de Las Fuentes L, Deswal A, Fleisher LA, Gentile F, Goldberger ZD, Hlatky MA, Joglar JA, Piano MR, Wijeysundera DN. Recent Innovations, Modifications, and Evolution of ACC/AHA Clinical Practice Guidelines: An Update for Our Constituencies: A Report of the American College of Cardiology/American Heart Association Task Force on Clinical Practice Guidelines. *Circulation*. 2019;139:e879–e886. doi: 10.1161/CIR.0000000000000651

Abbreviations

ACD	active compression-decompression
ACLS	advanced cardiovascular life support
ADC	apparent diffusion coefficient
AED	automated external defibrillator
AHA	American Heart Association
ALS	advanced life support
aOR	adjusted odds ratio
AV	atrioventricular
BLS	basic life support
COR	Class of Recommendation
CoSTR	International Consensus on Cardiopulmonary Resuscitation and Emergency Cardiovascular Care Science With Treatment Recommendations
CPR	cardiopulmonary resuscitation
CT	computed tomography
DWI	diffusion-weighted imaging
ECG	electrocardiogram
ECPR	extracorporeal cardiopulmonary resuscitation
EEG	electroencephalogram
EMS	emergency medical services
$ETCO_2$	(partial pressure of) end-tidal carbon dioxide
ETI	endotracheal intubation
GWR	gray-white ratio
ICU	intensive care unit
IHCA	in-hospital cardiac arrest
ILCOR	International Liaison Committee on Resuscitation
IO	intraosseous
ITD	impedance threshold device
IV	intravenous
LAST	local anesthetic systemic toxicity
LOE	Level of Evidence
MAP	mean arterial pressure
MRI	magnetic resonance imaging
NSE	neuron-specific enolase
OHCA	out-of-hospital cardiac arrest
$Paco_2$	arterial partial pressure of carbon dioxide
PCI	percutaneous coronary intervention
PE	pulmonary embolism
PMCD	perimortem cesarean delivery
pVT	pulseless ventricular tachycardia
RCT	randomized controlled trial
ROSC	return of spontaneous circulation
S100B	S100 calcium binding protein
SGA	supraglottic airway

(*Continued*)

SSEP	somatosensory evoked potential
STEMI	ST-segment elevation myocardial infarction
SVT	supraventricular tachycardia
TCA	tricyclic antidepressant
TOR	termination of resuscitation
TTM	targeted temperature management
VF	ventricular fibrillation
VT	ventricular tachycardia

MAJOR CONCEPTS

Overview Concepts of Adult Cardiac Arrest

Survival and recovery from adult cardiac arrest depend on a complex system working together to secure the best outcome for the victim. The main focus in adult cardiac arrest events includes rapid recognition, prompt provision of CPR, defibrillation of malignant shockable rhythms, and post-ROSC supportive care and treatment of underlying causes. This approach recognizes that most sudden cardiac arrest in adults is of cardiac cause, particularly myocardial infarction and electric disturbances. Arrests without a primary cardiac origin (eg, from respiratory failure, toxic ingestion, pulmonary embolism [PE], or drowning) are also common, however, and in such cases, treatment for reversible underlying causes is important for the rescuer to consider.[1] Some noncardiac etiologies may be particularly common in the in-hospital setting. Others, such as opioid overdose, are sharply on the rise in the out-of-hospital setting.[2] For any cardiac arrest, rescuers are instructed to call for help, perform CPR to restore coronary and cerebral blood flow, and apply an AED to directly treat ventricular fibrillation (VF) or ventricular tachycardia (VT), if present. Although the majority of resuscitation success is achieved by provision of high-quality CPR and defibrillation, other specific treatments for likely underlying causes may be helpful in some cases.

Adult Chain of Survival

The primary focus of cardiac arrest management for providers is the optimization of all critical steps required to improve outcomes. These include activation of the emergency response, provision of high-quality CPR and early defibrillation, ALS interventions, effective post-ROSC care including careful prognostication, and support during recovery and survivorship. All of these activities require organizational infrastructures to support the education, training, equipment, supplies, and communication that enable each survival. Thus, we recognize that each of these diverse aspects of care contributes to the ultimate functional survival of the cardiac arrest victim.

Resuscitation causes, processes, and outcomes are very different for OHCA and IHCA, which are reflected in their respective Chains of Survival (Figure 1). In OHCA, the care of the victim depends on community engagement and response. It is critical for community members to recognize cardiac arrest, phone 9-1-1 (or the local emergency response number), perform CPR

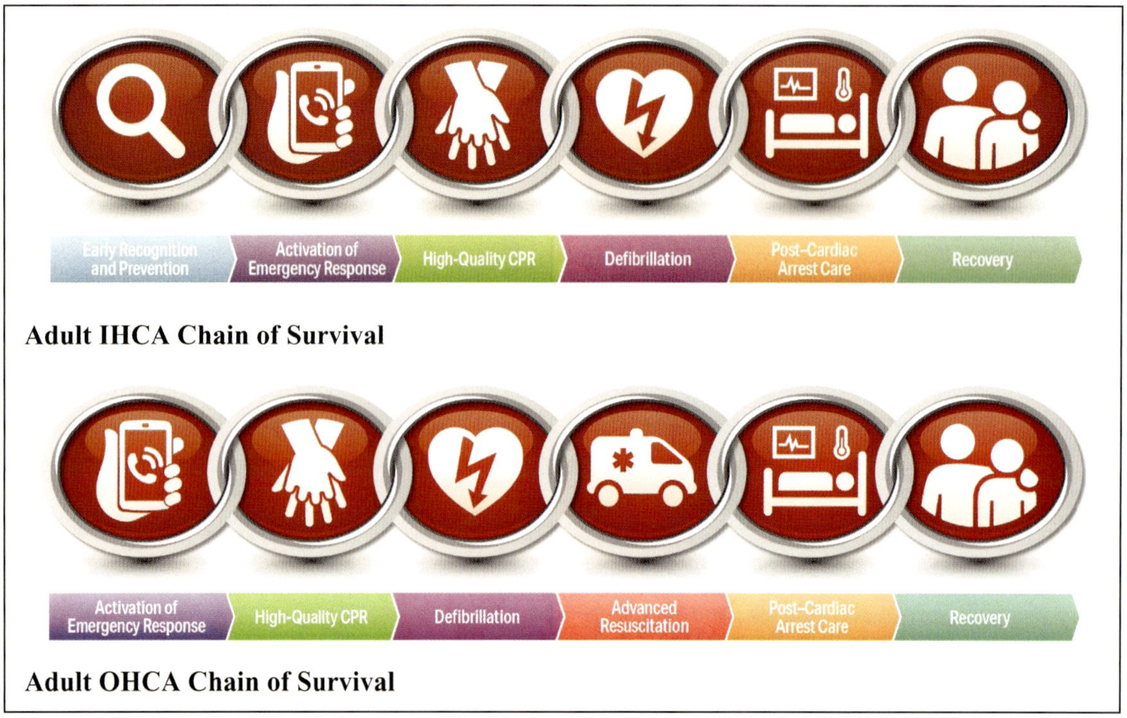
Early Recognition and Prevention
Activation of Emergency Response
High-Quality CPR
Defibrillation
Post-Cardiac Arrest Care
Recovery
Adult IHCA Chain of Survival
Activation of Emergency Response
High-Quality CPR
Defibrillation
Advanced Resuscitation
Post-Cardiac Arrest Care
Recovery
Adult OHCA Chain of Survival

Figure 1. 2020 American Heart Association Chains of Survival for IHCA and OHCA.
CPR indicates cardiopulmonary resuscitation; IHCA, in-hospital cardiac arrest; and OHCA, out-of-hospital cardiac arrest.

(including, for untrained lay rescuers, compression-only CPR), and use an AED.[3,4] Emergency medical personnel are then called to the scene, continue resuscitation, and transport the patient for stabilization and definitive management. In comparison, surveillance and prevention are critical aspects of IHCA. When an arrest occurs in the hospital, a strong multidisciplinary approach includes teams of medical professionals who respond, provide CPR, promptly defibrillate, begin ALS measures, and continue post-ROSC care. Outcomes from IHCA are overall superior to those from OHCA,[5] likely because of reduced delays in initiation of effective resuscitation.

The Adult OHCA and IHCA Chains of Survival have been updated to better highlight the evolution of systems of care and the critical role of recovery and survivorship with the addition of a new link. This Recovery link highlights the enormous recovery and survivorship journey, from the end of acute treatment for critical illness through multimodal rehabilitation (both short- and long-term), for both survivors and families after cardiac arrest. This new link acknowledges the need for the system of care to support recovery, discuss expectations, and provide plans that address treatment, surveillance, and rehabilitation for cardiac arrest survivors and their caregivers as they transition care from the hospital to home and return to role and social function.

REFERENCES

1. Lavonas EJ, Drennan IR, Gabrielli A, Heffner AC, Hoyte CO, Orkin AM, Sawyer KN, Donnino MW. Part 10: special circumstances of resuscitation: 2015 American Heart Association Guidelines Update for Cardiopulmonary Resuscitation and Emergency Cardiovascular Care. *Circulation*. 2015;132(suppl 2):S501–S518. doi: 10.1161/CIR.0000000000000264
2. Dezfulian C, Orkin AM, Maron BA, Elmer J, Girota S, Gladwin MT, Merchant RM, Panchal AR, Perman SM, Starks M, van Diepen S, Lavonas EJ; on behalf of the American Heart Association Council on Cardiopulmonary, Critical Care, Perioperative and Resuscitation; Council on Arteriosclerosis, Thrombosis and Vascular Biology; Council on Cardiovascular and Stroke Nursing; and Council on Clinical Cardiology. Opioid-associated out-of-hospital cardiac arrest: distinctive clinical features and implications for healthcare and public responses: a scientific statement from the American Heart Association. *Circulation*. In press.
3. Sayre MR, Berg RA, Cave DM, Page RL, Potts J, White RD; American Heart Association Emergency Cardiovascular Care Committee. Hands-only (compression-only) cardiopulmonary resuscitation: a call to action for bystander response to adults who experience out-of-hospital sudden cardiac arrest: a science advisory for the public from the American Heart Association Emergency Cardiovascular Care Committee. *Circulation*. 2008;117:2162–2167. doi: 10.1161/CIRCULATIONAHA.107.189380
4. Kleinman ME, Brennan EE, Goldberger ZD, Swor RA, Terry M, Bobrow BJ, Gazmuri RJ, Travers AH, Rea T. Part 5: adult basic life support and cardiopulmonary resuscitation quality: 2015 American Heart Association Guidelines Update for Cardiopulmonary Resuscitation and Emergency Cardiovascular Care. *Circulation*. 2015;132(suppl 2):S414–S435. doi: 10.1161/CIR.0000000000000259
5. Virani SS, Alonso A, Benjamin EJ, Bittencourt MS, Callaway CW, Carson AP, Chamberlain AM, Chang AR, Cheng S, Delling FN, et al: on behalf of the American Heart Association Council on Epidemiology and Prevention Statistics Committee and Stroke Statistics Subcommittee. Heart disease and stroke statistics—2020 update: a report from the American Heart Association. *Circulation*. 2020;141:e139–e596. doi: 10.1161/CIR.0000000000000757

SEQUENCE OF RESUSCITATION

Recognition of Cardiac Arrest

Recommendations for Recognition of Cardiac Arrest

COR	LOE	Recommendations
1	C-LD	1. If a victim is unconscious/unresponsive, with absent or abnormal breathing (ie, only gasping), the lay rescuer should assume the victim is in cardiac arrest.
1	C-LD	2. If a victim is unconscious/unresponsive, with absent or abnormal breathing (ie, only gasping), the healthcare provider should check for a pulse for no more than 10 s and, if no definite pulse is felt, should assume the victim is in cardiac arrest.

Synopsis

Lay rescuer CPR improves survival from cardiac arrest by 2- to 3-fold.[1] The benefit of providing CPR to a patient in cardiac arrest outweighs any potential risk of providing chest compressions to someone who is unconscious but not in cardiac arrest. It has been shown that the risk of injury from CPR is low in these patients.[2]

It has been shown previously that all rescuers may have difficulty detecting a pulse, leading to delays in CPR, or in some cases CPR not being performed at all for patients in cardiac arrest.[3] Recognition of cardiac arrest by lay rescuers, therefore, is determined on the basis of level of consciousness and the respiratory effort of the victim. Recognition of cardiac arrest by healthcare providers includes a pulse check, but the importance of not prolonging efforts to detect a pulse is emphasized.

Recommendation-Specific Supportive Text

1. Agonal breathing is characterized by slow, irregular gasping respirations that are ineffective for ventilation. Agonal breathing is described by lay rescuers with a variety of terms including, *abnormal breathing*, *snoring respirations*, and *gasping*.[4] Agonal breathing is common, reported as being present in up to 40% to 60% of victims of OHCA.[5] The presence of agonal breathing is cited as a common reason for lay rescuers to misdiagnose a patient as not being in cardiac arrest.[6] In patients who are unresponsive, with absent or abnormal breathing, lay rescuers should assume the patient is in cardiac arrest, call for help, and promptly initiate CPR. These 2 criteria (patient responsiveness and assessment of breathing) have been shown to rapidly identify a significant proportion of patients who are in cardiac arrest, allowing for immediate initiation of lay rescuer CPR. Further, initiation of chest compressions in patients who are unconscious

but not in cardiac arrest is associated with low rates of significant adverse events.[2] The adverse events noted included pain in the area of chest compressions (8.7%), bone fracture (ribs and clavicle) (1.7%), and rhabdomyolysis (0.3%), with no visceral injuries described.[2]

2. Protracted delays in CPR can occur when checking for a pulse at the outset of resuscitation efforts as well as between successive cycles of CPR. Healthcare providers often take too long to check for a pulse[7,8] and have difficulty determining if a pulse is present or absent.[7–9] There is no evidence, however, that checking for breathing, coughing, or movement is superior to a pulse check for detection of circulation.[10] Thus, healthcare providers are directed to quickly check for a pulse and to promptly start compressions when a pulse is not definitively palpated.[9,11]

This topic last received formal evidence review in 2010.[3]

REFERENCES

1. Sasson C, Rogers MA, Dahl J, Kellermann AL. Predictors of survival from out-of-hospital cardiac arrest: a systematic review and meta-analysis. *Circ Cardiovasc Qual Outcomes.* 2010;3:63–81. doi: 10.1161/CIRCOUTCOMES.109.889576
2. Olasveengen TM, Mancini ME, Perkins GD, Avis S, Brooks S, Castrén M, Chung SP, Considine J, Couper K, Escalante R, et al; on behalf of the Adult Basic Life Support Collaborators. Adult basic life support: 2020 International Consensus on Cardiopulmonary Resuscitation and Emergency Cardiovascular Care Science With Treatment Recommendations. *Circulation.* 2020;142(suppl 1):S41–S91. doi: 10.1161/CIR.0000000000000892
3. Berg RA, Hemphill R, Abella BS, Aufderheide TP, Cave DM, Hazinski MF, Lerner EB, Rea TD, Sayre MR, Swor RA. Part 5: adult basic life support: 2010 American Heart Association Guidelines for Cardiopulmonary Resuscitation and Emergency Cardiovascular Care. *Circulation.* 2010;122(suppl 3):S685–S705. doi: 10.1161/CIRCULATIONAHA.110.970939
4. Riou M, Ball S, Williams TA, Whiteside A, Cameron P, Fatovich DM, Perkins GD, Smith K, Bray J, Inoue M, O'Halloran KL, Bailey P, Brink D, Finn J. 'She's sort of breathing': What linguistic factors determine call-taker recognition of agonal breathing in emergency calls for cardiac arrest? *Resuscitation.* 2018;122:92–98. doi: 10.1016/j.resuscitation.2017.11.058
5. Fukushima H, Imanishi M, Iwami T, Seki T, Kawai Y, Norimoto K, Urisono Y, Hata M, Nishio K, Saeki K, Kurumatani N, Okuchi K. Abnormal breathing of sudden cardiac arrest victims described by laypersons and its association with emergency medical service dispatcher-assisted cardiopulmonary resuscitation instruction. *Emerg Med J.* 2015;32:314–317. doi: 10.1136/emermed-2013-203112
6. Brinkrolf P, Metelmann B, Scharte C, Zarbock A, Hahnenkamp K, Bohn A. Bystander-witnessed cardiac arrest is associated with reported agonal breathing and leads to less frequent bystander CPR. *Resuscitation.* 2018;127:114–118. doi: 10.1016/j.resuscitation.2018.04.017
7. Eberle B, Dick WF, Schneider T, Wisser G, Doetsch S, Tzanova I. Checking the carotid pulse check: diagnostic accuracy of first responders in patients with and without a pulse. *Resuscitation.* 1996;33:107–116. doi: 10.1016/s0300-9572(96)01016-7
8. Moule P. Checking the carotid pulse: diagnostic accuracy in students of the healthcare professions. *Resuscitation.* 2000;44:195–201. doi: 10.1016/s0300-9572(00)00139-8
9. Ochoa FJ, Ramalle-Gómara E, Carpintero JM, García A, Saralegui I. Competence of health professionals to check the carotid pulse. *Resuscitation.* 1998;37:173–175. doi: 10.1016/s0300-9572(98)00055-0
10. Perkins GD, Stephenson B, Hulme J, Monsieurs KG. Birmingham assessment of breathing study (BABS). *Resuscitation.* 2005;64:109–113. doi: 10.1016/j.resuscitation.2004.09.007
11. Mather C, O'Kelly S. The palpation of pulses. *Anaesthesia.* 1996;51:189–191. doi: 10.1111/j.1365-2044.1996.tb07713.x

Initiation of Resuscitation

Recommendations for Initiation of Resuscitation: Lay Rescuer (Untrained or Trained)

COR	LOE	Recommendations
1	B-NR	1. All lay rescuers should, at minimum, provide chest compressions for victims of cardiac arrest.
1	C-LD	2. After identifying a cardiac arrest, a lone responder should activate the emergency response system first and immediately begin CPR.
1	C-LD	3. We recommend that laypersons initiate CPR for presumed cardiac arrest, because the risk of harm to the patient is low if the patient is not in cardiac arrest.
2a	C-LD	4. For lay rescuers trained in CPR using chest compressions and ventilation (rescue breaths), it is reasonable to provide ventilation (rescue breaths) in addition to chest compressions for the adult in OHCA.

Synopsis

After cardiac arrest is recognized, the Chain of Survival continues with activation of the emergency response system and initiation of CPR. The prompt initiation of CPR is perhaps the most important intervention to improve survival and neurological outcomes. Ideally, activation of the emergency response system and initiation of CPR occur simultaneously. In the current era of widespread mobile device usage and accessibility, a lone responder can activate the emergency response system simultaneously with starting CPR by dialing for help, placing the phone on speaker mode to continue communication, and immediately commencing CPR. In the rare situation when a lone rescuer must leave the victim to dial EMS, the priority should be on prompt EMS activation followed by immediate return to the victim to initiate CPR.

Existing evidence suggests that the potential harm from CPR in a patient who has been incorrectly identified as having cardiac arrest is low.[1] Overall, the benefits of initiation of CPR in cardiac arrest outweigh the relatively low risk of injury for patients not in cardiac arrest. The initial phases of resuscitation once cardiac arrest is recognized are similar between lay responders and healthcare providers, with early CPR representing the priority. Lay rescuers may provide chest compression–only CPR to simplify the process and encourage CPR initiation, whereas healthcare providers may provide chest compressions and ventilation (Figures 2–4).

Recommendation-Specific Supportive Text

1. CPR is the single-most important intervention for a patient in cardiac arrest, and chest compressions should be provided promptly. Chest compressions are the most critical component of CPR, and a chest

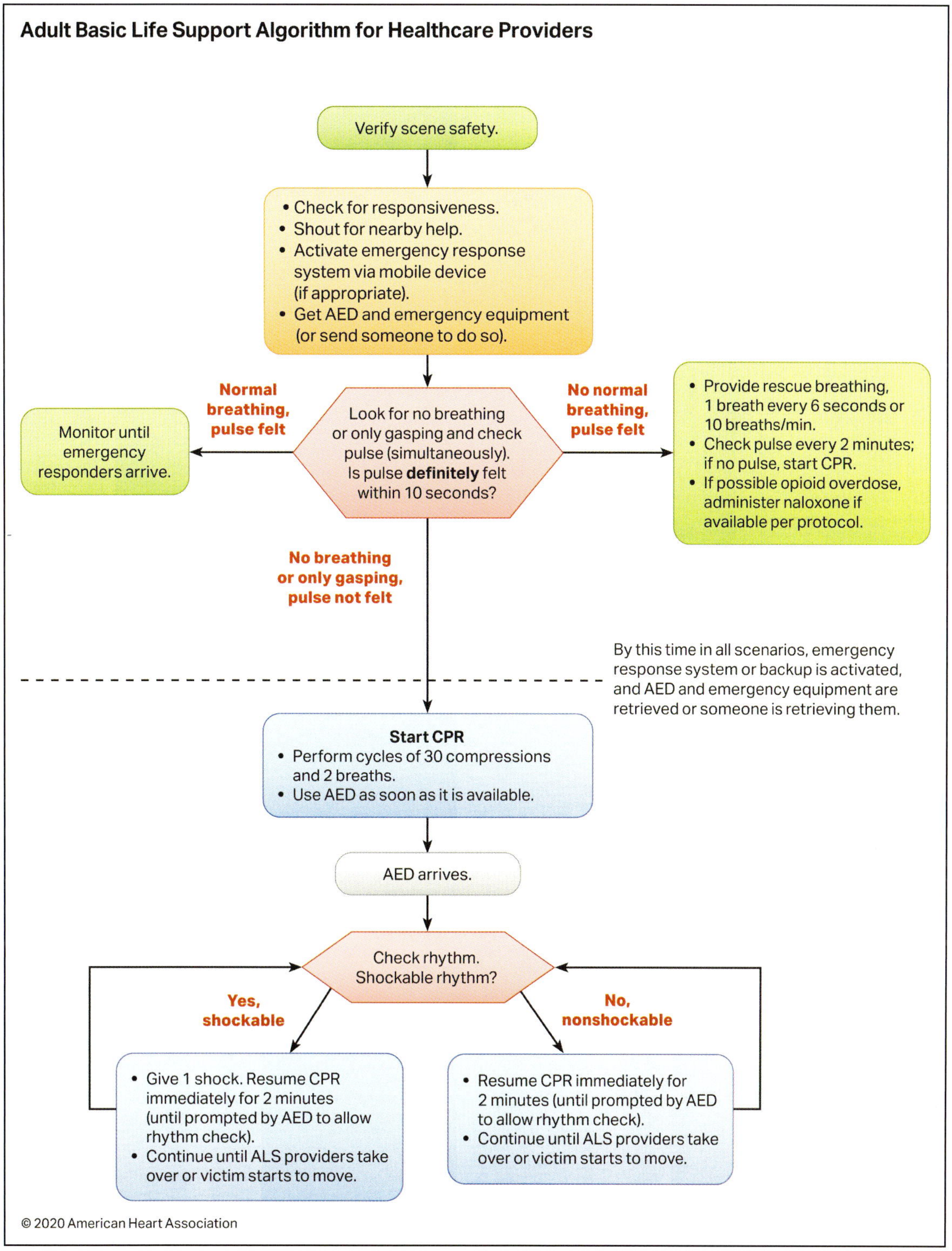
Adult Basic Life Support Algorithm for Healthcare Providers
Verify scene safety.
• Check for responsiveness.
• Shout for nearby help.
• Activate emergency response system via mobile device (if appropriate).
• Get AED and emergency equipment (or send someone to do so).
Look for no breathing or only gasping and check pulse (simultaneously). Is pulse definitely felt within 10 seconds?
Normal breathing, pulse felt
Monitor until emergency responders arrive.
No normal breathing, pulse felt
• Provide rescue breathing, 1 breath every 6 seconds or 10 breaths/min.
• Check pulse every 2 minutes; if no pulse, start CPR.
• If possible opioid overdose, administer naloxone if available per protocol.
No breathing or only gasping, pulse not felt
By this time in all scenarios, emergency response system or backup is activated, and AED and emergency equipment are retrieved or someone is retrieving them.
Start CPR
• Perform cycles of 30 compressions and 2 breaths.
• Use AED as soon as it is available.
AED arrives.
Check rhythm. Shockable rhythm?
Yes, shockable
• Give 1 shock. Resume CPR immediately for 2 minutes (until prompted by AED to allow rhythm check).
• Continue until ALS providers take over or victim starts to move.
No, nonshockable
• Resume CPR immediately for 2 minutes (until prompted by AED to allow rhythm check).
• Continue until ALS providers take over or victim starts to move.
© 2020 American Heart Association

Figure 2. Adult BLS Algorithm for Healthcare Providers.
AED indicates automated external defibrillator; ALS, advanced life support; BLS, basic life support; and CPR, cardiopulmonary resuscitation.

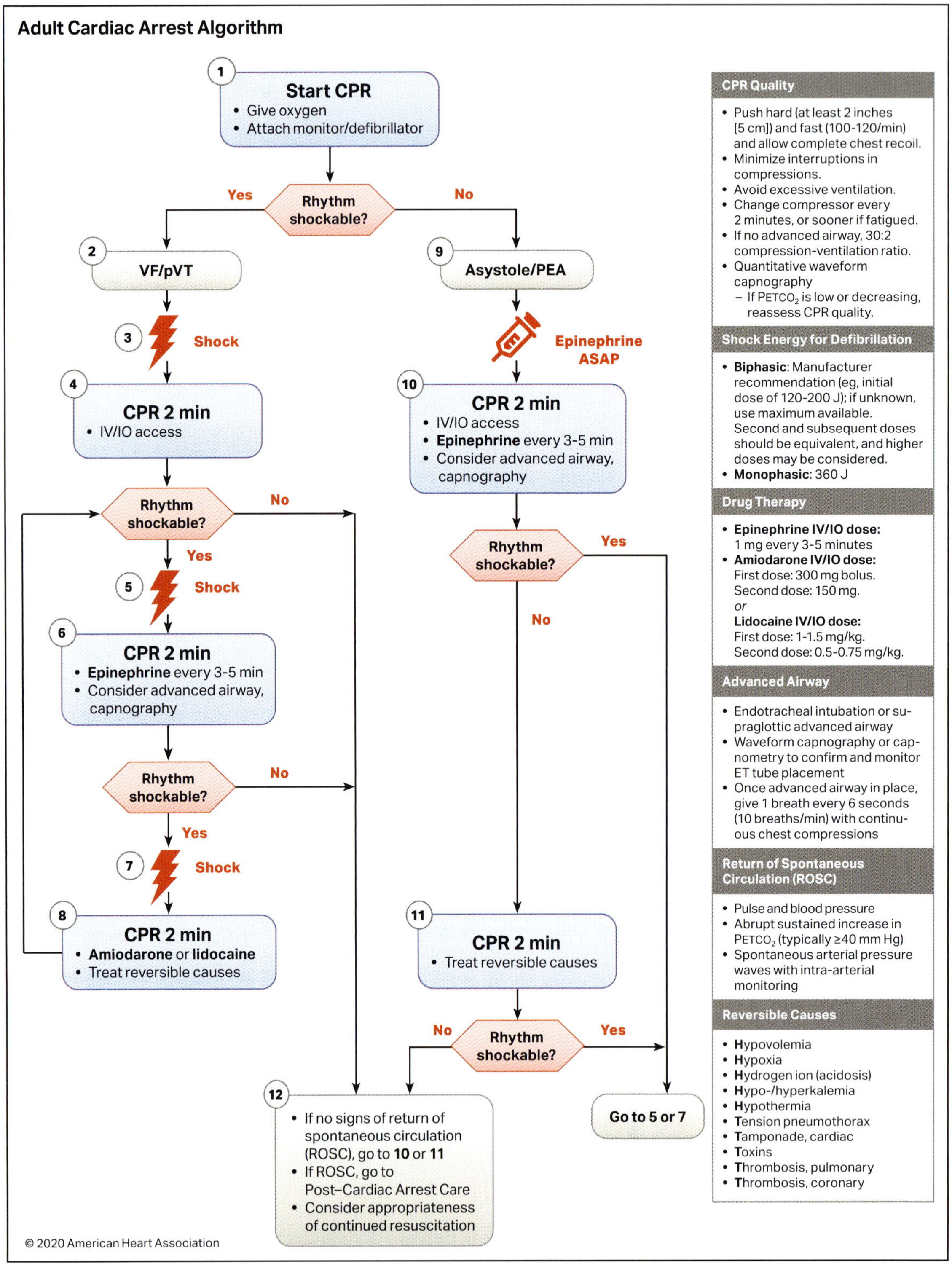

Figure 3. Adult Cardiac Arrest Algorithm.
CPR indicates cardiopulmonary resuscitation; ET, endotracheal; IO, intraosseous; IV, intravenous; PEA, pulseless electrical activity; pVT, pulseless ventricular tachycardia; and VF, ventricular fibrillation.

Adult Cardiac Arrest Circular Algorithm

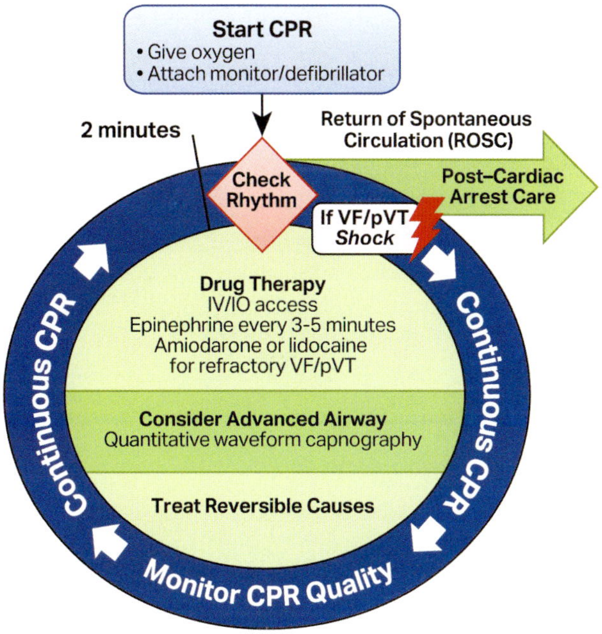

CPR Quality

- Push hard (at least 2 inches [5 cm]) and fast (100-120/min) and allow complete chest recoil.
- Minimize interruptions in compressions.
- Avoid excessive ventilation.
- Change compressor every 2 minutes, or sooner if fatigued.
- If no advanced airway, 30:2 compression-ventilation ratio.
- Quantitative waveform capnography
  – If P_{ETCO_2} is low or decreasing, reassess CPR quality.

Shock Energy for Defibrillation

- **Biphasic:** Manufacturer recommendation (eg, initial dose of 120-200 J); if unknown, use maximum available. Second and subsequent doses should be equivalent, and higher doses may be considered.
- **Monophasic:** 360 J

Drug Therapy

- **Epinephrine IV/IO dose:** 1 mg every 3-5 minutes
- **Amiodarone IV/IO dose:** First dose: 300 mg bolus. Second dose: 150 mg.
  or
- **Lidocaine IV/IO dose:** First dose: 1-1.5 mg/kg. Second dose: 0.5-0.75 mg/kg.

Advanced Airway

- Endotracheal intubation or supraglottic advanced airway
- Waveform capnography or capnometry to confirm and monitor ET tube placement
- Once advanced airway in place, give 1 breath every 6 seconds (10 breaths/min) with continuous chest compressions

Return of Spontaneous Circulation (ROSC)

- Pulse and blood pressure
- Abrupt sustained increase in P_{ETCO_2} (typically ≥40 mm Hg)
- Spontaneous arterial pressure waves with intra-arterial monitoring

Reversible Causes

- **H**ypovolemia
- **H**ypoxia
- **H**ydrogen ion (acidosis)
- **H**ypo-/hyperkalemia
- **H**ypothermia
- **T**ension pneumothorax
- **T**amponade, cardiac
- **T**oxins
- **T**hrombosis, pulmonary
- **T**hrombosis, coronary

Figure 4. Adult Cardiac Arrest Circular Algorithm.
CPR indicates cardiopulmonary resuscitation; ET, endotracheal; IO, intraosseous; IV, intravenous; pVT, pulseless ventricular tachycardia; and VF, ventricular fibrillation.

compression–only approach is appropriate if lay rescuers are untrained or unwilling to provide respirations. Beginning the CPR sequence with compressions minimized time to first chest compression.[2–4] Nationwide dissemination of chest compression–only CPR for lay rescuers was associated with an increase in the incidence of survival with favorable neurological outcome after OHCAs in Japan, likely due to an increase in lay rescuers providing CPR.[5] Chest compressions should be provided as soon as possible, without the need to remove the victim's clothing first.

2. The optimal timing of CPR initiation and emergency response system activation was evaluated by an ILCOR systematic review in 2020.[1] An observational study of over 17 000 OHCA events reported similar results from either a "call-first" strategy or a "CPR-first" strategy.[6] In the current era of ubiquitous mobile devices, ideally both the call to activate EMS and the initiation of CPR can occur simultaneously.
3. Four observational studies[7–10] reported outcomes from patients who were not in cardiac arrest and received CPR by lay rescuers. No serious harm from

CPR was found in patients when they were later determined not to have been in cardiac arrest.[1] This is in contrast to the significant risk of withholding CPR when a patient is in cardiac arrest, making the risk:benefit ratio strongly in favor of providing CPR for presumed cardiac arrest.

4. In some observational studies, improved outcomes have been noted in victims of cardiac arrest who received conventional CPR (compressions and ventilation) compared with those who received chest compressions only.[5,11,12] Other studies have reported no difference in outcomes for patients receiving conventional versus compression-only CPR.[11,13–21] Given the potential benefit of conventional CPR, if lay rescuers are appropriately trained, they should be encouraged to concurrently deliver ventilation with compressions. A thorough review of the data concerning the ratio of compressions to ventilation when performing conventional CPR is discussed in Ventilation and Compression-to-Ventilation Ratio.

These recommendations are supported by the *2020 ILCOR Consensus on CPR and Emergency Cardiovascular Care Science With Treatment Recommendations* (CoSTR).[1]

Recommmdendations for Initiation of Resuscitation: Healthcare Provider

COR	LOE	Recommendations
1	C-LD	1. A lone healthcare provider should commence with chest compressions rather than with ventilation.
2a	C-LD	2. It is reasonable for healthcare providers to perform chest compressions and ventilation for all adult patients in cardiac arrest from either a cardiac or noncardiac cause.

Recommendation-Specific Supportive Text

1. The *2010 Guidelines for CPR and Emergency Cardiovascular Care* included a major change for trained rescuers, who were instructed to begin the CPR sequence with chest compressions rather than with breaths (circulation, airway, and breathing versus airway, breathing, and circulation) to minimize the time to initiation of chest compressions. This approach is resupported by new literature, summarized in a 2020 ILCOR systematic review (Table 2).[1–4] In the recommended sequence, once chest compressions have been started, a single trained rescuer delivers rescue breaths by mouth to mask or by bag-mask device to provide oxygenation and ventilation. Manikin studies demonstrate that starting with chest compressions rather than with ventilation is associated with faster times to chest compressions,[3,23] rescue breaths,[4] and completion of the first CPR cycle.[4]
2. Healthcare providers are trained to deliver both compressions and ventilation. Delivery of chest compressions without assisted ventilation for prolonged periods could be less effective than conventional CPR (compressions plus ventilation) because arterial oxygen content decreases as CPR duration increases. This concern is especially pertinent in the setting of asphyxial cardiac arrest.[11] Healthcare providers, with their training and understanding, can realistically tailor the sequence of subsequent rescue actions to the most likely cause of arrest.

These recommendations are supported by the 2020 CoSTR for BLS.[1]

Table 2. Adult BLS Sequence[22]

Step	Lay Rescuer Not Trained	Lay Rescuer Trained	Healthcare Provider
1	Ensure scene safety.	Ensure scene safety.	Ensure scene safety.
2	Check for response.	Check for response.	Check for response.
3	Shout for nearby help. Phone or ask someone to phone 9-1-1 (the phone or caller with the phone remains at the victim's side, with the phone on speaker mode).	Shout for nearby help and activate the emergency response system (9-1-1, emergency response). If someone responds, ensure that the phone is at the side of the victim if at all possible.	Shout for nearby help/activate the resuscitation team; the provider can activate the resuscitation team at this time or after checking for breathing and pulse.
4	Follow the telecommunicator's* instructions.	Check for no breathing or only gasping; if none, begin CPR with compressions.	Check for no breathing or only gasping and check pulse (ideally simultaneously). Activation and retrieval of the AED/emergency equipment by the lone healthcare provider or by the second person sent by the rescuer must occur no later than immediately after the check for no normal breathing and no pulse identifies cardiac arrest.
5	Look for no breathing or only gasping, at the direction of the telecommunicator.	Answer the telecommunicator's questions, and follow the telecommunicator's instructions.	Immediately begin CPR, and use the AED/defibrillator when available.
6	Follow the telecommunicator's instructions.	Send the second person to retrieve an AED, if one is available.	When the second rescuer arrives, provide 2-rescuer CPR and use the AED/defibrillator.

AED indicates automated external defibrillator; BLS, basic life support; and CPR, cardiopulmonary resuscitation.
**Telecommunicator* and *dispatcher* are terms often used interchangeably.

Circulation. 2020;142(suppl 2):S366–S468. DOI: 10.1161/CIR.0000000000000916

REFERENCES

1. Olasveengen TM, Mancini ME, Perkins GD, Avis S, Brooks S, Castrén M, Chung SP, Considine J, Couper K, Escalante R, et al; on behalf of the Adult Basic Life Support Collaborators. Adult basic life support: 2020 International Consensus on Cardiopulmonary Resuscitation and Emergency Cardiovascular Care Science With Treatment Recommendations. *Circulation.* 2020;142(suppl 1):S41–S91. doi: 10.1161/CIR.0000000000000892
2. Lubrano R, Cecchetti C, Bellelli E, Gentile I, Loayza Levano H, Orsini F, Bertazzoni G, Messi G, Rugolotto S, Pirozzi N, Elli M. Comparison of times of intervention during pediatric CPR maneuvers using ABC and CAB sequences: a randomized trial. *Resuscitation.* 2012;83:1473–1477. doi: 10.1016/j.resuscitation.2012.04.011
3. Sekiguchi H, Kondo Y, Kukita I. Verification of changes in the time taken to initiate chest compressions according to modified basic life support guidelines. *Am J Emerg Med.* 2013;31:1248–1250. doi: 10.1016/j.ajem.2013.02.047
4. Marsch S, Tschan F, Semmer NK, Zobrist R, Hunziker PR, Hunziker S. ABC versus CAB for cardiopulmonary resuscitation: a prospective, randomized simulator-based trial. *Swiss Med Wkly.* 2013;143:w13856. doi: 10.4414/smw.2013.13856
5. Iwami T, Kitamura T, Kiyohara K, Kawamura T. Dissemination of Chest Compression-Only Cardiopulmonary Resuscitation and Survival After Out-of-Hospital Cardiac Arrest. *Circulation.* 2015;132:415–422. doi: 10.1161/CIRCULATIONAHA.114.014905
6. Kamikura T, Iwasaki H, Myojo Y, Sakagami S, Takei Y, Inaba H. Advantage of CPR-first over call-first actions for out-of-hospital cardiac arrests in nonelderly patients and of noncardiac aetiology. *Resuscitation.* 2015;96:37–45. doi: 10.1016/j.resuscitation.2015.06.027
7. White L, Rogers J, Bloomingdale M, Fahrenbruch C, Culley L, Subido C, Eisenberg M, Rea T. Dispatcher-assisted cardiopulmonary resuscitation: risks for patients not in cardiac arrest. *Circulation.* 2010;121:91–97. doi: 10.1161/CIRCULATIONAHA.109.872366
8. Haley KB, Lerner EB, Pirrallo RG, Croft H, Johnson A, Uihlein M. The frequency and consequences of cardiopulmonary resuscitation performed by bystanders on patients who are not in cardiac arrest. *Prehosp Emerg Care.* 2011;15:282–287. doi: 10.3109/10903127.2010.541981
9. Moriwaki Y, Sugiyama M, Tahara Y, Iwashita M, Kosuge T, Harunari N, Arata S, Suzuki N. Complications of bystander cardiopulmonary resuscitation for unconscious patients without cardiopulmonary arrest. *J Emerg Trauma Shock.* 2012;5:3–6. doi: 10.4103/0974-2700.93094
10. Tanaka Y, Nishi T, Takase K, Yoshita Y, Wato Y, Taniguchi J, Hamada Y, Inaba H. Survey of a protocol to increase appropriate implementation of dispatcher-assisted cardiopulmonary resuscitation for out-of-hospital cardiac arrest. *Circulation.* 2014;129:1751–1760. doi: 10.1161/CIRCULATIONAHA.113.004409
11. Kitamura T, Iwami T, Kawamura T, Nagao K, Tanaka H, Hiraide A; Implementation Working Group for All-Japan Utstein Registry of the Fire and Disaster Management Agency. Bystander-initiated rescue breathing for out-of-hospital cardiac arrests of noncardiac origin. *Circulation.* 2010;122:293–299. doi: 10.1161/CIRCULATIONAHA.109.926816
12. Ogawa T, Akahane M, Koike S, Tanabe S, Mizoguchi T, Imamura T. Outcomes of chest compression only CPR versus conventional CPR conducted by lay people in patients with out of hospital cardiopulmonary arrest witnessed by bystanders: nationwide population based observational study. *BMJ.* 2011;342:c7106. doi: 10.1136/bmj.c7106
13. Svensson L, Bohm K, Castrèn M, Pettersson H, Engerström L, Herlitz J, Rosenqvist M. Compression-only CPR or standard CPR in out-of-hospital cardiac arrest. *N Engl J Med.* 2010;363:434–442. doi: 10.1056/NEJMoa0908991
14. Rea TD, Fahrenbruch C, Culley L, Donohoe RT, Hambly C, Innes J, Bloomingdale M, Subido C, Romines S, Eisenberg MS. CPR with chest compression alone or with rescue breathing. *N Engl J Med.* 2010;363:423–433. doi: 10.1056/NEJMoa0908993
15. Iwami T, Kawamura T, Hiraide A, Berg RA, Hayashi Y, Nishiuchi T, Kajino K, Yonemoto N, Yukioka H, Sugimoto H, Kakuchi H, Sase K, Yokoyama H, Nonogi H. Effectiveness of bystander-initiated cardiac-only resuscitation for patients with out-of-hospital cardiac arrest. *Circulation.* 2007;116:2900–2907. doi: 10.1161/CIRCULATIONAHA.107.723411
16. Kitamura T, Iwami T, Kawamura T, Nagao K, Tanaka H, Berg RA, Hiraide A; Implementation Working Group for All-Japan Utstein Registry of the Fire and Disaster Management Agency. Time-dependent effectiveness of chest compression-only and conventional cardiopulmonary resuscitation for out-of-hospital cardiac arrest of cardiac origin. *Resuscitation.* 2011;82:3–9. doi: 10.1016/j.resuscitation.2010.09.468
17. Ong ME, Ng FS, Anushia P, Tham LP, Leong BS, Ong VY, Tiah L, Lim SH, Anantharaman V. Comparison of chest compression only and standard cardiopulmonary resuscitation for out-of-hospital cardiac arrest in Singapore. *Resuscitation.* 2008;78:119–126. doi: 10.1016/j.resuscitation.2008.03.012
18. SOS-KANTO Study Group. Cardiopulmonary resuscitation by bystanders with chest compression only (SOS-KANTO): an observational study. *Lancet.* 2007;369:920–926. doi: 10.1016/S0140-6736(07)60451-6
19. Bobrow BJ, Spaite DW, Berg RA, Stolz U, Sanders AB, Kern KB, Vadeboncoeur TF, Clark LL, Gallagher JV, Stapczynski JS, LoVecchio F, Mullins TJ, Humble WO, Ewy GA. Chest compression-only CPR by lay rescuers and survival from out-of-hospital cardiac arrest. *JAMA.* 2010;304:1447–1454. doi: 10.1001/jama.2010.1392
20. Olasveengen TM, Wik L, Steen PA. Standard basic life support vs. continuous chest compressions only in out-of-hospital cardiac arrest. *Acta Anaesthesiol Scand.* 2008;52:914–919. doi: 10.1111/j.1399-6576.2008.01723.x
21. Panchal AR, Bobrow BJ, Spaite DW, Berg RA, Stolz U, Vadeboncoeur TF, Sanders AB, Kern KB, Ewy GA. Chest compression-only cardiopulmonary resuscitation performed by lay rescuers for adult out-of-hospital cardiac arrest due to non-cardiac aetiologies. *Resuscitation.* 2013;84:435–439. doi: 10.1016/j.resuscitation.2012.07.038
22. Kleinman ME, Brennan EE, Goldberger ZD, Swor RA, Terry M, Bobrow BJ, Gazmuri RJ, Travers AH, Rea T. Part 5: adult basic life support and cardiopulmonary resuscitation quality: 2015 American Heart Association Guidelines Update for Cardiopulmonary Resuscitation and Emergency Cardiovascular Care. *Circulation.* 2015;132(suppl 2):S414–S435. doi: 10.1161/CIR.0000000000000259
23. Kobayashi M, Fujiwara A, Morita H, Nishimoto Y, Mishima T, Nitta M, Hayashi T, Hotta T, Hayashi Y, Hachisuka E, Sato K. A manikin-based observational study on cardiopulmonary resuscitation skills at the Osaka Senri medical rally. *Resuscitation.* 2008;78:333–339. doi: 10.1016/j.resuscitation.2008.03.230

Opening the Airway

Introduction

A patent airway is essential to facilitate proper ventilation and oxygenation. Although there is no high-quality evidence favoring one technique over another for establishment and maintenance of a patient's airway, rescuers should be aware of the advantages and disadvantages and maintain proficiency in the skills required for each technique. Rescuers should recognize that multiple approaches may be required to establish an adequate airway. Patients should be monitored constantly to verify airway patency and adequate ventilation and oxygenation. There are no studies comparing different strategies of opening the airway in cardiac arrest patients. Much of the evidence examining the effectiveness of airway strategies comes from radiographic and cadaver studies.

Recommendations for Opening the Airway

COR	LOE	Recommendations
1	C-EO	1. A healthcare provider should use the head tilt–chin lift maneuver to open the airway of a patient when no cervical spine injury is suspected.
1	C-EO	2. The trained lay rescuer who feels confident in performing both compressions and ventilation should open the airway using a head tilt–chin lift maneuver when no cervical spine injury is suspected.
2b	C-EO	3. The use of an airway adjunct (eg, oropharyngeal and/or nasopharyngeal airway) may be reasonable in unconscious (unresponsive) patients with no cough or gag reflex to facilitate delivery of ventilation with a bag-mask device.
2a	C-EO	4. In the presence of known or suspected basal skull fracture or severe coagulopathy, an oral airway is preferred compared with a nasopharyngeal airway.
3: No Benefit	C-LD	5. The routine use of cricoid pressure in adult cardiac arrest is not recommended.

Recommendation-Specific Supportive Text

1 and 2. The head tilt–chin lift has been shown to be effective in establishing an airway in noncardiac arrest and radiological studies.[2–5] No studies have compared head tilt–chin lift with other airway maneuvers to establish an airway during cardiac arrest.

3. Although there is no evidence examining the effectiveness of their use during cardiac arrest, oropharyngeal and nasopharyngeal airways can be used to maintain a patent airway and facilitate appropriate ventilation by preventing the tongue from occluding the airway. Incorrect placement, however, can cause an airway obstruction by displacing the tongue to the back of the oropharynx.[6,7]

4. The benefit of an oropharyngeal compared with a nasopharyngeal airway in the presence of a known or suspected basilar skull fracture or severe coagulopathy has not been assessed in clinical trials. However, an oral airway is preferred because of the risk of trauma with a nasopharyngeal airway. Multiple case reports have observed intracranial placement of nasopharyngeal airways in patients with basilar skull fractures.[8,9]

5. There is no evidence that cricoid pressure facilitates ventilation or reduces the risk of aspiration in cardiac arrest patients. There is some evidence that in non–cardiac arrest patients, cricoid pressure may protect against aspiration and gastric insufflation during bag-mask ventilation.[10–13] However, cricoid pressure may also impede ventilation and the placement of a supraglottic airway (SGA) or intubation,[14–20] and increase the risk of airway trauma during intubation.[21]

This topic last received formal evidence review in 2010.[22]

Recommendations for Opening the Airway After Head and Neck Trauma

COR	LOE	Recommendations
1	C-EO	1. In cases of suspected cervical spine injury, healthcare providers should open the airway by using a jaw thrust without head extension.
1	C-EO	2. In the setting of head and neck trauma, a head tilt–chin lift maneuver should be performed if the airway cannot be opened with a jaw thrust and airway adjunct insertion.
3: Harm	C-LD	3. In the setting of head and neck trauma, lay rescuers should not use immobilization devices because their use by untrained rescuers may be harmful.

Recommendation-Specific Supportive Text

1. Healthcare providers should consider the possibility of a spinal injury before opening the airway. If a spinal injury is suspected or cannot be ruled out, providers should open the airway by using a jaw thrust instead of head tilt–chin lift.[2]
2. Maintaining a patent airway and providing adequate ventilation and oxygenation are priorities during CPR. If a jaw thrust and/or insertion of an airway adjunct are ineffective in opening the airway and allowing ventilation to occur, a head tilt–chin lift may be the only way to open the airway. In these cases, this maneuver should be used even in cases of potential spinal injury because the need to open the airway outweighs the risk of further spinal damage in the cardiac arrest patient.
3. When spinal injury is suspected or cannot be ruled out, rescuers should maintain manual spinal motion restriction and not use immobilization

devices. Manual stabilization can decrease movement of the cervical spine during patient care while allowing for proper ventilation and airway control.[23,24] Spinal immobilization devices may make it more difficult to maintain airway patency[25,26] and provide adequate ventilation.

This topic last received formal evidence review in 2010.[22]

REFERENCES

1. Deleted in proof.
2. Elam JO, Greene DG, Schneider MA, Ruben HM, Gordon AS, Hustead RF, Benson DW, Clements JA, Ruben A. Head-tilt method of oral resuscitation. *JAMA*. 1960;172:812–815. doi: 10.1001/jama.1960.03020080042011
3. Guildner CW. Resuscitation—opening the airway: a comparative study of techniques for opening an airway obstructed by the tongue. *JACEP*. 1976;5:588–590. doi: 10.1016/s0361-1124(76)80217-1
4. Greene DG, Elam JO, Dobkin AB, Studley CL. Cinefluorographic study of hyperextension of the neck and upper airway patency. *JAMA*. 1961;176:570–573. doi: 10.1001/jama.1961.03040200006002
5. Ruben HM, Elam JO, Ruben AM, Greene DG. Investigation of upper airway problems in resuscitation. 1. Studies of pharyngeal x-rays and performance by laymen. *Anesthesiology*. 1961;22:271–279. doi: 10.1097/00000542-196103000-00017
6. Kim HJ, Kim SH, Min JY, Park WK. Determination of the appropriate oropharyngeal airway size in adults: Assessment using ventilation and an endoscopic view. *Am J Emerg Med*. 2017;35:1430–1434. doi: 10.1016/j.ajem.2017.04.029
7. Kim HJ, Kim SH, Min NH, Park WK. Determination of the appropriate sizes of oropharyngeal airways in adults: correlation with external facial measurements: A randomised crossover study. *Eur J Anaesthesiol*. 2016;33:936–942. doi: 10.1097/EJA.0000000000000439
8. Schade K, Borzotta A, Michaels A. Intracranial malposition of nasopharyngeal airway. *J Trauma*. 2000;49:967–968. doi: 10.1097/00005373-200011000-00032
9. Muzzi DA, Losasso TJ, Cucchiara RF. Complication from a nasopharyngeal airway in a patient with a basilar skull fracture. *Anesthesiology*. 1991;74:366–368. doi: 10.1097/00000542-199102000-00026
10. Salem MR, Wong AY, Mani M, Sellick BA. Efficacy of cricoid pressure in preventing gastric inflation during bag-mask ventilation in pediatric patients. *Anesthesiology*. 1974;40:96–98. doi: 10.1097/00000542-197401000-00026
11. Lawes EG, Campbell I, Mercer D. Inflation pressure, gastric insufflation and rapid sequence induction. *Br J Anaesth*. 1987;59:315–318. doi: 10.1093/bja/59.3.315
12. Petito SP, Russell WJ. The prevention of gastric inflation–a neglected benefit of cricoid pressure. *Anaesth Intensive Care*. 1988;16:139–143. doi: 10.1177/0310057X8801600202
13. Moynihan RJ, Brock-Utne JG, Archer JH, Feld LH, Kreitzman TR. The effect of cricoid pressure on preventing gastric insufflation in infants and children. *Anesthesiology*. 1993;78:652–656. doi: 10.1097/00000542-199304000-00007
14. Brimacombe J, White A, Berry A. Effect of cricoid pressure on ease of insertion of the laryngeal mask airway. *Br J Anaesth*. 1993;71:800–802. doi: 10.1093/bja/71.6.800
15. Allman KG. The effect of cricoid pressure application on airway patency. *J Clin Anesth*. 1995;7:197–199. doi: 10.1016/0952-8180(94)00048-9
16. Hartsilver EL, Vanner RG. Airway obstruction with cricoid pressure. *Anaesthesia*. 2000;55:208–211. doi: 10.1046/j.1365-2044.2000.01205.x
17. Hocking G, Roberts FL, Thew ME. Airway obstruction with cricoid pressure and lateral tilt. *Anaesthesia*. 2001;56:825–828. doi: 10.1046/j.1365-2044.2001.02133.x
18. Turgeon AF, Nicole PC, Trépanier CA, Marcoux S, Lessard MR. Cricoid pressure does not increase the rate of failed intubation by direct laryngoscopy in adults. *Anesthesiology*. 2005;102:315–319. doi: 10.1097/00000542-200502000-00012
19. Asai T, Goy RW, Liu EH. Cricoid pressure prevents placement of the laryngeal tube and laryngeal tube-suction II. *Br J Anaesth*. 2007;99:282–285. doi: 10.1093/bja/aem159
20. McNelis U, Syndercombe A, Harper I, Duggan J. The effect of cricoid pressure on intubation facilitated by the gum elastic bougie. *Anaesthesia*. 2007;62:456–459. doi: 10.1111/j.1365-2044.2007.05019.x
21. Carauna E, Chevret S, Pirracchio R. Effect of cricoid pressure on laryngeal view during prehospital tracheal intubation: a propensity-based analysis. *Emerg Med J*. 2017:132–137. doi: doi: 10.1136/emermed-2016-205715
22. Berg RA, Hemphill R, Abella BS, Aufderheide TP, Cave DM, Hazinski MF, Lerner EB, Rea TD, Sayre MR, Swor RA. Part 5: adult basic life support: 2010 American Heart Association Guidelines for Cardiopulmonary Resuscitation and Emergency Cardiovascular Care. *Circulation*. 2010;122(suppl 3):S685–S705. doi: 10.1161/CIRCULATIONAHA.110.970939
23. Majernick TG, Bieniek R, Houston JB, Hughes HG. Cervical spine movement during orotracheal intubation. *Ann Emerg Med*. 1986;15:417–420. doi: 10.1016/s0196-0644(86)80178-0
24. Lennarson PJ, Smith DW, Sawin PD, Todd MM, Sato Y, Traynelis VC. Cervical spinal motion during intubation: efficacy of stabilization maneuvers in the setting of complete segmental instability. *J Neurosurg*. 2001;94(suppl):265–270. doi: 10.3171/spi.2001.94.2.0265
25. Hastings RH, Wood PR. Head extension and laryngeal view during laryngoscopy with cervical spine stabilization maneuvers. *Anesthesiology*. 1994;80:825–831. doi: 10.1097/00000542-199404000-00015
26. Gerling MC, Davis DP, Hamilton RS, Morris GF, Vilke GM, Garfin SR, Hayden SR. Effects of cervical spine immobilization technique and laryngoscope blade selection on an unstable cervical spine in a cadaver model of intubation. *Ann Emerg Med*. 2000;36:293–300. doi: 10.1067/mem.2000.109442

Metrics for High-Quality CPR

Introduction

High-quality CPR is, along with defibrillation for those with shockable rhythms, the most important lifesaving intervention for a patient in cardiac arrest. The evidence for what constitutes optimal CPR continues to evolve as research emerges. A number of key components have been defined for high-quality CPR, including minimizing interruptions in chest compressions, providing compressions of adequate rate and depth, avoiding leaning on the chest between compressions, and avoiding excessive ventilation.[1] However, controlled studies are relatively lacking, and observational evidence is at times conflicting. The effect of individual CPR quality metrics or interventions is difficult to evaluate because so many happen concurrently and may interact with each other in their effect. Compression rate and compression depth, for example, have both been associated with better outcomes, yet these variables have been found to be inversely correlated with each other so that improving one may worsen the other.[1–3] CPR quality interventions are often applied in "bundles," making the benefit of any one specific measure difficult to ascertain. As more and more centers and EMS systems are using feedback devices and collecting data on CPR measures such as compression depth and chest compression fraction, these data will enable ongoing updates to these recommendations.

Recommendations for Positioning and Location for CPR		
COR	LOE	Recommendations
1	C-LD	1. When providing chest compressions, the rescuer should place the heel of one hand on the center (middle) of the victim's chest (the lower half of the sternum) and the heel of the other hand on top of the first so that the hands are overlapped.
1	C-EO	2. Resuscitation should generally be conducted where the victim is found, as long as high-quality CPR can be administered safely and effectively in that location.
2a	C-LD	3. It is preferred to perform CPR on a firm surface and with the victim in the supine position, when feasible.
2b	C-LD	4. When the victim cannot be placed in the supine position, it may be reasonable for rescuers to provide CPR with the victim in the prone position, particularly in hospitalized patients with an advanced airway in place.

Recommendation-Specific Supportive Text

1. A 2020 ILCOR systematic review identified 3 studies involving 57 total patients that investigated the effect of hand positioning on resuscitation process and outcomes.[4] Although no difference in resuscitation outcomes was noted, 2 studies found better physiological parameters (peak arterial pressure, mean arterial pressure [MAP], end-tidal carbon dioxide [$ETCO_2$]) when compression was performed over the lower third of the sternum compared with the middle of the sternum.[5,6] A third study found no difference.[7] Radiographic studies show the left ventricle is typically located inferior to the internipple line, corresponding with the lower half of the sternum.[8] However, hand placement inferior to the internipple line may result in compression over the xiphoid.[9] Although data from manikin studies conflict, it does not appear to matter whether the dominant or nondominant hand is placed in contact with the sternum.[10,11]
2. The primary considerations when determining if a victim needs to be moved before starting resuscitation are feasibility and safety of providing high-quality CPR in the location and position in which the victim is found. This is a separate question from the decision of if or when to transport a patient to the hospital with resuscitation ongoing.
3. The effectiveness of CPR appears to be maximized with the victim in a supine position and the rescuer kneeling beside the victim's chest (eg, out-of-hospital) or standing beside the bed (eg, in-hospital).[12] It is thought that optimal chest compressions are best delivered with the victim on a firm surface.[13,14] Manikin studies show generally acceptable thoracic compression with CPR performed on a hospital mattress.
4. An older systematic review identified 22 case reports of CPR being performed in the prone position (21 in the operating room, 1 in the intensive care unit [ICU]), with 10/22 patients surviving.[15] In a small case series of 6 patients with refractory IHCA, prone positioning with the use of a board with sandbag to compress the sternum improved hemodynamics during CPR but did not result in ROSC.[16] The efficacy of CPR in the prone position is not established, but the very limited evidence suggests it may be better than providing no CPR, when a patient cannot be placed in supine position, or until this can be done safely.

Recommendations 1, 2, and 3 are supported by the 2020 CoSTR for BLS.[4] Recommendation 4 last received formal evidence review in 2010.[17]

Recommendations for Compression Fraction and Pauses		
COR	LOE	Recommendations
1	C-LD	1. In adult cardiac arrest, total preshock and postshock pauses in chest compressions should be as short as possible.
1	C-LD	2. The healthcare provider should minimize the time taken to check for a pulse (no more than 10 s) during a rhythm check, and if the rescuer does not definitely feel a pulse, chest compressions should be resumed.
2a	B-R	3. When 2 or more rescuers are available, it is reasonable to switch chest compressors approximately every 2 min (or after about 5 cycles of compressions and ventilation at a ratio of 30:2) to prevent decreases in the quality of compressions.
2a	B-R	4. It is reasonable to immediately resume chest compressions after shock delivery for adults in cardiac arrest in any setting.
2a	C-LD	5. For adults in cardiac arrest receiving CPR without an advanced airway, it is reasonable to pause compressions to deliver 2 breaths, each given over 1 s.
2b	C-LD	6. In adult cardiac arrest, it may be reasonable to perform CPR with a chest compression fraction of at least 60%.

Recommendation-Specific Supportive Text

1. Observational evidence suggests improved outcomes with increased chest compression fraction in patients with shockable rhythms.[18,19] Specifically, studies have also reported increased ROSC with shorter perishock pauses.[20–22]
2. This recommendation is based on the overall principle of minimizing interruptions to CPR and maintaining a chest compression fraction of at least 60%, which studies have reported to be associated with better outcome.[18,19,23]

3. Chest compression depth begins to decrease after 90 to 120 seconds of CPR, although compression rates do not decrease significantly over that time window.[24] A randomized trial using manikins found no difference in the percentage of high-quality compressions when rotating every 1 minute compared with every 2 minutes.[25] Rotating the designated chest compressor every 2 minutes is sensible because this approach maintains chest compression quality and takes advantage of when CPR would ordinarily be paused for rhythm analysis.
4. Two RCTs enrolling more than 1000 patients did not find any increase in survival when pausing CPR to analyze rhythm after defibrillation.[26,27] Observational studies show decreased ROSC when chest compressions are not resumed immediately after shock.[28,29]
5. Because chest compression fraction of at least 60% is associated with better resuscitation outcomes, compression pauses for ventilation should be as short as possible.[18,19,23]
6. A 2015 systematic review reported significant heterogeneity among studies, with some studies, but not all, reporting better rates of survival to hospital discharge associated with higher chest compression fractions.[18,19,23] In 2 studies, higher chest compression fraction was associated with lower odds of survival.[2,30] Compression rate and depth and cointerventions such as defibrillation, airway management, and medications, are also important and may interact with chest compression fraction. High-performing EMS systems target at least 60%, with 80% or higher being a frequent goal.

Recommendations 1 and 4 are supported by the 2020 CoSTR for BLS.[4] Recommendations 2, 3, 5, and 6 last received formal evidence review in 2015.[31]

Recommendations for Compression Depth and Rate

COR	LOE	Recommendations
1	B-NR	1. During manual CPR, rescuers should perform chest compressions to a depth of at least 2 inches, or 5 cm, for an average adult while avoiding excessive chest compression depths (greater than 2.4 inches, or 6 cm).
2a	B-NR	2. In adult victims of cardiac arrest, it is reasonable for rescuers to perform chest compressions at a rate of 100 to 120/min.
2a	C-LD	3. It can be beneficial for rescuers to avoid leaning on the chest between compressions to allow complete chest wall recoil for adults in cardiac arrest.
2b	C-EO	4. It may be reasonable to perform chest compressions so that chest compression and recoil/relaxation times are approximately equal.

Recommendation-Specific Supportive Text

1. A 2020 ILCOR scoping review[32] identified 12 studies, including over 12 500 patients, looking at chest compression components. Several studies found better outcomes, including survival to hospital discharge and defibrillation success, when compression depth was at least 5 cm compared with less than 4 cm.[3,20,33,34]
2. The same review[32] identified 13 studies, involving 15 000 patients, that looked at compression rate. Results were somewhat inconsistent across studies, with only 3 observational studies in adults showing an association between higher compression rate and outcomes.[1,35,36] The only RCT identified included 292 patients and compared a rate of 100 to a rate of 120, finding no difference in outcomes.[37] There is no evidence to suggest altering the suggested compression rate of 100 to 120/min in adults. Three studies have reported that depth decreases as rate increases, highlighting the pitfalls of evaluating a single CPR quality metric in isolation.[1–3]
3. The ILCOR review[32] identified 2 observational studies that provided inconsistent results on the association between chest compression release velocity and survival, with 1 study finding no association and the other finding that faster release velocity was associated with increased survival.[38,39] Not allowing complete chest wall recoil has been associated with increased intrathoracic pressure and decreased coronary perfusion.[40,41]
4. CPR duty cycle refers to the proportion of time spent in compression relative to the total time of the compression plus decompression cycle. The 2010 Guidelines recommended a 50% duty cycle, in which the time spent in compression and decompression was equal, mainly on the basis of its perceived ease of being achieved in practice. Notably, in a clinical study in adults with out-of-hospital VF arrest (of whom 43% survived to hospital discharge), the mean duty cycle observed during resuscitation was 39%.[42] A study in children also found the mean duty cycle was 40%, suggesting that shorter duty cycles may be the norm in clinical practice.[43] Although many animal studies have observed higher blood flows and better outcomes when the duty cycle was less than 50%, the optimal duty cycle is not known. Currently, there is insufficient evidence to warrant a change from the existing recommendation, which remains a knowledge gap that requires further investigation.

Recommendations 1, 2, and 3 are supported by the 2020 CoSTR for BLS.[4] Recommendation 4 last received formal evidence review in 2010.[44]

Recommendations for CPR Feedback and Monitoring		
COR	LOE	Recommendations
2b	B-R	1. It may be reasonable to use audiovisual feedback devices during CPR for real-time optimization of CPR performance.
2b	C-LD	2. It may be reasonable to use physiological parameters such as arterial blood pressure or end-tidal CO_2 when feasible to monitor and optimize CPR quality.

Recommendation-Specific Supportive Text

1. A 2020 ILCOR systematic review found that most studies did not find a significant association between real-time feedback and improved patient outcomes.[4] However, no studies identified significant harm, and some demonstrated clinically important improvement in survival. One recent RCT reported a 25.6% increase in survival to hospital discharge from IHCA with audio feedback on compression depth and recoil (54% versus 28.4%; *P*<0.001).[45]
2. An analysis of data from the AHA's Get With The Guidelines-Resuscitation registry showed higher likelihood of ROSC (odds ratio, 1.22; 95% CI, 1.04–1.34; *P*=0.017) when CPR quality was monitored using either $ETCO_2$ or diastolic blood pressure.[46] An observational study in adult patients (IHCA and OHCA) reported that for every 10 mm compression depth increase, $ETCO_2$ increased 1.4 mm Hg.[47] A 2018 systematic review of $ETCO_2$ as a prognostic indicator for ROSC[48] found variability in cutoff values, but less than 10 mm Hg was generally associated with poor outcome and greater than 20 mm Hg had a stronger association with ROSC than a value of greater than 10 mm Hg. The combination of the association of higher $ETCO_2$ with ROSC and the finding that increased chest compression depth can increase $ETCO_2$ suggests that targeting compressions to a value of at least 10 mm Hg, and ideally 20 mm Hg or greater, may be useful. The validity and reliability of $ETCO_2$ in nonintubated patients is not well established. When available, invasive arterial blood pressure monitoring may also help assess and guide CPR efforts. The use of diastolic blood pressure monitoring during cardiac arrest was associated with higher ROSC,[46] but there are inadequate human data to suggest any specific pressure.

These recommendations are supported by the 2020 CoSTRs for BLS and ALS.[4,49]

REFERENCES

1. Idris AH, Guffey D, Pepe PE, Brown SP, Brooks SC, Callaway CW, Christenson J, Davis DP, Daya MR, Gray R, Kudenchuk PJ, Larsen J, Lin S, Menegazzi JJ, Sheehan K, Sopko G, Stiell I, Nichol G, Aufderheide TP; Resuscitation Outcomes Consortium Investigators. Chest compression rates and survival following out-of-hospital cardiac arrest. *Crit Care Med.* 2015;43:840–848. doi: 10.1097/CCM.0000000000000824
2. Vadeboncoeur T, Stolz U, Panchal A, Silver A, Venuti M, Tobin J, Smith G, Nunez M, Karamooz M, Spaite D, Bobrow B. Chest compression depth and survival in out-of-hospital cardiac arrest. *Resuscitation.* 2014;85:182–188. doi: 10.1016/j.resuscitation.2013.10.002
3. Stiell IG, Brown SP, Christenson J, Cheskes S, Nichol G, Powell J, Bigham B, Morrison LJ, Larsen J, Hess E, Vaillancourt C, Davis DP, Callaway CW; Resuscitation Outcomes Consortium (ROC) Investigators. What is the role of chest compression depth during out-of-hospital cardiac arrest resuscitation? *Crit Care Med.* 2012;40:1192–1198. doi: 10.1097/CCM.0b013e31823bc8bb
4. Olasveengen TM, Mancini ME, Perkins GD, Avis S, Brooks S, Castrén M, Chung SP, Considine J, Couper K, Escalante R, et al; on behalf of the Adult Basic Life Support Collaborators. Adult basic life support: 2020 International Consensus on Cardiopulmonary Resuscitation and Emergency Cardiovascular Care Science With Treatment Recommendations. *Circulation.* 2020;142(suppl 1):S41–S91. doi: 10.1161/CIR.0000000000000892
5. Cha KC, Kim HJ, Shin HJ, Kim H, Lee KH, Hwang SO. Hemodynamic effect of external chest compressions at the lower end of the sternum in cardiac arrest patients. *J Emerg Med.* 2013;44:691–697. doi: 10.1016/j.jemermed.2012.09.026
6. Orlowski JP. Optimum position for external cardiac compression in infants and young children. *Ann Emerg Med.* 1986;15:667–673. doi: 10.1016/s0196-0644(86)80423-1
7. Qvigstad E, Kramer-Johansen J, Tømte Ø, Skålhegg T, Sørensen Ø, Sunde K, Olasveengen TM. Clinical pilot study of different hand positions during manual chest compressions monitored with capnography. *Resuscitation.* 2013;84:1203–1207. doi: 10.1016/j.resuscitation.2013.03.010
8. Shin J, Rhee JE, Kim K. Is the inter-nipple line the correct hand position for effective chest compression in adult cardiopulmonary resuscitation? *Resuscitation.* 2007;75:305–310. doi: 10.1016/j.resuscitation.2007.05.003
9. Kusunoki S, Tanigawa K, Kondo T, Kawamoto M, Yuge O. Safety of the inter-nipple line hand position landmark for chest compression. *Resuscitation.* 2009;80:1175–1180. doi: 10.1016/j.resuscitation.2009.06.030
10. Nikandish R, Shahbazi S, Golabi S, Beygi N. Role of dominant versus non-dominant hand position during uninterrupted chest compression CPR by novice rescuers: a randomized double-blind crossover study. *Resuscitation.* 2008;76:256–260. doi: 10.1016/j.resuscitation.2007.07.032
11. Kundra P, Dey S, Ravishankar M. Role of dominant hand position during external cardiac compression. *Br J Anaesth.* 2000;84:491–493. doi: 10.1093/oxfordjournals.bja.a013475
12. Handley AJ, Handley JA. Performing chest compressions in a confined space. *Resuscitation.* 2004;61:55–61. doi: 10.1016/j.resuscitation.2003.11.012
13. Nishisaki A, Nysaether J, Sutton R, Maltese M, Niles D, Donoghue A, Bishnoi R, Helfaer M, Perkins GD, Berg R, Arbogast K, Nadkarni V. Effect of mattress deflection on CPR quality assessment for older children and adolescents. *Resuscitation.* 2009;80:540–545. doi: 10.1016/j.resuscitation.2009.02.006
14. Noordergraaf GJ, Paulussen IW, Venema A, van Berkom PF, Woerlee PH, Scheffer GJ, Noordergraaf A. The impact of compliant surfaces on in-hospital chest compressions: effects of common mattresses and a backboard. *Resuscitation.* 2009;80:546–552. doi: 10.1016/j.resuscitation.2009.03.023
15. Brown J, Rogers J, Soar J. Cardiac arrest during surgery and ventilation in the prone position: a case report and systematic review. *Resuscitation.* 2001;50:233–238. doi: 10.1016/s0300-9572(01)00362-8
16. Mazer SP, Weisfeldt M, Bai D, Cardinale C, Arora R, Ma C, Sciacca RR, Chong D, Rabbani LE. Reverse CPR: a pilot study of CPR in the prone position. *Resuscitation.* 2003;57:279–285. doi: 10.1016/s0300-9572(03)00037-6
17. Cave DM, Gazmuri RJ, Otto CW, Nadkarni VM, Cheng A, Brooks SC, Daya M, Sutton RM, Branson R, Hazinski MF. Part 7: CPR techniques and devices: 2010 American Heart Association Guidelines for Cardiopulmonary Resuscitation and Emergency Cardiovascular Care. *Circulation.* 2010;122:S720–728. doi: 10.1161/CIRCULATIONAHA.110.970970
18. Talikowska M, Tohira H, Finn J. Cardiopulmonary resuscitation quality and patient survival outcome in cardiac arrest: A systematic review and meta-analysis. *Resuscitation.* 2015;96:66–77. doi: 10.1016/j.resuscitation.2015.07.036
19. Christenson J, Andrusiek D, Everson-Stewart S, Kudenchuk P, Hostler D, Powell J, Callaway CW, Bishop D, Vaillancourt C, Davis D, Aufderheide TP, Idris A, Stouffer JA, Stiell I, Berg R; Resuscitation Outcomes Consortium Investigators. Chest compression fraction determines survival in patients with out-of-hospital ventricular fibrillation. *Circulation.* 2009;120:1241–1247. doi: 10.1161/CIRCULATIONAHA.109.852202
20. Edelson DP, Abella BS, Kramer-Johansen J, Wik L, Myklebust H, Barry AM, Merchant RM, Hoek TL, Steen PA, Becker LB. Effects of compression depth and pre-shock pauses predict defibrillation failure during cardiac arrest. *Resuscitation.* 2006;71:137–145. doi: 10.1016/j.resuscitation.2006.04.008

21. Eftestøl T, Sunde K, Steen PA. Effects of interrupting precordial compressions on the calculated probability of defibrillation success during out-of-hospital cardiac arrest. *Circulation.* 2002;105:2270–2273. doi: 10.1161/01.cir.0000016362.42586.fe
22. Cheskes S, Schmicker RH, Christenson J, Salcido DD, Rea T, Powell J, Edelson DP, Sell R, May S, Menegazzi JJ, Van Ottingham L, Olsufka M, Pennington S, Simonini J, Berg RA, Stiell I, Idris A, Bigham B, Morrison L; Resuscitation Outcomes Consortium (ROC) Investigators. Perishock pause: an independent predictor of survival from out-of-hospital shockable cardiac arrest. *Circulation.* 2011;124:58–66. doi: 10.1161/CIRCULATIONAHA.110.010736
23. Vaillancourt C, Everson-Stewart S, Christenson J, Andrusiek D, Powell J, Nichol G, Cheskes S, Aufderheide TP, Berg R, Stiell IG; Resuscitation Outcomes Consortium Investigators. The impact of increased chest compression fraction on return of spontaneous circulation for out-of-hospital cardiac arrest patients not in ventricular fibrillation. *Resuscitation.* 2011;82:1501–1507. doi: 10.1016/j.resuscitation.2011.07.011
24. Sugerman NT, Edelson DP, Leary M, Weidman EK, Herzberg DL, Vanden Hoek TL, Becker LB, Abella BS. Rescuer fatigue during actual in-hospital cardiopulmonary resuscitation with audiovisual feedback: a prospective multicenter study. *Resuscitation.* 2009;80:981–984. doi: 10.1016/j.resuscitation.2009.06.002
25. Manders S, Geijsel FE. Alternating providers during continuous chest compressions for cardiac arrest: every minute or every two minutes? *Resuscitation.* 2009;80:1015–1018. doi: 10.1016/j.resuscitation.2009.05.014
26. Jost D, Degrange H, Verret C, Hersan O, Banville IL, Chapman FW, Lank P, Petit JL, Fuilla C, Migliani R, et al; and the DEFI 2005 Work Group. DEFI 2005: a randomized controlled trial of the effect of automated external defibrillator cardiopulmonary resuscitation protocol on outcome from out-of-hospital cardiac arrest. *Circulation.* 2010;121:1614–1622. doi: 10.1161/CIRCULATIONAHA.109.878389
27. Beesems SG, Berdowski J, Hulleman M, Blom MT, Tijssen JG, Koster RW. Minimizing pre- and post-shock pauses during the use of an automatic external defibrillator by two different voice prompt protocols. A randomized controlled trial of a bundle of measures. *Resuscitation.* 2016;106:1–6. doi: 10.1016/j.resuscitation.2016.06.009
28. Rea TD, Helbock M, Perry S, Garcia M, Cloyd D, Becker L, Eisenberg M. Increasing use of cardiopulmonary resuscitation during out-of-hospital ventricular fibrillation arrest: survival implications of guideline changes. *Circulation.* 2006;114:2760–2765. doi: 10.1161/CIRCULATIONAHA.106.654715
29. Bobrow BJ, Clark LL, Ewy GA, Chikani V, Sanders AB, Berg RA, Richman PB, Kern KB. Minimally interrupted cardiac resuscitation by emergency medical services for out-of-hospital cardiac arrest. *JAMA.* 2008;299:1158–1165. doi: 10.1001/jama.299.10.1158
30. Cheskes S, Schmicker RH, Rea T, Powell J, Drennan IR, Kudenchuk P, Vaillancourt C, Conway W, Stiell I, Stub D, Davis D, Alexander N, Christenson J; Resuscitation Outcomes Consortium investigators. Chest compression fraction: A time dependent variable of survival in shockable out-of-hospital cardiac arrest. *Resuscitation.* 2015;97:129–135. doi: 10.1016/j.resuscitation.2015.07.003
31. Kleinman ME, Brennan EE, Goldberger ZD, Swor RA, Terry M, Bobrow BJ, Gazmuri RJ, Travers AH, Rea T. Part 5: adult basic life support and cardiopulmonary resuscitation quality: 2015 American Heart Association Guidelines Update for Cardiopulmonary Resuscitation and Emergency Cardiovascular Care. *Circulation.* 2015;132(suppl 2):S414–S435. doi: 10.1161/CIR.0000000000000259
32. Considine J, Gazmuri RJ, Perkins GD, Kudenchuk PJ, Olasveengen TM, Vaillancourt C, Nishiyama C, Hatanaka T, Mancini ME, Chung SP, Escalante-Kanashiro R, Morley P. Chest compression components (rate, depth, chest wall recoil and leaning): A scoping review. *Resuscitation.* 2020;146:188–202. doi: 10.1016/j.resuscitation.2019.08.042
33. Stiell IG, Brown SP, Nichol G, Cheskes S, Vaillancourt C, Callaway CW, Morrison LJ, Christenson J, Aufderheide TP, Davis DP, Free C, Hostler D, Stouffer JA, Idris AH; Resuscitation Outcomes Consortium Investigators. What is the optimal chest compression depth during out-of-hospital cardiac arrest resuscitation of adult patients? *Circulation.* 2014;130:1962–1970. doi: 10.1161/CIRCULATIONAHA.114.008671
34. Babbs CF, Kemeny AE, Quan W, Freeman G. A new paradigm for human resuscitation research using intelligent devices. *Resuscitation.* 2008;77:306–315. doi: 10.1016/j.resuscitation.2007.12.018
35. Kilgannon JH, Kirchhoff M, Pierce L, Aunchman N, Trzeciak S, Roberts BW. Association between chest compression rates and clinical outcomes following in-hospital cardiac arrest at an academic tertiary hospital. *Resuscitation.* 2017;110:154–161. doi: 10.1016/j.resuscitation.2016.09.015
36. Abella BS, Sandbo N, Vassilatos P, Alvarado JP, O'Hearn N, Wigder HN, Hoffman P, Tynus K, Vanden Hoek TL, Becker LB. Chest compression rates during cardiopulmonary resuscitation are suboptimal: a prospective study during in-hospital cardiac arrest. *Circulation.* 2005;111:428–434. doi: 10.1161/01.CIR.0000153811.84257.59
37. Hwang SO, Cha KC, Kim K, Jo YH, Chung SP, You JS, Shin J, Lee HJ, Park YS, Kim S, et al. A randomized controlled trial of compression rates during cardiopulmonary resuscitation. *J Korean Med Sci.* 2016;31:1491–1498. doi: 10.3346/jkms.2016.31.9.1491
38. Cheskes S, Common MR, Byers AP, Zhan C, Silver A, Morrison LJ. The association between chest compression release velocity and outcomes from out-of-hospital cardiac arrest. *Resuscitation.* 2015;86:38–43. doi: 10.1016/j.resuscitation.2014.10.020
39. Kovacs A, Vadeboncoeur TF, Stolz U, Spaite DW, Irisawa T, Silver A, Bobrow BJ. Chest compression release velocity: Association with survival and favorable neurologic outcome after out-of-hospital cardiac arrest. *Resuscitation.* 2015;92:107–114. doi: 10.1016/j.resuscitation.2015.04.026
40. Yannopoulos D, McKnite S, Aufderheide TP, Sigurdsson G, Pirrallo RG, Benditt D, Lurie KG. Effects of incomplete chest wall decompression during cardiopulmonary resuscitation on coronary and cerebral perfusion pressures in a porcine model of cardiac arrest. *Resuscitation.* 2005;64:363–372. doi: 10.1016/j.resuscitation.2004.10.009
41. Zuercher M, Hilwig RW, Ranger-Moore J, Nysaether J, Nadkarni VM, Berg MD, Kern KB, Sutton R, Berg RA. Leaning during chest compressions impairs cardiac output and left ventricular myocardial blood flow in piglet cardiac arrest. *Crit Care Med.* 2010;38:1141–1146. doi: 10.1097/CCM.0b013e3181ce1fe2
42. Johnson BV, Johnson B, Coult J, Fahrenbruch C, Blackwood J, Sherman L, Kudenchuk P, Sayre M, Rea T. Cardiopulmonary resuscitation duty cycle in out-of-hospital cardiac arrest. *Resuscitation.* 2015;87:86–90. doi: 10.1016/j.resuscitation.2014.11.008
43. Wolfe H, Morgan RW, Donoghue A, Niles DE, Kudenchuk P, Berg RA, Nadkarni VM, Sutton RM. Quantitative analysis of duty cycle in pediatric and adolescent in-hospital cardiac arrest. *Resuscitation.* 2016;106:65–69. doi: 10.1016/j.resuscitation.2016.06.003
44. Berg RA, Hemphill R, Abella BS, Aufderheide TP, Cave DM, Hazinski MF, Lerner EB, Rea TD, Sayre MR, Swor RA. Part 5: adult basic life support: 2010 American Heart Association Guidelines for Cardiopulmonary Resuscitation and Emergency Cardiovascular Care. *Circulation.* 2010;122(suppl 3):S685–S705. doi: 10.1161/CIRCULATIONAHA.110.970939
45. Goharani R, Vahedian-Azimi A, Farzanegan B, Bashar FR, Hajiesmaeili M, Shojaei S, Madani SJ, Gohari-Moghaddam K, Hatamian S, Mosavinasab SMM, Khoshfetrat M, Khabiri Khatir MA, Miller AC; MORZAK Collaborative. Real-time compression feedback for patients with in-hospital cardiac arrest: a multi-center randomized controlled clinical trial. *J Intensive Care.* 2019;7:5. doi: 10.1186/s40560-019-0357-5
46. Sutton RM, French B, Meaney PA, Topjian AA, Parshuram CS, Edelson DP, Schexnayder S, Abella BS, Merchant RM, Bembea M, Berg RA, Nadkarni VM; American Heart Association's Get With The Guidelines–Resuscitation Investigators. Physiologic monitoring of CPR quality during adult cardiac arrest: A propensity-matched cohort study. *Resuscitation.* 2016;106:76–82. doi: 10.1016/j.resuscitation.2016.06.018
47. Sheak KR, Wiebe DJ, Leary M, Babaeizadeh S, Yuen TC, Zive D, Owens PC, Edelson DP, Daya MR, Idris AH, Abella BS. Quantitative relationship between end-tidal carbon dioxide and CPR quality during both in-hospital and out-of-hospital cardiac arrest. *Resuscitation.* 2015;89:149–154. doi: 10.1016/j.resuscitation.2015.01.026
48. Paiva EF, Paxton JH, O'Neil BJ. The use of end-tidal carbon dioxide (ETCO2) measurement to guide management of cardiac arrest: A systematic review. *Resuscitation.* 2018;123:1–7. doi: 10.1016/j.resuscitation.2017.12.003
49. Berg KM, Soar J, Andersen LW, Böttiger BW, Cacciola S, Callaway CW, Couper K, Cronberg T, D'Arrigo S, Deakin CD, et al; on behalf of the Adult Advanced Life Support Collaborators. Adult advanced life support: 2020 International Consensus on Cardiopulmonary Resuscitation and Emergency Cardiovascular Care Science With Treatment Recommendations. *Circulation.* 2020;142(suppl 1):S92–S139. doi: 10.1161/CIR.0000000000000893

Ventilation and Compression-to-Ventilation Ratio

Introduction

The provision of rescue breaths for apneic patients with a pulse is essential. The relative contribution of assisted ventilation for patients in cardiac arrest is more controversial.

There is concern that delivery of chest compressions without assisted ventilation for prolonged periods could be less effective than conventional CPR (compressions plus breaths) because the arterial oxygen content will decrease as CPR duration increases. This concern is especially pertinent in the setting of asphyxial cardiac arrest. Much of the published research involves patients whose arrests were presumed to be of cardiac origin and in settings with short EMS response times. It is likely that a time threshold exists beyond which the absence of ventilation may be harmful, and the generalizability of the findings to all settings must be considered with caution.[1]

Once an advanced airway has been placed, delivering continuous chest compressions increases the compression fraction but makes it more difficult to deliver adequate ventilation. Simultaneous compressions and ventilation should be avoided,[2] but delivery of chest compressions without pausing for ventilation seems a reasonable option.[3] The use of SGAs adds to this complexity because efficiency of ventilation during cardiac arrest may be worse than when using an endotracheal tube, though this has not been borne out in recently published RCTs.[4,5]

Recommendations for Fundamentals of Ventilation During Cardiac Arrest

COR	LOE	Recommendations
2a	C-LD	1. For adults in cardiac arrest receiving ventilation, tidal volumes of approximately 500 to 600 mL, or enough to produce visible chest rise, are reasonable.
2a	C-EO	2. In patients without an advanced airway, it is reasonable to deliver breaths either by mouth or by using bag-mask ventilation.
2b	C-EO	3. When providing rescue breaths, it may be reasonable to give 1 breath over 1 s, take a "regular" (not deep) breath, and give a second rescue breath over 1 s.
3: Harm	C-LD	4. Rescuers should avoid excessive ventilation (too many breaths or too large a volume) during CPR.

Recommendation-Specific Supportive Text

1. Studies have reported that enough tidal volume to cause visible chest rise, or approximately 500 to 600 mL, provides adequate ventilation while minimizing the risk of overdistension or gastric insufflation.[6–9]
2. Both mouth-to-mouth rescue breathing and bag-mask ventilation provide oxygen and ventilation to the victim.[10] To provide mouth-to-mouth rescue breaths, open the victim's airway, pinch the victim's nose, create an airtight mouth-to-mouth seal, and provide a breath.
3. Taking a regular rather than a deep breath prevents the rescuer from getting dizzy or lightheaded and prevents overinflation of the victim's lungs. The most common cause of ventilation difficulty is an improperly opened airway,[11] so if the victim's chest does not rise with the first rescue breath, reposition the head by performing the head tilt–chin lift again and then give the second rescue breath. The recommendation for 1 second is to keep the pauses in CPR as brief as possible.
4. Excessive ventilation is unnecessary and can cause gastric inflation, regurgitation, and aspiration.[12,14] Excessive ventilation can also be harmful by increasing intrathoracic pressure, decreasing venous return to the heart, and diminishing cardiac output and survival.[14]

This topic last received formal evidence review in 2010.[15]

Recommendations for Ventilation During Cardiac Arrest: Special Situations

COR	LOE	Recommendations
2a	C-LD	1. It is reasonable for a rescuer to use mouth-to-nose ventilation if ventilation through the victim's mouth is impossible or impractical.
2b	C-EO	2. For a victim with a tracheal stoma who requires rescue breathing, either mouth-to-stoma or face mask (pediatric preferred)–to–stoma ventilation may be reasonable.

Recommendation-Specific Supportive Text

1. Mouth-to-nose ventilation may be necessary if ventilation through the victim's mouth is impossible because of trauma, positioning, or difficulty obtaining a seal. A case series suggests that mouth-to-nose ventilation in adults is feasible, safe, and effective.[16]
2. Effective ventilation of the patient with a tracheal stoma may require ventilation through the stoma, either by using mouth-to-stoma rescue breaths or by use of a bag-mask technique that creates a tight seal over the stoma with a round, pediatric face mask. There is no published evidence on the safety, effectiveness, or feasibility of mouth-to-stoma ventilation. One study of patients with laryngectomies showed that a pediatric face mask created a better peristomal seal than a standard ventilation mask.[17]

This topic last received formal evidence review in 2010.[15]

Recommendation for Ventilation in Patients With Spontaneous Circulation (Respiratory Arrest)

COR	LOE	Recommendation
2b	C-LD	1. If an adult victim with spontaneous circulation (ie, strong and easily palpable pulses) requires support of ventilation, it may be reasonable for the healthcare provider to give rescue breaths at a rate of about 1 breath every 6 s, or about 10 breaths per minute.

Recommendation-Specific Supportive Text

1. Since the last review in 2010 of rescue breathing in adult patients, there has been no evidence to support a change in previous recommendations. A study in critically ill patients who required ventilatory support found that bag-mask ventilation at a rate of 10 breaths per minute decreased hypoxic events before intubation.[18]

This topic last received formal evidence review in 2010.[15]

Recommendations for Compression-to-Ventilation Ratio: ALS		
COR	LOE	Recommendations
2a	B-R	1. Before placement of an advanced airway (supraglottic airway or tracheal tube), it is reasonable for healthcare providers to perform CPR with cycles of 30 compressions and 2 breaths.
2b	B-R	2. It may be reasonable for EMS providers to use a rate of 10 breaths per minute (1 breath every 6 s) to provide asynchronous ventilation during continuous chest compressions before placement of an advanced airway.
2b	C-LD	3. If an advanced airway is in place, it may be reasonable for the provider to deliver 1 breath every 6 s (10 breaths/min) while continuous chest compressions are being performed.
2b	C-LD	4. It may be reasonable to initially use minimally interrupted chest compressions (ie, delayed ventilation) for witnessed shockable OHCA as part of a bundle of care.

Recommendation-Specific Supportive Text

1. A 2017 ILCOR systematic review found that a ratio of 30 compressions to 2 breaths was associated with better survival than alternate ratios, a recommendation that was reaffirmed by the AHA in 2018.[19,20] Most of these studies examined "bundles" of cardiac arrest care, making it impossible to know if the improvement was due to the compression-to-ventilation ratio itself. This ratio is supported by a large OHCA RCT in which the use of 30:2 (with a pause in compressions of less than 5 seconds) was at least as good as continuous chest compressions.[21]
2. In a large trial, survival and survival with favorable neurological outcome were similar in a group of patients with OHCA treated with ventilations at a rate of 10/min without pausing compressions, compared with a 30:2 ratio before intubation.[21]
3. A 2017 systematic review identified 1 observational human study and 10 animal studies comparing different ventilation rates after advanced airway placement.[22] No clear benefit from a rate of 10 was identified, but no other rate was found to be superior. A 2017 ILCOR systematic review did not identify any new evidence to alter this recommendation, which was reiterated in the "2017 AHA Focused Update on Adult BLS and CPR Quality: An Update to the AHA Guidelines for CPR and Emergency Cardiovascular Care."[19,20]
4. A 2017 ILCOR systematic review concluded that although the evidence from observational studies supporting the use of bundles of care including minimally interrupted chest compressions was of very low certainty (primarily unadjusted results), systems already using such an approach may continue to do so.[19]

These recommendations are supported by the 2017 focused update on adult BLS and CPR quality guidelines.[20]

REFERENCES

1. Kleinman ME, Brennan EE, Goldberger ZD, Swor RA, Terry M, Bobrow BJ, Gazmuri RJ, Travers AH, Rea T. Part 5: adult basic life support and cardiopulmonary resuscitation quality: 2015 American Heart Association Guidelines Update for Cardiopulmonary Resuscitation and Emergency Cardiovascular Care. *Circulation.* 2015;132(suppl 2):S414–S435. doi: 10.1161/CIR.0000000000000259
2. Krischer JP, Fine EG, Weisfeldt ML, Guerci AD, Nagel E, Chandra N. Comparison of prehospital conventional and simultaneous compression-ventilation cardiopulmonary resuscitation. *Crit Care Med.* 1989;17:1263–1269. doi: 10.1097/00003246-198912000-00005
3. Jabre P, Penaloza A, Pinero D, Duchateau FX, Borron SW, Javaudin F, Richard O, de Longueville D, Bouilleau G, Devaud ML, Heidet M, Lejeune C, Fauroux S, Greingor JL, Manara A, Hubert JC, Guihard B, Vermylen O, Lievens P, Auffret Y, Maisondieu C, Huet S, Claessens B, Lapostolle F, Javaud N, Reuter PG, Baker E, Vicaut E, Adnet F. Effect of Bag-Mask Ventilation vs Endotracheal Intubation During Cardiopulmonary Resuscitation on Neurological Outcome After Out-of-Hospital Cardiorespiratory Arrest: A Randomized Clinical Trial. *JAMA.* 2018;319:779–787. doi: 10.1001/jama.2018.0156
4. Benger JR, Kirby K, Black S, Brett SJ, Clout M, Lazaroo MJ, Nolan JP, Reeves BC, Robinson M, Scott LJ, Smartt H, South A, Stokes EA, Taylor J, Thomas M, Voss S, Wordsworth S, Rogers CA. Effect of a Strategy of a Supraglottic Airway Device vs Tracheal Intubation During Out-of-Hospital Cardiac Arrest on Functional Outcome: The AIRWAYS-2 Randomized Clinical Trial. *JAMA.* 2018;320:779–791. doi: 10.1001/jama.2018.11597
5. Wang HE, Schmicker RH, Daya MR, Stephens SW, Idris AH, Carlson JN, Colella MR, Herren H, Hansen M, Richmond NJ, Puyana JCJ, Aufderheide TP, Gray RE, Gray PC, Verkest M, Owens PC, Brienza AM, Sternig KJ, May SJ, Sopko GR, Weisfeldt ML, Nichol G. Effect of a Strategy of Initial Laryngeal Tube Insertion vs Endotracheal Intubation on 72-Hour Survival in Adults With Out-of-Hospital Cardiac Arrest: A Randomized Clinical Trial. *JAMA.* 2018;320:769–778. doi: 10.1001/jama.2018.7044
6. Wenzel V, Keller C, Idris AH, Dörges V, Lindner KH, Brimacombe JR. Effects of smaller tidal volumes during basic life support ventilation in patients with respiratory arrest: good ventilation, less risk? *Resuscitation.* 1999;43:25–29. doi: 10.1016/s0300-9572(99)00118-5
7. Baskett P, Nolan J, Parr M. Tidal volumes which are perceived to be adequate for resuscitation. *Resuscitation.* 1996;31:231–234. doi: 10.1016/0300-9572(96)00994-x
8. Dörges V, Ocker H, Hagelberg S, Wenzel V, Idris AH, Schmucker P. Smaller tidal volumes with room-air are not sufficient to ensure adequate oxygenation during bag-valve-mask ventilation. *Resuscitation.* 2000;44:37–41. doi: 10.1016/s0300-9572(99)00161-6
9. Dörges V, Ocker H, Hagelberg S, Wenzel V, Schmucker P. Optimisation of tidal volumes given with self-inflatable bags without additional oxygen. *Resuscitation.* 2000;43:195–199. doi: 10.1016/s0300-9572(99)00148-3
10. Wenzel V, Idris AH, Banner MJ, Fuerst RS, Tucker KJ. The composition of gas given by mouth-to-mouth ventilation during CPR. *Chest.* 1994;106:1806–1810. doi: 10.1378/chest.106.6.1806
11. Safar P, Escarraga LA, Chang F. Upper airway obstruction in the unconscious patient. *J Appl Physiol.* 1959;14:760–764. doi: 10.1152/jappl.1959.14.5.760

12. Berg MD, Idris AH, Berg RA. Severe ventilatory compromise due to gastric distention during pediatric cardiopulmonary resuscitation. *Resuscitation.* 1998;36:71–73. doi: 10.1016/s0300-9572(97)00077-4
13. Deleted in proof.
14. Aufderheide TP, Sigurdsson G, Pirrallo RG, Yannopoulos D, McKnite S, von Briesen C, Sparks CW, Conrad CJ, Provo TA, Lurie KG. Hyperventilation-induced hypotension during cardiopulmonary resuscitation. *Circulation.* 2004;109:1960–1965. doi: 10.1161/01.CIR.0000126594.79136.61
15. Berg RA, Hemphill R, Abella BS, Aufderheide TP, Cave DM, Hazinski MF, Lerner EB, Rea TD, Sayre MR, Swor RA. Part 5: adult basic life support: 2010 American Heart Association Guidelines for Cardiopulmonary Resuscitation and Emergency Cardiovascular Care. *Circulation.* 2010;122(suppl 3):S685–S705. doi: 10.1161/CIRCULATIONAHA.110.970939
16. Ruben H. The immediate treatment of respiratory failure. *Br J Anaesth.* 1964;36:542–549. doi: 10.1093/bja/36.9.542
17. Bhalla RK, Corrigan A, Roland NJ. Comparison of two face masks used to deliver early ventilation to laryngectomized patients. *Ear Nose Throat J.* 2004;83:414, 416.
18. Casey JD, Janz DR, Russell DW, Vonderhaar DJ, Joffe AM, Dischert KM, Brown RM, Zouk AN, Gulati S, Heideman BE, et al; and the PreVent Investigators and the Pragmatic Critical Care Research Group. Bag-mask ventilation during tracheal intubation of critically ill adults. *N Engl J Med.* 2019;380:811–821. doi: 10.1056/NEJMoa1812405
19. Ashoor HM, Lillie E, Zarin W, Pham B, Khan PA, Nincic V, Yazdi F, Ghassemi M, Ivory J, Cardoso R, Perkins GD, de Caen AR, Tricco AC; ILCOR Basic Life Support Task Force. Effectiveness of different compression-to-ventilation methods for cardiopulmonary resuscitation: A systematic review. *Resuscitation.* 2017;118:112–125. doi: 10.1016/j.resuscitation.2017.05.032
20. Kleinman ME, Goldberger ZD, Rea T, Swor RA, Bobrow BJ, Brennan EE, Terry M, Hemphill R, Gazmuri RJ, Hazinski MF, Travers AH. 2017 American Heart Association Focused Update on Adult Basic Life Support and Cardiopulmonary Resuscitation Quality: An Update to the American Heart Association Guidelines for Cardiopulmonary Resuscitation and Emergency Cardiovascular Care. *Circulation.* 2018;137:e7–e13. doi: 10.1161/CIR.0000000000000539
21. Nichol G, Leroux B, Wang H, Callaway CW, Sopko G, Weisfeldt M, Stiell I, Morrison LJ, Aufderheide TP, Cheskes S, Christenson J, Kudenchuk P, Vaillancourt C, Rea TD, Idris AH, Colella R, Isaacs M, Straight R, Stephens S, Richardson J, Condle J, Schmicker RH, Egan D, May S, Ornato JP; ROC Investigators. Trial of Continuous or Interrupted Chest Compressions during CPR. *N Engl J Med.* 2015;373:2203–2214. doi: 10.1056/NEJMoa1509139
22. Vissers G, Soar J, Monsieurs KG. Ventilation rate in adults with a tracheal tube during cardiopulmonary resuscitation: A systematic review. *Resuscitation.* 2017;119:5–12. doi: 10.1016/j.resuscitation.2017.07.018

Defibrillation

Introduction

Along with CPR, early defibrillation is critical to survival when sudden cardiac arrest is caused by VF or pulseless VT (pVT).[1,2] Defibrillation is most successful when administered as soon as possible after onset of VF/VT and a reasonable immediate treatment when the interval from onset to shock is very brief. Conversely, when VF/VT is more protracted, depletion of the heart's energy reserves can compromise the efficacy of defibrillation unless replenished by a prescribed period of CPR before the rhythm analysis. Minimizing disruptions in CPR surrounding shock administration is also a high priority.

Currently marketed defibrillators use proprietary shock waveforms that differ in their electric characteristics. These deliver different peak currents even at the same programmed energy setting, making comparisons of shock efficacy between devices challenging. Energy setting specifications for cardioversion also differ between defibrillators. Refer to the device manufacturer's recommended energy for a particular waveform.

Technologies are now in development to diagnose the underlying cardiac rhythm during ongoing CPR and to derive prognostic information from the ventricular waveform that can help guide patient management. These still require further testing and validation before routine use.

Recommendations for Defibrillation Indication, Type, and Energy

COR	LOE	Recommendations
1	B-NR	1. Defibrillators (using biphasic or monophasic waveforms) are recommended to treat tachyarrhythmias requiring a shock.
2a	B-R	2. Based on their greater success in arrhythmia termination, defibrillators using biphasic waveforms are preferred over monophasic defibrillators for treatment of tachyarrhythmias.
2a	B-NR	3. A single shock strategy is reasonable in preference to stacked shocks for defibrillation in the setting of unmonitored cardiac arrest.
2a	C-LD	4. It is reasonable that selection of fixed versus escalating energy levels for subsequent shocks for presumed shock-refractory arrhythmias be based on the specific manufacturer's instructions for that waveform. If this is not known, defibrillation at the maximal dose may be considered.
2b	B-R	5. If using a defibrillator capable of escalating energies, higher energy for second and subsequent shocks may be considered for presumed shock-refractory arrhythmias.
2b	C-LD	6. In the absence of conclusive evidence that one biphasic waveform is superior to another in termination of VF, it is reasonable to use the manufacturer's recommended energy dose for the first shock. If this is not known, defibrillation at the maximal dose may be considered.

Recommendation-Specific Supportive Text

1. Emergent electric cardioversion and defibrillation are highly effective at terminating VF/VT and other tachyarrhythmias. No shock waveform has distinguished itself as achieving a consistently higher rate of ROSC or survival. Biphasic and monophasic shock waveforms are likely equivalent in their clinical outcome efficacy.[3]
2. No shock waveform has proved to be superior in improving the rate of ROSC or survival. However, biphasic waveform defibrillators (which deliver pulses of opposite polarity) expose patients to a much lower peak electric current with equivalent or greater efficacy for terminating atrial[4] and ventricular tachyarrhythmias than monophasic (single polarity) defibrillators do.[5–10,13] These potential differences in safety and efficacy favor preferential use of a biphasic defibrillator, when available.

 Circulation. 2020;142(suppl 2):S366–S468. DOI: 10.1161/CIR.0000000000000916

Biphasic defibrillators have largely replaced monophasic shock defibrillators, which are no longer manufactured.

3. The rationale for a single shock strategy, in which CPR is immediately resumed after the first shock rather than after serial "stacked" shocks (if required) is based on a number of considerations. These include the high success rate of the first shock with biphasic waveforms (lessening the need for successive shocks), the declining success of immediate second and third serial shocks when the first shock has failed,[14] and the protracted interruption in CPR required for a series of stacked shocks. A single shock strategy results in shorter interruptions in CPR and a significantly improved survival to hospital admission and discharge (although not 1-year survival) compared with serial "stacked" shocks.[15–17] It is unknown whether stacked shocks or single shocks are more effective in settings of a monitored witnessed arrest (for example, see the section on Cardiac Arrest After Cardiac Surgery).
4. Regardless of waveform, successful defibrillation requires that a shock be of sufficient energy to terminate VF/VT. In cases where the initial shock fails to terminate VF/VT, subsequent shocks may be effective when repeated at the same or an escalating energy setting.[18,19] An optimal energy setting for first or subsequent biphasic defibrillation, whether fixed or escalating, has not been identified, and its selection can be based on the defibrillator's manufacturer specification.
5. There is no conclusive evidence of superiority of one biphasic shock waveform over another for defibrillation.[20] Given the variability in electric characteristics between proprietary biphasic waveforms, it is reasonable to use the energy settings specified by the manufacturer for that specific device. If a manufacturer's specified energy setting for defibrillation is not known at the time of intended use, the maximum dose setting for that device may be considered.
6. Commercially available defibrillators either provide fixed energy settings or allow for escalating energy settings; both approaches are highly effective in terminating VF/VT.[18] An optimal energy setting for first or subsequent biphasic defibrillation, whether fixed or escalating, has not been identified and is best deferred to the defibrillator's manufacturer. A randomized trial comparing fixed 150 J biphasic defibrillation with escalating higher shock energies (200–300–360 J) observed similar rates of successful defibrillation and conversion to an organized rhythm after the first shock. However, among patients who required multiple shocks, escalating shock energy resulted in a significantly higher rate of conversion to an organized rhythm, although overall survival did not differ between the 2 treatment groups.[19] When VF/VT is refractory to the first shock, an equivalent or higher energy setting than the first shock may be considered. As yet, there is no conclusive evidence of superiority of one biphasic shock waveform over another for defibrillation.[20] It is reasonable to use the energy settings specified by the manufacturer for that specific device. If a manufacturer's specified energy setting for defibrillation is not known at the time of intended use, the maximum dose setting for that device may be considered.

Recommendations 1, 2, and 6 last received formal evidence review in 2015.[21] Recommendations 3, 4, and 5 are supported by the 2020 CoSTR for BLS.[22]

Recommendation for Pads for Defibrillation

COR	LOE	Recommendation
2a	C-LD	1. It is reasonable to place defibrillation paddles or pads on the exposed chest in an anterolateral or anteroposterior position, and to use a paddle or pad electrode diameter more than 8 cm in adults.

Recommendation-Specific Supportive Text

1. Anterolateral, anteroposterior, anterior-left infrascapular, and anterior-right infrascapular electrode placements are comparably effective for treating supraventricular and ventricular arrhythmias.[24–28] A larger pad/paddle size (within the limits of 8–12 cm in diameter) lowers transthoracic impedance.[29,30] Self-adhesive pads have largely replaced defibrillation paddles in clinical practice. Before pad placement, remove all clothing and jewelry from the chest.

This recommendation is supported by a 2020 ILCOR scoping review, which found no new information to update the 2010 recommendations.[22,31]

Recommendation for Automatic- Versus Manual-Mode Defibrillation

COR	LOE	Recommendation
2b	C-LD	1. It may be reasonable to use a defibrillator in manual mode as compared with automatic mode depending on the skill set of the operator.

Recommendation-Specific Supportive Text

1. AEDs are highly accurate in their detection of shockable arrhythmias but require a pause in CPR for automated rhythm analysis.[32,33] Manual defibrillation can result in a shorter hands-off period for rhythm confirmation in operators with a sufficient skill for rapid and reliable rhythm interpretation.[34,35]

This recommendation is supported by a 2020 ILCOR scoping review,[22] which found no new information to update the 2010 recommendations.[31]

Recommendations for CPR Before Defibrillation		
COR	**LOE**	**Recommendations**
1	C-LD	1. CPR is recommended until a defibrillator or AED is applied.
2a	B-R	2. In unmonitored cardiac arrest, it is reasonable to provide a brief prescribed period of CPR while a defibrillator is being obtained and readied for use before initial rhythm analysis and possible defibrillation.
2a	C-LD	3. Immediate defibrillation is reasonable for provider-witnessed or monitored VF/pVT of short duration when a defibrillator is already applied or immediately available.

Recommendation-Specific Supportive Text

1. CPR is the single-most important intervention for a patient in cardiac arrest and should be provided until a defibrillator is applied to minimize interruptions in compressions.
2. When VF/VT has been present for more than a few minutes, myocardial reserves of oxygen and other energy substrates are rapidly depleted. If replenished by a period of CPR before shock, defibrillation success improves significantly.[1,2,36,37] Because no differences in outcome were seen in studies comparing short (typically approximately about 30 seconds) with prolonged (up to 3 minutes) periods of CPR preceding the initial rhythm analysis, a brief period of CPR while the defibrillator is readied for use may be sufficient in unmonitored cardiac arrest.[38–40] Even in monitored arrests, it can take time to attach pads, power on a defibrillator, and charge the capacitor before shock delivery, during which there is good reason to administer CPR.
3. Early defibrillation improves outcome from cardiac arrest.[41–43] When VF is of short duration, myocardial reserves of oxygen and other energy substrates are likely to remain intact. During this early electric phase, the rhythm is most responsive to defibrillation.[44,45] Thus, if the onset of VF is monitored or witnessed with a defibrillator that is already applied, or to which there is immediate access, it is reasonable to administer a shock as soon as possible. Interim CPR should be provided if there is any delay in obtaining or readying the defibrillator for use.

Recommendations 1 and 2 are supported by the 2020 CoSTR for BLS.[22] Recommendation 3 last received formal evidence review in 2010.[46]

Recommendation for Anticipatory Defibrillator Charging		
COR	**LOE**	**Recommendation**
2b	C-EO	1. It may be reasonable to charge a manual defibrillator during chest compressions either before or after a scheduled rhythm analysis.

Recommendation-Specific Supportive Text

1. There are differing approaches to charging a manual defibrillator during resuscitation. It is not uncommon for chest compressions to be paused for rhythm detection and continue to be withheld while the defibrillator is charged and prepared for shock delivery. This approach results in a protracted hands-off period before shock. Precharging the defibrillator during ongoing chest compressions shortens the hands-off chest time surrounding defibrillation, without evidence of harm.[47] Although no study has directly evaluated the effect of precharging itself on cardiac arrest outcome, shorter perishock pauses (which could result from such a strategy) are associated with improved survival from VF arrest.[48] Two approaches are reasonable: either charging the defibrillator before a rhythm check or resuming compressions briefly after a rhythm check while the defibrillator charges. Either approach may reduce no-flow time.[49,50]

This recommendation is supported by the 2020 CoSTR for ALS.[51]

Recommendation for Postshock Rhythm Check		
COR	**LOE**	**Recommendation**
2b	C-LD	1. It may be reasonable to immediately resume chest compressions after shock administration rather than pause CPR to perform a postshock rhythm check in cardiac arrest patients.

Recommendation-Specific Supportive Text

1. Immediate resumption of chest compressions after shock results in a shorter perishock pause and improves the overall hands-on time (chest compression fraction) during resuscitation, which is associated with improved survival from VF arrest.[16,48] Even when successful, defibrillation is often followed by a variable (and sometimes protracted) period of asystole or pulseless electrical activity, during which providing CPR while awaiting a return of rhythm and pulse is advisable. Whether resumption of CPR immediately after shock might reinduce VF/VT is controversial.[52–54] This potential concern has not been borne out by any evidence of worsened survival from such a strategy. Should there be physiological evidence of return of circulation such as an arterial waveform or abrupt rise in $ETCO_2$ after shock, a pause of chest compressions briefly for confirmatory rhythm analysis may be warranted.

This recommendation is supported by the 2020 CoSTR for BLS.[22]

Recommendations for Ancillary Defibrillator Technologies		
COR	LOE	Recommendations
2b	C-LD	1. The value of artifact-filtering algorithms for analysis of electrocardiogram (ECG) rhythms during chest compressions has not been established.
2b	C-LD	2. The value of VF waveform analysis to guide the acute management of adults with cardiac arrest has not been established.

Recommendation-Specific Supportive Text

1. CPR obscures interpretation of the underlying rhythm because of the artifact created by chest compressions on the ECG. This makes it difficult to plan the next step of care and can potentially delay or even misdirect drug therapies if given empirically (blindly) based on the patient's presumed, but not actual, underlying rhythm. Time taken for rhythm analysis also disrupts CPR. Artifact-filtering and other innovative techniques to disclose the underlying rhythm beneath ongoing CPR can surmount these challenges and minimize interruptions in chest compressions while offering a diagnostic advantage to better direct therapies.[55–60] Despite the theoretical advantages, no study has evaluated these technologies in a real-time clinical setting or validated their clinical effectiveness compared to current resuscitation strategies. At present, filtering algorithms are strictly used for visual (manual) rhythm interpretation and not for automated VF/VT rhythm detection in AEDs during ongoing CPR. This added potential application remains untested. Recognizing the need for further clinical research, a 2020 ILCOR systematic review recommended against adopting artifact-filtering algorithms for rhythm analysis during CPR at the present time.[51] The writing group also endorses the need for further investigation and clinical validation before these technologies are adopted into clinical practice.
2. The electric characteristics of the VF waveform are known to change over time.[61] VF waveform analysis may be of value in predicting the success of defibrillation or other therapies during the course of resuscitation.[62–64] The prospect of basing therapies on a prognostic analysis of the VF waveform in real-time is an exciting and developing avenue of new research. However, the validity, reliability, and clinical effectiveness of an approach that prompts or withholds shock or other therapies on the basis of predictive analyses is currently uncertain. The only prospective clinical trial comparing a standard shock-first protocol with a waveform analysis-guided shock algorithm observed no differences in outcome.[65] The consensus of the writing group is that there is currently insufficient evidence to support the routine use of waveform analysis to guide resuscitation care, but it is an area in which further research with clinical validation is needed and encouraged.

Recommendation 1 is supported by the 2020 CoSTR for ALS.[51] Recommendation 2 is supported by a 2020 ILCOR evidence update,[51] which found no new information to update the 2010 recommendations.[66]

Recommendation for Double Sequential Defibrillation		
COR	LOE	Recommendation
2b	C-LD	1. The usefulness of double sequential defibrillation for refractory shockable rhythm has not been established.

Recommendation-Specific Supportive Text

1. There is limited evidence examining double sequential defibrillation in clinical practice. A number of case reports have shown good outcomes in patients who received double sequential defibrillation. However, these case reports are subject to publication bias and should not be used to support its effectiveness.[67] A handful of observational studies demonstrated no difference in outcomes (ROSC, survival, neurological outcome) with the use of double sequential defibrillation compared with standard defibrillation.[68–71] These studies should also be interpreted with caution, because the use of double sequential defibrillation was not protocolized and was often used late in the resuscitation after standard resuscitation was unsuccessful. Published reports also do not distinguish the application of double sequential defibrillation for truly shock-refractory (incessant) VF versus VF that recurs during the period of CPR after a successful shock, which is the more common clinical scenario.[3,7] A 2020 ILCOR systematic review found no evidence to support double sequential defibrillation and recommended against its routine use compared with standard defibrillation.[51] A recent pilot RCT (not included in the systematic review) of 152 patients who remained in VF after at least 3 shocks found higher rates of VF termination and ROSC with double sequential defibrillation or alternative defibrillator pad placement compared with standard defibrillation but was not powered for these outcomes and did not report patient survival.[72] A number of unanswered questions remain about double sequential defibrillation, including intershock timing, pad positioning, technique, and the possibility of harm with increased energy and defibrillator damage.[73,74] It is premature for double sequential defibrillation to be incorporated into routine clinical practice given the lack of evidence. Its usefulness should be explored in the context of clinical

trials. An ongoing RCT (NCT04080986) may provide answers to some of these questions.

This recommendation is supported by the 2020 CoSTR for ALS.[51]

REFERENCES

1. Larsen MP, Eisenberg MS, Cummins RO, Hallstrom AP. Predicting survival from out-of-hospital cardiac arrest: a graphic model. *Ann Emerg Med.* 1993;22:1652–1658. doi: 10.1016/s0196-0644(05)81302-2
2. Swor RA, Jackson RE, Cynar M, Sadler E, Basse E, Boji B, Rivera-Rivera EJ, Maher A, Grubb W, Jacobson R. Bystander CPR, ventricular fibrillation, and survival in witnessed, unmonitored out-of-hospital cardiac arrest. *Ann Emerg Med.* 1995;25:780–784. doi: 10.1016/s0196-0644(95)70207-5
3. Kudenchuk PJ, Cobb LA, Copass MK, Olsufka M, Maynard C, Nichol G. Transthoracic incremental monophasic versus biphasic defibrillation by emergency responders (TIMBER): a randomized comparison of monophasic with biphasic waveform ascending energy defibrillation for the resuscitation of out-of-hospital cardiac arrest due to ventricular fibrillation. *Circulation.* 2006;114:2010–2018. doi: 10.1161/CIRCULATIONAHA.106.636506
4. Inácio JF, da Rosa Mdos S, Shah J, Rosário J, Vissoci JR, Manica AL, Rodrigues CG. Monophasic and biphasic shock for transthoracic conversion of atrial fibrillation: systematic review and network meta-analysis. *Resuscitation.* 2016;100:66–75. doi: 10.1016/j.resuscitation.2015.12.009
5. Higgins SL, O'Grady SG, Banville I, Chapman FW, Schmitt PW, Lank P, Walker RG, Ilina M. Efficacy of lower-energy biphasic shocks for transthoracic defibrillation: a follow-up clinical study. *Prehosp Emerg Care.* 2004;8:262–267. doi: 10.1016/j.prehos.2004.02.002
6. Didon JP, Fontaine G, White RD, Jekova I, Schmid JJ, Cansell A. Clinical experience with a low-energy pulsed biphasic waveform in out-of-hospital cardiac arrest. *Resuscitation.* 2008;76:350–353. doi: 10.1016/j.resuscitation.2007.08.010
7. van Alem AP, Chapman FW, Lank P, Hart AA, Koster RW. A prospective, randomised and blinded comparison of first shock success of monophasic and biphasic waveforms in out-of-hospital cardiac arrest. *Resuscitation.* 2003;58:17–24. doi: 10.1016/s0300-9572(03)00106-0
8. Morrison LJ, Dorian P, Long J, Vermeulen M, Schwartz B, Sawadsky B, Frank J, Cameron B, Burgess R, Shield J, Bagley P, Mausz V, Brewer JE, Lerman BB; Steering Committee, Central Validation Committee, Safety and Efficacy Committee. Out-of-hospital cardiac arrest rectilinear biphasic to monophasic damped sine defibrillation waveforms with advanced life support intervention trial (ORBIT). *Resuscitation.* 2005;66:149–157. doi: 10.1016/j.resuscitation.2004.11.031
9. Schneider T, Martens PR, Paschen H, Kuisma M, Wolcke B, Gliner BE, Russell JK, Weaver WD, Bossaert L, Chamberlain D. Multicenter, randomized, controlled trial of 150-J biphasic shocks compared with 200- to 360-J monophasic shocks in the resuscitation of out-of-hospital cardiac arrest victims. Optimized Response to Cardiac Arrest (ORCA) Investigators. *Circulation.* 2000;102:1780–1787. doi: 10.1161/01.cir.102.15.1780
10. White RD, Hankins DG, Bugliosi TF. Seven years' experience with early defibrillation by police and paramedics in an emergency medical services system. *Resuscitation.* 1998;39:145–151. doi: 10.1016/s0300-9572(98)00135-x
11. Deleted in proof.
12. Deleted in proof.
13. Leng CT, Paradis NA, Calkins H, Berger RD, Lardo AC, Rent KC, Halperin HR. Resuscitation after prolonged ventricular fibrillation with use of monophasic and biphasic waveform pulses for external defibrillation. *Circulation.* 2000;101:2968–2974. doi: 10.1161/01.cir.101.25.2968
14. Koster RW, Walker RG, Chapman FW. Recurrent ventricular fibrillation during advanced life support care of patients with prehospital cardiac arrest. *Resuscitation.* 2008;78:252–257. doi: 10.1016/j.resuscitation.2008.03.231
15. Bobrow BJ, Clark LL, Ewy GA, Chikani V, Sanders AB, Berg RA, Richman PB, Kern KB. Minimally interrupted cardiac resuscitation by emergency medical services for out-of-hospital cardiac arrest. *JAMA.* 2008;299:1158–1165. doi: 10.1001/jama.299.10.1158
16. Rea TD, Helbock M, Perry S, Garcia M, Cloyd D, Becker L, Eisenberg M. Increasing use of cardiopulmonary resuscitation during out-of-hospital ventricular fibrillation arrest: survival implications of guideline changes. *Circulation.* 2006;114:2760–2765. doi: 10.1161/CIRCULATIONAHA.106.654715
17. Jost D, Degrange H, Verret C, Hersan O, Banville IL, Chapman FW, Lank P, Petit JL, Fuilla C, Migliani R, et al; and the DEFI 2005 Work Group. DEFI 2005: a randomized controlled trial of the effect of automated external defibrillator cardiopulmonary resuscitation protocol on outcome from out-of-hospital cardiac arrest. *Circulation.* 2010;121:1614–1622. doi: 10.1161/CIRCULATIONAHA.109.878389
18. Hess EP, Russell JK, Liu PY, White RD. A high peak current 150-J fixed-energy defibrillation protocol treats recurrent ventricular fibrillation (VF) as effectively as initial VF. *Resuscitation.* 2008;79:28–33. doi: 10.1016/j.resuscitation.2008.04.028
19. Stiell IG, Walker RG, Nesbitt LP, Chapman FW, Cousineau D, Christenson J, Bradford P, Sookram S, Berringer R, Lank P, Wells GA. BIPHASIC Trial: a randomized comparison of fixed lower versus escalating higher energy levels for defibrillation in out-of-hospital cardiac arrest. *Circulation.* 2007;115:1511–1517. doi: 10.1161/CIRCULATIONAHA.106.648204
20. Morrison LJ, Henry RM, Ku V, Nolan JP, Morley P, Deakin CD. Single-shock defibrillation success in adult cardiac arrest: a systematic review. *Resuscitation.* 2013;84:1480–1486. doi: 10.1016/j.resuscitation.2013.07.008
21. Link MS, Berkow LC, Kudenchuk PJ, Halperin HR, Hess EP, Moitra VK, Neumar RW, O'Neil BJ, Paxton JH, Silvers SM, et al. Part 7: adult advanced cardiovascular life support: 2015 American Heart Association Guidelines Update for Cardiopulmonary Resuscitation and Emergency Cardiovascular Care. *Circulation.* 2015;132(suppl 2):S444–S464. doi: 10.1161/CIR.0000000000000261
22. Olasveengen TM, Mancini ME, Perkins GD, Avis S, Brooks S, Castrén M, Chung SP, Considine J, Couper K, Escalante R, et al; on behalf of the Adult Basic Life Support Collaborators. Adult basic life support: 2020 International Consensus on Cardiopulmonary Resuscitation and Emergency Cardiovascular Care Science With Treatment Recommendations. *Circulation.* 2020;142(suppl 1):S41–S91. doi: 10.1161/CIR.0000000000000892
23. Deleted in proof.
24. Boodhoo L, Mitchell AR, Bordoli G, Lloyd G, Patel N, Sulke N. DC cardioversion of persistent atrial fibrillation: a comparison of two protocols. *Int J Cardiol.* 2007;114:16–21. doi: 10.1016/j.ijcard.2005.11.108
25. Brazdzionyte J, Babarskiene RM, Stanaitiene G. Anterior-posterior versus anterior-lateral electrode position for biphasic cardioversion of atrial fibrillation. *Medicina (Kaunas).* 2006;42:994–998.
26. Chen CJ, Guo GB. External cardioversion in patients with persistent atrial fibrillation: a reappraisal of the effects of electrode pad position and transthoracic impedance on cardioversion success. *Jpn Heart J.* 2003;44:921–932. doi: 10.1536/jhj.44.921
27. Stanaitiene G, Babarskiene RM. [Impact of electrical shock waveform and paddle positions on efficacy of direct current cardioversion for atrial fibrillation]. *Medicina (Kaunas).* 2008;44:665–672.
28. Krasteva V, Matveev M, Mudrov N, Prokopova R. Transthoracic impedance study with large self-adhesive electrodes in two conventional positions for defibrillation. *Physiol Meas.* 2006;27:1009–1022. doi: 10.1088/0967-3334/27/10/007
29. Kerber RE, Grayzel J, Hoyt R, Marcus M, Kennedy J. Transthoracic resistance in human defibrillation. Influence of body weight, chest size, serial shocks, paddle size and paddle contact pressure. *Circulation.* 1981;63:676–682. doi: 10.1161/01.cir.63.3.676
30. Connell PN, Ewy GA, Dahl CF, Ewy MD. Transthoracic impedance to defibrillator discharge. Effect of electrode size and electrode-chest wall interface. *J Electrocardiol.* 1973;6:313–31M. doi: 10.1016/s0022-0736(73)80053-6
31. Jacobs I, Sunde K, Deakin CD, Hazinski MF, Kerber RE, Koster RW, Morrison LJ, Nolan JP, Sayre MR, Defibrillation Chapter C. Part 6: Defibrillation: 2010 International Consensus on Cardiopulmonary Resuscitation and Emergency Cardiovascular Care Science With Treatment Recommendations. *Circulation.* 2010;122 (Suppl 2):S325–337. doi: 10.1161/CIRCULATIONAHA.110.971010
32. Loma-Osorio P, Nunez M, Aboal J, Bosch D, Batlle P, Ruiz de Morales E, Ramos R, Brugada J, Onaga H, Morales A, et al. The Girona Territori Cardioprotegit Project: performance evaluation of public defibrillators. *Rev Esp Cardiol (Engl Ed).* 2018;71:79–85. doi: 10.1016/j.rec.2017.04.011
33. Zijlstra JA, Bekkers LE, Hulleman M, Beesems SG, Koster RW. Automated external defibrillator and operator performance in out-of-hospital cardiac arrest. *Resuscitation.* 2017;118:140–146. doi: 10.1016/j.resuscitation.2017.05.017
34. Kramer-Johansen J, Edelson DP, Abella BS, Becker LB, Wik L, Steen PA. Pauses in chest compression and inappropriate shocks: a comparison of manual and semi-automatic defibrillation attempts. *Resuscitation.* 2007;73:212–220. doi: 10.1016/j.resuscitation.2006.09.006
35. Cheskes S, Hillier M, Byers A, Verbeek PR, Drennan IR, Zhan C, Morrison LJ. The association between manual mode defibrillation, pre-shock pause duration and appropriate shock delivery when employed by basic life

support paramedics during out-of-hospital cardiac arrest. *Resuscitation.* 2015;90:61–66. doi: 10.1016/j.resuscitation.2015.02.022

36. Eftestøl T, Wik L, Sunde K, Steen PA. Effects of cardiopulmonary resuscitation on predictors of ventricular fibrillation defibrillation success during out-of-hospital cardiac arrest. *Circulation.* 2004;110:10–15. doi: 10.1161/01.CIR.0000133323.15565.75
37. Holmberg M, Holmberg S, Herlitz J. Incidence, duration and survival of ventricular fibrillation in out-of-hospital cardiac arrest patients in sweden. *Resuscitation.* 2000;44:7–17. doi: 10.1016/s0300-9572(99)00155-0
38. Baker PW, Conway J, Cotton C, Ashby DT, Smyth J, Woodman RJ, Grantham H; Clinical Investigators. Defibrillation or cardiopulmonary resuscitation first for patients with out-of-hospital cardiac arrests found by paramedics to be in ventricular fibrillation? A randomised control trial. *Resuscitation.* 2008;79:424–431. doi: 10.1016/j.resuscitation.2008.07.017
39. Jacobs IG, Finn JC, Oxer HF, Jelinek GA. CPR before defibrillation in out-of-hospital cardiac arrest: a randomized trial. *Emerg Med Australas.* 2005;17:39–45. doi: 10.1111/j.1742-6723.2005.00694.x
40. Stiell IG, Nichol G, Leroux BG, Rea TD, Ornato JP, Powell J, Christenson J, Callaway CW, Kudenchuk PJ, Aufderheide TP, Idris AH, Daya MR, Wang HE, Morrison LJ, Davis D, Andrusiek D, Stephens S, Cheskes S, Schmicker RH, Fowler R, Vaillancourt C, Hostler D, Zive D, Pirrallo RG, Vilke GM, Sopko G, Weisfeldt M; ROC Investigators. Early versus later rhythm analysis in patients with out-of-hospital cardiac arrest. *N Engl J Med.* 2011;365:787–797. doi: 10.1056/NEJMoa1010076
41. Bircher NG, Chan PS, Xu Y; American Heart Association's Get With The Guidelines–Resuscitation Investigators. Delays in Cardiopulmonary Resuscitation, Defibrillation, and Epinephrine Administration All Decrease Survival in In-hospital Cardiac Arrest. *Anesthesiology.* 2019;130:414–422. doi: 10.1097/ALN.0000000000002563
42. Valenzuela TD, Roe DJ, Nichol G, Clark LL, Spaite DW, Hardman RG. Outcomes of rapid defibrillation by security officers after cardiac arrest in casinos. *N Engl J Med.* 2000;343:1206–1209. doi: 10.1056/NEJM200010263431701
43. White RD, Asplin BR, Bugliosi TF, Hankins DG. High discharge survival rate after out-of-hospital ventricular fibrillation with rapid defibrillation by police and paramedics. *Ann Emerg Med.* 1996;28:480–485. doi: 10.1016/s0196-0644(96)70109-9
44. Weisfeldt ML, Becker LB. Resuscitation after cardiac arrest: a 3-phase time-sensitive model. *JAMA.* 2002;288:3035–3038. doi: 10.1001/jama.288.23.3035
45. Kern KB, Garewal HS, Sanders AB, Janas W, Nelson J, Sloan D, Tacker WA, Ewy GA. Depletion of myocardial adenosine triphosphate during prolonged untreated ventricular fibrillation: effect on defibrillation success. *Resuscitation.* 1990;20:221–229. doi: 10.1016/0300-9572(90)90005-y
46. Link MS, Atkins DL, Passman RS, Halperin HR, Samson RA, White RD, Cudnik MT, Berg MD, Kudenchuk PJ, Kerber RE. Part 6: electrical therapies: automated external defibrillators, defibrillation, cardioversion, and pacing: 2010 American Heart Association Guidelines for Cardiopulmonary Resuscitation and Emergency Cardiovascular Care. *Circulation.* 2010;122(suppl 3):S706–S719. doi: 10.1161/CIRCULATIONAHA.110.970954
47. Edelson DP, Robertson-Dick BJ, Yuen TC, Eilevstjønn J, Walsh D, Bareis CJ, Vanden Hoek TL, Abella BS. Safety and efficacy of defibrillator charging during ongoing chest compressions: a multi-center study. *Resuscitation.* 2010;81:1521–1526. doi: 10.1016/j.resuscitation.2010.07.014
48. Cheskes S, Schmicker RH, Christenson J, Salcido DD, Rea T, Powell J, Edelson DP, Sell R, May S, Menegazzi JJ, Van Ottingham L, Olsufka M, Pennington S, Simonini J, Berg RA, Stiell I, Idris A, Bigham B, Morrison L; Resuscitation Outcomes Consortium (ROC) Investigators. Perishock pause: an independent predictor of survival from out-of-hospital shockable cardiac arrest. *Circulation.* 2011;124:58–66. doi: 10.1161/CIRCULATIONAHA.110.010736
49. Hansen LK, Folkestad L, Brabrand M. Defibrillator charging before rhythm analysis significantly reduces hands-off time during resuscitation: a simulation study. *Am J Emerg Med.* 2013;31:395–400. doi: 10.1016/j.ajem.2012.08.029
50. Kemper M, Zech A, Lazarovici M, Zwissler B, Prückner S, Meyer O. Defibrillator charging before rhythm analysis causes peri-shock pauses exceeding guideline recommended maximum 5 s: A randomized simulation trial. *Anaesthesist.* 2019;68:546–554. doi: 10.1007/s00101-019-0623-x
51. Berg KM, Soar J, Andersen LW, Böttiger BW, Cacciola S, Callaway CW, Couper K, Cronberg T, D'Arrigo S, Deakin CD, et al; on behalf of the Adult Advanced Life Support Collaborators. Adult advanced life support: 2020 International Consensus on Cardiopulmonary Resuscitation and Emergency Cardiovascular Care Science With Treatment Recommendations. *Circulation.* 2020;142(suppl 1):S92–S139. doi: 10.1161/CIR.0000000000000893
52. Berdowski J, ten Haaf M, Tijssen JG, Chapman FW, Koster RW. Time in recurrent ventricular fibrillation and survival after out-of-hospital cardiac arrest. *Circulation.* 2010;122:1101–1108. doi: 10.1161/CIRCULATIONAHA.110.958173
53. Hess EP, White RD. Ventricular fibrillation is not provoked by chest compression during post-shock organized rhythms in out-of-hospital cardiac arrest. *Resuscitation.* 2005;66:7–11. doi: 10.1016/j.resuscitation.2005.01.011
54. Berdowski J, Tijssen JG, Koster RW. Chest compressions cause recurrence of ventricular fibrillation after the first successful conversion by defibrillation in out-of-hospital cardiac arrest. *Circ Arrhythm Electrophysiol.* 2010;3:72–78. doi: 10.1161/CIRCEP.109.902114
55. Li Y, Bisera J, Tang W, Weil MH. Automated detection of ventricular fibrillation to guide cardiopulmonary resuscitation. *Crit Pathw Cardiol.* 2007;6:131–134. doi: 10.1097/HPC.0b013e31813429b0
56. Tan Q, Freeman GA, Geheb F, Bisera J. Electrocardiographic analysis during uninterrupted cardiopulmonary resuscitation. *Crit Care Med.* 2008;36(11 Suppl):S409–S412. doi: 10.1097/ccm.0b013e31818a7fbf
57. Li Y, Bisera J, Weil MH, Tang W. An algorithm used for ventricular fibrillation detection without interrupting chest compression. *IEEE Trans Biomed Eng.* 2012;59:78–86. doi: 10.1109/TBME.2011.2118755
58. Babaeizadeh S, Firoozabadi R, Han C, Helfenbein ED. Analyzing cardiac rhythm in the presence of chest compression artifact for automated shock advisory. *J Electrocardiol.* 2014;47:798–803. doi: 10.1016/j.jelectrocard.2014.07.021
59. Fumagalli F, Silver AE, Tan Q, Zaidi N, Ristagno G. Cardiac rhythm analysis during ongoing cardiopulmonary resuscitation using the Analysis During Compressions with Fast Reconfirmation technology. *Heart Rhythm.* 2018;15:248–255. doi: 10.1016/j.hrthm.2017.09.003
60. Hu Y, Tang H, Liu C, Jing D, Zhu H, Zhang Y, Yu X, Zhang G, Xu J. The performance of a new shock advisory algorithm to reduce interruptions during CPR. *Resuscitation.* 2019;143:1–9. doi: 10.1016/j.resuscitation.2019.07.026
61. Asano Y, Davidenko JM, Baxter WT, Gray RA, Jalife J. Optical mapping of drug-induced polymorphic arrhythmias and torsade de pointes in the isolated rabbit heart. *J Am Coll Cardiol.* 1997;29:831–842. doi: 10.1016/s0735-1097(96)00588-8
62. Callaway CW, Sherman LD, Mosesso VN Jr, Dietrich TJ, Holt E, Clarkson MC. Scaling exponent predicts defibrillation success for out-of-hospital ventricular fibrillation cardiac arrest. *Circulation.* 2001;103:1656–1661. doi: 10.1161/01.cir.103.12.1656
63. Coult J, Blackwood J, Sherman L, Rea TD, Kudenchuk PJ, Kwok H. Ventricular Fibrillation Waveform Analysis During Chest Compressions to Predict Survival From Cardiac Arrest. *Circ Arrhythm Electrophysiol.* 2019;12:e006924. doi: 10.1161/CIRCEP.118.006924
64. Coult J, Kwok H, Sherman L, Blackwood J, Kudenchuk PJ, Rea TD. Ventricular fibrillation waveform measures combined with prior shock outcome predict defibrillation success during cardiopulmonary resuscitation. *J Electrocardiol.* 2018;51:99–106. doi: 10.1016/j.jelectrocard.2017.07.016
65. Freese JP, Jorgenson DB, Liu PY, Innes J, Matallana L, Nammi K, Donohoe RT, Whitbread M, Silverman RA, Prezant DJ. Waveform analysis-guided treatment versus a standard shock-first protocol for the treatment of out-of-hospital cardiac arrest presenting in ventricular fibrillation: results of an international randomized, controlled trial. *Circulation.* 2013;128:995–1002. doi: 10.1161/CIRCULATIONAHA.113.003273
66. Neumar RW, Otto CW, Link MS, Kronick SL, Shuster M, Callaway CW, Kudenchuk PJ, Ornato JP, McNally B, Silvers SM, et al. Part 8: adult advanced cardiovascular life support: 2010 American Heart Association Guidelines for Cardiopulmonary Resuscitation and Emergency Cardiovascular Care. *Circulation.* 2010;122:S729–S767. doi: 10.1161/CIRCULATIONAHA.110.970988
67. Clemency BM, Pastwik B, Gillen D. Double sequential defibrillation and the tyranny of the case study. *Am J Emerg Med.* 2019;37:792–793. doi: 10.1016/j.ajem.2018.09.002
68. Beck LR, Ostermayer DG, Ponce JN, Srinivasan S, Wang HE. Effectiveness of Prehospital Dual Sequential Defibrillation for Refractory Ventricular Fibrillation and Ventricular Tachycardia Cardiac Arrest. *Prehosp Emerg Care.* 2019;23:597–602. doi: 10.1080/10903127.2019.1584256
69. Mapp JG, Hans AJ, Darrington AM, Ross EM, Ho CC, Miramontes DA, Harper SA, Wampler DA; Prehospital Research and Innovation in Military and Expeditionary Environments (PRIME) Research Group. Prehospital Double Sequential Defibrillation: A Matched Case-Control Study. *Acad Emerg Med.* 2019;26:994–1001. doi: 10.1111/acem.13672

70. Ross EM, Redman TT, Harper SA, Mapp JG, Wampler DA, Miramontes DA. Dual defibrillation in out-of-hospital cardiac arrest: A retrospective cohort analysis. *Resuscitation.* 2016;106:14–17. doi: 10.1016/j.resuscitation.2016.06.011
71. Emmerson AC, Whitbread M, Fothergill RT. Double sequential defibrillation therapy for out-of-hospital cardiac arrests: The London experience. *Resuscitation.* 2017;117:97–101. doi: 10.1016/j.resuscitation.2017.06.011
72. Cheskes S, Dorian P, Feldman M, McLeod S, Scales DC, Pinto R, Turner L, Morrison LJ, Drennan IR, Verbeek PR. Double sequential external defibrillation for refractory ventricular fibrillation: the DOSE VF pilot randomized controlled trial. *Resuscitation.* 2020;150:178–184. doi: 10.1016/j.resuscitation.2020.02.010
73. Gerstein NS, McLean AR, Stecker EC, Schulman PM. External Defibrillator Damage Associated With Attempted Synchronized Dual-Dose Cardioversion. *Ann Emerg Med.* 2018;71:109–112. doi: 10.1016/j.annemergmed.2017.04.005
74. Kudenchuk PJ. Shocking insights on double defibrillation: How, when and why not? *Resuscitation.* 2019;140:209–210. doi: 10.1016/j.resuscitation.2019.05.022

Other Electric or Pseudo-Electric Therapies for Cardiac Arrest

Introduction

In addition to defibrillation, several alternative electric and pseudoelectrical therapies have been explored as possible treatment options during cardiac arrest. Transcutaneous pacing has been studied during cardiac arrest with bradyasystolic cardiac rhythm. The theory is that the heart will respond to electric stimuli by producing myocardial contraction and generating forward movement of blood, but clinical trials have not shown pacing to improve patient outcomes.

Other pseudoelectrical therapies, such as cough CPR, fist or percussion pacing, and precordial thump have all been described as temporizing measures in select patients who are either periarrest or in the initial seconds of witnessed cardiac arrest (before losing consciousness in the case of cough CPR) when definitive therapy is not readily available. Precordial thump is a single, sharp, high-velocity impact (or "punch") to the middle sternum by the ulnar aspect of a tightly clenched fist. The force from a precordial thump is intended to transmit electric energy to the heart, similar to a low-energy shock, in hope of terminating the underlying tachyarrhythmia.

Fist (or percussion) pacing is the delivery of a serial, rhythmic, relatively low-velocity impact to the sternum by a closed fist.[1] Fist pacing is administered in an attempt to stimulate an electric impulse sufficient to cause myocardial depolarization. Cough CPR is described as repeated deep breaths followed immediately by a cough every few seconds in an attempt to increase aortic and intracardiac pressures, providing transient hemodynamic support before a loss of consciousness.

Recommendation for Electric Pacing

COR	LOE	Recommendation
3: No Benefit	B-R	1. Electric pacing is not recommended for routine use in established cardiac arrest.

Recommendation-Specific Supportive Text

1. Existing evidence, including observational and quasi-RCT data, suggests that pacing by a transcutaneous, transvenous, or transmyocardial approach in cardiac arrest does not improve the likelihood of ROSC or survival, regardless of the timing of pacing administration in established asystole, location of arrest (in-hospital or out-of-hospital), or primary cardiac rhythm (asystole, pulseless electrical activity).[2–6] Protracted interruptions in chest compressions while the success of pacing is assessed can also be detrimental to survival. It is not known whether the timing of pacing initiation may influence pacing success such that pacing may be useful in the initial seconds of select cases of witnessed, monitored cardiac arrest (see the section on Cardiac Arrest After Cardiac Surgery). If pacing is attempted during cardiac arrest related to the special circumstances described above, providers are cautioned against its performance at the expense of high-quality CPR, particularly when assessing electric and mechanical capture.

This topic last underwent formal evidence review in 2010.[7]

Recommendations for Precordial Thump

COR	LOE	Recommendations
2b	B-NR	1. The precordial thump may be considered at the onset of a rescuer-witnessed, monitored, unstable ventricular tachyarrhythmia when a defibrillator is not immediately ready for use and is performed without delaying CPR or shock delivery.
3: No Benefit	C-LD	2. The precordial thump should not be used routinely for established cardiac arrest.

Recommendation-Specific Supportive Text

1 and 2. The intent of precordial thump is to transmit the mechanical force of the "thump" to the heart as electric energy analogous to a pacing stimulus or very low-energy shock (depending on its force) and is referred to as *electromechanical transduction*.[1] There is no evidence that the use of precordial thump during routine cardiac arrest care in the out-of-hospital or in-hospital settings improves rates of ROSC or survival to hospital discharge.[8–12] It may be beneficial only at the very early onset of VT when the arrhythmia is most vulnerable to lower-energy termination such as in responder-witnessed, monitored events, or in a controlled laboratory environment, but even then it is rarely effective.[13] Although there are case reports of success without evidence of harm from a precordial thump,[9,14,15] if fortuitously administered on the electrically vulnerable portion of an organized rhythm (T wave), the thump (like an unsynchronized shock) risks

acceleration or conversion of the rhythm to VF,[16–19] analogous to commotio cordis.[20] Thus, although the thump may be useful as a single brief intervention under specific circumstances (ie, when a cardiac arrest is witnessed by the responder and monitor-confirmed to be due to VF/VT and a defibrillator is not readily available for use), it should not delay CPR or deployment of a defibrillator.

These recommendations are supported by the 2020 CoSTR for BLS.[21]

Recommendation for Fist/Percussion Pacing

COR	LOE	Recommendation
2b	C-LD	1. Fist (percussion) pacing may be considered as a temporizing measure in exceptional circumstances such as witnessed, monitored in-hospital arrest (eg, cardiac catheterization laboratory) for bradyasystole before a loss of consciousness and if performed without delaying definitive therapy.

Recommendation-Specific Supportive Text

1. Fist, or percussion, pacing is administered with the goal of stimulating an electric impulse sufficient to cause depolarization and contraction of the myocardium, resulting in a pulse. There are a number of case reports and case series that examined the use of fist pacing during asystolic or "life-threatening bradycardic" events[1,22–25] showing favorable outcomes of survival[22] and ROSC.[23] None of these studies, however, were controlled or comparative, and it is not known if the use of fist pacing itself improves rates of ROSC or survival compared with standard therapy. There is no role for fist pacing in patients in cardiac arrest.

This recommendation is supported by the 2020 CoSTR for BLS.[21]

Recommendation for Cough CPR

COR	LOE	Recommendation
2b	C-LD	1. "Cough" CPR may be considered as a temporizing measure for the witnessed, monitored onset of a hemodynamically significant tachyarrhythmia or bradyarrhythmia before a loss of consciousness without delaying definitive therapy.

Recommendation-Specific Supportive Text

1. It is important to underscore that while cough CPR by definition cannot be used for an unconscious patient, it can be harmful in any setting if diverting time, effort, and attention from performing high-quality CPR. Cough CPR is described as a repetitive deep inspiration followed by a cough every few seconds before the loss of consciousness. It is feasible only at the onset of a hemodynamically significant arrhythmia in a cooperative, conscious patient who has ideally been previously instructed on its performance, and as a bridge to definitive care. There are no studies comparing cough CPR to standard resuscitation care. Limited evidence from case reports and case series demonstrates transient increases in aortic and intracardiac pressure with the use of cough CPR at the onset of tachyarrhythmias or bradyarrhythmias in conscious patients.[10,26–28] These studies suffer from considerable selection bias and lack of comparison groups, and do not control for the confounding effect of other treatments, making them hard to interpret.

This recommendation is supported by the 2020 CoSTR for BLS.[21]

REFERENCES

1. Tucker KJ, Shaburihvili TS, Gedevanishvili AT. Manual external (fist) pacing during high-degree atrioventricular block: a lifesaving intervention. *Am J Emerg Med*. 1995;13:53–54. doi: 10.1016/0735-6757(95)90243-0
2. Sherbino J, Verbeek PR, MacDonald RD, Sawadsky BV, McDonald AC, Morrison LJ. Prehospital transcutaneous cardiac pacing for symptomatic bradycardia or bradyasystolic cardiac arrest: a systematic review. *Resuscitation*. 2006;70:193–200. doi: 10.1016/j.resuscitation.2005.11.019
3. White JD, Brown CG. Immediate transthoracic pacing for cardiac asystole in an emergency department setting. *Am J Emerg Med*. 1985;3:125–128. doi: 10.1016/0735-6757(85)90034-8
4. Hedges JR, Syverud SA, Dalsey WC, Feero S, Easter R, Shultz B. Prehospital trial of emergency transcutaneous cardiac pacing. *Circulation*. 1987;76:1337–1343. doi: 10.1161/01.cir.76.6.1337
5. Barthell E, Troiano P, Olson D, Stueven HA, Hendley G. Prehospital external cardiac pacing: a prospective, controlled clinical trial. *Ann Emerg Med*. 1988;17:1221–1226. doi: 10.1016/s0196-0644(88)80074-x
6. Cummins RO, Graves JR, Larsen MP, Hallstrom AP, Hearne TR, Ciliberti J, Nicola RM, Horan S. Out-of-hospital transcutaneous pacing by emergency medical technicians in patients with asystolic cardiac arrest. *N Engl J Med*. 1993;328:1377–1382. doi: 10.1056/NEJM199305133281903
7. Neumar RW, Otto CW, Link MS, Kronick SL, Shuster M, Callaway CW, Kudenchuk PJ, Ornato JP, McNally B, Silvers SM, et al. Part 8: adult advanced cardiovascular life support: 2010 American Heart Association Guidelines for Cardiopulmonary Resuscitation and Emergency Cardiovascular Care. *Circulation*. 2010;122:S729–S767. doi: 10.1161/CIRCULATIONAHA.110.970988
8. Nehme Z, Andrew E, Bernard SA, Smith K. Treatment of monitored out-of-hospital ventricular fibrillation and pulseless ventricular tachycardia utilising the precordial thump. *Resuscitation*. 2013;84:1691–1696. doi: 10.1016/j.resuscitation.2013.08.011
9. Pellis T, Kette F, Lovisa D, Franceschino E, Magagnin L, Mercante WP, Kohl P. Utility of pre-cordial thump for treatment of out of hospital cardiac arrest: a prospective study. *Resuscitation*. 2009;80:17–23. doi: 10.1016/j.resuscitation.2008.10.018
10. Caldwell G, Millar G, Quinn E, Vincent R, Chamberlain DA. Simple mechanical methods for cardioversion: defence of the precordial thump and cough version. *BMJ. (Clin Res Ed)*. 1985;291:627–630. doi: 10.1136/bmj.291.6496.627
11. Gertsch M, Hottinger S, Hess T. Serial chest thumps for the treatment of ventricular tachycardia in patients with coronary artery disease. *Clin Cardiol*. 1992;15:181–188. doi: 10.1002/clc.4960150309
12. Rajagopalan RS, Appu KS, Sultan SK, Jagannadhan TG, Nityanandan K, Sethuraman S. Precordial thump in ventricular tachycardia. *J Assoc Physicians India*. 1971;19:725–729.
13. Haman L, Parizek P, Vojacek J. Precordial thump efficacy in termination of induced ventricular arrhythmias. *Resuscitation*. 2009;80:14–16. doi: 10.1016/j.resuscitation.2008.07.022
14. Befeler B. Mechanical stimulation of the heart: its therapeutic value in tachyarrhythmias. *Chest*. 1978;73:832–838. doi: 10.1378/chest.73.6.832
15. Volkmann H, Klumbies A, Kühnert H, Paliege R, Dannberg G, Siegert K. [Terminating ventricular tachycardias by mechanical heart stimulation with precordial thumps]. *Z Kardiol*. 1990;79:717–724.

16. Morgera T, Baldi N, Chersevani D, Medugno G, Camerini F. Chest thump and ventricular tachycardia. *Pacing Clin Electrophysiol.* 1979;2:69–75. doi: 10.1111/j.1540-8159.1979.tb05178.x
17. Krijne R. Rate acceleration of ventricular tachycardia after a precordial chest thump. *Am J Cardiol.* 1984;53:964–965. doi: 10.1016/0002-9149(84)90539-3
18. Sclarovsky S, Kracoff OH, Agmon J. Acceleration of ventricular tachycardia induced by a chest thump. *Chest.* 1981;80:596–599. doi: 10.1378/chest.80.5.596
19. Yakaitis RW, Redding JS. Precordial thumping during cardiac resuscitation. *Crit Care Med.* 1973;1:22–26. doi: 10.1097/00003246-197301000-00004
20. Link MS, Maron BJ, Wang PJ, VanderBrink BA, Zhu W, Estes NA III. Upper and lower limits of vulnerability to sudden arrhythmic death with chest-wall impact (commotio cordis). *J Am Coll Cardiol.* 2003;41:99–104. doi: 10.1016/s0735-1097(02)02669-4
21. Olasveengen TM, Mancini ME, Perkins GD, Avis S, Brooks S, Castrén M, Chung SP, Considine J, Couper K, Escalante R, et al; on behalf of the Adult Basic Life Support Collaborators. Adult basic life support: 2020 International Consensus on Cardiopulmonary Resuscitation and Emergency Cardiovascular Care Science With Treatment Recommendations. *Circulation.* 2020;142(suppl 1):S41–S91. doi: 10.1161/CIR.0000000000000892
22. Klumbies A, Paliege R, Volkmann H. [Mechanical emergency stimulation in asystole and extreme bradycardia]. *Z Gesamte Inn Med.* 1988;43:348–352.
23. Iseri LT, Allen BJ, Baron K, Brodsky MA. Fist pacing, a forgotten procedure in bradyasystolic cardiac arrest. *Am Heart J.* 1987;113:1545–1550. doi: 10.1016/0002-8703(87)90697-1
24. Paliege R, Volkmann H, Klumbies A. The fist as a pacemaker for the heart—investigations about the mechanical stimulation of the heart in case of emergency. *Deutsche Gesundheitswesen Zeitschrift für Klinische Medizin.* 1982;37:1094–1100.
25. Scherf D, Bornemann C. Thumping of the precordium in ventricular standstill. *Am J Cardiol.* 1960;5:30–40. doi: 10.1016/0002-9149(60)90006-0
26. Petelenz T, Iwiński J, Chlebowczyk J, Czyz Z, Flak Z, Fiutowski L, Zaorski K, Petelenz T, Zeman S. Self–administered cough cardiopulmonary resuscitation (c-CPR) in patients threatened by MAS events of cardiovascular origin. *Wiad Lek.* 1998;51:326–336.
27. Niemann JT, Rosborough J, Hausknecht M, Brown D, Criley JM. Cough-CPR: documentation of systemic perfusion in man and in an experimental model: a "window" to the mechanism of blood flow in external CPR. *Crit Care Med.* 1980;8:141–146. doi: 10.1097/00003246-198003000-00011
28. Marozsán I, Albared JL, Szatmáry LJ. Life-threatening arrhythmias stopped by cough. *Cor Vasa.* 1990;32:401–408.

Vascular Access

Recommendations for Vascular Access in Cardiac Arrest Management

COR	LOE	Recommendations
2a	B-NR	1. It is reasonable for providers to first attempt establishing intravenous access for drug administration in cardiac arrest.
2b	B-NR	2. Intraosseous access may be considered if attempts at intravenous access are unsuccessful or not feasible.
2b	C-LD	3. In appropriately trained providers, central venous access may be considered if attempts to establish intravenous and intraosseous access are unsuccessful or not feasible.
2b	C-LD	4. Endotracheal drug administration may be considered when other access routes are not available.

Synopsis

The traditional approach for giving emergency pharmacotherapy is by the peripheral IV route. However, obtaining IV access under emergent conditions can prove to be challenging based on patient characteristics and operator experience leading to delay in pharmacological treatments.

Alternatives to IV access for acute drug administration include IO, central venous, intracardiac, and endotracheal routes. Intracardiac drug administration was discouraged in the *2000 AHA Guidelines for CPR and Emergency Cardiovascular Care* given its highly specialized skill set, potential morbidity, and other available options for access.[1,2] Endotracheal drug administration results in low blood concentrations and unpredictable pharmacological effect and has also largely fallen into disuse given other access options. Central venous access is primarily used in the hospital setting because it requires appropriate training to acquire and maintain the needed skill set.

IO access has grown in popularity given the relative ease and speed with which it can be achieved, a higher successful placement rate compared with IV cannulation, and the relatively low procedural risk. However, the efficacy of IV versus IO drug administration in cardiac arrest remains to be elucidated.

Recommendation-Specific Supportive Text

1. The peripheral IV route has been the traditional approach to vascular access for emergency drug and fluid administration during resuscitation. The pharmacokinetic properties, acute effects, and clinical efficacy of emergency drugs have primarily been described when given intravenously.[3–6] The IV route has precedence, is usually accessible, and affords a potentially more predictable drug response, making it a reasonable initial approach for vascular access.
2. The paucity of information on the efficacy of IO drug administration during CPR was acknowledged in 2010, but since then the IO route has grown in popularity. IO access is increasingly implemented as a first-line approach for emergent vascular access. A 2020 ILCOR systematic review[7] comparing IV versus IO (principally pretibial placement) drug administration during cardiac arrest found the IV route was associated with better clinical outcomes compared with IO in 5 retrospective studies.[8–12] There were significant concerns for bias, particularly due to the fact that need for IO placement may indicate patient or arrest characteristics that are also risk factors for poor outcome. Subgroup analyses of IV versus IO route from 2 RCTs were also included in this systematic review. In these, no statistically significant effect modification by route of administration was identified. Point estimates favored IV access except for the outcome of ROSC in the PARAMEDIC2 trial, where the effect of epinephrine was similar regardless of route.[13,14] Site specificity may also be an issue with IO administration, because IO access

was nearly always pretibial in these studies. On the basis of these results, the writing group concluded that establishing a peripheral IV remains a reasonable initial approach, but IO access may be considered when an IV is not successful or feasible. Further research is needed to assess the efficacy of drugs delivered intravenously as compared with intraosseously (tibial and humeral).

3. Drug administration by central venous access (by internal jugular or subclavian vein) achieves higher peak concentrations and more rapid circulation times than drugs administered by peripheral IV do,[15–17] but there are currently no data comparing clinical outcomes between these access routes. Central access is associated with higher morbidity, takes time to perform, and may also require interruption of CPR. Current use of this approach is largely in the hospital and may be considered by skilled providers when IV and IO access are not successful or feasible.
4. Endotracheal drug administration is regarded as the least-preferred route of drug administration because it is associated with unpredictable (but generally low) drug concentrations[18–20] and lower rates of ROSC and survival.[21]

Recommendations 1 and 2 are supported by the 2020 CoSTR for ALS.[22] Recommendations 3 and 4 last received formal evidence review in 2010.[20]

REFERENCES

1. The American Heart Association in collaboration with the International Liaison Committee on Resuscitation. Guidelines 2000 for Cardiopulmonary Resuscitation and Emergency Cardiovascular Care. Part 6: advanced cardiovascular life support: section 6: pharmacology II: agents to optimize cardiac output and blood pressure. *Circulation*. 2000;102(suppl):I129–I135.
2. Aitkenhead AR. Drug administration during CPR: what route? *Resuscitation*. 1991;22:191–195. doi: 10.1016/0300-9572(91)90011-m
3. Collinsworth KA, Kalman SM, Harrison DC. The clinical pharmacology of lidocaine as an antiarrhythymic drug. *Circulation*. 1974;50:1217–1230. doi: 10.1161/01.cir.50.6.1217
4. Greenblatt DJ, Bolognini V, Koch-Weser J, Harmatz JS. Pharmacokinetic approach to the clinical use of lidocaine intravenously. *JAMA*. 1976;236:273–277.
5. Riva E, Gerna M, Latini R, Giani P, Volpi A, Maggioni A. Pharmacokinetics of amiodarone in man. *J Cardiovasc Pharmacol*. 1982;4:264–269. doi: 10.1097/00005344-198203000-00015
6. Orlowski JP, Porembka DT, Gallagher JM, Lockrem JD, VanLente F. Comparison study of intraosseous, central intravenous, and peripheral intravenous infusions of emergency drugs. *Am J Dis Child*. 1990;144:112–117. doi: 10.1001/archpedi.1990.02150250124049
7. Granfeldt A, Avis SR, Lind PC, Holmberg MJ, Kleinman M, Maconochie I, Hsu CH, Fernanda de Almeida M, Wang TL, Neumar RW, Andersen LW. Intravenous vs. intraosseous administration of drugs during cardiac arrest: A systematic review. *Resuscitation*. 2020;149:150–157. doi: 10.1016/j.resuscitation.2020.02.025
8. Feinstein BA, Stubbs BA, Rea T, Kudenchuk PJ. Intraosseous compared to intravenous drug resuscitation in out-of-hospital cardiac arrest. *Resuscitation*. 2017;117:91–96. doi: 10.1016/j.resuscitation.2017.06.014
9. Kawano T, Grunau B, Scheuermeyer FX, Gibo K, Fordyce CB, Lin S, Stenstrom R, Schlamp R, Jenneson S, Christenson J. Intraosseous Vascular Access Is Associated With Lower Survival and Neurologic Recovery Among Patients With Out-of-Hospital Cardiac Arrest. *Ann Emerg Med*. 2018;71:588–596. doi: 10.1016/j.annemergmed.2017.11.015
10. Clemency B, Tanaka K, May P, Innes J, Zagroba S, Blaszak J, Hostler D, Cooney D, McGee K, Lindstrom H. Intravenous vs. intraosseous access and return of spontaneous circulation during out of hospital cardiac arrest. *Am J Emerg Med*. 2017;35:222–226. doi: 10.1016/j.ajem.2016.10.052
11. Nguyen L, Suarez S, Daniels J, Sanchez C, Landry K, Redfield C. Effect of Intravenous Versus Intraosseous Access in Prehospital Cardiac Arrest. *Air Med J*. 2019;38:147–149. doi: 10.1016/j.amj.2019.02.005
12. Mody P, Brown SP, Kudenchuk PJ, Chan PS, Khera R, Ayers C, Pandey A, Kern KB, de Lemos JA, Link MS, Idris AH. Intraosseous versus intravenous access in patients with out-of-hospital cardiac arrest: Insights from the resuscitation outcomes consortium continuous chest compression trial. *Resuscitation*. 2019;134:69–75. doi: 10.1016/j.resuscitation.2018.10.031
13. Daya MR, Leroux BG, Dorian P, Rea TD, Newgard CD, Morrison LJ, Lupton JR, Menegazzi JJ, Ornato JP, Sopko G, Christenson J, Idris A, Mody P, Vilke GM, Herdeman C, Barbic D, Kudenchuk PJ; Resuscitation Outcomes Consortium Investigators. Survival After Intravenous Versus Intraosseous Amiodarone, Lidocaine, or Placebo in Out-of-Hospital Shock-Refractory Cardiac Arrest. *Circulation*. 2020;141:188–198. doi: 10.1161/CIRCULATIONAHA.119.042240
14. Nolan JP, Deakin CD, Ji C, Gates S, Rosser A, Lall R, Perkins GD. Intraosseous versus intravenous administration of adrenaline in patients with out-of-hospital cardiac arrest: a secondary analysis of the PARAMEDIC2 placebo-controlled trial [published online January 30, 2020]. *Intensive Care Med*. 2020:Epub ahead of print. doi: 10.1007/s00134-019-05920-7
15. Barsan WG, Levy RC, Weir H. Lidocaine levels during CPR: differences after peripheral venous, central venous, and intracardiac injections. *Ann Emerg Med*. 1981;10:73–78. doi: 10.1016/s0196-0644(81)80339-3
16. Kuhn GJ, White BC, Swetnam RE, Mumey JF, Rydesky MF, Tintinalli JE, Krome RL, Hoehner PJ. Peripheral vs central circulation times during CPR: a pilot study. *Ann Emerg Med*. 1981;10:417–419. doi: 10.1016/s0196-0644(81)80308-3
17. Emerman CL, Pinchak AC, Hancock D, Hagen JF. Effect of injection site on circulation times during cardiac arrest. *Crit Care Med*. 1988;16:1138–1141. doi: 10.1097/00003246-198811000-00011
18. Schüttler J, Bartsch A, Ebeling BJ, Hörnchen U, Kulka P, Sühling B, Stoeckel H. [Endobronchial administration of adrenaline in preclinical cardiopulmonary resuscitation]. *Anasth Intensivther Notfallmed*. 1987;22:63–68.
19. Hörnchen U, Schüttler J, Stoeckel H, Eichelkraut W, Hahn N. Endobronchial instillation of epinephrine during cardiopulmonary resuscitation. *Crit Care Med*. 1987;15:1037–1039. doi: 10.1097/00003246-198711000-00009
20. Neumar RW, Otto CW, Link MS, Kronick SL, Shuster M, Callaway CW, Kudenchuk PJ, Ornato JP, McNally B, Silvers SM, et al. Part 8: adult advanced cardiovascular life support: 2010 American Heart Association Guidelines for Cardiopulmonary Resuscitation and Emergency Cardiovascular Care. *Circulation*. 2010;122:S729–S767. doi: 10.1161/CIRCULATIONAHA.110.970988
21. Niemann JT, Stratton SJ, Cruz B, Lewis RJ. Endotracheal drug administration during out-of-hospital resuscitation: where are the survivors? *Resuscitation*. 2002;53:153–157. doi: 10.1016/s0300-9572(02)00004-7
22. Berg KM, Soar J, Andersen LW, Böttiger BW, Cacciola S, Callaway CW, Couper K, Cronberg T, D'Arrigo S, Deakin CD, et al; on behalf of the Adult Advanced Life Support Collaborators. Adult advanced life support: 2020 International Consensus on Cardiopulmonary Resuscitation and Emergency Cardiovascular Care Science With Treatment Recommendations. *Circulation*. 2020;142(suppl 1):S92–S139. doi: 10.1161/CIR.0000000000000893

Vasopressor Medications During Cardiac Arrest

Recommendations for Vasopressor Management in Cardiac Arrest		
COR	**LOE**	**Recommendations**
1	B-R	1. We recommend that epinephrine be administered for patients in cardiac arrest.
2a	B-R	2. Based on the protocols used in clinical trials, it is reasonable to administer epinephrine 1 mg every 3 to 5 min for cardiac arrest.
2a	C-LD	3. With respect to timing, for cardiac arrest with a nonshockable rhythm, it is reasonable to administer epinephrine as soon as feasible.
2b	C-LD	4. With respect to timing, for cardiac arrest with a shockable rhythm, it may be reasonable to administer epinephrine after initial defibrillation attempts have failed.
2b	C-LD	5. Vasopressin alone or vasopressin in combination with epinephrine may be considered in cardiac arrest but offers no advantage as a substitute for epinephrine in cardiac arrest.
3: No Benefit	B-R	6. High-dose epinephrine is not recommended for routine use in cardiac arrest.

Synopsis

Epinephrine has been hypothesized to have beneficial effects during cardiac arrest primarily because of its α-adrenergic effects, leading to increased coronary and cerebral perfusion pressure during CPR. Conversely, the β-adrenergic effects may increase myocardial oxygen demand, reduce subendocardial perfusion, and may be proarrhythmic. Two randomized, placebo-controlled trials, enrolling over 8500 patients, evaluated the efficacy of epinephrine for OHCA.[1,2] A systematic review and meta-analysis of these and other studies[3] concluded that epinephrine significantly increased ROSC and survival to hospital discharge. Epinephrine did not lead to increased survival with favorable or unfavorable neurological outcome at 3 months, although both of these outcomes occurred slightly more frequently in the epinephrine group.[2] Observational data suggest better outcomes when epinephrine is given sooner, and the low survival with favorable neurological outcome in the available trials may be due in part to the median time of 21 minutes from arrest to receipt of epinephrine. This time delay is a consistent issue in OHCA trials. Time to drug in IHCA is generally much shorter, and the effect of epinephrine on outcomes in the IHCA population may therefore be different. No trials to date have found any benefit of either higher-dose epinephrine or other vasopressors over standard-dose epinephrine during CPR.

Recommendation-Specific Supportive Text

1. The suggestion to administer epinephrine was strengthened to a recommendation based on a systematic review and meta-analysis,[3] which included results of 2 randomized trials of epinephrine for OHCA, 1 of which included over 8000 patients,[1,2] showing that epinephrine increased ROSC and survival. At 3 months, the time point felt to be most meaningful for neurological recovery, there was a nonsignificant increase in survivors with both favorable and unfavorable neurological outcome in the epinephrine group.[2] Any drug that increases the rate of ROSC and survival, but is given after several minutes of downtime, will likely increase both favorable and unfavorable neurological outcome. Determining the likelihood of favorable or unfavorable neurological outcome at the time of arrest is currently not feasible. Therefore, continuing to use a drug that has been shown to increase survival, while focusing our broader efforts on shortening time to drug for all patients so that more survivors will have a favorable neurological outcome, seems the most beneficial approach.
2. The existing trials have used a protocol of 1 mg every 3 to 5 minutes. Operationally, administering epinephrine every second cycle of CPR, after the initial dose, may also be reasonable.
3. Of 16 observational studies on timing in the recent systematic review, all found an association between earlier epinephrine and ROSC for patients with nonshockable rhythms, although improvements in survival were not universally seen.[3]
4. For shockable rhythms, trial protocols have directed that epinephrine be given after the third shock. The literature supports prioritizing defibrillation and CPR initially and giving epinephrine if initial attempts with CPR and defibrillation are not successful.[3]
5. The recent systematic review[3] found no difference in outcomes in trials comparing vasopressin alone or vasopressin combined with epinephrine to epinephrine alone for cardiac arrest, although these studies were underpowered.
6. Multiple RCTs have compared high-dose with standard-dose epinephrine, and although some have shown higher rates of ROSC with high-dose epinephrine, none have shown improvement in survival to discharge or any longer-term outcomes.[4–11]

These recommendations are supported by the "2019 AHA Focused Update on Advanced Cardiovascular Life Support: Use of Advanced Airways, Vasopressors, and Extracorporeal CPR During Cardiac Arrest: An Update to the AHA Guidelines for CPR and Emergency Cardiovascular Care."[12]

REFERENCES

1. Jacobs IG, Finn JC, Jelinek GA, Oxer HF, Thompson PL. Effect of adrenaline on survival in out-of-hospital cardiac arrest: a randomised double-blind placebo-controlled trial. *Resuscitation.* 2011;82:1138–1143. doi: 10.1016/j.resuscitation.2011.06.029
2. Perkins GD, Ji C, Deakin CD, Quinn T, Nolan JP, Scomparin C, Regan S, Long J, Slowther A, Pocock H, Black JJM, Moore F, Fothergill RT, Rees N, O'Shea L, Docherty M, Gunson I, Han K, Charlton K, Finn J, Petrou S, Stallard N, Gates S, Lall R; PARAMEDIC2 Collaborators. A Randomized Trial of Epinephrine in Out-of-Hospital Cardiac Arrest. *N Engl J Med.* 2018;379:711–721. doi: 10.1056/NEJMoa1806842
3. Holmberg MJ, Issa MS, Moskowitz A, Morley P, Welsford M, Neumar RW, Paiva EF, Coker A, Hansen CK, Andersen LW, Donnino MW, Berg KM; International Liaison Committee on Resuscitation Advanced Life Support Task Force Collaborators. Vasopressors during adult cardiac arrest: A systematic review and meta-analysis. *Resuscitation.* 2019;139:106–121. doi: 10.1016/j.resuscitation.2019.04.008
4. Brown CG, Martin DR, Pepe PE, Stueven H, Cummins RO, Gonzalez E, Jastremski M. A comparison of standard-dose and high-dose epinephrine in cardiac arrest outside the hospital. The Multicenter High-Dose Epinephrine Study Group. *N Engl J Med.* 1992;327:1051–1055. doi: 10.1056/NEJM199210083271503
5. Choux C, Gueugniaud PY, Barbieux A, Pham E, Lae C, Dubien PY, Petit P. Standard doses versus repeated high doses of epinephrine in cardiac arrest outside the hospital. *Resuscitation.* 1995;29:3–9. doi: 10.1016/0300-9572(94)00810-3
6. Gueugniaud PY, Mols P, Goldstein P, Pham E, Dubien PY, Deweerdt C, Vergnion M, Petit P, Carli P. A comparison of repeated high doses and repeated standard doses of epinephrine for cardiac arrest outside the hospital. European Epinephrine Study Group. *N Engl J Med.* 1998;339:1595–1601. doi: 10.1056/NEJM199811263392204
7. Lindner KH, Ahnefeld FW, Prengel AW. Comparison of standard and high-dose adrenaline in the resuscitation of asystole and electromechanical dissociation. *Acta Anaesthesiol Scand.* 1991;35:253–256. doi: 10.1111/j.1399-6576.1991.tb03283.x
8. Lipman J, Wilson W, Kobilski S, Scribante J, Lee C, Kraus P, Cooper J, Barr J, Moyes D. High-dose adrenaline in adult in-hospital asystolic cardiopulmonary resuscitation: a double-blind randomised trial. *Anaesth Intensive Care.* 1993;21:192–196. doi: 10.1177/0310057X9302100210
9. Sherman BW, Munger MA, Foulke GE, Rutherford WF, Panacek EA. High-dose versus standard-dose epinephrine treatment of cardiac arrest after failure of standard therapy. *Pharmacotherapy.* 1997;17:242–247.
10. Stiell IG, Hebert PC, Weitzman BN, Wells GA, Raman S, Stark RM, Higginson LA, Ahuja J, Dickinson GE. High-dose epinephrine in adult cardiac arrest. *N Engl J Med.* 1992;327:1045–1050. doi: 10.1056/NEJM199210083271502
11. Callaham M, Madsen CD, Barton CW, Saunders CE, Pointer J. A randomized clinical trial of high-dose epinephrine and norepinephrine vs standard-dose epinephrine in prehospital cardiac arrest. *JAMA.* 1992;268:2667–2672.
12. Panchal AR, Berg KM, Hirsch KG, Kudenchuk PJ, Del Rios M, Cabañas JG, Link MS, Kurz MC, Chan PS, Morley PT, et al. 2019 American Heart Association focused update on advanced cardiovascular life support: use of advanced airways, vasopressors, and extracorporeal cardiopulmonary resuscitation during cardiac arrest: an update to the American Heart Association guidelines for cardiopulmonary resuscitation and emergency cardiovascular care. *Circulation.* 2019;140:e881–e894. doi: 10.1161/CIR.0000000000000732

Nonvasopressor Medications During Cardiac Arrest

Recommendations for Nonvasopressor Medications

COR	LOE	Recommendations
2b	B-R	1. Amiodarone or lidocaine may be considered for VF/pVT that is unresponsive to defibrillation.
2b	C-LD	2. For patients with OHCA, use of steroids during CPR is of uncertain benefit.
3: No Benefit	B-NR	3. Routine administration of calcium for treatment of cardiac arrest is not recommended.
3: No Benefit	B-R	4. Routine use of sodium bicarbonate is not recommended for patients in cardiac arrest.
3: No Benefit	B-R	5. The routine use of magnesium for cardiac arrest is not recommended.

Synopsis

Pharmacological treatment of cardiac arrest is typically deployed when CPR with or without attempted defibrillation fails to achieve ROSC. This may include vasopressor agents such as epinephrine (discussed in Vasopressor Medications During Cardiac Arrest) as well as drugs without direct hemodynamic effects ("nonpressors") such as antiarrhythmic medications, magnesium, sodium bicarbonate, calcium, or steroids (discussed here). Although theoretically attractive and of some proven benefit in animal studies, none of the latter therapies has been definitively proved to improve overall survival after cardiac arrest, although some may have possible benefit in selected populations and/or special circumstances.

Recommendations for the treatment of cardiac arrest due to hyperkalemia, including the use of calcium and sodium bicarbonate, are presented in Electrolyte Abnormalities. Recommendations for management of torsades de pointes are also presented in Torsades de Pointes.

Recommendation-Specific Supportive Text

1. Administration of amiodarone or lidocaine to patients with OHCA was last formally reviewed in 2018[1] and demonstrated improved survival to hospital admission but did not improve overall survival to hospital discharge or survival with good neurological outcome.[1,2] However, amiodarone and lidocaine each significantly improved survival to hospital discharge in a prespecified subgroup of patients with bystander-witnessed arrest, potentially arguing for a

time-dependent benefit and a group for whom these drugs may be more useful. Other antiarrhythmic agents were not specifically addressed in the most recent evidence review and merit further evaluation. These include bretylium tosylate, which was recently reintroduced in the United States for treatment of immediately life-threatening ventricular arrhythmias but without any new information on its effectiveness or safety.[3] Sotalol requires administration as a slow infusion, rendering it impractical to use in cardiac arrest.[4] Similar limitations also apply to procainamide, although it has been given by rapid infusion as a second-line agent in cardiac arrest, with uncertain benefit.[5] The efficacy of antiarrhythmic drugs when given in combination for cardiac arrest has not been systematically addressed and remains a knowledge gap. The role of prophylactic antiarrhythmic medications on ROSC after successful defibrillation is also uncertain. Though not associated with improved survival to hospital discharge, lidocaine decreased the recurrence of VF/pVT when administered prophylactically after successful defibrillation and ROSC.[6] The "2018 AHA Focused Update on Advanced Cardiovascular Life Support Use of Antiarrhythmic Drugs During and Immediately After Cardiac Arrest: An Update to the AHA Guidelines for CPR and Emergency Cardiovascular Care"[1] concluded that lidocaine use could be considered in specific circumstances (such as during EMS transport) when treatment of recurrent VF/pVT might be compromised. There is no evidence addressing the use of other antiarrhythmic drugs for this specific indication.

2. Two randomized trials from the same center reported improved survival and neurological outcome when steroids were bundled in combination with vasopressin and epinephrine during cardiac arrest and also administered after successful resuscitation from cardiac arrest.[7,8] However, nonrandomized studies of strictly intra-arrest corticosteroid administration, in addition to standard resuscitation, show mixed outcomes.[9,10] Due to the only studies suggesting benefit being from a single center with a bundled intervention, and observational data having conflicting results, whether steroids are beneficial during cardiac arrest remains unclear. At least 1 trial attempting to validate the findings of Mentzelopoulos et al is ongoing (NCT03640949).
3. Since last addressed by the 2010 Guidelines, a 2013 systematic review found little evidence to support the routine use of calcium in undifferentiated cardiac arrest, though the evidence is very weak due to lack of clinical trials and the tendency to use calcium as a "last resort" medication in refractory cardiac arrest.[11] Administration of calcium in special circumstances such as hyperkalemia and calcium blocker overdose is addressed in Electrolyte Abnormalities and in Toxicity: β-Adrenergic Blockers and Calcium Channel Blockers.
4. Clinical trials and observational studies since the 2010 Guidelines have yielded no new evidence that routine administration of sodium bicarbonate improves outcomes from undifferentiated cardiac arrest and evidence suggests that it may worsen survival and neurological recovery.[12–14] Use of sodium bicarbonate in special circumstances such as hyperkalemia and drug overdose is addressed in Electrolyte Abnormalities and in Toxicity: Sodium Channel Blockers, Including Tricyclic Antidepressants.
5. Magnesium's role as an antiarrhythmic agent was last addressed by the 2018 focused update on advanced cardiovascular life support (ACLS) guidelines.[1] RCTs have not found it to improve ROSC, survival, or neurological outcome regardless of the presenting cardiac arrest rhythm,[15–18] nor useful for monomorphic VT.[19] There are anecdotal reports and small case series attesting to magnesium's efficacy in the treatment of torsades de pointes (See Torsades de Pointes).

Recommendations 1 and 5 are supported by the 2018 focused update on ACLS guidelines.[1] Recommendation 2 last received formal evidence review in 2015.[20] Recommendations 3 and 4 last received formal evidence review in 2010.[21]

REFERENCES

1. Panchal AR, Berg KM, Kudenchuk PJ, Del Rios M, Hirsch KG, Link MS, Kurz MC, Chan PS, Cabañas JG, Morley PT, Hazinski MF, Donnino MW. 2018 American Heart Association Focused Update on Advanced Cardiovascular Life Support Use of Antiarrhythmic Drugs During and Immediately After Cardiac Arrest: An Update to the American Heart Association Guidelines for Cardiopulmonary Resuscitation and Emergency Cardiovascular Care. *Circulation*. 2018;138:e740–e749. doi: 10.1161/CIR.0000000000000613
2. Kudenchuk PJ, Brown SP, Daya M, Rea T, Nichol G, Morrison LJ, Leroux B, Vaillancourt C, Wittwer L, Callaway CW, Christenson J, Egan D, Ornato JP, Weisfeldt ML, Stiell IG, Idris AH, Aufderheide TP, Dunford JV, Colella MR, Vilke GM, Brienza AM, Desvigne-Nickens P, Gray PC, Gray R, Seals N, Straight R, Dorian P; Resuscitation Outcomes Consortium Investigators. Amiodarone, Lidocaine, or Placebo in Out-of-Hospital Cardiac Arrest. *N Engl J Med*. 2016;374:1711–1722. doi: 10.1056/NEJMoa1514204
3. Chowdhury A, Fernandes B, Melhuish TM, White LD. Antiarrhythmics in Cardiac Arrest: A Systematic Review and Meta-Analysis. *Heart Lung Circ*. 2018;27:280–290. doi: 10.1016/j.hlc.2017.07.004
4. Batul SA, Gopinathannair R. Intravenous Sotalol - Reintroducing a Forgotten Agent to the Electrophysiology Therapeutic Arsenal. *J Atr Fibrillation*. 2017;9:1499. doi: 10.4022/jafib.1499
5. Markel DT, Gold LS, Allen J, Fahrenbruch CE, Rea TD, Eisenberg MS, Kudenchuk PJ. Procainamide and survival in ventricular fibrillation out-of-hospital cardiac arrest. *Acad Emerg Med*. 2010;17:617–623. doi: 10.1111/j.1553-2712.2010.00763.x
6. Kudenchuk PJ, Newell C, White L, Fahrenbruch C, Rea T, Eisenberg M. Prophylactic lidocaine for post resuscitation care of patients

with out-of-hospital ventricular fibrillation cardiac arrest. *Resuscitation.* 2013;84:1512–1518. doi: 10.1016/j.resuscitation.2013.05.022

7. Mentzelopoulos SD, Zakynthinos SG, Tzoufi M, Katsios N, Papastylianou A, Gkisioti S, Stathopoulos A, Kollintza A, Stamataki E, Roussos C. Vasopressin, epinephrine, and corticosteroids for in-hospital cardiac arrest. *Arch Intern Med.* 2009;169:15–24. doi: 10.1001/archinternmed.2008.509
8. Mentzelopoulos SD, Malachias S, Chamos C, Konstantopoulos D, Ntaidou T, Papastylianou A, Kolliantzaki I, Theodoridi M, Ischaki H, Makris D, Zakynthinos E, Zintzaras E, Sourlas S, Aloizos S, Zakynthinos SG. Vasopressin, steroids, and epinephrine and neurologically favorable survival after in-hospital cardiac arrest: a randomized clinical trial. *JAMA.* 2013;310:270–279. doi: 10.1001/jama.2013.7832
9. Tsai MS, Chuang PY, Yu PH, Huang CH, Tang CH, Chang WT, Chen WJ. Glucocorticoid use during cardiopulmonary resuscitation may be beneficial for cardiac arrest. *Int J Cardiol.* 2016;222:629–635. doi: 10.1016/j.ijcard.2016.08.017
10. Tsai MS, Huang CH, Chang WT, Chen WJ, Hsu CY, Hsieh CC, Yang CW, Chiang WC, Ma MH, Chen SC. The effect of hydrocortisone on the outcome of out-of-hospital cardiac arrest patients: a pilot study. *Am J Emerg Med.* 2007;25:318–325. doi: 10.1016/j.ajem.2006.12.007
11. Kette F, Ghuman J, Parr M. Calcium administration during cardiac arrest: a systematic review. *Eur J Emerg Med.* 2013;20:72–78. doi: 10.1097/MEJ.0b013e328358e336
12. Vukmir RB, Katz L; Sodium Bicarbonate Study Group. Sodium bicarbonate improves outcome in prolonged prehospital cardiac arrest. *Am J Emerg Med.* 2006;24:156–161. doi: 10.1016/j.ajem.2005.08.016
13. Ahn S, Kim YJ, Sohn CH, Seo DW, Lim KS, Donnino MW, Kim WY. Sodium bicarbonate on severe metabolic acidosis during prolonged cardiopulmonary resuscitation: a double-blind, randomized, placebo-controlled pilot study. *J Thorac Dis.* 2018;10:2295–2302. doi: 10.21037/jtd.2018.03.124
14. Kawano T, Grunau B, Scheuermeyer FX, Gibo K, Dick W, Fordyce CB, Dorian P, Stenstrom R, Straight R, Christenson J. Prehospital sodium bicarbonate use could worsen long term survival with favorable neurological recovery among patients with out-of-hospital cardiac arrest. *Resuscitation.* 2017;119:63–69. doi: 10.1016/j.resuscitation.2017.08.008
15. Fatovich DM, Prentice DA, Dobb GJ. Magnesium in cardiac arrest (the magic trial). *Resuscitation.* 1997;35:237–241. doi: 10.1016/s0300-9572(97)00062-2
16. Allegra J, Lavery R, Cody R, Birnbaum G, Brennan J, Hartman A, Horowitz M, Nashed A, Yablonski M. Magnesium sulfate in the treatment of refractory ventricular fibrillation in the prehospital setting. *Resuscitation.* 2001;49:245–249. doi: 10.1016/s0300-9572(00)00375-0
17. Hassan TB, Jagger C, Barnett DB. A randomised trial to investigate the efficacy of magnesium sulphate for refractory ventricular fibrillation. *Emerg Med J.* 2002;19:57–62.
18. Thel MC, Armstrong AL, McNulty SE, Califf RM, O'Connor CM. Randomised trial of magnesium in in-hospital cardiac arrest. Duke Internal Medicine Housestaff. *Lancet.* 1997;350:1272–1276. doi: 10.1016/s0140-6736(97)05048-4
19. Manz M, Jung W, Lüderitz B. Effect of magnesium on sustained ventricular tachycardia [in German]. *Herz.* 1997;22(suppl 1):51–55. doi: 10.1007/bf03042655
20. Link MS, Berkow LC, Kudenchuk PJ, Halperin HR, Hess EP, Moitra VK, Neumar RW, O'Neil BJ, Paxton JH, Silvers SM, et al. Part 7: adult advanced cardiovascular life support: 2015 American Heart Association Guidelines Update for Cardiopulmonary Resuscitation and Emergency Cardiovascular Care. *Circulation.* 2015;132(suppl 2):S444–S464. doi: 10.1161/CIR.0000000000000261
21. Neumar RW, Otto CW, Link MS, Kronick SL, Shuster M, Callaway CW, Kudenchuk PJ, Ornato JP, McNally B, Silvers SM, et al. Part 8: adult advanced cardiovascular life support: 2010 American Heart Association Guidelines for Cardiopulmonary Resuscitation and Emergency Cardiovascular Care. *Circulation.* 2010;122:S729–S767. doi: 10.1161/CIRCULATIONAHA.110.970988

Adjuncts to CPR

Recommendations for Adjuncts to CPR

COR	LOE	Recommendations
2b	C-LD	1. If an experienced sonographer is present and use of ultrasound does not interfere with the standard cardiac arrest treatment protocol, then ultrasound may be considered as an adjunct to standard patient evaluation, although its usefulness has not been well established.
2b	C-LD	2. When supplemental oxygen is available, it may be reasonable to use the maximal feasible inspired oxygen concentration during CPR.
2b	C-LD	3. An abrupt increase in end-tidal CO_2 may be used to detect ROSC during compressions or when a rhythm check reveals an organized rhythm.
2b	C-EO	4. Routine measurement of arterial blood gases during CPR has uncertain value.
2b	C-EO	5. Arterial pressure monitoring by arterial line may be used to detect ROSC during chest compressions or when a rhythm check reveals an organized rhythm.

Synopsis

Although the vast majority of cardiac arrest trials have been conducted in OHCA, IHCA comprises almost half of the arrests that occur in the United States annually, and many OHCA resuscitations continue into the emergency department. IHCA patients often have invasive monitoring devices in place such as central venous or arterial lines, and personnel to perform advanced procedures such as arterial blood gas analysis or point-of-care ultrasound are often present. Advanced monitoring such as $ETCO_2$ monitoring is being increasingly used. Determining the utility of such physiological monitoring or diagnostic procedures is important. High-quality CPR, defibrillation when appropriate, vasopressors and/or antiarrhythmics, and airway management remain the cornerstones of cardiac arrest resuscitation, but some emerging data suggest that incorporating patient-specific imaging and physiological data into our approach to resuscitation holds some promise. See Metrics for High-Quality CPR for recommendations on physiological monitoring during CPR. More research in this area is clearly needed.

Recommendation-Specific Supportive Text

1. Point-of-care cardiac ultrasound can identify cardiac tamponade or other potentially reversible causes of cardiac arrest and identify cardiac motion in pulseless electrical activity.[1,2] However,

cardiac ultrasound is also associated with longer interruptions in chest compressions.[3] A single small RCT found no improvement in outcomes with the use of cardiac ultrasound during CPR.[4]

2. No adult human studies directly compare levels of inspired oxygen concentration during CPR. A small number of studies has shown that higher Pao_2 during CPR is associated with ROSC, but this is likely due to differences in patients or resuscitation quality.[5–7]
3. Observational studies have found that increases in $ETCO_2$ of more than 10 mm Hg may indicate ROSC, although no specific cutoff value indicative of ROSC has been identified.[8]
4. Arterial Po_2 and Pco_2 values are dependent on cardiac output and ventilation and therefore will depend on both patient characteristics and CPR quality. One small study found wide discrepancies in blood gases between mixed venous and arterial samples during CPR and concluded that arterial samples are not accurate during resuscitation.[9]
5. If an arterial line is in place, an abrupt increase in diastolic pressure or the presence of an arterial waveform during a rhythm check showing an organized rhythm may indicate ROSC.

Recommendations 1, 3, and 5 last received formal evidence review in 2015.[10] . Recommendation 2 last received formal evidence review in 2015,[10] with an evidence update completed in 2020.[11] Recommendation 4 last received formal evidence review in 2010.[12]

REFERENCES

1. Breitkreutz R, Price S, Steiger HV, Seeger FH, Ilper H, Ackermann H, Rudolph M, Uddin S, Weigand MA, Müller E, Walcher F; Emergency Ultrasound Working Group of the Johann Wolfgang Goethe-University Hospital, Frankfurt am Main. Focused echocardiographic evaluation in life support and peri-resuscitation of emergency patients: a prospective trial. *Resuscitation.* 2010;81:1527–1533. doi: 10.1016/j.resuscitation.2010.07.013
2. Gaspari R, Weekes A, Adhikari S, Noble VE, Nomura JT, Theodoro D, Woo M, Atkinson P, Blehar D, Brown SM, Caffery T, Douglass E, Fraser J, Haines C, Lam S, Lanspa M, Lewis M, Liebmann O, Limkakeng A, Lopez F, Platz E, Mendoza M, Minnigan H, Moore C, Novik J, Rang L, Scruggs W, Raio C. Emergency department point-of-care ultrasound in out-of-hospital and in-ED cardiac arrest. *Resuscitation.* 2016;109:33–39. doi: 10.1016/j.resuscitation.2016.09.018
3. Clattenburg EJ, Wroe P, Brown S, Gardner K, Losonczy L, Singh A, Nagdev A. Point-of-care ultrasound use in patients with cardiac arrest is associated prolonged cardiopulmonary resuscitation pauses: A prospective cohort study. *Resuscitation.* 2018;122:65–68. doi: 10.1016/j.resuscitation.2017.11.056
4. Chardoli M, Heidari F, Rabiee H, Sharif-Alhoseini M, Shokoohi H, Rahimi-Movaghar V. Echocardiography integrated ACLS protocol versus conventional cardiopulmonary resuscitation in patients with pulseless electrical activity cardiac arrest. *Chin J Traumatol.* 2012;15:284–287.
5. Spindelboeck W, Schindler O, Moser A, Hausler F, Wallner S, Strasser C, Haas J, Gemes G, Prause G. Increasing arterial oxygen partial pressure during cardiopulmonary resuscitation is associated with improved rates of hospital admission. *Resuscitation.* 2013;84:770–775. doi: 10.1016/j.resuscitation.2013.01.012
6. Spindelboeck W, Gemes G, Strasser C, Toescher K, Kores B, Metnitz P, Haas J, Prause G. Arterial blood gases during and their dynamic changes after cardiopulmonary resuscitation: A prospective clinical study. *Resuscitation.* 2016;106:24–29. doi: 10.1016/j.resuscitation.2016.06.013
7. Patel JK, Schoenfeld E, Parikh PB, Parnia S. Association of Arterial Oxygen Tension During In-Hospital Cardiac Arrest With Return of Spontaneous Circulation and Survival. *J Intensive Care Med.* 2018;33:407–414. doi: 10.1177/0885066616658420
8. Sandroni C, De Santis P, D'Arrigo S. Capnography during cardiac arrest. *Resuscitation.* 2018;132:73–77. doi: 10.1016/j.resuscitation.2018.08.018
9. Weil MH, Rackow EC, Trevino R, Grundler W, Falk JL, Griffel MI. Difference in acid-base state between venous and arterial blood during cardiopulmonary resuscitation. *N Engl J Med.* 1986;315:153–156. doi: 10.1056/NEJM198607173150303
10. Link MS, Berkow LC, Kudenchuk PJ, Halperin HR, Hess EP, Moitra VK, Neumar RW, O'Neil BJ, Paxton JH, Silvers SM, et al. Part 7: adult advanced cardiovascular life support: 2015 American Heart Association Guidelines Update for Cardiopulmonary Resuscitation and Emergency Cardiovascular Care. *Circulation.* 2015;132(suppl 2):S444–S464. doi: 10.1161/CIR.0000000000000261
11. Berg KM, Soar J, Andersen LW, Böttiger BW, Cacciola S, Callaway CW, Couper K, Cronberg T, D'Arrigo S, Deakin CD, et al; on behalf of the Adult Advanced Life Support Collaborators. Adult advanced life support: 2020 International Consensus on Cardiopulmonary Resuscitation and Emergency Cardiovascular Care Science With Treatment Recommendations. *Circulation.* 2020;142(suppl 1):S92–S139. doi: 10.1161/CIR.0000000000000893
12. Neumar RW, Otto CW, Link MS, Kronick SL, Shuster M, Callaway CW, Kudenchuk PJ, Ornato JP, McNally B, Silvers SM, et al. Part 8: adult advanced cardiovascular life support: 2010 American Heart Association Guidelines for Cardiopulmonary Resuscitation and Emergency Cardiovascular Care. *Circulation.* 2010;122:S729–S767. doi: 10.1161/CIRCULATIONAHA.110.970988

Termination of Resuscitation

Recommendations for Termination of Resuscitation

COR	LOE	Recommendations
1	B-NR	1. If termination of resuscitation (TOR) is being considered, BLS EMS providers should use the BLS termination of resuscitation rule where ALS is not available or may be significantly delayed.
2a	B-NR	2. It is reasonable for prehospital ALS providers to use the adult ALS TOR rule to terminate resuscitation efforts in the field for adult victims of OHCA.
2a	B-NR	3. In a tiered ALS- and BLS-provider system, the use of the BLS TOR rule can avoid confusion at the scene of a cardiac arrest without compromising diagnostic accuracy.
2b	C-LD	4. In intubated patients, failure to achieve an end-tidal CO_2 of greater than 10 mm Hg by waveform capnography after 20 min of ALS resuscitation may be considered as a component of a multimodal approach to decide when to end resuscitative efforts, but it should not be used in isolation.
3: No Benefit	C-LD	5. We suggest against the use of point-of-care ultrasound for prognostication during CPR.
3: Harm	C-EO	6. In nonintubated patients, a specific end-tidal CO_2 cutoff value at any time during CPR should not be used as an indication to end resuscitative efforts.

Synopsis

OHCA is a resource-intensive condition most often associated with low rates of survival. It is important for EMS providers to be able to differentiate patients in whom continued resuscitation is futile from patients with a chance of survival who should receive continued resuscitation and transportation to hospital. This will aid in both resource utilization and optimizing a patient's chance for survival. Using a validated TOR rule will help ensure accuracy in determining futile patients (Figures 5 and 6). *Futility* is often defined as less than 1% chance of survival,[1] suggesting that for a TOR rule to be valid it should demonstrate high accuracy for predicting futility with the lower confidence limit greater than 99% on external validation.

Recommendation-Specific Supportive Text

1. The BLS TOR rule recommends TOR when all of the following criteria apply before moving to the ambulance for transport: (1) arrest was not witnessed by EMS providers or first responder; (2) no ROSC obtained; and (3) no shocks were delivered. In a recent meta-analysis of 7 published studies (33 795 patients), only 0.13% (95% CI, 0.03%–0.58%) of patients who fulfilled the BLS termination criteria survived to hospital discharge.[3]
2. The ALS TOR rule recommends TOR when all of the following criteria apply before moving to the ambulance for transport: (1) arrest was not witnessed; (2) no bystander CPR was provided; (3) no ROSC after full ALS care in the field; and (4) no AED shocks were delivered. In a recent meta-analysis of 2 published studies (10 178 patients), only 0.01% (95% CI, 0.00%–0.07%) of patients who fulfilled the ALS termination criteria survived to hospital discharge.[3]
3. The BLS TOR rule, otherwise known as the *universal TOR rule* (arrest not witnessed by EMS providers; no shock delivered; no ROSC), has been prospectively validated in combined BLS and ALS systems.[4] Although the rule did not have adequate specificity after 6 minutes of resuscitation (false-positive rate: 2.1%) it did achieve better than 99% specificity after approximately 15 minutes of attempted resuscitation, while still reducing transportation by half. A retrospective analysis found that application of the universal TOR at 20 minutes of resuscitation was able to predict futility, identifying over 99% of survivors and patients with good neurological outcome.[5]
4. In intubated patients, an $ETCO_2$ measurement less than 10 mm Hg indicates low to no blood flow. Several small studies provide evidence showing that an $ETCO_2$ less than 10 mm Hg after 20 minutes of ALS resuscitation is strongly but not perfectly predictive of futility.[6–9] These small observational studies suffer from high risk of bias. Alternative $ETCO_2$ thresholds and timepoints have been proposed. The use of $ETCO_2$ alone to predict patient outcome needs to be validated in a large prospective study.
5. A recent systematic review found that no sonographic finding had consistently high sensitivity for clinical outcomes to be used as the sole criterion to terminate cardiac arrest resuscitation.[10] Although some findings demonstrated higher ranges of sensitivity and/or specificity, studies examining the use of point-of-care ultrasound during cardiac arrest demonstrate varying results and are hindered by significant bias. There is considerable heterogeneity between studies in terms of timing and application of point-of-care ultrasound as well as inconsistent definitions and terminology in terms of cardiac motion. Further there is little research examining the interrater reliability of ultrasound findings during cardiac arrest.[11,12] In addition, see Adjuncts to CPR for ultrasound as an adjunct to CPR.

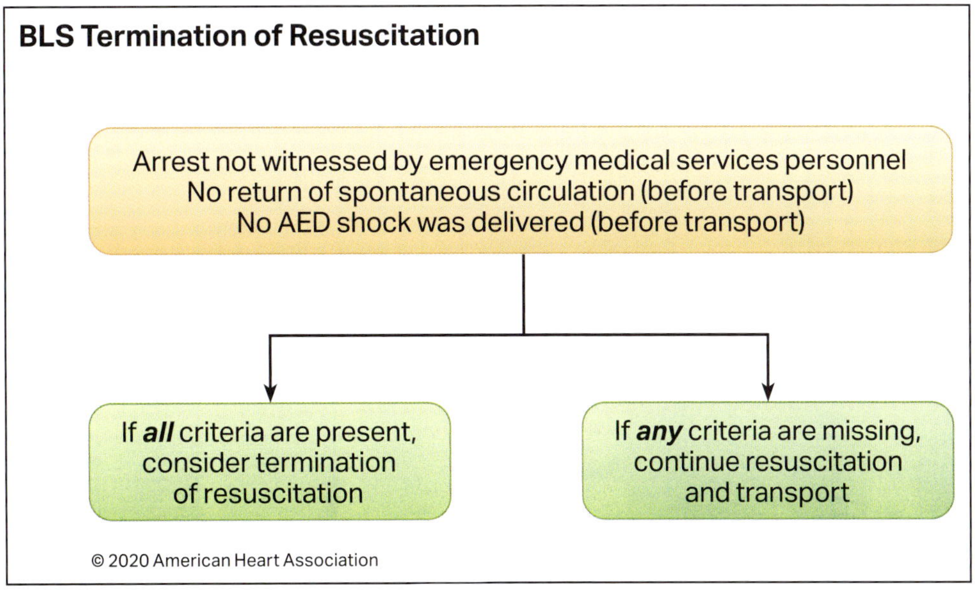

BLS Termination of Resuscitation
Arrest not witnessed by emergency medical services personnel
No return of spontaneous circulation (before transport)
No AED shock was delivered (before transport)
If *all* criteria are present, consider termination of resuscitation
If *any* criteria are missing, continue resuscitation and transport
© 2020 American Heart Association

Figure 5. Adult basic life support termination of resuscitation rule.[2]
AED indicates automated external defibrillator; and BLS, basic life support.

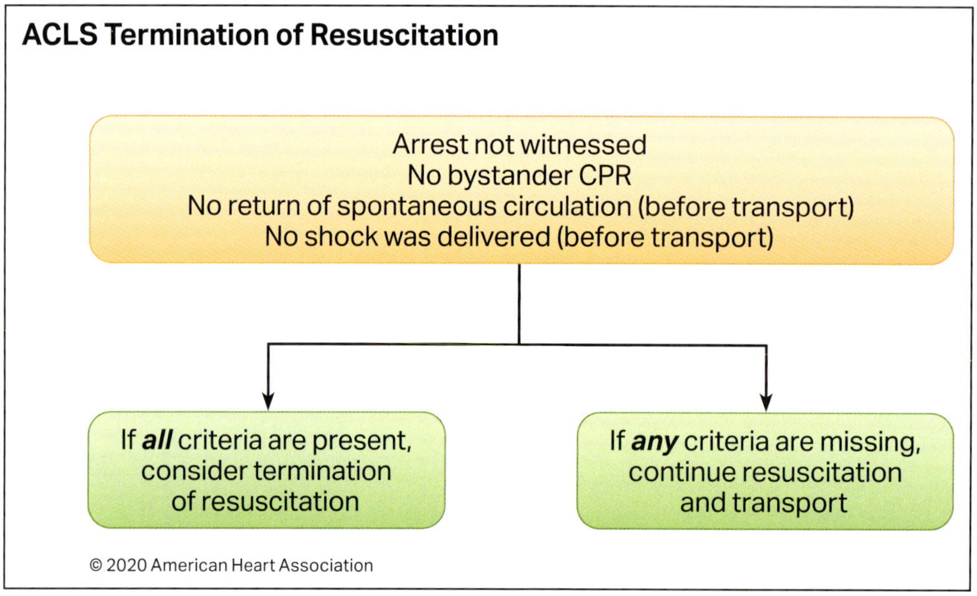
ACLS Termination of Resuscitation
Arrest not witnessed
No bystander CPR
No return of spontaneous circulation (before transport)
No shock was delivered (before transport)
If all criteria are present, consider termination of resuscitation
If any criteria are missing, continue resuscitation and transport
© 2020 American Heart Association

Figure 6. Adult advanced life support termination of resuscitation rule.[2]
ACLS indicates advanced cardiovascular life support; and CPR, cardiopulmonary resuscitation.

6. No studies were found that specifically examined the use of $ETCO_2$ in cardiac arrest patients without an advanced airway. It is not known whether $ETCO_2$ values during bag-mask ventilation are as reliable as those with an advanced airway in place. Because of the lack of evidence, there is nothing to support using any cutoff value of $ETCO_2$ for decisions about TOR in a nonintubated patient.

Recommendations 1, 2, 3, and 5 are supported by the 2020 CoSTRs for BLS and ALS.[13,14] Recommendations 4 and 6 last received formal evidence review in 2015.[15]

REFERENCES

1. Schneiderman LJ. Defining Medical Futility and Improving Medical Care. *J Bioeth Inq.* 2011;8:123–131. doi: 10.1007/s11673-011-9293-3
2. Morrison LJ, Kierzek G, Diekema DS, Sayre MR, Silvers SM, Idris AH, Mancini ME. Part 3: ethics: 2010 American Heart Association Guidelines for Cardiopulmonary Resuscitation and Emergency Cardiovascular Care. *Circulation.* 2010;122(suppl 3):S665–S675. doi: 10.1161/CIRCULATIONAHA.110.970905
3. Ebell MH, Vellinga A, Masterson S, Yun P. Meta-analysis of the accuracy of termination of resuscitation rules for out-of-hospital cardiac arrest. *Emerg Med J.* 2019;36:479–484. doi: 10.1136/emermed-2018-207833
4. Grunau B, Taylor J, Scheuermeyer FX, Stenstrom R, Dick W, Kawano T, Barbic D, Drennan I, Christenson J. External Validation of the Universal Termination of Resuscitation Rule for Out-of-Hospital Cardiac Arrest in British Columbia. *Ann Emerg Med.* 2017;70:374–381.e1. doi: 10.1016/j.annemergmed.2017.01.030
5. Drennan IR, Case E, Verbeek PR, Reynolds JC, Goldberger ZD, Jasti J, Charleston M, Herren H, Idris AH, Leslie PR, Austin MA, Xiong Y, Schmicker RH, Morrison LJ; Resuscitation Outcomes Consortium Investigators. A comparison of the universal TOR Guideline to the absence of prehospital ROSC and duration of resuscitation in predicting futility from out-of-hospital cardiac arrest. *Resuscitation.* 2017;111:96–102. doi: 10.1016/j.resuscitation.2016.11.021
6. Ahrens T, Schallom L, Bettorf K, Ellner S, Hurt G, O'Mara V, Ludwig J, George W, Marino T, Shannon W. End-tidal carbon dioxide measurements as a prognostic indicator of outcome in cardiac arrest. *Am J Crit Care.* 2001;10:391–398.
7. Levine RL, Wayne MA, Miller CC. End-tidal carbon dioxide and outcome of out-of-hospital cardiac arrest. *N Engl J Med.* 1997;337:301–306. doi: 10.1056/NEJM199707313370503
8. Wayne MA, Levine RL, Miller CC. Use of end-tidal carbon dioxide to predict outcome in prehospital cardiac arrest. *Ann Emerg Med.* 1995;25:762–767. doi: 10.1016/s0196-0644(95)70204-0
9. Akinci E, Ramadan H, Yuzbasioglu Y, Coskun F. Comparison of end-tidal carbon dioxide levels with cardiopulmonary resuscitation success presented to emergency department with cardiopulmonary arrest. *Pak J Med Sci.* 2014;30:16–21. doi: 10.12669/pjms.301.4024
10. Reynolds JC, Mahmoud SI, Nicholson T, Drennan IR, Berg K, O'Neil BJ, Welsford M; on behalf of the Advanced Life Support Task Force of the International Liaison Committee on Resuscitation. Prognostication with point-of-care echocardiography during cardiac arrest: a systematic review. *Resuscitation.* 2020:In press.
11. Flato UA, Paiva EF, Carballo MT, Buehler AM, Marco R, Timerman A. Echocardiography for prognostication during the resuscitation of intensive care unit patients with non-shockable rhythm cardiac arrest. *Resuscitation.* 2015;92:1–6. doi: 10.1016/j.resuscitation.2015.03.024
12. Gaspari R, Weekes A, Adhikari S, Noble VE, Nomura JT, Theodoro D, Woo M, Atkinson P, Blehar D, Brown SM, Caffery T, Douglass E, Fraser J, Haines C, Lam S, Lanspa M, Lewis M, Liebmann O, Limkakeng A, Lopez F, Platz E, Mendoza M, Minnigan H, Moore C, Novik J, Rang L, Scruggs W, Raio C. Emergency department point-of-care ultrasound in out-of-hospital and in-ED cardiac arrest. *Resuscitation.* 2016;109:33–39. doi: 10.1016/j.resuscitation.2016.09.018
13. Olasveengen TM, Mancini ME, Perkins GD, Avis S, Brooks S, Castrén M, Chung SP, Considine J, Couper K, Escalante R, et al; on behalf of the Adult Basic Life Support Collaborators. Adult basic life support: 2020 International Consensus on Cardiopulmonary Resuscitation and Emergency Cardiovascular Care Science With Treatment Recommendations. *Circulation.* 2020;142(suppl 1):S41–S91. doi: 10.1161/CIR.0000000000000892
14. Berg KM, Soar J, Andersen LW, Böttiger BW, Cacciola S, Callaway CW, Couper K, Cronberg T, D'Arrigo S, Deakin CD, et al; on behalf of the Adult Advanced Life Support Collaborators. Adult advanced life support: 2020 International Consensus on Cardiopulmonary Resuscitation and Emergency Cardiovascular Care Science With Treatment Recommendations. *Circulation.* 2020;142(suppl 1):S92–S139. doi: 10.1161/CIR.0000000000000893
15. Link MS, Berkow LC, Kudenchuk PJ, Halperin HR, Hess EP, Moitra VK, Neumar RW, O'Neil BJ, Paxton JH, Silvers SM, et al. Part 7: adult advanced cardiovascular life support: 2015 American Heart Association Guidelines Update for Cardiopulmonary Resuscitation and Emergency Cardiovascular Care. *Circulation.* 2015;132(suppl 2):S444–S464. doi: 10.1161/CIR.0000000000000261

ADVANCED TECHNIQUES AND DEVICES FOR RESUSCITATION

Advanced Airway Placement

Introduction

Airway management during cardiac arrest usually commences with a basic strategy such as bag-mask ventilation. In addition, it may be helpful for providers to master an advanced airway strategy as well as a second (backup) strategy for use if they are unable to establish the first-choice airway adjunct. Because placement of an advanced airway may result in interruption of chest compressions, a malpositioned device, or undesirable hyperventilation, providers should carefully weigh these risks against the potential benefits of an advanced airway. The 2019 focused update on ACLS guidelines addressed the use of advanced airways in cardiac arrest and noted that either bag-mask ventilation or an advanced airway strategy may be considered during CPR for adult cardiac arrest in any setting.[1] Outcomes from advanced airway and bag-mask ventilation interventions are highly dependent on the skill set and experience of the provider (Figure 7). Thus, the ultimate decision of the use, type, and timing of an advanced airway will require consideration of a host of patient and provider characteristics that are not easily defined

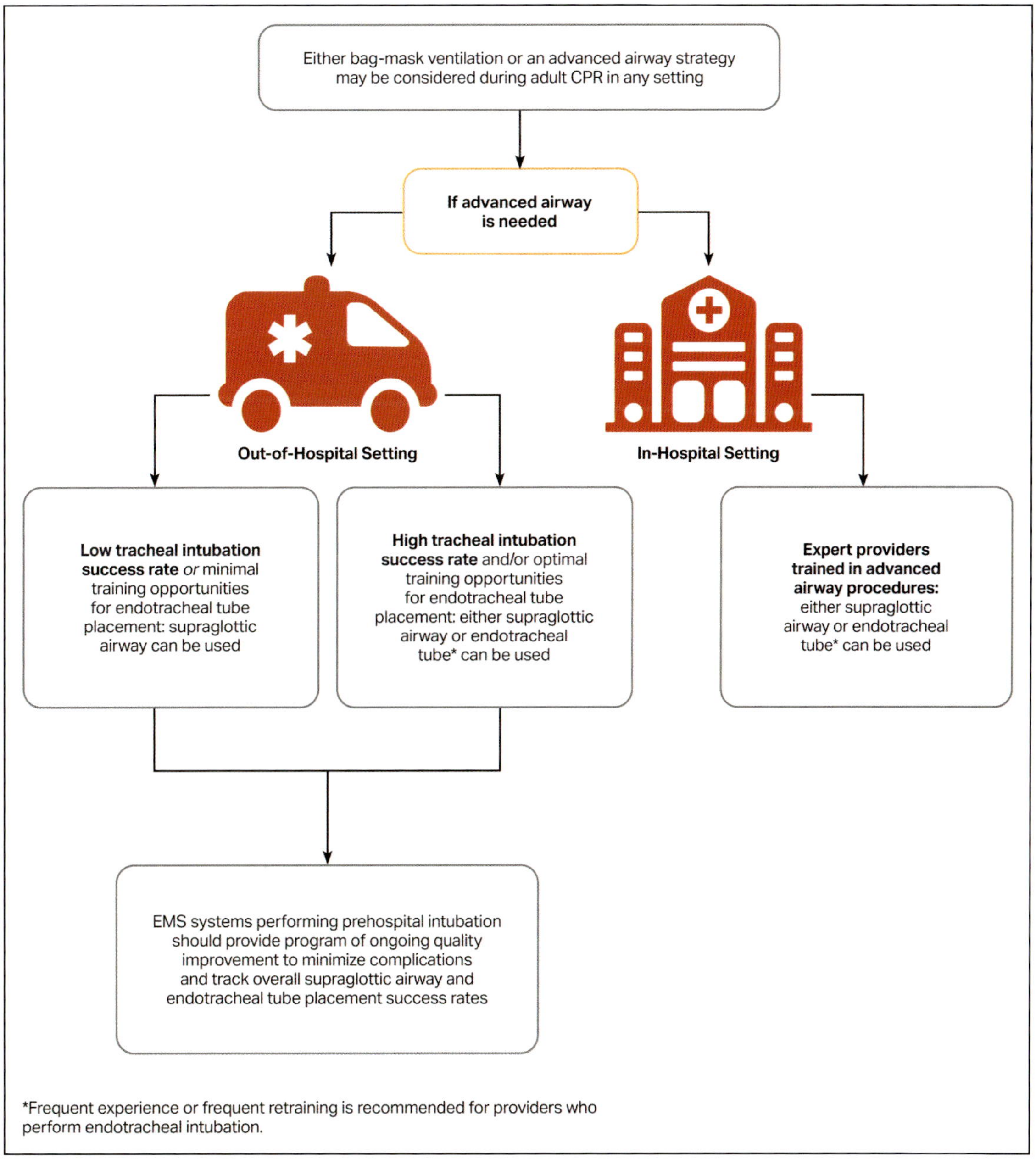

Figure 7. Schematic representation of ALS recommendations for use of advanced airways during CPR.
ALS indicates advanced life support; CPR, cardiopulmonary resuscitation; and EMS, emergency medical services.

in a global recommendation. Important considerations for determining airway management strategies is provider airway management skill and experience, frequent retraining for providers, and ongoing quality improvement to minimize airway management complications.

Recommendation for Advanced Airway Interventions During Cardiac Arrest		
COR	LOE	Recommendation
2b	B-R	1. Either bag-mask ventilation or an advanced airway strategy may be considered during CPR for adult cardiac arrest in any setting depending on the situation and skill set of the provider.

Recommendation-Specific Supportive Text

1. One large RCT in OHCA comparing bag-mask ventilation with endotracheal intubation (ETI) in a physician-based EMS system showed no significant benefit for either technique for 28-day survival or survival with favorable neurological outcome.[2] The success rate of ETI in this study was 98%, suggesting a relatively optimal setting for the potential success of ETI as an intervention. Further research is required to determine equivalence or superiority between the 2 approaches for acute airway management.

These recommendations are supported by the 2019 focused update on ACLS guidelines.[1]

Recommendations for Choice of Advanced Airway Device: Endotracheal Intubation Versus Supraglottic Airway		
COR	LOE	Recommendations
2a	B-R	1. If an advanced airway is used, a supraglottic airway can be used for adults with OHCA in settings with low tracheal intubation success rates or minimal training opportunities for endotracheal tube placement.
2a	B-R	2. If an advanced airway is used, either a supraglottic airway or endotracheal intubation can be used for adults with OHCA in settings with high tracheal intubation success rates or optimal training opportunities for endotracheal tube placement.
2a	B-R	3. If an advanced airway is used in the in-hospital setting by expert providers trained in these procedures, either a supraglottic airway or an endotracheal tube placement can be used.

Recommendation-Specific Supportive Text

1, 2, and 3. One RCT in OHCA comparing SGA (with iGel) to ETI in a non–physician-based EMS system (ETI success, 69%) found no difference in survival or survival with favorable neurological outcome at hospital discharge.[3] A second RCT in OHCA comparing SGA (with laryngeal tube) with ETI in a non–physician-based EMS system (ETI success, 52%) found both better survival to hospital discharge and better survival to hospital discharge with good neurological outcome in the patients managed with SGA.[4] These results are challenging to contextualize because they both allowed for provider deviation from protocol based on clinical judgment. Additionally, precise thresholds for high or low tracheal intubation success rates have not been identified, though guidance can be taken from the existing clinical trials. Thus, it is difficult to understand the potential benefit (or harm), per individual, that drove the decision to place the specific advanced airway device. The decision on placement of an advanced airway requires an understanding of patient and provider characteristics that are not easily defined in a global recommendation. Because of a paucity of studies on advanced airway management for IHCA, the IHCA recommendations are extrapolated from OHCA data. Based on these issues, there is a need for further research specifically on the interface between patient factors and the experience, training, tools, and skills of the provider. Given these reasons, a recommendation for SGA in preference to ETI would be premature.

These recommendations are supported by the 2019 focused update on ACLS guidelines.[1]

Recommendations for Advanced Airway Placement Considerations		
COR	LOE	Recommendations
1	B-NR	1. Frequent experience or frequent retraining is recommended for providers who perform endotracheal intubation.
1	C-LD	2. If advanced airway placement will interrupt chest compressions, providers may consider deferring insertion of the airway until the patient fails to respond to initial CPR and defibrillation attempts or obtains ROSC.
1	C-LD	3. Continuous waveform capnography is recommended in addition to clinical assessment as the most reliable method of confirming and monitoring correct placement of an endotracheal tube.
1	C-EO	4. EMS systems that perform prehospital intubation should provide a program of ongoing quality improvement to minimize complications and track overall supraglottic airway and endotracheal tube placement success rates.

Recommendation-Specific Supportive Text

1. To maintain provider skills from initial training, frequent retraining is important.[5,6] However, future research will need to address the specific type, amount, and duration between training experiences.
2. Although an advanced airway can be placed without interrupting chest compressions,[7] unfortunately, such interruptions still occur. Therefore,

providers should weigh the potential benefits of an advanced airway with the benefits of maintaining a high chest compression fraction.[8–10]

3. In a small clinical trial and several observational studies, waveform capnography was 100% specific for confirming endotracheal tube position during cardiac arrest.[11–13]The sensitivity of waveform capnography decreases after a prolonged cardiac arrest.[11–13] The use of waveform capnography to assess the placement of other advanced airways (eg, Combitube, laryngeal mask airway) has not been studied.
4. The rationale for tracking the overall success rate for systems performing ETI is to make informed decisions as to whether practice should allow for ETI, move toward SGA, or simply use bag-mask ventilation for patients in cardiac arrest; recommendations will vary depending on the overall success rate in a given system.

These recommendations are supported by the 2019 focused update on ACLS guidelines.[1]

REFERENCES

1. Panchal AR, Berg KM, Hirsch KG, Kudenchuk PJ, Del Rios M, Cabañas JG, Link MS, Kurz MC, Chan PS, Morley PT, et al. 2019 American Heart Association focused update on advanced cardiovascular life support: use of advanced airways, vasopressors, and extracorporeal cardiopulmonary resuscitation during cardiac arrest: an update to the American Heart Association guidelines for cardiopulmonary resuscitation and emergency cardiovascular care. *Circulation.* 2019;140:e881–e894. doi: 10.1161/CIR.0000000000000732
2. Jabre P, Penaloza A, Pinero D, Duchateau FX, Borron SW, Javaudin F, Richard O, de Longueville D, Bouilleau G, Devaud ML, Heidet M, Lejeune C, Fauroux S, Greingor JL, Manara A, Hubert JC, Guihard B, Vermylen O, Lievens P, Auffret Y, Maisondieu C, Huet S, Claessens B, Lapostolle F, Javaud N, Reuter PG, Baker E, Vicaut E, Adnet F. Effect of Bag-Mask Ventilation vs Endotracheal Intubation During Cardiopulmonary Resuscitation on Neurological Outcome After Out-of-Hospital Cardiorespiratory Arrest: A Randomized Clinical Trial. *JAMA.* 2018;319:779–787. doi: 10.1001/jama.2018.0156
3. Benger JR, Kirby K, Black S, Brett SJ, Clout M, Lazaroo MJ, Nolan JP, Reeves BC, Robinson M, Scott LJ, Smartt H, South A, Stokes EA, Taylor J, Thomas M, Voss S, Wordsworth S, Rogers CA. Effect of a Strategy of a Supraglottic Airway Device vs Tracheal Intubation During Out-of-Hospital Cardiac Arrest on Functional Outcome: The AIRWAYS-2 Randomized Clinical Trial. *JAMA.* 2018;320:779–791. doi: 10.1001/jama.2018.11597
4. Wang HE, Schmicker RH, Daya MR, Stephens SW, Idris AH, Carlson JN, Colella MR, Herren H, Hansen M, Richmond NJ, Puyana JCJ, Aufderheide TP, Gray RE, Gray PC, Verkest M, Owens PC, Brienza AM, Sternig KJ, May SJ, Sopko GR, Weisfeldt ML, Nichol G. Effect of a Strategy of Initial Laryngeal Tube Insertion vs Endotracheal Intubation on 72-Hour Survival in Adults With Out-of-Hospital Cardiac Arrest: A Randomized Clinical Trial. *JAMA.* 2018;320:769–778. doi: 10.1001/jama.2018.7044
5. Wong ML, Carey S, Mader TJ, Wang HE; American Heart Association National Registry of Cardiopulmonary Resuscitation Investigators. Time to invasive airway placement and resuscitation outcomes after inhospital cardiopulmonary arrest. *Resuscitation.* 2010;81:182–186. doi: 10.1016/j.resuscitation.2009.10.027
6. Warner KJ, Carlbom D, Cooke CR, Bulger EM, Copass MK, Sharar SR. Paramedic training for proficient prehospital endotracheal intubation. *Prehosp Emerg Care.* 2010;14:103–108. doi: 10.3109/10903120903144858
7. Gatward JJ, Thomas MJ, Nolan JP, Cook TM. Effect of chest compressions on the time taken to insert airway devices in a manikin. *Br J Anaesth.* 2008;100:351–356. doi: 10.1093/bja/aem364
8. Talikowska M, Tohira H, Finn J. Cardiopulmonary resuscitation quality and patient survival outcome in cardiac arrest: A systematic review and meta-analysis. *Resuscitation.* 2015;96:66–77. doi: 10.1016/j.resuscitation.2015.07.036
9. Vaillancourt C, Everson-Stewart S, Christenson J, Andrusiek D, Powell J, Nichol G, Cheskes S, Aufderheide TP, Berg R, Stiell IG; Resuscitation Outcomes Consortium Investigators. The impact of increased chest compression fraction on return of spontaneous circulation for out-of-hospital cardiac arrest patients not in ventricular fibrillation. *Resuscitation.* 2011;82:1501–1507. doi: 10.1016/j.resuscitation.2011.07.011
10. Christenson J, Andrusiek D, Everson-Stewart S, Kudenchuk P, Hostler D, Powell J, Callaway CW, Bishop D, Vaillancourt C, Davis D, Aufderheide TP, Idris A, Stouffer JA, Stiell I, Berg R; Resuscitation Outcomes Consortium Investigators. Chest compression fraction determines survival in patients with out-of-hospital ventricular fibrillation. *Circulation.* 2009;120:1241–1247. doi: 10.1161/CIRCULATIONAHA.109.852202
11. Grmec S. Comparison of three different methods to confirm tracheal tube placement in emergency intubation. *Intensive Care Med.* 2002;28:701–704. doi: 10.1007/s00134-002-1290-x
12. Takeda T, Tanigawa K, Tanaka H, Hayashi Y, Goto E, Tanaka K. The assessment of three methods to verify tracheal tube placement in the emergency setting. *Resuscitation.* 2003;56:153–157. doi: 10.1016/s0300-9572(02)00345-3
13. Tanigawa K, Takeda T, Goto E, Tanaka K. Accuracy and reliability of the self-inflating bulb to verify tracheal intubation in out-of-hospital cardiac arrest patients. *Anesthesiology.* 2000;93:1432–1436. doi: 10.1097/00000542-200012000-00015

Alternative CPR Techniques and Devices

Introduction

Many alternatives and adjuncts to conventional CPR have been developed. These include mechanical CPR, impedance threshold devices (ITD), active compression-decompression (ACD) CPR, and interposed abdominal compression CPR. Many of these techniques and devices require specialized equipment and training.

Mechanical CPR devices deliver automated chest compressions, thereby eliminating the need for manual chest compressions. There are 2 different types of mechanical CPR devices: a load-distributing compression band that compresses the entire thorax circumferentially and a pneumatic piston device that compresses the chest in an anteroposterior direction. A recent systematic review of 11 RCTs (overall moderate to low certainty of evidence) found no evidence of improved survival with good neurological outcome with mechanical CPR compared with manual CPR in either OHCA or IHCA.[1] Given the perceived logistic advantages related to limited personnel and safety during patient transport, mechanical CPR remains popular among some providers and systems.

ACD-CPR is performed by using a handheld device with a suction cup applied to the midsternum, actively lifting up the chest during decompressions, thereby enhancing the negative intrathoracic pressure generated by chest recoil and increasing venous return and cardiac output during the next chest compression. The ITD is a pressure-sensitive valve attached to an advanced airway or face mask that limits air entry into the lungs during the decompression phase of CPR, enhancing the negative intrathoracic pressure generated during chest wall recoil and improving venous return and cardiac output during CPR.

There are many alternative CPR techniques being used, and many are unproven. As an example, there is insufficient evidence concerning the cardiac arrest bundle of care with the inclusion of "heads-up" CPR to provide a recommendation concerning its use.[2] Further investigation in this and other alternative CPR techniques is best explored in the context of formal controlled clinical research.

Recommendations for Mechanical CPR Devices

COR	LOE	Recommendations
2b	C-LD	1. The use of mechanical CPR devices may be considered in specific settings where the delivery of high-quality manual compressions may be challenging or dangerous for the provider, as long as rescuers strictly limit interruptions in CPR during deployment and removal of the device.
3: No Benefit	B-R	2. The routine use of mechanical CPR devices is not recommended.

Recommendation-Specific Supportive Text

1 and 2. Studies of mechanical CPR devices have not demonstrated a benefit when compared with manual CPR, with a suggestion of worse neurological outcome in some studies. In the ASPIRE trial (1071 patients), use of the load-distributing band device was associated with similar odds of survival to hospital discharge (adjusted odds ratio [aOR], 0.56; CI, 0.31–1.00; *P*=0.06), and worse survival with good neurological outcome (3.1% versus 7.5%; *P*=0.006), compared with manual CPR.[3] In the CIRC trial (n=4231), use of load-distributing band–CPR resulted in statistically equivalent rates of survival to hospital discharge (aOR, 1.06; CI, 0.83–1.37) and survival with good neurological outcome (aOR, 0.80; CI, 0.47–1.37).[4] In the PARAMEDIC trial (n=4470), use of a mechanical piston device produced similar rates of 30-day survival (aOR, 0.86; CI, 0.64–1.15), and worse survival with good neurological outcome (aOR, 0.72; CI, 0.52–0.99), compared with manual CPR.[5] In the LINC trial (n=2589), survival with good neurological outcome was similar in both groups (8.3% versus 7.8%; risk difference, 0.55%; 95% CI, −1.5% to 2.6%).[6]

Acknowledging these data, the use of mechanical CPR devices by trained personnel may be beneficial in settings where reliable, high-quality manual compressions are not possible or may cause risk to personnel (ie, limited personnel, moving ambulance, angiography suite, prolonged resuscitation, or with concerns for infectious disease exposure).

This topic last received formal evidence review in 2015.[7]

Recommendations for Active Compression-Decompression CPR and Impedance Threshold Devices

COR	LOE	Recommendations
2b	B-NR	1. The effectiveness of active compression-decompression CPR is uncertain. Active compression-decompression CPR might be considered for use when providers are adequately trained and monitored.
2b	C-LD	2. The combination of active compression-decompression CPR and impedance threshold device may be reasonable in settings with available equipment and properly trained personnel.
3: No Benefit	A	3. The routine use of the impedance threshold device as an adjunct during conventional CPR is not recommended.

Recommendation-Specific Supportive Text

1. A 2013 Cochrane review of 10 trials comparing ACD-CPR with standard CPR found no differences in mortality and neurological function in adults with OHCA or IHCA.[8] An important added consideration with this modality is that of increased rescuer fatigue, which could impair the overall quality of CPR.
2. ACD-CPR and ITD may act synergistically to enhance venous return during chest decompression and improve blood flow to vital organs during CPR. The ResQTrial demonstrated that ACD plus ITD was associated with improved survival to hospital discharge with favorable neurological function for OHCA compared with standard CPR, though this study was limited by a lack of blinding, different CPR feedback elements between the study arms (ie, cointervention), lack of CPR quality assessment, and early TOR.[9,10] The *2015 AHA Guidelines Update for CPR and Emergency Cardiovascular Care*[7] evaluated this topic and noted that though a large RCT of low-quality demonstrated benefit of its use, additional trials were needed to confirm the results because of study limitations noted. Thus, ACD-CPR plus ITD was not recommended in previous versions of the AHA Guidelines. However, in settings where the equipment and trained personnel are available, ACD-CPR plus ITD could be an alternative to standard CPR.
3. In the PRIMED study (n=8178), the use of the ITD (compared with a sham device) did not significantly improve survival to hospital discharge or survival with good neurological function in patients with OHCA.[11] Despite the addition of a post hoc analysis of the PRIMED trial for ITD,[12] the routine use of the ITD as an adjunct during conventional CPR is not recommended.

This topic last received formal evidence review in 2015.[7]

Recommendation for Alternative CPR Techniques		
COR	**LOE**	**Recommendation**
2b	B-NR	1. Interposed abdominal compression CPR may be considered during in-hospital resuscitation when sufficient personnel trained in its use are available.

Recommendation-Specific Supportive Text

1. Interposed abdominal compression CPR is a 3-rescuer technique that includes conventional chest compressions combined with alternating abdominal compressions. The dedicated rescuer who provides manual abdominal compressions will compress the abdomen midway between the xiphoid and the umbilicus during the relaxation phase of chest compression. This topic was last reviewed in 2010 and identified 2 randomized trials, interposed abdominal compression CPR performed by trained rescuers improved short-term survival[13] and survival to hospital discharge,[14] compared with conventional CPR for adult IHCA. One RCT of adult OHCA[15] did not show any survival advantage to interposed abdominal compression CPR. More evaluation is needed to further define the routine use of this technique.

This topic last received formal evidence review in 2010.[16]

REFERENCES

1. Wang PL, Brooks SC. Mechanical versus manual chest compressions for cardiac arrest. *Cochrane Database Syst Rev.* 2018;8:CD007260. doi: 10.1002/14651858.CD007260.pub4
2. Pepe PE, Scheppke KA, Antevy PM, Crowe RP, Millstone D, Coyle C, Prusansky C, Garay S, Ellis R, Fowler RL, Moore JC. Confirming the Clinical Safety and Feasibility of a Bundled Methodology to Improve Cardiopulmonary Resuscitation Involving a Head-Up/Torso-Up Chest Compression Technique. *Crit Care Med.* 2019;47:449–455. doi: 10.1097/CCM.0000000000003608
3. Hallstrom A, Rea TD, Sayre MR, Christenson J, Anton AR, Mosesso VN Jr, Van Ottingham L, Olsufka M, Pennington S, White LJ, Yahn S, Husar J, Morris MF, Cobb LA. Manual chest compression vs use of an automated chest compression device during resuscitation following out-of-hospital cardiac arrest: a randomized trial. *JAMA.* 2006;295:2620–2628. doi: 10.1001/jama.295.22.2620
4. Wik L, Olsen JA, Persse D, Sterz F, Lozano M Jr, Brouwer MA, Westfall M, Souders CM, Malzer R, van Grunsven PM, Travis DT, Whitehead A, Herken UR, Lerner EB. Manual vs. integrated automatic load-distributing band CPR with equal survival after out of hospital cardiac arrest. The randomized CIRC trial. *Resuscitation.* 2014;85:741–748. doi: 10.1016/j.resuscitation.2014.03.005
5. Perkins GD, Lall R, Quinn T, Deakin CD, Cooke MW, Horton J, Lamb SE, Slowther AM, Woollard M, Carson A, Smyth M, Whitfield R, Williams A, Pocock H, Black JJ, Wright J, Han K, Gates S; PARAMEDIC trial collaborators. Mechanical versus manual chest compression for out-of-hospital cardiac arrest (PARAMEDIC): a pragmatic, cluster randomised controlled trial. *Lancet.* 2015;385:947–955. doi: 10.1016/S0140-6736(14)61886-9
6. Rubertsson S, Lindgren E, Smekal D, Östlund O, Silfverstolpe J, Lichtveld RA, Boomars R, Ahlstedt B, Skoog G, Kastberg R, et al. Mechanical chest compressions and simultaneous defibrillation vs conventional cardiopulmonary resuscitation in out-of-hospital cardiac arrest: the LINC randomized trial. *JAMA.* 2014;311:53–61. doi: 10.1001/jama.2013.282538
7. Brooks SC, Anderson ML, Bruder E, Daya MR, Gaffney A, Otto CW, Singer AJ, Thiagarajan RR, Travers AH. Part 6: alternative techniques and ancillary devices for cardiopulmonary resuscitation: 2015 American Heart Association Guidelines Update for Cardiopulmonary Resuscitation and Emergency Cardiovascular Care. *Circulation.* 2015;132(suppl 2):S436–S443. doi: 10.1161/CIR.0000000000000260
8. Lafuente-Lafuente C, Melero-Bascones M. Active chest compression-decompression for cardiopulmonary resuscitation. *Cochrane Database Syst Rev.* 2013:CD002751. doi: 10.1002/14651858.CD002751.pub3
9. Aufderheide TP, Frascone RJ, Wayne MA, Mahoney BD, Swor RA, Domeier RM, Olinger ML, Holcomb RG, Tupper DE, Yannopoulos D, Lurie KG. Standard cardiopulmonary resuscitation versus active compression-decompression cardiopulmonary resuscitation with augmentation of negative intrathoracic pressure for out-of-hospital cardiac arrest: a randomised trial. *Lancet.* 2011;377:301–311. doi: 10.1016/S0140-6736(10)62103-4
10. Frascone RJ, Wayne MA, Swor RA, Mahoney BD, Domeier RM, Olinger ML, Tupper DE, Setum CM, Burkhart N, Klann L, Salzman JG, Wewerka SS, Yannopoulos D, Lurie KG, O'Neil BJ, Holcomb RG, Aufderheide TP. Treatment of non-traumatic out-of-hospital cardiac arrest with active compression decompression cardiopulmonary resuscitation plus an impedance threshold device. *Resuscitation.* 2013;84:1214–1222. doi: 10.1016/j.resuscitation.2013.05.002
11. Aufderheide TP, Nichol G, Rea TD, Brown SP, Leroux BG, Pepe PE, Kudenchuk PJ, Christenson J, Daya MR, Dorian P, Callaway CW, Idris AH, Andrusiek D, Stephens SW, Hostler D, Davis DP, Dunford JV, Pirrallo RG, Stiell IG, Clement CM, Craig A, Van Ottingham L, Schmidt TA, Wang HE, Weisfeldt ML, Ornato JP, Sopko G; Resuscitation Outcomes Consortium (ROC) Investigators. A trial of an impedance threshold device in out-of-hospital cardiac arrest. *N Engl J Med.* 2011;365:798–806. doi: 10.1056/NEJMoa1010821
12. Sugiyama A, Duval S, Nakamura Y, Yoshihara K, Yannopoulos D. Impedance Threshold Device Combined With High-Quality Cardiopulmonary Resuscitation Improves Survival With Favorable Neurological Function After Witnessed Out-of-Hospital Cardiac Arrest. *Circ J.* 2016;80:2124–2132. doi: 10.1253/circj.CJ-16-0449
13. Sack JB, Kesselbrenner MB, Jarrad A. Interposed abdominal compression-cardiopulmonary resuscitation and resuscitation outcome during asystole and electromechanical dissociation. *Circulation.* 1992;86:1692–1700. doi: 10.1161/01.cir.86.6.1692
14. Sack JB, Kesselbrenner MB, Bregman D. Survival from in-hospital cardiac arrest with interposed abdominal counterpulsation during cardiopulmonary resuscitation. *JAMA.* 1992;267:379–385.
15. Mateer JR, Stueven HA, Thompson BM, Aprahamian C, Darin JC. Pre-hospital IAC-CPR versus standard CPR: paramedic resuscitation of cardiac arrests. *Am J Emerg Med.* 1985;3:143–146. doi: 10.1016/0735-6757(85)90038-5
16. Cave DM, Gazmuri RJ, Otto CW, Nadkarni VM, Cheng A, Brooks SC, Daya M, Sutton RM, Branson R, Hazinski MF. Part 7: CPR techniques and devices: 2010 American Heart Association Guidelines for Cardiopulmonary Resuscitation and Emergency Cardiovascular Care. *Circulation.* 2010;122:S720–728. doi: 10.1161/CIRCULATIONAHA.110.970970

Extracorporeal CPR

Recommendation for Extracorporeal CPR		
COR	**LOE**	**Recommendation**
2b	C-LD	1. There is insufficient evidence to recommend the routine use of extracorporeal CPR (ECPR) for patients with cardiac arrest. ECPR may be considered for select cardiac arrest patients for whom the suspected cause of the cardiac arrest is potentially reversible during a limited period of mechanical cardiorespiratory support.

Synopsis

ECPR refers to the initiation of cardiopulmonary bypass during the resuscitation of a patient in cardiac arrest. This involves the cannulation of a large vein and artery and initiation of venoarterial extracorporeal circulation and membrane oxygenation (ECMO) (Figure 8). The goal of ECPR is to support end organ perfusion while potentially reversible

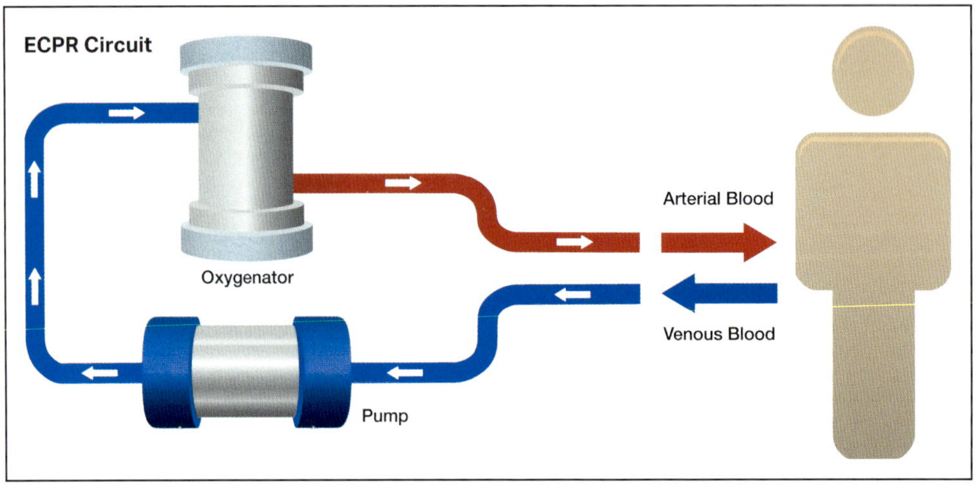

Figure 8. Schematic depiction of components of extracorporeal membrane oxygenator circuit as used for ECPR.
Components include venous cannula, a pump, an oxygenator, and an arterial cannula. ECPR indicates extracorporeal cardiopulmonary resuscitation.

conditions are addressed. ECPR is a complex intervention that requires a highly trained team, specialized equipment, and multidisciplinary support within a healthcare system. The 2019 focused update on ACLS guidelines[1] addressed the use of ECPR for cardiac arrest and noted that there is insufficient evidence to recommend the routine use of ECPR in cardiac arrest. However, ECPR may be considered if there is a potentially reversible cause of an arrest that would benefit from temporary cardiorespiratory support. One important consideration is the selection of patients for ECPR and further research is needed to define patients who would most benefit from the intervention. Furthermore, the resource intensity required to begin and maintain an ECPR program should be considered in the context of strengthening other links in the Chain of Survival. Additional investigations are necessary to evaluate cost-effectiveness, resource allocation, and ethics surrounding the routine use of ECPR in resuscitation.

Recommendation-Specific Supportive Text

1. There are no RCTs on the use of ECPR for OHCA or IHCA. Fifteen observational studies were identified for OHCA that varied in inclusion criteria, ECPR settings, and study design, with the majority of studies reporting improved neurological outcome associated with ECPR.[2] For ECPR use in the in-hospital setting, all studies were assessed as having very serious risk of bias (primarily due to confounding) and the overall certainty of evidence was rated as very low for all outcomes.[2] In 3 studies, ECPR was not associated with beneficial effects for short- or long-term neurological outcomes,[3–5] while 1 study[6] did report associated short- and long-term neurological outcome benefit. Despite many studies reporting favorable outcomes with the use of ECPR, the vast majority of the studies are from single centers with varying inclusion criteria and settings, with decisions to perform ECPR made on a case-by-case basis. While there is currently no evidence to clearly define what should constitute "selected patients," most of the studies analyzed included younger patients with fewer comorbidities. More data are clearly needed from studies of higher methodologic quality, including randomized trials.

These recommendations are supported by the 2019 focused update on ACLS guidelines.[1]

REFERENCES

1. Panchal AR, Berg KM, Hirsch KG, Kudenchuk PJ, Del Rios M, Cabañas JG, Link MS, Kurz MC, Chan PS, Morley PT, et al. 2019 American Heart Association focused update on advanced cardiovascular life support: use of advanced airways, vasopressors, and extracorporeal cardiopulmonary resuscitation during cardiac arrest: an update to the American Heart Association guidelines for cardiopulmonary resuscitation and emergency cardiovascular care. *Circulation*. 2019;140:e881–e894. doi: 10.1161/CIR.0000000000000732
2. Holmberg MJ, Geri G, Wiberg S, Guerguerian AM, Donnino MW, Nolan JP, Deakin CD, Andersen LW; International Liaison Committee on Resuscitation's (ILCOR) Advanced Life Support and Pediatric Task Forces. Extracorporeal cardiopulmonary resuscitation for cardiac arrest: A systematic review. *Resuscitation*. 2018;131:91–100. doi: 10.1016/j.resuscitation.2018.07.029
3. Blumenstein J, Leick J, Liebetrau C, Kempfert J, Gaede L, Groß S, Krug M, Berkowitsch A, Nef H, Rolf A, Arlt M, Walther T, Hamm CW, Möllmann H. Extracorporeal life support in cardiovascular patients with observed refractory in-hospital cardiac arrest is associated with favourable short and long-term outcomes: A propensity-matched analysis. *Eur Heart J Acute Cardiovasc Care*. 2016;5:13–22. doi: 10.1177/2048872615612454
4. Chen YS, Lin JW, Yu HY, Ko WJ, Jerng JS, Chang WT, Chen WJ, Huang SC, Chi NH, Wang CH, Chen LC, Tsai PR, Wang SS, Hwang JJ, Lin FY. Cardiopulmonary resuscitation with assisted extracorporeal life-support versus conventional cardiopulmonary resuscitation in adults with in-hospital cardiac arrest: an observational study and propensity analysis. *Lancet*. 2008;372:554–561. doi: 10.1016/S0140-6736(08)60958-7
5. Lin JW, Wang MJ, Yu HY, Wang CH, Chang WT, Jerng JS, Huang SC, Chou NK, Chi NH, Ko WJ, Wang YC, Wang SS, Hwang JJ, Lin FY, Chen YS. Comparing the survival between extracorporeal rescue and conventional resuscitation in adult in-hospital cardiac arrests: propensity analysis of three-year data. *Resuscitation*. 2010;81:796–803. doi: 10.1016/j.resuscitation.2010.03.002
6. Shin TG, Choi JH, Jo IJ, Sim MS, Song HG, Jeong YK, Song YB, Hahn JY, Choi SH, Gwon HC, Jeon ES, Sung K, Kim WS, Lee YT. Extracorporeal cardiopulmonary resuscitation in patients with inhospital cardiac arrest: A comparison with conventional cardiopulmonary resuscitation. *Crit Care Med*. 2011;39:1–7. doi: 10.1097/CCM.0b013e3181feb339

SPECIFIC ARRHYTHMIA MANAGEMENT

Wide-Complex Tachycardia

Recommendations for Pharmacological Management of Hemodynamically Stable Wide-Complex Tachycardia

COR	LOE	Recommendations
2b	B-NR	1. In hemodynamically stable patients, IV adenosine may be considered for treatment and aiding rhythm diagnosis when the cause of the regular, monomorphic rhythm cannot be determined.
2b	B-R	2. Administration of IV amiodarone, procainamide, or sotalol may be considered for the treatment of wide-complex tachycardia.
3: Harm	B-NR	3. Verapamil should not be administered for any wide-complex tachycardia unless known to be of supraventricular origin and not being conducted by an accessory pathway.
3: Harm	C-LD	4. Adenosine should not be administered for hemodynamically unstable, irregularly irregular, or polymorphic wide-complex tachycardias.

Synopsis

A *wide-complex tachycardia* is defined as a rapid rhythm (generally 150 beats/min or more when attributable to an arrhythmia) with a QRS duration of 0.12 seconds or more. It can represent any aberrantly conducted supraventricular tachycardia (SVT), including paroxysmal SVT caused by atrioventricular (AV) reentry, aberrantly conducted atrial fibrillation, atrial flutter, or ectopic atrial tachycardia. A wide-complex tachycardia can also be caused by any of these supraventricular arrhythmias when conducted by an accessory pathway (called *pre-excited arrhythmias*). Conversely, a wide-complex tachycardia can also be due to VT or a rapid ventricular paced rhythm in patients with a pacemaker.

Initial management of wide-complex tachycardia requires a rapid assessment of the patient's hemodynamic stability. Unstable patients require immediate electric cardioversion. If hemodynamically stable, a presumptive rhythm diagnosis should be attempted by obtaining a 12-lead ECG to evaluate the tachycardia's features. This includes identifying P waves and their relationship to QRS complexes and (in the case of patients with a pacemaker) pacing spikes preceding QRS complexes.

A wide-complex tachycardia can be regular or irregularly irregular and have uniform (monomorphic) or differing (polymorphic) QRS complexes from beat to beat. Each of these features can also be useful in making a presumptive rhythm diagnosis. An irregularly irregular wide-complex tachycardia with monomorphic QRS complexes suggests atrial fibrillation with aberrancy, whereas pre-excited atrial fibrillation or polymorphic VT are likely when QRS complexes change in their configuration from beat to beat. Conversely, a regular wide-complex tachycardia could represent monomorphic VT or an aberrantly conducted reentrant paroxysmal SVT, ectopic atrial tachycardia, or atrial flutter. Distinguishing between these rhythm etiologies is the key to proper drug selection for treatment. While hemodynamically stable rhythms afford an opportunity for evaluation and pharmacological treatment, the need for prompt electric cardioversion should be anticipated in the event the arrhythmia proves unresponsive to these measures or rapid decompensation occurs. A more detailed approach to rhythm management is found elsewhere.[1–3]

Recommendation-Specific Supportive Text

1. Before embarking on empirical drug therapy, obtaining a 12-lead ECG and/or seeking expert consultation for diagnosis is encouraged, if available. If a regular wide-complex tachycardia is suspected to be paroxysmal SVT, vagal maneuvers can be considered before initiating pharmacological therapies (see Regular Narrow-Complex Tachycardia). Adenosine is an ultra–short-acting drug that is effective in terminating regular tachycardias when caused by AV reentry. Adenosine will not typically terminate atrial arrhythmias (such as atrial flutter or atrial tachycardia) but will transiently slow the ventricular rate by blocking conduction of P waves through the AV node, afford their recognition, and help establish the rhythm diagnosis. While ineffective in terminating ventricular arrhythmias, adenosine's relatively short-lived effect on blood pressure makes it less likely to destabilize monomorphic VT in an otherwise hemodynamically stable patient. These features make adenosine relatively safe for treating a hemodynamically stable, regular, monomorphic wide-complex tachycardia of unknown type[4] and as an aid in rhythm diagnosis, although its use is not completely without risk.[5,6]
2. IV antiarrhythmic medications may be considered in stable patients with wide-complex tachycardia, particularly if suspected to be VT or having failed adenosine. Because of their longer duration of action, antiarrhythmic agents may also be useful to prevent recurrences of wide-complex tachycardia. Lidocaine is not included as a treatment option for undifferentiated wide-complex tachycardia because it is a relatively "narrow-spectrum" drug that is ineffective for SVT, probably because its kinetic properties are less effective for VT at hemodynamically tolerated rates than amiodarone, procainamide, or sotalol are.[7–10] In contrast, amiodarone, procainamide, and sotalol are "broader-spectrum" antiarrhythmics than lidocaine and can treat both SVT and VT, but they can

cause hypotension. Since the 2010 Guidelines, a new branded bioequivalent formulation of amiodarone has become available for IV infusion with less hypotensive effects than the older generic formulation.[11] There are few direct comparisons of efficacy between amiodarone, procainamide, and sotalol themselves,[12] which the writing group felt were insufficient to favor one of these drugs over another, apart from cautioning about their use in patients with long QT, amiodarone in suspected pre-excited arrhythmias, or giving these drugs in combination without prior expert consultation. Any of these drugs can also worsen wide-complex tachycardia, converting it to an arrhythmia that is more rapid, less hemodynamically stable, or more malignant, such that availability of a defibrillator is encouraged when these drugs are administered.[13]

3. Verapamil is a calcium channel blocking agent that slows AV node conduction, shortens the refractory period of accessory pathways, and acts as a negative inotrope and vasodilator. Its effects are mediated by a different mechanism and are longer lasting than adenosine. Though effective for treating a wide-complex tachycardia known to be of supraventricular origin and not involving accessory pathway conduction, verapamil's negative inotropic and hypotensive effects can destabilize VT[14] and accelerate pre-excited atrial fibrillation and flutter.[15] Similar concerns may also apply to other drugs commonly used to treat SVTs, such as diltiazem and β-adrenergic blockers, which are not addressed in this recommendation and require evidence review.
4. The combination of adenosine's short-lived slowing of AV node conduction, shortening of refractoriness in the myocardium and accessory pathways, and hypotensive effects make it unsuitable in hemodynamically unstable patients and for treating irregularly irregular and polymorphic wide-complex tachycardias. Adenosine only transiently slows irregularly irregular rhythms, such as atrial fibrillation, rendering it unsuitable for their management. The drug's hypotensive and tissue refractoriness–shortening effects can accelerate ventricular rates in polymorphic VT and, when atrial fibrillation or flutter are conducted by an accessory pathway, risk degeneration to VF.[16] Thus, the drug is not recommended in hemodynamically unstable patients or for treating irregularly irregular or polymorphic wide-complex tachycardias.

This topic last received formal evidence review in 2010.[17]

Recommendation for Electric Management of Hemodynamically Stable Wide-Complex Tachycardia

COR	LOE	Recommendation
2a	C-LD	1. If pharmacological therapy is unsuccessful for the treatment of a hemodynamically stable wide-complex tachycardia, cardioversion or seeking urgent expert consultation is reasonable.

Recommendation-Specific Supportive Text

1. When available, expert consultation can be helpful to assist in the diagnosis and management of treatment-refractory wide-complex tachycardia. Electric cardioversion can be useful either as first-line treatment or for drug-refractory wide-complex tachycardia due to reentry rhythms (such as atrial fibrillation, atrial flutter, AV reentry, and VT). However, electric cardioversion may not be effective for automatic tachycardias (such as ectopic atrial tachycardias), entails risks associated with sedation, and does not prevent recurrences of the wide-complex tachycardia. Notably, when the QRS complex is of uniform morphology, shock synchronized to the QRS is encouraged because this minimizes the risk of provoking VF by a mistimed shock during the vulnerable period of the cardiac cycle (T wave).[18] In contrast, polymorphic wide-complex tachycardias cannot be synchronized reliably because of the differing characteristics of each QRS complex, and require high-energy defibrillation.[19]

This topic last received formal evidence review in 2010.[17]

REFERENCES

1. Al-Khatib SM, Stevenson WG, Ackerman MJ, Bryant WJ, Callans DJ, Curtis AB, Deal BJ, Dickfeld T, Field ME, Fonarow GC, et al. 2017 AHA/ACC/HRS guideline for management of patients with ventricular arrhythmias and the prevention of sudden cardiac death: A report of the American College of Cardiology/American Heart Association Task Force on Clinical Practice Guidelines and the Heart Rhythm Society. *Circulation.* 2018;138:e272–e391. doi: 10.1161/CIR.0000000000000549
2. Page RL, Joglar JA, Caldwell MA, Calkins H, Conti JB, Deal BJ, Estes NA III, Field ME, Goldberger ZD, Hammill SC, Indik JH, Lindsay BD, Olshansky B, Russo AM, Shen WK, Tracy CM, Al-Khatib SM; Evidence Review Committee Chair‡. 2015 ACC/AHA/HRS Guideline for the Management of Adult Patients With Supraventricular Tachycardia: A Report of the American College of Cardiology/American Heart Association Task Force on Clinical Practice Guidelines and the Heart Rhythm Society. *Circulation.* 2016;133:e506–e574. doi: 10.1161/CIR.0000000000000311
3. January CT, Wann LS, Calkins H, Chen LY, Cigarroa JE, Cleveland JC Jr, Ellinor PT, Ezekowitz MD, Field ME, Furie KL, Heidenreich PA, Murray KT, Shea JB, Tracy CM, Yancy CW. 2019 AHA/ACC/HRS Focused Update of the 2014 AHA/ACC/HRS Guideline for the Management of Patients With Atrial Fibrillation: A Report of the American College of Cardiology/American Heart Association Task Force on Clinical Practice Guidelines and the Heart Rhythm Society in Collaboration With the Society of Thoracic Surgeons. *Circulation.* 2019;140:e125–e151. doi: 10.1161/CIR.0000000000000665
4. Marill KA, Wolfram S, Desouza IS, Nishijima DK, Kay D, Setnik GS, Stair TO, Ellinor PT. Adenosine for wide-complex tachycardia: efficacy and safety. *Crit Care Med.* 2009;37:2512–2518. doi: 10.1097/CCM.0b013e3181a93661

5. Shah CP, Gupta AK, Thakur RK, Hayes OW, Mehrotra A, Lokhandwala YY. Adenosine-induced ventricular fibrillation. *Indian Heart J.* 2001;53:208–210.
6. Parham WA, Mehdirad AA, Biermann KM, Fredman CS. Case report: adenosine induced ventricular fibrillation in a patient with stable ventricular tachycardia. *J Interv Card Electrophysiol.* 2001;5:71–74. doi: 10.1023/a:1009810025584
7. Josephson ME. Lidocaine and sustained monomorphic ventricular tachycardia: fact or fiction. *Am J Cardiol.* 1996;78:82–83. doi: 10.1016/s0002-9149(96)00271-8
8. Somberg JC, Bailin SJ, Haffajee CI, Paladino WP, Kerin NZ, Bridges D, Timar S, Molnar J; Amio-Aqueous Investigators. Intravenous lidocaine versus intravenous amiodarone (in a new aqueous formulation) for incessant ventricular tachycardia. *Am J Cardiol.* 2002;90:853–859. doi: 10.1016/s0002-9149(02)02707-8
9. Gorgels AP, van den Dool A, Hofs A, Mulleneers R, Smeets JL, Vos MA, Wellens HJ. Comparison of procainamide and lidocaine in terminating sustained monomorphic ventricular tachycardia. *Am J Cardiol.* 1996;78:43–46. doi: 10.1016/s0002-9149(96)00224-x
10. Ho DS, Zecchin RP, Richards DA, Uther JB, Ross DL. Double-blind trial of lignocaine versus sotalol for acute termination of spontaneous sustained ventricular tachycardia. *Lancet.* 1994;344:18–23. doi: 10.1016/s0140-6736(94)91048-0
11. Cushing DJ, Cooper WD, Gralinski MR, Lipicky RJ. The hypotensive effect of intravenous amiodarone is sustained throughout the maintenance infusion period. *Clin Exp Pharmacol Physiol.* 2010;37:358–361. doi: 10.1111/j.1440-1681.2009.05303.x
12. Ortiz M, Martín A, Arribas F, Coll-Vinent B, Del Arco C, Peinado R, Almendral J; PROCAMIO Study Investigators. Randomized comparison of intravenous procainamide vs. intravenous amiodarone for the acute treatment of tolerated wide QRS tachycardia: the PROCAMIO study. *Eur Heart J.* 2017;38:1329–1335. doi: 10.1093/eurheartj/ehw230
13. Friedman PL, Stevenson WG. Proarrhythmia. *Am J Cardiol.* 1998;82:50N–58N. doi: 10.1016/s0002-9149(98)00586-4
14. Buxton AE, Marchlinski FE, Doherty JU, Flores B, Josephson ME. Hazards of intravenous verapamil for sustained ventricular tachycardia. *Am J Cardiol.* 1987;59:1107–1110. doi: 10.1016/0002-9149(87)90857-5
15. Gulamhusein S, Ko P, Carruthers SG, Klein GJ. Acceleration of the ventricular response during atrial fibrillation in the Wolff-Parkinson-White syndrome after verapamil. *Circulation.* 1982;65:348–354. doi: 10.1161/01.cir.65.2.348
16. Gupta AK, Shah CP, Maheshwari A, Thakur RK, Hayes OW, Lokhandwala YY. Adenosine induced ventricular fibrillation in Wolff-Parkinson-White syndrome. *Pacing Clin Electrophysiol.* 2002;25(4 Pt 1):477–480. doi: 10.1046/j.1460-9592.2002.00477.x
17. Neumar RW, Otto CW, Link MS, Kronick SL, Shuster M, Callaway CW, Kudenchuk PJ, Ornato JP, McNally B, Silvers SM, et al. Part 8: adult advanced cardiovascular life support: 2010 American Heart Association Guidelines for Cardiopulmonary Resuscitation and Emergency Cardiovascular Care. *Circulation.* 2010;122:S729–S767. doi: 10.1161/CIRCULATIONAHA.110.970988
18. Trohman RG, Parrillo JE. Direct current cardioversion: indications, techniques, and recent advances. *Crit Care Med.* 2000;28(suppl):N170–N173. doi: 10.1097/00003246-200010001-00010
19. Dell'Orfano JT, Naccarelli GV. Update on external cardioversion and defibrillation. *Curr Opin Cardiol.* 2001;16:54–57. doi: 10.1097/00001573-200101000-00008

Torsades de Pointes

Synopsis

Polymorphic VT refers to a wide-complex tachycardia of ventricular origin with differing configurations of the QRS complex from beat to beat. However, the most critical feature in the diagnosis and treatment of polymorphic VT is not the morphology of rhythm but rather what is known (or suspected) about the patient's underlying QT interval. Torsades de pointes is a form of polymorphic VT that is associated with a prolonged heart rate–corrected QT interval when the rhythm is normal and VT is not present. The risk for developing *torsades* increases when the corrected QT interval is greater than 500 milliseconds and accompanied by bradycardia.[1] Torsades can be due to an inherited genetic abnormality[2] and can also be caused by drugs and electrolyte imbalances that cause lengthening of the QT interval.[3]

Conversely, polymorphic VT not associated with a long QT is most often due to acute myocardial ischemia.[4,5] Other potential causes include catecholaminergic polymorphic VT, a genetic abnormality in which polymorphic VT is provoked by exercise or emotion in the absence of QT prolongation[6]; "short QT" syndrome, a form of polymorphic VT associated with an unusually short QT interval (corrected QT interval less than 330–370 milliseconds)[7,8]; and bidirectional VT seen in digitalis toxicity in which the axis of alternate QRS complexes shifts by 180 degrees.[9] Supportive data for the acute pharmacological treatment of polymorphic VT, with and without long corrected QT interval, is largely based on case reports and case series, because no RCTs exist.

Recommendation for Electric Treatment of Polymorphic VT

COR	LOE	Recommendation
1	B-NR	1. Immediate defibrillation is recommended for sustained, hemodynamically unstable polymorphic VT.

Recommendation-Specific Supportive Text

1. Regardless of the underlying QT interval, all forms of polymorphic VT tend to be hemodynamically and electrically unstable. They may repeatedly recur and remit spontaneously, become sustained, or degenerate to VF, for which electric shock may be required. When the QRS complex of a VT is of uniform morphology, electric cardioversion with the shock synchronized to the QRS minimizes the risk of provoking VF by a mistimed shock during the vulnerable period of the cardiac cycle (T wave).[10] In contrast, polymorphic VT cannot be synchronized reliably because of the differing characteristics of each QRS complex and requires high-energy unsynchronized defibrillation.[11] While effective in terminating polymorphic VT, electric shock may not prevent its recurrence, for which pharmacological therapies are often required and the primary focus of the ensuing recommendations

This topic last received formal evidence review in 2010.[12]

Recommendation for Pharmacological Treatment of Polymorphic VT Associated With a Long QT Interval (Torsades De Pointes)

COR	LOE	Recommendation
2b	C-LD	1. Magnesium may be considered for treatment of polymorphic VT associated with a long QT interval (torsades de pointes).

Recommendation-Specific Supportive Text

1. Torsades de pointes typically presents in a recurring pattern of self-terminating, hemodynamically unstable polymorphic VT in context of a known or suspected long QT abnormality, often with an associated bradycardia. Immediate defibrillation is the treatment of choice when torsades is sustained or degenerates to VF. However, termination of torsades by shock does not prevent its recurrence, which requires additional measures. In small case series, IV magnesium has been effective in suppressing and preventing recurrences of *torsades*.[13–16] Magnesium is believed to suppress early afterdepolarizations, which are fluctuations in the myocardial action potential that can trigger the salvos of VT seen in torsades.[17] Correcting any electrolyte abnormalities, particularly hypokalemia, is also advisable. *Torsades* is not treatable with antiarrhythmic medications, which can themselves prolong the QT interval and promote the arrhythmia. When given acutely, β-adrenergic blockers can also precipitate torsades by causing or worsening bradycardia. In patients with bradycardia or pause-precipitated torsades, expert consultation is best sought for additional measures such as overdrive pacing or isoproterenol,[18–20] if needed. The use of magnesium in torsades de pointes was addressed by the 2010 Guidelines and updated in a 2018 focused update on ACLS guidelines,[21] with an interim evidence review that identified no new information that would modify previous recommendations.

This topic last received formal evidence review in 2010.[12]

Recommendations for Pharmacological Treatment of Polymorphic VT Not Associated With a Long QT Interval

COR	LOE	Recommendations
2b	C-LD	1. IV lidocaine, amiodarone, and measures to treat myocardial ischemia may be considered to treat polymorphic VT in the absence of a prolonged QT interval.
3: No Benefit	C-LD	2. We do not recommend routine use of magnesium for the treatment of polymorphic VT with a normal QT interval.

Recommendation-Specific Supportive Text

1. Polymorphic VT that is not associated with QT prolongation is often triggered by acute myocardial ischemia and infarction,[4,5] often rapidly degenerates into VF, and is treated similarly to other ventricular arrhythmias (VT and VF). However, termination of polymorphic VT with defibrillation may not prevent its recurrence, which often requires additional measures. No RCTs have been performed to determine the best practice for pharmacological management of polymorphic VT. However measures to treat myocardial ischemia (eg, β-adrenergic blockers or emergent coronary intervention) as well as lidocaine and amiodarone may be effective[22–29] in concert with defibrillation when the arrhythmia is sustained. β-Adrenergic blockers have also been shown to reduce the incidence of ventricular arrhythmias in acute coronary syndromes.[30,31] Expert consultation is advisable when other causes of polymorphic VT are suspected, for which β-adrenergic blockers and antiarrhythmics may also have efficacy.[6,32] This topic was last addressed by the 2010 Guidelines, with an interim evidence update that identified no new information that would modify previous recommendations. Newer defined diagnostic entities causing polymorphic VT merit future evidence evaluation.
2. In the absence of long QT, magnesium has not been shown to be effective in the treatment of polymorphic VT [13] or to afford benefit in the acute management of other ventricular tachyarrhythmias.[16]

These recommendations are supported by the 2018 focused update on ACLS guidelines.[21]

REFERENCES

1. Chan A, Isbister GK, Kirkpatrick CM, Dufful SB. Drug-induced QT prolongation and torsades de pointes: evaluation of a QT nomogram. *QJM.* 2007;100:609–615. doi: 10.1093/qjmed/hcm072
2. Saprungruang A, Khongphatthanayothin A, Mauleekoonphairoj J, Wandee P, Kanjanauthai S, Bhuiyan ZA, Wilde AAM, Poovorawan Y. Genotype and clinical characteristics of congenital long QT syndrome in Thailand. *Indian Pacing Electrophysiol J.* 2018;18:165–171. doi: 10.1016/j.ipej.2018.07.007
3. Drew BJ, Ackerman MJ, Funk M, Gibler WB, Kligfield P, Menon V, Philippides GJ, Roden DM, Zareba W; American Heart Association Acute Cardiac Care Committee of the Council on Clinical Cardiology; Council on Cardiovascular Nursing; American College of Cardiology Foundation. Prevention of torsade de pointes in hospital settings: a scientific statement from the American Heart Association and the American College of Cardiology Foundation. *J Am Coll Cardiol.* 2010;55:934–947. doi: 10.1016/j.jacc.2010.01.001
4. Pogwizd SM, Corr PB. Electrophysiologic mechanisms underlying arrhythmias due to reperfusion of ischemic myocardium. *Circulation.* 1987;76:404–426. doi: 10.1161/01.cir.76.2.404
5. Wolfe CL, Nibley C, Bhandari A, Chatterjee K, Scheinman M. Polymorphous ventricular tachycardia associated with acute myocardial infarction. *Circulation.* 1991;84:1543–1551. doi: 10.1161/01.cir.84.4.1543
6. Liu N, Ruan Y, Priori SG. Catecholaminergic polymorphic ventricular tachycardia. *Prog Cardiovasc Dis.* 2008;51:23–30. doi: 10.1016/j.pcad.2007.10.005
7. Cross B, Homoud M, Link M, Foote C, Garlitski AC, Weinstock J, Estes NA III. The short QT syndrome. *J Interv Card Electrophysiol.* 2011;31:25–31. doi: 10.1007/s10840-011-9566-0
8. Gollob MH, Redpath CJ, Roberts JD. The short QT syndrome: proposed diagnostic criteria. *J Am Coll Cardiol.* 2011;57:802–812. doi: 10.1016/j.jacc.2010.09.048
9. Chapman M, Hargreaves M, Schneider H, Royle M. Bidirectional ventricular tachycardia associated with digoxin toxicity and with normal digoxin levels. *Heart Rhythm.* 2014;11:1222–1225. doi: 10.1016/j.hrthm.2014.03.050
10. Trohman RG, Parrillo JE. Direct current cardioversion: indications, techniques, and recent advances. *Crit Care Med.* 2000;28(suppl):N170–N173. doi: 10.1097/00003246-200010001-00010
11. Dell'Orfano JT, Naccarelli GV. Update on external cardioversion and defibrillation. *Curr Opin Cardiol.* 2001;16:54–57. doi: 10.1097/00001573-200101000-00008

12. Neumar RW, Otto CW, Link MS, Kronick SL, Shuster M, Callaway CW, Kudenchuk PJ, Ornato JP, McNally B, Silvers SM, et al. Part 8: adult advanced cardiovascular life support: 2010 American Heart Association Guidelines for Cardiopulmonary Resuscitation and Emergency Cardiovascular Care. *Circulation.* 2010;122:S729–S767. doi: 10.1161/CIRCULATIONAHA.110.970988
13. Tzivoni D, Banai S, Schuger C, Benhorin J, Keren A, Gottlieb S, Stern S. Treatment of torsade de pointes with magnesium sulfate. *Circulation.* 1988;77:392–397. doi: 10.1161/01.cir.77.2.392
14. Tzivoni D, Keren A, Cohen AM, Loebel H, Zahavi I, Chenzbraun A, Stern S. Magnesium therapy for torsades de pointes. *Am J Cardiol.* 1984;53:528–530. doi: 10.1016/0002-9149(84)90025-0
15. Hoshino K, Ogawa K, Hishitani T, Isobe T, Etoh Y. Successful uses of magnesium sulfate for torsades de pointes in children with long QT syndrome. *Pediatr Int.* 2006;48:112–117. doi: 10.1111/j.1442-200X.2006.02177.x
16. Manz M, Jung W, Lüderitz B. Effect of magnesium on sustained ventricular tachycardia [in German]. *Herz.* 1997;22(suppl 1):51–55. doi: 10.1007/bf03042655
17. Baker WL. Treating arrhythmias with adjunctive magnesium: identifying future research directions. *Eur Heart J Cardiovasc Pharmacother.* 2017;3:108–117. doi: 10.1093/ehjcvp/pvw028
18. DiSegni E, Klein HO, David D, Libhaber C, Kaplinsky E. Overdrive pacing in quinidine syncope and other long QT-interval syndromes. *Arch Intern Med.* 1980;140:1036–1040.
19. Damiano BP, Rosen MR. Effects of pacing on triggered activity induced by early afterdepolarizations. *Circulation.* 1984;69:1013–1025. doi: 10.1161/01.cir.69.5.1013
20. Suarez K, Mack R, Hardegree EL, Chiles C, Banchs JE, Gonzalez MD. Isoproterenol suppresses recurrent torsades de pointes in a patient with long QT syndrome type 2. *HeartRhythm Case Rep.* 2018;4:576–579. doi: 10.1016/j.hrcr.2018.08.013
21. Panchal AR, Berg KM, Kudenchuk PJ, Del Rios M, Hirsch KG, Link MS, Kurz MC, Chan PS, Cabañas JG, Morley PT, Hazinski MF, Donnino MW. 2018 American Heart Association Focused Update on Advanced Cardiovascular Life Support Use of Antiarrhythmic Drugs During and Immediately After Cardiac Arrest: An Update to the American Heart Association Guidelines for Cardiopulmonary Resuscitation and Emergency Cardiovascular Care. *Circulation.* 2018;138:e740–e749. doi: 10.1161/CIR.0000000000000613
22. Vrana M, Pokorny J, Marcian P, Fejfar Z. Class I and III antiarrhythmic drugs for prevention of sudden cardiac death and management of postmyocardial infarction arrhythmias. A review. *Biomed Pap Med Fac Univ Palacky Olomouc Czech Repub.* 2013;157:114–124. doi: 10.5507/bp.2013.030
23. Nalliah CJ, Zaman S, Narayan A, Sullivan J, Kovoor P. Coronary artery reperfusion for ST elevation myocardial infarction is associated with shorter cycle length ventricular tachycardia and fewer spontaneous arrhythmias. *Europace.* 2014;16:1053–1060. doi: 10.1093/europace/eut307
24. Brady W, Meldon S, DeBehnke D. Comparison of prehospital monomorphic and polymorphic ventricular tachycardia: prevalence, response to therapy, and outcome. *Ann Emerg Med.* 1995;25:64–70. doi: 10.1016/s0196-0644(95)70357-8
25. Brady WJ, DeBehnke DJ, Laundrie D. Prevalence, therapeutic response, and outcome of ventricular tachycardia in the out-of-hospital setting: a comparison of monomorphic ventricular tachycardia, polymorphic ventricular tachycardia, and torsades de pointes. *Acad Emerg Med.* 1999;6:609–617. doi: 10.1111/j.1553-2712.1999.tb00414.x
26. Luqman N, Sung RJ, Wang CL, Kuo CT. Myocardial ischemia and ventricular fibrillation: pathophysiology and clinical implications. *Int J Cardiol.* 2007;119:283–290. doi: 10.1016/j.ijcard.2006.09.016
27. Gorenek B, Lundqvist CB, Terradellas JB, Camm AJ, Hindricks G, Huber K, Kirchhof P, Kuck KH, Kudaiberdieva G, Lin T, Raviele A, Santini M, Tilz RR, Valgimigli M, Vos MA, Vrints C, Zeymer U. Cardiac arrhythmias in acute coronary syndromes: position paper from the joint EHRA, ACCA, and EAPCI task force. *Eur Heart J Acute Cardiovasc Care.* 2015;4:386. doi: 10.1177/2048872614550583
28. Carmeliet E. Cardiac ionic currents and acute ischemia: from channels to arrhythmias. *Physiol Rev.* 1999;79:917–1017. doi: 10.1152/physrev.1999.79.3.917
29. Steg PG, James SK, Atar D, Badano LP, Blömstrom-Lundqvist C, Borger MA, Di Mario C, Dickstein K, Ducrocq G, Fernandez-Aviles F, et al; and the Task Force on the management of ST-segment elevation acute myocardial infarction of the European Society of Cardiology. ESC Guidelines for the management of acute myocardial infarction in patients presenting with ST-segment elevation. *Eur Heart J.* 2012;33:2569–2619. doi: 10.1093/eurheartj/ehs215
30. Al-Khatib SM, Stevenson WG, Ackerman MJ, Bryant WJ, Callans DJ, Curtis AB, Deal BJ, Dickfeld T, Field ME, Fonarow GC, et al. 2017 AHA/ACC/HRS guideline for management of patients with ventricular arrhythmias and the prevention of sudden cardiac death: A report of the American College of Cardiology/American Heart Association Task Force on Clinical Practice Guidelines and the Heart Rhythm Society. *Circulation.* 2018;138:e272–e391. doi: 10.1161/CIR.0000000000000549
31. Chatterjee S, Chaudhuri D, Vedanthan R, Fuster V, Ibanez B, Bangalore S, Mukherjee D. Early intravenous beta-blockers in patients with acute coronary syndrome—a meta-analysis of randomized trials. *Int J Cardiol.* 2013;168:915–921. doi: 10.1016/j.ijcard.2012.10.050
32. Van Houzen NE, Alsheikh-Ali AA, Garlitski AC, Homoud MK, Weinstock J, Link MS, Estes NA III. Short QT syndrome review. *J Interv Card Electrophysiol.* 2008;23:1–5. doi: 10.1007/s10840-008-9201-x

Regular Narrow-Complex Tachycardia

Introduction

Management of SVTs is the subject of a recent joint treatment guideline from the AHA, the American College of Cardiology, and the Heart Rhythm Society.[1]

Narrow-complex tachycardia represents a range of tachyarrhythmias originating from a circuit or focus involving the atria or the AV node. Clinicians must determine if the tachycardia is narrow-complex or wide-complex tachycardia and if it has a regular or irregular rhythm. For patients with a sinus tachycardia (heart rate greater than 100/min, P waves), no specific drug treatment is needed, and clinicians should focus on identification and treatment of the underlying cause of the tachycardia (fever, dehydration, pain). If the patient presents with SVT, the primary goal of treatment is to quickly identify and treat patients who are hemodynamically unstable (ischemic chest pain, altered mental status, shock, hypotension, acute heart failure) or symptomatic due to the arrhythmia. Synchronized cardioversion or drugs or both may be used to control unstable or symptomatic regular narrow-complex tachycardia. The available evidence suggests no appreciable differences in success or major adverse event rates between calcium channel blockers and adenosine.[2]

In patients with narrow-complex tachycardia who are refractory to the measures described, this may indicate a more complicated rhythm abnormality for which expert consultation may be advisable.

Recommendations for Electric Therapies for Regular Narrow-Complex Tachycardia

COR	LOE	Recommendations
1	B-NR	1. Synchronized cardioversion is recommended for acute treatment in patients with hemodynamically unstable SVT.
1	B-NR	2. Synchronized cardioversion is recommended for acute treatment in patients with hemodynamically stable SVT when vagal maneuvers and pharmacological therapy is ineffective or contraindicated.

Recommendation-Specific Supportive Text

1 and 2. Management of hemodynamically unstable patients with SVT must start with prompt restoration of sinus rhythm through the use of cardioversion. Cardioversion has been shown to be both safe and effective in the prehospital setting for hemodynamically unstable patients with SVT who had failed to respond to vagal maneuvers and IV pharmacological therapies.[3] Cardioversion is advised in patients who present with hypotension, acutely altered mental status, signs of shock, chest pain, or acute heart failure. Though rare, cardioversion may also be necessary in stable patients with SVT. Most stable patients with SVT have high conversion success rates of 80% to 98% with pharmacological management (eg, adenosine, diltiazem).[4,5] However, if drugs fail to restore sinus rhythm, cardioversion is safe and effective for stable patients after adequate sedation and anesthesia.

These recommendations are supported by the "2015 ACC/AHA/HRS Guideline for the Management of Adult Patients With SVT: A Report of the American College of Cardiology/AHA Task Force on Clinical Practice Guidelines and the Heart Rhythm Society."[6]

Recommendations for Pharmacological Therapies for Regular Narrow-Complex Tachycardia

COR	LOE	Recommendations
1	B-R	1. Vagal maneuvers are recommended for acute treatment in patients with SVT at a regular rate.
1	B-R	2. Adenosine is recommended for acute treatment in patients with SVT at a regular rate.
2a	B-R	3. IV diltiazem or verapamil can be effective for acute treatment in patients with hemodynamically stable SVT at a regular rate.
2a	C-LD	4. IV β-adrenergic blockers are reasonable for acute treatment in patients with hemodynamically stable SVT at a regular rate.

Recommendation-Specific Supportive Text

1. Success rates for the Valsalva maneuver in terminating SVT range from 19% to 54%.[7] Augmenting the Valsalva maneuver with passive leg raise is more effective.[8] Caution is advised when deploying carotid massage in older patients given the potential thromboembolic risk.
2. The 2015 American College of Cardiology, AHA, and Heart Rhythm Society Guidelines evaluated and recommended adenosine as a first-line treatment for regular SVT because of its effectiveness, extremely short half-life, and favorable side-effect profile.[6] A Cochrane systematic review of 7 RCTs (622 patients) found similar rates of conversion to sinus rhythm with adenosine or calcium channel blockers (90% versus 93%) and no significant difference in hypotension.[2] Adenosine may have profound effects in post–heart transplant patients and can cause severe bronchospasm in asthma patients.
3. Treatment of hemodynamically stable patients with IV diltiazem or verapamil have been shown to convert SVT to normal sinus rhythm in 64% to 98% of patients.[4,9–11] These agents are particularly useful in patients who cannot tolerate β-adrenergic blockers or who have recurrent SVT after treatment with adenosine. Caution should be taken to administer these medications slowly to decrease the potential for hypotension.[11] Diltiazem and verapamil are not appropriate in the setting of suspected systolic heart failure.[6]
4. Evidence for the effectiveness of β-adrenergic blockers in terminating SVT is limited. In a trial that compared esmolol with diltiazem, diltiazem was more effective in terminating SVT.[5] Nonetheless, β-adrenergic blockers are generally safe, and it is reasonable to use them to terminate SVT in hemodynamically stable patients.[6]

These recommendations are supported by the 2015 American College of Cardiology, AHA, and Heart Rhythm Society Guidelines for the Management of Adult Patients With SVT.[6]

REFERENCES

1. Page RL, Joglar JA, Caldwell MA, Calkins H, Conti JB, Deal BJ, Estes NAM 3rd, Field ME, Goldberger ZD, Hammill SC, Indik JH, Lindsay BD, Olshansky B, Russo AM, Shen WK, Tracy CM, Al-Khatib SM. 2015 ACC/AHA/HRS Guideline for the Management of Adult Patients With Supraventricular Tachycardia: A Report of the American College of Cardiology/American Heart Association Task Force on Clinical Practice Guidelines and the Heart Rhythm Society. *J Am Coll Cardiol.* 2016;67:e27–e115. doi: 10.1016/j.jacc.2015.08.856
2. Alabed S, Sabouni A, Providencia R, Atallah E, Qintar M, Chico TJ. Adenosine versus intravenous calcium channel antagonists for supraventricular tachycardia. *Cochrane Database Syst Rev.* 2017;10:CD005154. doi: 10.1002/14651858.CD005154.pub4
3. Roth A, Elkayam I, Shapira I, Sander J, Malov N, Kehati M, Golovner M. Effectiveness of prehospital synchronous direct-current cardioversion for supraventricular tachyarrhythmias causing unstable hemodynamic states. *Am J Cardiol.* 2003;91:489–491. doi: 10.1016/s0002-9149(02)03257-5
4. Brady WJ Jr, DeBehnke DJ, Wickman LL, Lindbeck G. Treatment of out-of-hospital supraventricular tachycardia: adenosine vs verapamil. *Acad Emerg Med.* 1996;3:574–585. doi: 10.1111/j.1553-2712.1996.tb03467.x
5. Gupta A, Naik A, Vora A, Lokhandwala Y. Comparison of efficacy of intravenous diltiazem and esmolol in terminating supraventricular tachycardia. *J Assoc Physicians India.* 1999;47:969–972.
6. Page RL, Joglar JA, Caldwell MA, Calkins H, Conti JB, Deal BJ, Estes NA III, Field ME, Goldberger ZD, Hammill SC, Indik JH, Lindsay BD, Olshansky B, Russo AM, Shen WK, Tracy CM, Al-Khatib SM; Evidence Review Committee Chair‡. 2015 ACC/AHA/HRS Guideline for the Management of Adult Patients With Supraventricular Tachycardia: A Report of the American College of Cardiology/American Heart Association Task Force on Clinical Practice Guidelines and the Heart Rhythm Society. *Circulation.* 2016;133:e506–e574. doi: 10.1161/CIR.0000000000000311
7. Smith GD, Fry MM, Taylor D, Morgans A, Cantwell K. Effectiveness of the Valsalva Manoeuvre for reversion of supraventricular tachycardia. *Cochrane Database Syst Rev.* 2015:Cd009502. doi: 10.1002/14651858.CD009502.pub3

8. Appelboam A, Reuben A, Mann C, Gagg J, Ewings P, Barton A, Lobban T, Dayer M, Vickery J, Benger J; REVERT trial collaborators. Postural modification to the standard Valsalva manoeuvre for emergency treatment of supraventricular tachycardias (REVERT): a randomised controlled trial. *Lancet.* 2015;386:1747–1753. doi: 10.1016/S0140-6736(15)61485-4
9. Lim SH, Anantharaman V, Teo WS, Chan YH. Slow infusion of calcium channel blockers compared with intravenous adenosine in the emergency treatment of supraventricular tachycardia. *Resuscitation.* 2009;80:523–528. doi: 10.1016/j.resuscitation.2009.01.017
10. Madsen CD, Pointer JE, Lynch TG. A comparison of adenosine and verapamil for the treatment of supraventricular tachycardia in the prehospital setting. *Ann Emerg Med.* 1995;25:649–655. doi: 10.1016/s0196-0644(95)70179-6
11. Lim SH, Anantharaman V, Teo WS. Slow-infusion of calcium channel blockers in the emergency management of supraventricular tachycardia. *Resuscitation.* 2002;52:167–174. doi: 10.1016/s0300-9572(01)00459-2

Atrial Fibrillation or Flutter With Rapid Ventricular Response

Introduction

Atrial fibrillation is an SVT consisting of disorganized atrial electric activation and uncoordinated atrial contraction. Atrial flutter is an SVT with a macroreentrant circuit resulting in rapid atrial activation but intermittent ventricular response. These arrhythmias are common and often coexist, and their treatment recommendations are similar.

Treatment of atrial fibrillation/flutter depends on the hemodynamic stability of the patient as well as prior history of arrhythmia, comorbidities, and responsiveness to medication. Hemodynamically unstable patients and those with rate-related ischemia should receive urgent electric cardioversion. Hemodynamically stable patients can be treated with a rate-control or rhythm-control strategy. Rate control is more common in the emergency setting, using IV administration of a nondihydropyridine calcium channel antagonist (eg, diltiazem, verapamil) or a β-adrenergic blocker (eg, metoprolol, esmolol). While amiodarone is typically considered a rhythm-control agent, it can effectively reduce ventricular rate with potential use in patients with congestive heart failure where β-adrenergic blockers may not be tolerated and nondihydropyridine calcium channel antagonists are contraindicated. Long-term anticoagulation may be necessary for patients at risk for thromboembolic events based on their CHA_2DS_2-VASc score. The choice of anticoagulation is beyond the scope of these guidelines.

The rhythm-control strategy (sometimes called *chemical cardioversion*) includes antiarrhythmic medications given to convert the rhythm to sinus and/or prevent recurrent atrial fibrillation/flutter (Table 3). Patient selection, evaluation, timing, drug selection, and anticoagulation for patients undergoing rhythm control are beyond the scope of these guidelines and are presented elsewhere.[1,2]

The management of patients with preexcitation syndromes (aka Wolff-Parkinson-White) is covered in the Wide-Complex Tachycardia section.

Recommendations for Electric Therapies for Atrial Fibrillation/Flutter

COR	LOE	Recommendations
1	C-LD	1. Hemodynamically unstable patients with atrial fibrillation or atrial flutter with rapid ventricular response should receive electric cardioversion.
1	C-LD	2. Urgent direct-current cardioversion of new-onset atrial fibrillation in the setting of acute coronary syndrome is recommended for patients with hemodynamic compromise, ongoing ischemia, or inadequate rate control.
2a	C-LD	3. For synchronized cardioversion of atrial fibrillation using biphasic energy, an initial energy of 120 to 200 J is reasonable, depending on the specific biphasic defibrillator being used.
2b	C-LD	4. For synchronized cardioversion of atrial flutter using biphasic energy, an initial energy of 50 to 100 J may be reasonable, depending on the specific biphasic defibrillator being used.

Recommendation-Specific Supportive Text

1 and 2. Uncontrolled tachycardia may impair ventricular filling, cardiac output, and coronary perfusion while increasing myocardial oxygen demand. While an expeditious trial of medications and/or fluids may be appropriate in some cases, unstable patients or patients with ongoing cardiac ischemia with atrial fibrillation or atrial flutter need to be cardioverted promptly.[1–3] When making the decision for cardioversion, one should also consider whether the arrhythmia is the cause of the tachycardia. Potential exacerbation of rapid ventricular response by secondary causes (eg, sepsis) should be considered and may inform initial attempts at hemodynamic stabilization with pharmacotherapy. There are few data addressing these strategies in hemodynamically unstable patients. However, studies demonstrating hemodynamic benefits of successful cardioversion have been published.[4,5] In addition, risks of hypotension and hypoperfusion with use of negative inotropes have been demonstrated even in normotensive patients.[6–8] Hemodynamically unstable patients and those with ongoing cardiac ischemia are likely to benefit from the improved hemodynamic status associated with restoration of sinus rhythm and avoidance of hypotension caused by the alternative pharmacological therapies. Depending on the clinical scenario, patients cardioverted from atrial fibrillation or atrial flutter of 48 hours' duration or longer are candidates for anticoagulation. Details about anticoagulation selection can be found elsewhere.[2]

Table 3. IV Medications Commonly Used for Acute Rate Control in Atrial Fibrillation and Atrial Flutter[18]

Medication	Bolus Dose	Infusion Rate	Notes
Nondihydropyridine Calcium Channel Blockers			
Diltiazem	0.25 mg/kg IV bolus over 2 min	5–10 mg/h	Avoid in hypotension, heart failure, cardiomyopathy, and acute coronary syndromes
Verapamil	0.075–0.15 mg/kg IV bolus over 2 min; may give an additional dose after 30 min if no response	0.005 mg/kg per min	Avoid in hypotension, heart failure, cardiomyopathy, acute and coronary syndromes
β-Adrenergic Blockers			
Metoprolol	2.5–5 mg over 2 min, up to 3 doses		Avoid in decompensated heart failure
Esmolol	500 μg/kg IV over 1 min	50–300 μg/kg per min	Short duration of action; avoid in decompensated heart failure
Propranolol	1 mg IV over 1 min, up to 3 doses		Avoid in decompensated heart failure
Other Medications			
Amiodarone	300 mg IV over 1 h	10–50 mg/h over 24 h	Multiple dosing schemes exist for amiodarone
Digoxin	0.25 mg IV, repeated to maximum dose 1.5 mg over 24 h		Typically used as adjunctive therapy with another option from above; caution in patients with renal impairment

IV indicates intravenous.

3 and 4. The electric energy required to successfully cardiovert a patient from atrial fibrillation or atrial flutter to sinus rhythm varies and is generally less in patients with new-onset arrhythmia, thin body habitus, and when biphasic waveform shocks are delivered.[9–15] Obese patients may require greater energy.[16] If initial cardioversion is unsuccessful, energy is increased in subsequent attempts. Less energy is generally required for atrial flutter than for atrial fibrillation.[11] Higher energies of 200 J or more are associated with improved first shock success and decreased total energy delivery. In addition, a retrospective analysis found that lower energy shocks were associated with higher risk of cardioversion-induced VF.[17] Previous guidelines included a comparison of monophasic and biphasic waveforms. This recommendation now focuses primarily on biphasic waveforms. Recommended energy levels vary with different devices, reducing the validity of generalized recommendations. This topic requires further study with a comprehensive systematic review to better understand the optimal electric doses with current devices. The writing group assessment of the LOE as C-LD is consistent with the limited evidence using modern devices and energy waveforms.

These recommendations are supported by the "2014 AHA/ACC/HRS Guideline for the Management of Patients With Atrial Fibrillation: A Report of the American College of Cardiology/AHA Task Force on Practice Guidelines and the Heart Rhythm Society"[18] as well as the focused update of those guidelines published in 2019.[2]

Recommendations for Medical Therapies for Atrial Fibrillation/Flutter

COR	LOE	Recommendations
1	B-NR	1. IV administration of a β-adrenergic blocker or nondihydropyridine calcium channel antagonist is recommended to slow the ventricular heart rate in the acute setting in patients with atrial fibrillation or atrial flutter with rapid ventricular response without preexcitation.
2a	B-NR	2. IV amiodarone can be useful for rate control in critically ill patients with atrial fibrillation with rapid ventricular response without preexcitation.
3: Harm	C-LD	3. In patients with atrial fibrillation and atrial flutter in the setting of preexcitation, digoxin, nondihydropyridine calcium channel antagonists, β-adrenergic blockers, and IV amiodarone should not be administered because they may increase the ventricular response and result in VF.
3: Harm	C-EO	4. Nondihydropyridine calcium channel antagonists and IV β-adrenergic blockers should not be used in patients with left ventricular systolic dysfunction and decompensated heart failure because these may lead to further hemodynamic compromise.

Recommendation-Specific Supportive Text

1 and 2. Clinical trial evidence shows that nondihydropyridine calcium channel antagonists (eg, diltiazem, verapamil), β-adrenergic blockers (eg, esmolol, propranolol), amiodarone, and digoxin are all effective for rate control in patients with atrial fibrillation/flutter.[6–8,19–23] Calcium channel blockers may be more effective than amiodarone, and cause more hypotension.[6] Digoxin is rarely used in the acute setting because of slow onset of effect.[1,2]

Circulation. 2020;142(suppl 2):S366–S468. DOI: 10.1161/CIR.0000000000000916

3. Based on limited case reports and small case series, there is concern that patients with concomitant preexcitation and atrial fibrillation or atrial flutter may develop VF in response to accelerated ventricular response after the administration of AV nodal blocking agents such as digoxin, nondihydropyridine calcium channel antagonists, β-adrenergic blockers, or IV amiodarone.[24–27] In this setting, cardioversion is recommended as the most appropriate management.
4. Because of their negative inotropic effect, nondihydropyridine calcium channel antagonists (eg, diltiazem, verapamil) may further decompensate patients with left ventricular systolic dysfunction and symptomatic heart failure. They may be used in patients with heart failure with preserved ejection fraction. β-Adrenergic blockers may be used in compensated patients with cardiomyopathy; however, they should be used with caution or avoided altogether in patients with decompensated heart failure. This recommendation is based on expert consensus and pathophysiologic rationale.[2,18,28] β-Adrenergic blockers may be used in patients with chronic obstructive pulmonary disease because multiple studies have shown no negative effects.[29]

These recommendations are supported by 2014 AHA, American College of Cardiology, and Heart Rhythm Society Guideline for the Management of Patients With Atrial Fibrillation[18] as well as the focused update of those guidelines published in 2019.[2]

REFERENCES

1. January CT, Wann LS, Alpert JS, Calkins H, Cigarroa JE, Cleveland JC Jr, Conti JB, Ellinor PT, Ezekowitz MD, Field ME, Murray KT, Sacco RL, Stevenson WG, Tchou PJ, Tracy CM, Yancy CW; ACC/AHA Task Force Members. 2014 AHA/ACC/HRS guideline for the management of patients with atrial fibrillation: executive summary: a report of the American College of Cardiology/American Heart Association Task Force on practice guidelines and the Heart Rhythm Society. *Circulation.* 2014;130:2071–2104. doi: 10.1161/CIR.0000000000000040
2. January CT, Wann LS, Calkins H, Chen LY, Cigarroa JE, Cleveland JC Jr, Ellinor PT, Ezekowitz MD, Field ME, Furie KL, Heidenreich PA, Murray KT, Shea JB, Tracy CM, Yancy CW. 2019 AHA/ACC/HRS Focused Update of the 2014 AHA/ACC/HRS Guideline for the Management of Patients With Atrial Fibrillation: A Report of the American College of Cardiology/American Heart Association Task Force on Clinical Practice Guidelines and the Heart Rhythm Society in Collaboration With the Society of Thoracic Surgeons. *Circulation.* 2019;140:e125–e151. doi: 10.1161/CIR.0000000000000665
3. McMurray J, Køber L, Robertson M, Dargie H, Colucci W, Lopez-Sendon J, Remme W, Sharpe DN, Ford I. Antiarrhythmic effect of carvedilol after acute myocardial infarction: results of the Carvedilol Post-Infarct Survival Control in Left Ventricular Dysfunction (CAPRICORN) trial. *J Am Coll Cardiol.* 2005;45:525–530. doi: 10.1016/j.jacc.2004.09.076
4. DeMaria AN, Lies JE, King JF, Miller RR, Amsterdam EA, Mason DT. Echographic assessment of atrial transport, mitral movement, and ventricular performance following electroversion of supraventricular arrhythmias. *Circulation.* 1975;51:273–282. doi: 10.1161/01.cir.51.2.273
5. Raymond RJ, Lee AJ, Messineo FC, Manning WJ, Silverman DI. Cardiac performance early after cardioversion from atrial fibrillation. *Am Heart J.* 1998;136:435–442. doi: 10.1016/s0002-8703(98)70217-0
6. Delle Karth G, Geppert A, Neunteufl T, Priglinger U, Haumer M, Gschwandtner M, Siostrzonek P, Heinz G. Amiodarone versus diltiazem for rate control in critically ill patients with atrial tachyarrhythmias. *Crit Care Med.* 2001;29:1149–1153. doi: 10.1097/00003246-200106000-00011
7. Platia EV, Michelson EL, Porterfield JK, Das G. Esmolol versus verapamil in the acute treatment of atrial fibrillation or atrial flutter. *Am J Cardiol.* 1989;63:925–929. doi: 10.1016/0002-9149(89)90141-0
8. Ellenbogen KA, Dias VC, Plumb VJ, Heywood JT, Mirvis DM. A placebo-controlled trial of continuous intravenous diltiazem infusion for 24-hour heart rate control during atrial fibrillation and atrial flutter: a multicenter study. *J Am Coll Cardiol.* 1991;18:891–897. doi: 10.1016/0735-1097(91)90743-s
9. Glover BM, Walsh SJ, McCann CJ, Moore MJ, Manoharan G, Dalzell GW, McAllister A, McClements B, McEneaney DJ, Trouton TG, Mathew TP, Adgey AA. Biphasic energy selection for transthoracic cardioversion of atrial fibrillation. The BEST AF Trial. *Heart.* 2008;94:884–887. doi: 10.1136/hrt.2007.120782
10. Inácio JF, da Rosa Mdos S, Shah J, Rosário J, Vissoci JR, Manica AL, Rodrigues CG. Monophasic and biphasic shock for transthoracic conversion of atrial fibrillation: systematic review and network meta-analysis. *Resuscitation.* 2016;100:66–75. doi: 10.1016/j.resuscitation.2015.12.009
11. Gallagher MM, Guo XH, Poloniecki JD, Guan Yap Y, Ward D, Camm AJ. Initial energy setting, outcome and efficiency in direct current cardioversion of atrial fibrillation and flutter. *J Am Coll Cardiol.* 2001;38:1498–1504. doi: 10.1016/s0735-1097(01)01540-6
12. Scholten M, Szili-Torok T, Klootwijk P, Jordaens L. Comparison of monophasic and biphasic shocks for transthoracic cardioversion of atrial fibrillation. *Heart.* 2003;89:1032–1034. doi: 10.1136/heart.89.9.1032
13. Page RL, Kerber RE, Russell JK, Trouton T, Waktare J, Gallik D, Olgin JE, Ricard P, Dalzell GW, Reddy R, Lazzara R, Lee K, Carlson M, Halperin B, Bardy GH; BiCard Investigators. Biphasic versus monophasic shock waveform for conversion of atrial fibrillation: the results of an international randomized, double-blind multicenter trial. *J Am Coll Cardiol.* 2002;39:1956–1963. doi: 10.1016/s0735-1097(02)01898-3
14. Reisinger J, Gstrein C, Winter T, Zeindlhofer E, Höllinger K, Mori M, Schiller A, Winter A, Geiger H, Siostrzonek P. Optimization of initial energy for cardioversion of atrial tachyarrhythmias with biphasic shocks. *Am J Emerg Med.* 2010;28:159–165. doi: 10.1016/j.ajem.2008.10.028
15. Alatawi F, Gurevitz O, White RD, Ammash NM, Malouf JF, Bruce CJ, Moon BS, Rosales AG, Hodge D, Hammill SC, Gersh BJ, Friedman PA. Prospective, randomized comparison of two biphasic waveforms for the efficacy and safety of transthoracic biphasic cardioversion of atrial fibrillation. *Heart Rhythm.* 2005;2:382–387. doi: 10.1016/j.hrthm.2004.12.024
16. Voskoboinik A, Moskovitch J, Plunkett G, Bloom J, Wong G, Nalliah C, Prabhu S, Sugumar H, Paramasweran R, McLellan A, et al. Cardioversion of atrial fibrillation in obese patients: Results from the Cardioversion-BMI randomized controlled trial. *J Cardiovasc Electrophysiol.* 2019;30:155–161. doi: 10.1111/jce.13786
17. Gallagher MM, Yap YG, Padula M, Ward DE, Rowland E, Camm AJ. Arrhythmic complications of electrical cardioversion: relationship to shock energy. *Int J Cardiol.* 2008;123:307–312. doi: 10.1016/j.ijcard.2006.12.014
18. January CT, Wann LS, Alpert JS, Calkins H, Cigarroa JE, Cleveland JC Jr, Conti JB, Ellinor PT, Ezekowitz MD, Field ME, et al. 2014 AHA/ACC/HRS guideline for the management of patients with atrial fibrillation: a report of the American College of Cardiology/American Heart Association Task Force on practice guidelines and the Heart Rhythm Society. *Circulation.* 2014;130:e199–e267. doi: 10.1161/CIR.0000000000000041
19. Abrams J, Allen J, Allin D, Anderson J, Anderson S, Blanski L, Chadda K, DiBianco R, Favrot L, Gonzalez J. Efficacy and safety of esmolol vs propranolol in the treatment of supraventricular tachyarrhythmias: a multicenter double-blind clinical trial. *Am Heart J.* 1985;110:913–922. doi: 10.1016/0002-8703(85)90185-1
20. Siu CW, Lau CP, Lee WL, Lam KF, Tse HF. Intravenous diltiazem is superior to intravenous amiodarone or digoxin for achieving ventricular rate control in patients with acute uncomplicated atrial fibrillation. *Crit Care Med.* 2009;37:2174–9; quiz 2180. doi: 10.1097/CCM.0b013e3181a02f56
21. Clemo HF, Wood MA, Gilligan DM, Ellenbogen KA. Intravenous amiodarone for acute heart rate control in the critically ill patient with atrial tachyarrhythmias. *Am J Cardiol.* 1998;81:594–598. doi: 10.1016/s0002-9149(97)00962-4
22. Hou ZY, Chang MS, Chen CY, Tu MS, Lin SL, Chiang HT, Woosley RL. Acute treatment of recent-onset atrial fibrillation and flutter with a tailored dosing regimen of intravenous amiodarone. A randomized, digoxin-controlled study. *Eur Heart J.* 1995;16:521–528. doi: 10.1093/oxfordjournals.eurheartj.a060945

23. Salerno DM, Dias VC, Kleiger RE, Tschida VH, Sung RJ, Sami M, Giorgi LV. Efficacy and safety of intravenous diltiazem for treatment of atrial fibrillation and atrial flutter. The Diltiazem-Atrial Fibrillation/Flutter Study Group. *Am J Cardiol.* 1989;63:1046–1051. doi: 10.1016/0002-9149(89)90076-3
24. Gulamhusein S, Ko P, Carruthers SG, Klein GJ. Acceleration of the ventricular response during atrial fibrillation in the Wolff-Parkinson-White syndrome after verapamil. *Circulation.* 1982;65:348–354. doi: 10.1161/01.cir.65.2.348
25. Jacob AS, Nielsen DH, Gianelly RE. Fatal ventricular fibrillation following verapamil in Wolff-Parkinson-White syndrome with atrial fibrillation. *Ann Emerg Med.* 1985;14:159–160. doi: 10.1016/s0196-0644(85)81080-5
26. Boriani G, Biffi M, Frabetti L, Azzolini U, Sabbatani P, Bronzetti G, Capucci A, Magnani B. Ventricular fibrillation after intravenous amiodarone in Wolff-Parkinson-White syndrome with atrial fibrillation. *Am Heart J.* 1996;131:1214–1216. doi: 10.1016/s0002-8703(96)90098-8
27. Kim RJ, Gerling BR, Kono AT, Greenberg ML. Precipitation of ventricular fibrillation by intravenous diltiazem and metoprolol in a young patient with occult Wolff-Parkinson-White syndrome. *Pacing Clin Electrophysiol.* 2008;31:776–779. doi: 10.1111/j.1540-8159.2008.01086.x
28. Yancy CW, Jessup M, Bozkurt B, Butler J, Casey DE Jr, Drazner MH, Fonarow GC, Geraci SA, Horwich T, Januzzi JL, et al; on behalf of the American College of Cardiology Foundation/American Heart Association Task Force on Practice Guidelines. 2013 ACCF/AHA guideline for the management of heart failure: a report of the American College of Cardiology Foundation/American Heart Association Task Force on practice guidelines. *Circulation.* 2013;128:e240–e327. doi: 10.1161/CIR.0b013e31829e8776
29. Salpeter S, Ormiston T, Salpeter E. Cardioselective beta-blockers for chronic obstructive pulmonary disease. *Cochrane Database Syst Rev.* 2005:CD003566. doi: 10.1002/14651858.CD003566.pub2

Bradycardia

Introduction

Bradycardia is generally defined as a heart rate less than 60/min. Bradycardia can be a normal finding, especially for athletes or during sleep. When bradycardia occurs secondary to a pathological cause, it can lead to decreased cardiac output with resultant hypotension and tissue hypoperfusion. The clinical manifestations of bradycardia can range from an absence of symptoms to symptomatic bradycardia (bradycardia associated with acutely altered mental status, ischemic chest discomfort, acute heart failure, hypotension, or other signs of shock that persist despite adequate airway and breathing). The cause of the bradycardia may dictate the severity of the presentation. For example, patients with severe hypoxia and impending respiratory failure may suddenly develop a profound bradycardia that leads to cardiac arrest if not addressed immediately. In contrast, a patient who develops third-degree heart block but is otherwise well compensated might experience relatively low blood pressure but otherwise be stable. Therefore, the management of bradycardia will depend on both the underlying cause and severity of the clinical presentation. In 2018, the AHA, American College of Cardiology, and Heart Rhythm Society published an extensive guideline on the evaluation and management of stable and unstable bradycardia.[2] This guideline focuses exclusively on symptomatic bradycardia in the ACLS setting and maintains consistency with the 2018 guideline.

Recommendations for Initial Management of Bradycardia

COR	LOE	Recommendations
1	C-EO	1. In patients presenting with acute symptomatic bradycardia, evaluation and treatment of reversible causes is recommended.
2a	B-NR	2. In patients with acute bradycardia associated with hemodynamic compromise, administration of atropine is reasonable to increase heart rate.
2b	C-LD	3. If bradycardia is unresponsive to atropine, IV adrenergic agonists with rate-accelerating effects (eg, epinephrine) or transcutaneous pacing may be effective while the patient is prepared for emergent transvenous temporary pacing if required.
2b	C-EO	4. Immediate pacing might be considered in unstable patients with high-degree AV block when IV/IO access is not available.

Recommendation-Specific Supportive Text

1. Symptomatic bradycardia may be caused by a number of potentially reversible or treatable causes, including structural heart disease, increased vagal tone, hypoxemia, myocardial ischemia, or medications.[2] Bradycardia may be difficult to resolve until the underlying cause is treated, making evaluation of underlying cause imperative, simultaneous with emergent treatments for stabilization.
2. Atropine has been shown to be effective for the treatment of symptomatic bradycardia in both observational studies and in 1 limited RCT.[3–7]
3. If atropine is ineffective, either alternative agents to increase heart rate and blood pressure or transcutaneous pacing are reasonable next steps. For medical management of a periarrest patient, epinephrine has gained popularity, including IV infusion and utilization of "push-dose" administration for acute bradycardia and hypotension. Studies on push-dose epinephrine for bradycardia specifically are lacking, although limited data support its use for hypotension.[8] Use of push-dose vasopressor requires careful attention to correct dosing. Medication errors leading to adverse effects have been reported.[9] Dopamine infusion can also increase heart rate.[10] There are limited studies comparing medications to transcutaneous pacing for the treatment of bradycardia. A randomized feasibility study in patients failing atropine compared dopamine to transcutaneous pacing and found no difference in survival to discharge.[10] Whether to trial transcutaneous pacing, epinephrine, dopamine, or other vasoactive agent will likely therefore depend on clinician experience and resources available.
4. For severe symptomatic bradycardia causing shock, if no IV or IO access is available, immediate transcutaneous pacing while access is being

pursued may be undertaken. A 2006 systematic review involving 7 studies of transcutaneous pacing for symptomatic bradycardia and bradyasystolic cardiac arrest in the prehospital setting did not find a benefit from pacing compared with standard ACLS, although a subgroup analysis from 1 trial suggested a possible benefit in patients with symptomatic bradycardia.[11]

These recommendations are supported by the "2018 ACC/AHA/HRS Guideline on the Evaluation and Management of Patients With Bradycardia and Cardiac Conduction Delay: A Report of the American College of Cardiology/AHA Task Force on Clinical Practice Guidelines and the Heart Rhythm Society."[2]

Recommendation for Transvenous Pacing for Bradycardia		
COR	LOE	Recommendation
2a	C-LD	1. In patients with persistent hemodynamically unstable bradycardia refractory to medical therapy, temporary transvenous pacing is reasonable to increase heart rate and improve symptoms.

Recommendation-Specific Supportive Text

1. When bradycardia is refractory to medical management and results in severe symptoms, the reasonable next step is placement of a temporary pacing catheter for transvenous pacing. Limited evidence for this intervention consists largely of observational studies, many of which have focused on indications and the relatively high complication rate (including bloodstream infections and pneumothorax, among others).[12–14] However, when the heart rate does not improve with medications and shock persists, transvenous pacing can improve the heart rate and symptoms until more definitive treatment (correction of underlying cause or permanent pacemaker placement) can be implemented.

These recommendations are supported by the 2018 American College of Cardiology, AHA, and Heart Rhythm Society guideline on the evaluation and management of patients with bradycardia and cardiac conduction delay.[2]

REFERENCES

1. Deleted in proof.
2. Kusumoto FM, Schoenfeld MH, Barrett C, Edgerton JR, Ellenbogen KA, Gold MR, Goldschlager NF, Hamilton RM, Joglar JA, Kim RJ, Lee R, Marine JE, McLeod CJ, Oken KR, Patton KK, Pellegrini CN, Selzman KA, Thompson A, Varosy PD. 2018 ACC/AHA/HRS Guideline on the Evaluation and Management of Patients With Bradycardia and Cardiac Conduction Delay: A Report of the American College of Cardiology/American Heart Association Task Force on Clinical Practice Guidelines and the Heart Rhythm Society. *Circulation.* 2019;140:e382–e482. doi: 10.1161/CIR.0000000000000628
3. Smith I, Monk TG, White PF. Comparison of transesophageal atrial pacing with anticholinergic drugs for the treatment of intraoperative bradycardia. *Anesth Analg.* 1994;78:245–252. doi: 10.1213/00000539-199402000-00009
4. Brady WJ, Swart G, DeBehnke DJ, Ma OJ, Aufderheide TP. The efficacy of atropine in the treatment of hemodynamically unstable bradycardia and atrioventricular block: prehospital and emergency department considerations. *Resuscitation.* 1999;41:47–55. doi: 10.1016/s0300-9572(99)00032-5
5. Chadda KD, Lichstein E, Gupta PK, Kourtesis P. Effects of atropine in patients with bradyarrhythmia complicating myocardial infarction. Usefulness of an optimum dose for overdrive. *Am J Med.* 1977;63:503–510. doi: 10.1016/0002-9343(77)90194-2
6. Swart G, Brady WJ Jr, DeBehnke DJ, MA OJ, Aufderheide TP. Acute myocardial infarction complicated by hemodynamically unstable bradyarrhythmia: prehospital and ED treatment with atropine. *Am J Emerg Med.* 1999;17:647–652. doi: 10.1016/s0735-6757(99)90151-1
7. Chadda KD, Lichstein E, Gupta PK, Choy R. Bradycardia-hypotension syndrome in acute myocardial infarction. Reappraisal of the overdrive effects of atropine. *Am J Med.* 1975;59:158–164. doi: 10.1016/0002-9343(75)90349-6
8. Nawrocki PS, Poremba M, Lawner BJ. Push Dose Epinephrine Use in the Management of Hypotension During Critical Care Transport. *Prehosp Emerg Care.* 2020;24:188–195. doi: 10.1080/10903127.2019.1588443
9. Cole JB, Knack SK, Karl ER, Horton GB, Satpathy R, Driver BE. Human Errors and Adverse Hemodynamic Events Related to "Push Dose Pressors" in the Emergency Department. *J Med Toxicol.* 2019;15:276–286. doi: 10.1007/s13181-019-00716-z
10. Morrison LJ, Long J, Vermeulen M, Schwartz B, Sawadsky B, Frank J, Cameron B, Burgess R, Shield J, Bagley P, Mausz V, Brewer JE, Dorian P. A randomized controlled feasibility trial comparing safety and effectiveness of prehospital pacing versus conventional treatment: 'PrePACE'. *Resuscitation.* 2008;76:341–349. doi: 10.1016/j.resuscitation.2007.08.008
11. Sherbino J, Verbeek PR, MacDonald RD, Sawadsky BV, McDonald AC, Morrison LJ. Prehospital transcutaneous cardiac pacing for symptomatic bradycardia or bradyasystolic cardiac arrest: a systematic review. *Resuscitation.* 2006;70:193–200. doi: 10.1016/j.resuscitation.2005.11.019
12. Ferguson JD, Banning AP, Bashir Y. Randomised trial of temporary cardiac pacing with semirigid and balloon-flotation electrode catheters. *Lancet.* 1997;349:1883. doi: 10.1016/S0140-6736(97)24026-2
13. McCann P. A review of temporary cardiac pacing wires. *Indian Pacing Electrophysiol J.* 2007;7:40–49.
14. Jou YL, Hsu HP, Tuan TC, Wang KL, Lin YJ, Lo LW, Hu YF, Kong CW, Chang SL, Chen SA. Trends of temporary pacemaker implant and underlying disease substrate. *Pacing Clin Electrophysiol.* 2010;33:1475–1484. doi: 10.1111/j.1540-8159.2010.02893.x

Care After ROSC

Postresuscitation Care

Introduction

Post–cardiac arrest care is a critical component of the Chain of Survival. What defines optimal hospital care for patients with ROSC after cardiac arrest is not completely known, but there is increasing interest in identifying and optimizing practices that are likely to improve outcomes. The systemic impact of the ischemia-reperfusion injury caused by cardiac arrest and subsequent resuscitation requires post–cardiac arrest care to simultaneously support the multiple organ systems that are affected. After initial stabilization, care of critically ill postarrest patients hinges on hemodynamic support, mechanical ventilation, temperature management, diagnosis and treatment of underlying causes, diagnosis and treatment of seizures, vigilance for and treatment of infection, and management of the critically ill state of the patient. Many cardiac arrest patients who survive the initial event will eventually die because of withdrawal of life-sustaining treatment in the setting of neurological injury. This cause of death is especially prominent in those with OHCA but is also frequent after IHCA.[1,2] Thus, much of postarrest care focuses on mitigating injury to the brain. Possible contributors to this goal include optimization of cerebral perfusion pressure, management of oxygen and carbon dioxide levels, control of core body temperature, and detection and treatment of seizures (Figure 9). Cardiac arrest results in heterogeneous injury; thus, death can also result from multiorgan dysfunction or shock. In light of the complexity of postarrest patients, a multidisciplinary team with expertise in cardiac arrest care is preferred, and the development of multidisciplinary protocols is critical to optimize survival and neurological outcome.

Key topics in postresuscitation care that are not covered in this section, but are discussed later, are targeted temperature management (TTM) (Targeted Temperature Management), percutaneous coronary intervention (PCI) in cardiac arrest (PCI After Cardiac Arrest), neuroprognostication (Neuroprognostication), and recovery (Recovery).

Recommendations for Considerations in the Early Postresuscitation Period

COR	LOE	Recommendations
1	B-NR	1. A comprehensive, structured, multidisciplinary system of care should be implemented in a consistent manner for the treatment of post–cardiac arrest patients.
1	B-NR	2. A 12-lead ECG should be obtained as soon as feasible after ROSC to determine whether acute ST-segment elevation is present.
2a	C-EO	3. To avoid hypoxia in adults with ROSC in the immediate postarrest period, it is reasonable to use the highest available oxygen concentration until the arterial oxyhemoglobin saturation or the partial pressure of arterial oxygen can be measured reliably.

Recommendation-Specific Supportive Text

1. Observational studies evaluating the utility of cardiac receiving centers suggest that a strong system of care may represent a logical clinical link between successful resuscitation and ultimate survival.[3] Although data are limited, taken together with experience from regionalized approaches to other emergencies such as trauma, stroke, and ST-segment elevation acute myocardial infarction, consistent implementation of a system of care to manage cardiac arrest patients may improve outcomes.
2. Patients with 12-lead identification of ST-segment elevation myocardial infarction (STEMI) should have coronary angiography for possible PCI, highlighting the importance of obtaining an ECG for diagnostic purposes.[4] However, multiple studies have reported that absence of ST-segment elevations does not rule out an intervenable coronary lesion.[5–7]
3. Several RCTs have compared a titrated approach to oxygen administration with an approach of administering 100% oxygen in the first 1 to 2 hours after ROSC.[8–10] All of these were conducted in the prehospital setting. However, these trials only titrated oxygen once an oxygen saturation could be measured with a pulse oximeter. No studies have investigated titration of oxygen in patients for whom oxygen saturation (by pulse oximeter) or partial pressure of oxygen in the blood (by arterial blood gas) cannot be measured. The recommendation to administer 100% oxygen until measurement of this vital sign is possible is therefore based on physiology and the expert opinion that hypoxia could worsen end-organ damage and should be avoided.

Recommendation 1 is supported by the 2019 focused update on ACLS guidelines.[3] Recommendation 2 last received formal evidence review in 2015.[4] Recommendation 3 is supported by the 2020 CoSTR for ALS.[11]

Recommendation for Blood Pressure Management After ROSC

COR	LOE	Recommendation
2a	B-NR	1. It is preferable to avoid hypotension by maintaining a systolic blood pressure of at least 90 mm Hg and a mean arterial pressure of at least 65 mm Hg in the postresuscitation period.

Recommendation-Specific Supportive Text

1. Hypotension may worsen brain and other organ injury after cardiac arrest by decreasing oxygen delivery to tissues. The optimal MAP target after ROSC, however, is not clear. This topic was previously reviewed by ILCOR in 2015,[12] and a detailed evidence update was conducted by the Australia and New Zealand Council of Resuscitation on behalf of ILCOR for 2020.[11] Several observational studies have found that postresuscitation hypotension is associated with worse survival and neurological outcome.[13–19] One study found no association between higher MAP during TTM treatment and outcome, although shock at admission was associated with poor outcome.[20] Definitions of *hypotension* vary between studies, with systolic blood pressure of 90 mm Hg and MAP of 65 mm Hg being common cutoffs used. Two RCTs conducted since 2015 compared a lower blood pressure target (standard care or MAP greater than 65 mm Hg in one study and MAP 65–75 mm Hg in the other) with a higher target (MAP 85–100 in one study and MAP 80–100 mm Hg in the other).[21,22] Both studies failed to detect any difference in survival or survival with favorable neurological

Adult Post–Cardiac Arrest Care Algorithm

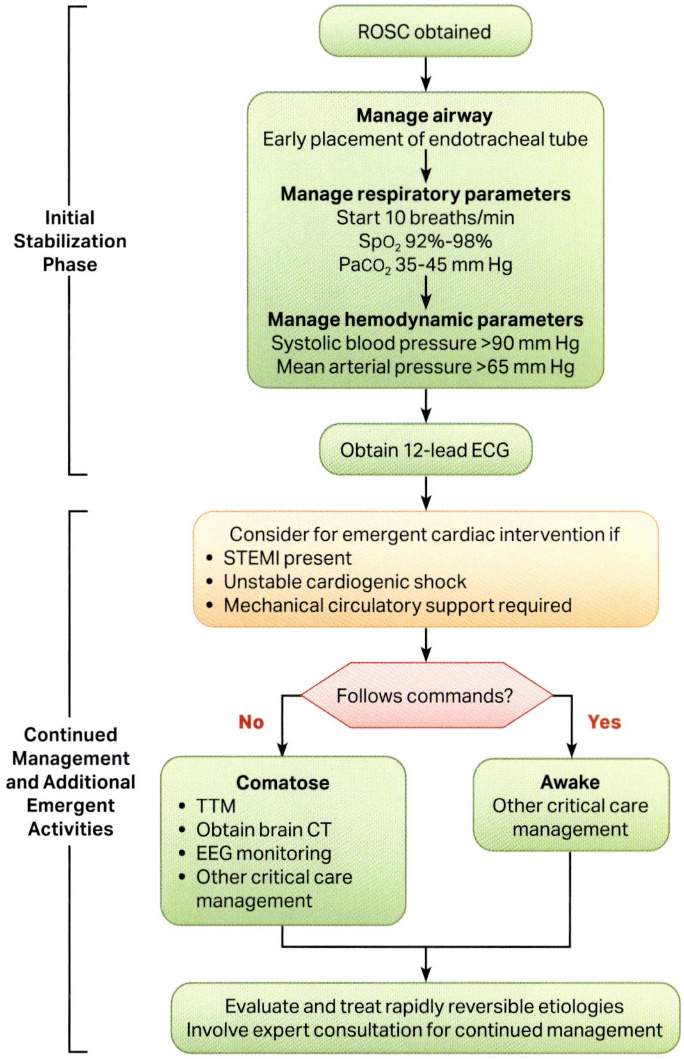

Initial Stabilization Phase
ROSC obtained
Manage airway
Early placement of endotracheal tube
Manage respiratory parameters
Start 10 breaths/min
SpO_2 92%-98%
$PaCO_2$ 35-45 mm Hg
Manage hemodynamic parameters
Systolic blood pressure >90 mm Hg
Mean arterial pressure >65 mm Hg
Obtain 12-lead ECG
Continued Management and Additional Emergent Activities
Consider for emergent cardiac intervention if
• STEMI present
• Unstable cardiogenic shock
• Mechanical circulatory support required
Follows commands?
No
Yes
Comatose
• TTM
• Obtain brain CT
• EEG monitoring
• Other critical care management
Awake
Other critical care management
Evaluate and treat rapidly reversible etiologies
Involve expert consultation for continued management

Initial Stabilization Phase

Resuscitation is ongoing during the post-ROSC phase, and many of these activities can occur concurrently. However, if prioritization is necessary, follow these steps:

- Airway management: Waveform capnography or capnometry to confirm and monitor endotracheal tube placement
- Manage respiratory parameters: Titrate FIO_2 for SpO_2 92%-98%; start at 10 breaths/min; titrate to $PaCO_2$ of 35-45 mm Hg
- Manage hemodynamic parameters: Administer crystalloid and/or vasopressor or inotrope for goal systolic blood pressure >90 mm Hg or mean arterial pressure >65 mm Hg

Continued Management and Additional Emergent Activities

These evaluations should be done concurrently so that decisions on targeted temperature management (TTM) receive high priority as cardiac interventions.

- Emergent cardiac intervention: Early evaluation of 12-lead electrocardiogram (ECG); consider hemodynamics for decision on cardiac intervention
- TTM: If patient is not following commands, start TTM as soon as possible; begin at 32-36°C for 24 hours by using a cooling device with feedback loop
- Other critical care management
  - Continuously monitor core temperature (esophageal, rectal, bladder)
  - Maintain normoxia, normocapnia, euglycemia
  - Provide continuous or intermittent electroencephalogram (EEG) monitoring
  - Provide lung-protective ventilation

H's and T's

Hypovolemia
Hypoxia
Hydrogen ion (acidosis)
Hypokalemia/**h**yperkalemia
Hypothermia
Tension pneumothorax
Tamponade, cardiac
Toxins
Thrombosis, pulmonary
Thrombosis, coronary

Figure 9. Adult Post–Cardiac Arrest Care Algorithm.
CT indicates computed tomography; ROSC, return of spontaneous circulation; and STEMI, ST-segment elevation myocardial infarction.

outcome, although neither study was appropriately powered for these outcomes. One trial did find improvement in cerebral oxygenation with higher MAP,[21] which is a proposed mechanism for the benefit effect of higher MAP in hypoxic ischemic encephalopathy. A recent observational study comparing outcomes in patients with MAP 70 to 90 mm Hg to those with MAP greater than 90 mm Hg also found that higher MAP was associated with better neurological outcome.[23] Although some of these data suggest targeting a MAP of 80 mm Hg or higher in those at risk for neurological injury after cardiac arrest might be beneficial, this remains unproven.

These recommendations are supported by the 2015 Guidelines Update[24] and a 2020 evidence update.[11]

Recommendations for Oxygenation and Ventilation After ROSC

COR	LOE	Recommendations
1	B-NR	1. We recommend avoiding hypoxemia in all patients who remain comatose after ROSC.
2b	B-R	2. Once reliable measurement of peripheral blood oxygen saturation is available, avoiding hyperoxemia by titrating the fraction of inspired oxygen to target an oxygen saturation of 92% to 98% may be reasonable in patients who remain comatose after ROSC.
2b	B-R	3. Maintaining the arterial partial pressure of carbon dioxide ($Paco_2$) within a normal physiological range (generally 35–45 mm Hg) may be reasonable in patients who remain comatose after ROSC.

Recommendation-Specific Supportive Text

1. In a 2020 ILCOR systematic review,[11] 1 observational study reported that hypoxemia after return of circulation was associated with worse outcome.[25] This was not seen in other studies,[26–28] and all studies were at high risk of bias. This recommendation is therefore based primarily on the physiological rationale that hypoxia increases the risk of end-organ damage, and the fact that hypoxemia is the best available surrogate for hypoxia.
2. There are some physiological basis and preclinical data for hyperoxemia leading to increased inflammation and exacerbating brain injury in postarrest patients.[29] A 2020 ILCOR systematic review[11] identified 5 RCTs comparing a titrated or lower oxygen administration strategy with usual care or a higher oxygen administration strategy in postarrest patients: 3 in the prehospital setting and 2 in the ICU setting.[8–10,30,31] Overall, these trials found no difference in clinical outcomes, but all were underpowered for these outcomes. A recent large RCT compared usual care with aggressive avoidance of hyperoxemia in mechanically ventilated critically ill patients and found no difference between groups in the overall cohort but increased survival in the intervention arm in the subgroup of 164 postarrest patients.[32] Observational data are inconsistent and very limited by confounding.[11] Three RCTs on this topic are ongoing (NCT03138005, NCT03653325, NCT03141099). The suggested range of 92% to 98% is intended as a practical approximation of the normal range.
3. Two RCTs compared a strategy of targeting high-normal $Paco_2$ (44–46 mm Hg) with one targeting low-normal $Paco_2$ (33–35 mm Hg)[31] and a strategy targeting moderate hypercapnia ($Paco_2$ 50–55 mm Hg) compared with normocapnia ($Paco_2$ 35–45 mm Hg).[33] Neither trial found a difference in any clinical outcomes. Results across 6 observational studies were inconsistent, and all studies were limited by significant risk of bias.[25,34–38] There is a large ongoing RCT addressing this question (NCT03114033).

These recommendations are supported by the 2020 CoSTR for ALS.[11]

Recommendations for Seizure Diagnosis and Management

COR	LOE	Recommendations
1	C-LD	1. We recommend treatment of clinically apparent seizures in adult post–cardiac arrest survivors.
1	C-LD	2. We recommend promptly performing and interpreting an electroencephalogram (EEG) for the diagnosis of seizures in all comatose patients after ROSC.
2b	C-LD	3. The treatment of nonconvulsive seizures (diagnosed by EEG only) may be considered.
2b	C-LD	4. The same anticonvulsant regimens used for the treatment of seizures caused by other etiologies may be considered for seizures detected after cardiac arrest.
3: No Benefit	B-R	5. Seizure prophylaxis in adult post–cardiac arrest survivors is not recommended.

Recommendation-Specific Supportive Text

1. A 2020 ILCOR systematic review[11] identified no controlled studies comparing treatment of seizures with no treatment of seizures in this population. In spite of the lack of evidence, untreated clinically apparent seizure activity is thought to be potentially harmful to the brain, and treatment of seizures is recommended in other settings[39] and likely also warranted after cardiac arrest.
2. The writing group acknowledged that there is no direct evidence that EEG to detect nonconvulsive seizures improves outcomes. This recommendation is based on the fact that nonconvulsive seizures are common in postarrest patients and that the presence of seizures may

be important prognostically, although whether treatment of nonconvulsive seizures affects outcome in this setting remains uncertain. An ILCOR systematic review done for 2020 did not specifically address the timing and method of obtaining EEGs in postarrest patients who remain unresponsive. Data on the relative benefit of continuous versus intermittent EEG are limited. One study found no difference in survival with good neurological outcome at 3 months in patients monitored with routine (one to two 20-minute EEGs over 24 hours) versus continuous (for 18–24 hours) EEG.[40]

3. Nonconvulsive seizures are common after cardiac arrest. Whether treatment of seizure activity on EEG that is not associated with clinically evident seizures affects outcome is currently unknown. A randomized trial investigating this question is ongoing (NCT02056236).
4. The 2020 CoSTR recommends that seizures be treated when diagnosed in postarrest patients.[11] No specific agent was recommended. However, the CoSTR described 2 retrospective studies suggesting valproate, levetiracetam, and fosphenytoin may all be effective, with fosphenytoin found to be associated with more hypotension in 1 study.[41,42] Common sedatives such as propofol and midazolam have also been found to be effective in suppressing seizure activity after cardiac arrest.[43–45]
5. A 2020 ILCOR systematic review[11] identified 2 RCTs comparing seizure prophylaxis with no seizure prophylaxis in comatose postarrest patients.[46,47] Neither study found any difference in occurrence of seizures or survival with favorable neurological outcome between groups.

These recommendations are supported by the 2020 CoSTR for ALS.[11]

Recommendations for Other Postresuscitation Care		
COR	**LOE**	**Recommendations**
2b	B-R	1. The benefit of any specific target range of glucose management is uncertain in adults with ROSC after cardiac arrest.
2b	B-R	2. The routine use of prophylactic antibiotics in postarrest patients is of uncertain benefit.
2b	B-R	3. The effectiveness of agents to mitigate neurological injury in patients who remain comatose after ROSC is uncertain.
2b	B-R	4. The routine use of steroids for patients with shock after ROSC is of uncertain value.

Recommendation-Specific Supportive Text

1. One small RCT from 2007,[48] found no difference in survival between strict and moderate glucose control. In the absence of other evidence specific to cardiac arrest, it seems reasonable to manage blood glucose levels in postarrest patients with the same approach used for the general critically ill population, namely using insulin therapy when needed to maintain a blood glucose of 150 to 180 mg/dL.[49]
2. A 2020 ILCOR systematic review found 2 RCTs and a small number of observational studies evaluating the effect of prophylactic antibiotics on outcomes in postarrest patients.[11,50] The RCTs found no difference in survival or neurological outcome.[51,52] One RCT[51] did find lower incidence of early pneumonia in those who received prophylactic antibiotics, but this did not translate to a difference in other outcomes. When data from the 2 RCTs were pooled, there was no overall difference in infections.[51,52]
3. The topic of neuroprotective agents was last reviewed in detail in 2010. Multiple agents, including magnesium, coenzyme Q10 (ubiquinol), exanatide, xenon gas, methylphenidate, and amantadine, have been considered as possible agents to either mitigate neurological injury or facilitate patient awakening. This work has been largely observational,[53–57] although randomized trials have been conducted on coenzyme Q10, xenon gas, and exanatide.[58–60] A small trial on the effect of coenzyme Q10 reported better survival in those receiving coenzyme Q10, but there was no significant difference in favorable neurological outcome and these findings have yet to be validated.[58] One additional coenzyme Q10 trial was recently completed but results are not yet available (NCT02934555). None of the other studies identified have been able to show a difference in any clinical outcomes with use of any of the agents studied.
4. Since this topic was last updated in detail in 2015, at least 2 randomized trials have been completed on the effect of steroids on shock and other outcomes after ROSC, only 1 of which has been published to date.[61] In this study, shock reversal and other outcomes did not differ between groups. A large retrospective observational study did find that steroid use after cardiac arrest was associated with survival.[62] Steroid use for septic shock has been evaluated extensively, with a recent trial of over 1200 patients finding improved survival in those treated with steroids.[63] A trial enrolling 3800 patients did not find a mortality benefit, although time to discharge from ICU and time to shock reversal were both shorter in the steroid group.[64] Taken together, there is no definitive evidence of benefit from steroids after ROSC. However, the data in sepsis suggest that some patients with severe shock may benefit from steroids and that

the co-occurrence of sepsis and cardiac arrest is important to consider.

Recommendation 1 last received formal evidence review in 2010 and is supported by the "Guidelines for the Use of an Insulin Infusion for the Management of Hyperglycemia in Critically Ill Patients" from the Society for Critical Care Medicine.[49] Recommendation 2 is supported by the 2020 CoSTR for ALS.[11] Recommendations 3 and 4 last received formal evidence review in 2015.[24]

REFERENCES

1. Witten L, Gardner R, Holmberg MJ, Wiberg S, Moskowitz A, Mehta S, Grossestreuer AV, Yankama T, Donnino MW, Berg KM. Reasons for death in patients successfully resuscitated from out-of-hospital and in-hospital cardiac arrest. *Resuscitation.* 2019;136:93–99. doi: 10.1016/j.resuscitation.2019.01.031
2. Laver S, Farrow C, Turner D, Nolan J. Mode of death after admission to an intensive care unit following cardiac arrest. *Intensive Care Med.* 2004;30:2126–2128. doi: 10.1007/s00134-004-2425-z
3. Panchal AR, Berg KM, Cabanas JG, Kurz MC, Link MS, Del Rios M, Hirsch KG, Chan PS, Hazinski MF, Morley PT, et al. 2019 American Heart Association focused update on systems of care: dispatcher-assisted cardiopulmonary resuscitation and cardiac arrest centers: an update to the American Heart Association Guidelines for Cardiopulmonary Resuscitation and Emergency Cardiovascular Care. *Circulation.* 2019;140:e895–e903. doi: 10.1161/CIR.0000000000000733
4. Levine GN, Bates ER, Blankenship JC, Bailey SR, Bittl JA, Cercek B, Chambers CE, Ellis SG, Guyton RA, Hollenberg SM, Khot UN, Lange RA, Mauri L, Mehran R, Moussa ID, Mukherjee D, Ting HH, O'Gara PT, Kushner FG, Ascheim DD, Brindis RG, Casey DE Jr, Chung MK, de Lemos JA, Diercks DB, Fang JC, Franklin BA, Granger CB, Krumholz HM, Linderbaum JA, Morrow DA, Newby LK, Ornato JP, Ou N, Radford MJ, Tamis-Holland JE, Tommaso CL, Tracy CM, Woo YJ, Zhao DX. 2015 ACC/AHA/SCAI Focused Update on Primary Percutaneous Coronary Intervention for Patients With ST-Elevation Myocardial Infarction: An Update of the 2011 ACCF/AHA/SCAI Guideline for Percutaneous Coronary Intervention and the 2013 ACCF/AHA Guideline for the Management of ST-Elevation Myocardial Infarction. *Circulation.* 2016;133:1135–1147. doi: 10.1161/CIR.0000000000000336
5. Stær-Jensen H, Nakstad ER, Fossum E, Mangschau A, Eritsland J, Draegni T, Jacobsen D, Sunde K, Andersen GO. Post-resuscitation ECG for selection of patients for immediate coronary angiography in out-of-hospital cardiac arrest. *Circ Cardiovasc Interv.* 2015;8 doi: 10.1161/CIRCINTERVENTIONS.115.002784
6. Zanuttini D, Armellini I, Nucifora G, Grillo MT, Morocutti G, Carchietti E, Trillò G, Spedicato L, Bernardi G, Proclemer A. Predictive value of electrocardiogram in diagnosing acute coronary artery lesions among patients with out-of-hospital-cardiac-arrest. *Resuscitation.* 2013;84:1250–1254. doi: 10.1016/j.resuscitation.2013.04.023
7. Sideris G, Voicu S, Dillinger JG, Stratiev V, Logeart D, Broche C, Vivien B, Brun PY, Deye N, Capan D, Aout M, Megarbane B, Baud FJ, Henry P. Value of post-resuscitation electrocardiogram in the diagnosis of acute myocardial infarction in out-of-hospital cardiac arrest patients. *Resuscitation.* 2011;82:1148–1153. doi: 10.1016/j.resuscitation.2011.04.023
8. Kuisma M, Boyd J, Voipio V, Alaspää A, Roine RO, Rosenberg P. Comparison of 30 and the 100% inspired oxygen concentrations during early post-resuscitation period: a randomised controlled pilot study. *Resuscitation.* 2006;69:199–206. doi: 10.1016/j.resuscitation.2005.08.010
9. Bray JE, Hein C, Smith K, Stephenson M, Grantham H, Finn J, Stub D, Cameron P, Bernard S; EXACT Investigators. Oxygen titration after resuscitation from out-of-hospital cardiac arrest: A multi-centre, randomised controlled pilot study (the EXACT pilot trial). *Resuscitation.* 2018;128:211–215. doi: 10.1016/j.resuscitation.2018.04.019
10. Thomas M, Voss S, Benger J, Kirby K, Nolan JP. Cluster randomised comparison of the effectiveness of 100% oxygen versus titrated oxygen in patients with a sustained return of spontaneous circulation following out of hospital cardiac arrest: a feasibility study. PROXY: post ROSC OXYgenation study. *BMC Emerg Med.* 2019;19:16. doi: 10.1186/s12873-018-0214-1
11. Berg KM, Soar J, Andersen LW, Böttiger BW, Cacciola S, Callaway CW, Couper K, Cronberg T, D'Arrigo S, Deakin CD, et al; on behalf of the Adult Advanced Life Support Collaborators. Adult advanced life support: 2020 International Consensus on Cardiopulmonary Resuscitation and Emergency Cardiovascular Care Science With Treatment Recommendations. *Circulation.* 2020;142(suppl 1):S92–S139. doi: 10.1161/CIR.0000000000000893
12. Soar J, Nolan JP, Böttiger BW, Perkins GD, Lott C, Carli P, Pellis T, Sandroni C, Skrifvars MB, Smith GB, Sunde K, Deakin CD; Adult advanced life support section Collaborators. European Resuscitation Council Guidelines for Resuscitation 2015: Section 3. Adult advanced life support. *Resuscitation.* 2015;95:100–147. doi: 10.1016/j.resuscitation.2015.07.016
13. Trzeciak S, Jones AE, Kilgannon JH, Milcarek B, Hunter K, Shapiro NI, Hollenberg SM, Dellinger P, Parrillo JE. Significance of arterial hypotension after resuscitation from cardiac arrest. *Crit Care Med.* 2009;37:2895–903; quiz 2904. doi: 10.1097/ccm.0b013e3181b01d8c
14. Chiu YK, Lui CT, Tsui KL. Impact of hypotension after return of spontaneous circulation on survival in patients of out-of-hospital cardiac arrest. *Am J Emerg Med.* 2018;36:79–83. doi: 10.1016/j.ajem.2017.07.019
15. Bray JE, Bernard S, Cantwell K, Stephenson M, Smith K; and the VACAR Steering Committee. The association between systolic blood pressure on arrival at hospital and outcome in adults surviving from out-of-hospital cardiac arrests of presumed cardiac aetiology. *Resuscitation.* 2014;85:509–515. doi: 10.1016/j.resuscitation.2013.12.005
16. Russo JJ, Di Santo P, Simard T, James TE, Hibbert B, Couture E, Marbach J, Osborne C, Ramirez FD, Wells GA, Labinaz M, Le May MR; from the CAPITAL study group. Optimal mean arterial pressure in comatose survivors of out-of-hospital cardiac arrest: An analysis of area below blood pressure thresholds. *Resuscitation.* 2018;128:175–180. doi: 10.1016/j.resuscitation.2018.04.028
17. Laurikkala J, Wilkman E, Pettilä V, Kurola J, Reinikainen M, Hoppu S, Ala-Kokko T, Tallgren M, Tiainen M, Vaahersalo J, Varpula T, Skrifvars MB; FINNRESUSCI Study Group. Mean arterial pressure and vasopressor load after out-of-hospital cardiac arrest: Associations with one-year neurologic outcome. *Resuscitation.* 2016;105:116–122. doi: 10.1016/j.resuscitation.2016.05.026
18. Annoni F, Dell'Anna AM, Franchi F, Creteur J, Scolletta S, Vincent JL, Taccone FS. The impact of diastolic blood pressure values on the neurological outcome of cardiac arrest patients. *Resuscitation.* 2018;130:167–173. doi: 10.1016/j.resuscitation.2018.07.017
19. Janiczek JA, Winger DG, Coppler P, Sabedra AR, Murray H, Pinsky MR, Rittenberger JC, Reynolds JC, Dezfulian C. Hemodynamic Resuscitation Characteristics Associated with Improved Survival and Shock Resolution After Cardiac Arrest. *Shock.* 2016;45:613–619. doi: 10.1097/SHK.0000000000000554
20. Young MN, Hollenbeck RD, Pollock JS, Giuseffi JL, Wang L, Harrell FE, McPherson JA. Higher achieved mean arterial pressure during therapeutic hypothermia is not associated with neurologically intact survival following cardiac arrest. *Resuscitation.* 2015;88:158–164. doi: 10.1016/j.resuscitation.2014.12.008
21. Ameloot K, De Deyne C, Eertmans W, Ferdinande B, Dupont M, Palmers PJ, Petit T, Nuyens P, Maeremans J, Vundelinckx J, Vanhaverbeke M, Belmans A, Peeters R, Demaerel P, Lemmens R, Dens J, Janssens S. Early goal-directed haemodynamic optimization of cerebral oxygenation in comatose survivors after cardiac arrest: the Neuroprotect post-cardiac arrest trial. *Eur Heart J.* 2019;40:1804–1814. doi: 10.1093/eurheartj/ehz120
22. Jakkula P, Pettilä V, Skrifvars MB, Hästbacka J, Loisa P, Tiainen M, Wilkman E, Toppila J, Koskue T, Bendel S, Birkelund T, Laru-Sompa R, Valkonen M, Reinikainen M; COMACARE study group. Targeting low-normal or high-normal mean arterial pressure after cardiac arrest and resuscitation: a randomised pilot trial. *Intensive Care Med.* 2018;44:2091–2101. doi: 10.1007/s00134-018-5446-8
23. Roberts BW, Kilgannon JH, Hunter BR, Puskarich MA, Shea L, Donnino M, Jones C, Fuller BM, Kline JA, Jones AE, Shapiro NI, Abella BS, Trzeciak S. Association Between Elevated Mean Arterial Blood Pressure and Neurologic Outcome After Resuscitation From Cardiac Arrest: Results From a Multicenter Prospective Cohort Study. *Crit Care Med.* 2019;47:93–100. doi: 10.1097/CCM.0000000000003474
24. Callaway CW, Donnino MW, Fink EL, Geocadin RG, Golan E, Kern KB, Leary M, Meurer WJ, Peberdy MA, Thompson TM, et al. Part 8: post–cardiac arrest care: 2015 American Heart Association Guidelines Update for Cardiopulmonary Resuscitation and Emergency Cardiovascular Care. *Circulation.* 2015;132(suppl 2):S465–482. doi: 10.1161/cir.0000000000000262

25. Wang HE, Prince DK, Drennan IR, Grunau B, Carlbom DJ, Johnson N, Hansen M, Elmer J, Christenson J, Kudenchuk P, Aufderheide T, Weisfeldt M, Idris A, Trzeciak S, Kurz M, Rittenberger JC, Griffiths D, Jasti J, May S; Resuscitation Outcomes Consortium (ROC) Investigators. Post-resuscitation arterial oxygen and carbon dioxide and outcomes after out-of-hospital cardiac arrest. *Resuscitation.* 2017;120:113–118. doi: 10.1016/j.resuscitation.2017.08.244
26. Ebner F, Ullén S, Åneman A, Cronberg T, Mattsson N, Friberg H, Hassager C, Kjærgaard J, Kuiper M, Pelosi P, Undén J, Wise MP, Wetterslev J, Nielsen N. Associations between partial pressure of oxygen and neurological outcome in out-of-hospital cardiac arrest patients: an explorative analysis of a randomized trial. *Crit Care.* 2019;23:30. doi: 10.1186/s13054-019-2322-z
27. Humaloja J, Litonius E, Efendijev I, Folger D, Raj R, Pekkarinen PT, Skrifvars MB. Early hyperoxemia is not associated with cardiac arrest outcome. *Resuscitation.* 2019;140:185–193. doi: 10.1016/j.resuscitation.2019.04.035
28. Johnson NJ, Dodampahala K, Rosselot B, Perman SM, Mikkelsen ME, Goyal M, Gaieski DF, Grossestreuer AV. The Association Between Arterial Oxygen Tension and Neurological Outcome After Cardiac Arrest. *Ther Hypothermia Temp Manag.* 2017;7:36–41. doi: 10.1089/ther.2016.0015
29. Pilcher J, Weatherall M, Shirtcliffe P, Bellomo R, Young P, Beasley R. The effect of hyperoxia following cardiac arrest - A systematic review and meta-analysis of animal trials. *Resuscitation.* 2012;83:417–422. doi: 10.1016/j.resuscitation.2011.12.021
30. Young P, Bailey M, Bellomo R, Bernard S, Dicker B, Freebairn R, Henderson S, Mackle D, McArthur C, McGuinness S, Smith T, Swain A, Weatherall M, Beasley R. HyperOxic Therapy OR NormOxic Therapy after out-of-hospital cardiac arrest (HOT OR NOT): a randomised controlled feasibility trial. *Resuscitation.* 2014;85:1686–1691. doi: 10.1016/j.resuscitation.2014.09.011
31. Jakkula P, Reinikainen M, Hästbacka J, Loisa P, Tiainen M, Pettilä V, Toppila J, Lähde M, Bäcklund M, Okkonen M, et al; and the COMACARE study group. Targeting two different levels of both arterial carbon dioxide and arterial oxygen after cardiac arrest and resuscitation: a randomised pilot trial. *Intensive Care Med.* 2018;44:2112–2121. doi: 10.1007/s00134-018-5453-9
32. Mackle D, Bellomo R, Bailey M, Beasley R, Deane A, Eastwood G, Finfer S, Freebairn R, King V, Linke N, et al; and the ICU-ROX Investigators the Australian New Zealand Intensive Care Society Clinical Trials Group. Conservative oxygen therapy during mechanical ventilation in the ICU. *N Engl J Med.* 2020;382:989–998. doi: 10.1056/NEJMoa1903297
33. Eastwood GM, Schneider AG, Suzuki S, Peck L, Young H, Tanaka A, Mårtensson J, Warrillow S, McGuinness S, Parke R, Gilder E, Mccarthy L, Galt P, Taori G, Eliott S, Lamac T, Bailey M, Harley N, Barge D, Hodgson CL, Morganti-Kossmann MC, Pébay A, Conquest A, Archer JS, Bernard S, Stub D, Hart GK, Bellomo R. Targeted therapeutic mild hypercapnia after cardiac arrest: A phase II multi-centre randomised controlled trial (the CCC trial). *Resuscitation.* 2016;104:83–90. doi: 10.1016/j.resuscitation.2016.03.023
34. Vaahersalo J, Bendel S, Reinikainen M, Kurola J, Tiainen M, Raj R, Pettilä V, Varpula T, Skrifvars MB; FINNRESUSCI Study Group. Arterial blood gas tensions after resuscitation from out-of-hospital cardiac arrest: associations with long-term neurologic outcome. *Crit Care Med.* 2014;42:1463–1470. doi: 10.1097/CCM.0000000000000228
35. Hope Kilgannon J, Hunter BR, Puskarich MA, Shea L, Fuller BM, Jones C, Donnino M, Kline JA, Jones AE, Shapiro NI, Abella BS, Trzeciak S, Roberts BW. Partial pressure of arterial carbon dioxide after resuscitation from cardiac arrest and neurological outcome: A prospective multi-center protocol-directed cohort study. *Resuscitation.* 2019;135:212–220. doi: 10.1016/j.resuscitation.2018.11.015
36. Roberts BW, Kilgannon JH, Chansky ME, Mittal N, Wooden J, Trzeciak S. Association between postresuscitation partial pressure of arterial carbon dioxide and neurological outcome in patients with post-cardiac arrest syndrome. *Circulation.* 2013;127:2107–2113. doi: 10.1161/CIRCULATIONAHA.112.000168
37. von Auenmueller KI, Christ M, Sasko BM, Trappe HJ. The Value of Arterial Blood Gas Parameters for Prediction of Mortality in Survivors of Out-of-hospital Cardiac Arrest. *J Emerg Trauma Shock.* 2017;10:134–139. doi: 10.4103/JETS.JETS_146_16
38. Ebner F, Harmon MBA, Aneman A, Cronberg T, Friberg H, Hassager C, Juffermans N, Kjærgaard J, Kuiper M, Mattsson N, Pelosi P, Ullén S, Undén J, Wise MP, Nielsen N. Carbon dioxide dynamics in relation to neurological outcome in resuscitated out-of-hospital cardiac arrest patients: an exploratory Target Temperature Management Trial substudy. *Crit Care.* 2018;22:196. doi: 10.1186/s13054-018-2119-5
39. Glauser T, Shinnar S, Gloss D, Alldredge B, Arya R, Bainbridge J, Bare M, Bleck T, Dodson WE, Garrity L, Jagoda A, Lowenstein D, Pellock J, Riviello J, Sloan E, Treiman DM. Evidence-Based Guideline: Treatment of Convulsive Status Epilepticus in Children and Adults: Report of the Guideline Committee of the American Epilepsy Society. *Epilepsy Curr.* 2016;16:48–61. doi: 10.5698/1535-7597-16.1.48
40. Fatuzzo D, Beuchat I, Alvarez V, Novy J, Oddo M, Rossetti AO. Does continuous EEG influence prognosis in patients after cardiac arrest? *Resuscitation.* 2018;132:29–32. doi: 10.1016/j.resuscitation.2018.08.023
41. Solanki P, Coppler PJ, Kvaløy JT, Baldwin MA, Callaway CW, Elmer J; Pittsburgh Post-Cardiac Arrest Service. Association of antiepileptic drugs with resolution of epileptiform activity after cardiac arrest. *Resuscitation.* 2019;142:82–90. doi: 10.1016/j.resuscitation.2019.07.007
42. Kapur J, Elm J, Chamberlain JM, Barsan W, Cloyd J, Lowenstein D, Shinnar S, Conwit R, Meinzer C, Cock H, Fountain N, Connor JT, Silbergleit R; NETT and PECARN Investigators. Randomized Trial of Three Anticonvulsant Medications for Status Epilepticus. *N Engl J Med.* 2019;381:2103–2113. doi: 10.1056/NEJMoa1905795
43. Thömke F, Weilemann SL. Poor prognosis despite successful treatment of postanoxic generalized myoclonus. *Neurology.* 2010;74:1392–1394. doi: 10.1212/WNL.0b013e3181dad5b9
44. Aicua RI, Rapun I, Novy J, Solari D, Oddo M, Rossetti AO. Early Lance-Adams syndrome after cardiac arrest: prevalence, time to return to awareness, and outcome in a large cohort. *Resuscitation.* 2017;115:169–172. doi: 10.1016/j.resuscitation.2017.03.020
45. Koutroumanidis M, Sakellariou D. Low frequency nonevolving generalized periodic epileptiform discharges and the borderland of hypoxic nonconvulsive status epilepticus in comatose patients after cardiac arrest. *Epilepsy Behav.* 2015;49:255–262. doi: 10.1016/j.yebeh.2015.04.060
46. Brain Resuscitation Clinical Trial I Study Group. Randomized clinical study of thiopental loading in comatose survivors of cardiac arrest. *N Engl J Med.* 1986;314:397–403. doi: 10.1056/nejm198602133140701
47. Longstreth WT Jr, Fahrenbruch CE, Olsufka M, Walsh TR, Copass MK, Cobb LA. Randomized clinical trial of magnesium, diazepam, or both after out-of-hospital cardiac arrest. *Neurology.* 2002;59:506–514. doi: 10.1212/wnl.59.4.506
48. Oksanen T, Skrifvars MB, Varpula T, Kuitunen A, Pettilä V, Nurmi J, Castrén M. Strict versus moderate glucose control after resuscitation from ventricular fibrillation. *Intensive Care Med.* 2007;33:2093–2100. doi: 10.1007/s00134-007-0876-8
49. Jacobi J, Bircher N, Krinsley J, Agus M, Braithwaite SS, Deutschman C, Freire AX, Geehan D, Kohl B, Nasraway SA, Rigby M, Sands K, Schallom L, Taylor B, Umpierrez G, Mazuski J, Schunemann H. Guidelines for the use of an insulin infusion for the management of hyperglycemia in critically ill patients. *Crit Care Med.* 2012;40:3251–3276. doi: 10.1097/CCM.0b013e3182653269
50. Couper K, Laloo R, Field R, Perkins GD, Thomas M, Yeung J. Prophylactic antibiotic use following cardiac arrest: A systematic review and meta-analysis. *Resuscitation.* 2019;141:166–173. doi: 10.1016/j.resuscitation.2019.04.047
51. François B, Cariou A, Clere-Jehl R, Dequin PF, Renon-Carron F, Daix T, Guitton C, Deye N, Legriel S, Plantefève G, Quenot JP, Desachy A, Kamel T, Bedon-Carte S, Diehl JL, Chudeau N, Karam E, Durand-Zaleski I, Giraudeau B, Vignon P, Le Gouge A; CRICS-TRIGGERSEP Network and the ANTHARTIC Study Group. Prevention of Early Ventilator-Associated Pneumonia after Cardiac Arrest. *N Engl J Med.* 2019;381:1831–1842. doi: 10.1056/NEJMoa1812379
52. Ribaric SF, Turel M, Knafelj R, Gorjup V, Stanic R, Gradisek P, Cerovic O, Mirkovic T, Noc M. Prophylactic versus clinically-driven antibiotics in comatose survivors of out-of-hospital cardiac arrest-A randomized pilot study. *Resuscitation.* 2017;111:103–109. doi: 10.1016/j.resuscitation.2016.11.025
53. Pearce A, Lockwood C, van den Heuvel C, Pearce J. The use of therapeutic magnesium for neuroprotection during global cerebral ischemia associated with cardiac arrest and cardiac surgery in adults: a systematic review. *JBI Database System Rev Implement Rep.* 2017;15:86–118. doi: 10.11124/JBISRIR-2016-003236
54. Perucki WH, Hiendlmayr B, O'Sullivan DM, Gunaseelan AC, Fayas F, Fernandez AB. Magnesium Levels and Neurologic Outcomes in Patients Undergoing Therapeutic Hypothermia After Cardiac Arrest. *Ther Hypothermia Temp Manag.* 2018;8:14–17. doi: 10.1089/ther.2017.0016
55. Suzuki M, Hatakeyama T, Nakamura R, Saiki T, Kamisasanuki T, Sugiki D, Matsushima H. Serum Magnesium Levels and Neurological Outcomes in Patients Undergoing Targeted Temperature Management After Cardiac Arrest. *J Emerg Nurs.* 2020;46:59–65. doi: 10.1016/j.jen.2019.10.006
56. Cocchi MN, Giberson B, Berg K, Salciccioli JD, Naini A, Buettner C, Akuthota P, Gautam S, Donnino MW. Coenzyme Q10 levels are low and

associated with increased mortality in post-cardiac arrest patients. *Resuscitation.* 2012;83:991–995. doi: 10.1016/j.resuscitation.2012.03.023
57. Reynolds JC, Rittenberger JC, Callaway CW. Methylphenidate and amantadine to stimulate reawakening in comatose patients resuscitated from cardiac arrest. *Resuscitation.* 2013;84:818–824. doi: 10.1016/j.resuscitation.2012.11.014
58. Damian MS, Ellenberg D, Gildemeister R, Lauermann J, Simonis G, Sauter W, Georgi C. Coenzyme Q10 combined with mild hypothermia after cardiac arrest: a preliminary study. *Circulation.* 2004;110:3011–3016. doi: 10.1161/01.CIR.0000146894.45533.C2
59. Laitio R, Hynninen M, Arola O, Virtanen S, Parkkola R, Saunavaara J, Roine RO, Grönlund J, Ylikoski E, Wennervirta J, Bäcklund M, Silvasti P, Nukarinen E, Tiainen M, Saraste A, Pietilä M, Airaksinen J, Valanne L, Martola J, Silvennoinen H, Scheinin H, Harjola VP, Niiranen J, Korpi K, Varpula M, Inkinen O, Olkkola KT, Maze M, Vahlberg T, Laitio T. Effect of Inhaled Xenon on Cerebral White Matter Damage in Comatose Survivors of Out-of-Hospital Cardiac Arrest: A Randomized Clinical Trial. *JAMA.* 2016;315:1120–1128. doi: 10.1001/jama.2016.1933
60. Wiberg S, Hassager C, Schmidt H, Thomsen JH, Frydland M, Lindholm MG, Høfsten DE, Engstrøm T, Køber L, Møller JE, Kjaergaard J. Neuroprotective Effects of the Glucagon-Like Peptide-1 Analog Exenatide After Out-of-Hospital Cardiac Arrest: A Randomized Controlled Trial. *Circulation.* 2016;134:2115–2124. doi: 10.1161/CIRCULATIONAHA.116.024088
61. Donnino MW, Andersen LW, Berg KM, Chase M, Sherwin R, Smithline H, Carney E, Ngo L, Patel PV, Liu X, Cutlip D, Zimetbaum P, Cocchi MN; Collaborating Authors from the Beth Israel Deaconess Medical Center's Center for Resuscitation Science Research Group. Corticosteroid therapy in refractory shock following cardiac arrest: a randomized, double-blind, placebo-controlled, trial. *Crit Care.* 2016;20:82. doi: 10.1186/s13054-016-1257-x
62. Tsai MS, Chuang PY, Huang CH, Tang CH, Yu PH, Chang WT, Chen WJ. Postarrest Steroid Use May Improve Outcomes of Cardiac Arrest Survivors. *Crit Care Med.* 2019;47:167–175. doi: 10.1097/CCM.0000000000003468
63. Annane D, Renault A, Brun-Buisson C, Megarbane B, Quenot JP, Siami S, Cariou A, Forceville X, Schwebel C, Martin C, Timsit JF, Misset B, Ali Benali M, Colin G, Souweine B, Asehnoune K, Mercier E, Chimot L, Charpentier C, François B, Boulain T, Petitpas F, Constantin JM, Dhonneur G, Baudin F, Combes A, Bohé J, Loriferne JF, Amathieu R, Cook F, Slama M, Leroy O, Capellier G, Dargent A, Hissem T, Maxime V, Bellissant E; CRICS-TRIGGERSEP Network. Hydrocortisone plus Fludrocortisone for Adults with Septic Shock. *N Engl J Med.* 2018;378:809–818. doi: 10.1056/NEJMoa1705716
64. Venkatesh B, Finfer S, Cohen J, Rajbhandari D, Arabi Y, Bellomo R, Billot L, Correa M, Glass P, Harward M, et al; on behalf of the ADRENAL Trial Investigators and the Australian–New Zealand Intensive Care Society Clinical Trials Group. Adjunctive glucocorticoid therapy in patients with septic shock. *N Engl J Med.* 2018;378:797–808. doi: 10.1056/NEJMoa1705835

Targeted Temperature Management

Introduction

TTM between 32°C and 36°C for at least 24 hours is currently recommended for all cardiac rhythms in both OHCA and IHCA. Multiple randomized trials have been performed in various domains of TTM and were summarized in a systematic review published in 2015.[1] Subsequent to the 2015 recommendations, additional randomized trials have evaluated TTM for nonshockable rhythms as well as TTM duration. Many of these were reviewed in an evidence update provided in the 2020 COSTR for ALS.[2] Many uncertainties within the topic of TTM remain, including whether temperature should vary on the basis of patient characteristics, how long TTM should be maintained, and how quickly it should be started. An updated systematic review on several aspects of this important topic is needed once currently ongoing clinical trials have been completed.

Recommendations for Indications for TTM		
COR	**LOE**	**Recommendations**
1	B-R	1. We recommend TTM for adults who do not follow commands after ROSC from OHCA with any initial rhythm.
1	B-R	2. We recommend TTM for adults who do not follow commands after ROSC from IHCA with initial nonshockable rhythm.
1	B-NR	3. We recommend TTM for adults who do not follow commands after ROSC from IHCA with initial shockable rhythm.

Recommendation-Specific Supportive Text

1. Two RCTs of patients with OHCA with an initially shockable rhythm published in 2002 reported benefit from mild hypothermia when compared with no temperature management.[1,3,4] A more recent trial comparing a target temperature of 33°C to 37°C in patients (IHCA and OHCA) with initial nonshockable rhythm also found better outcomes in those treated with a temperature of 33°C.[5] A large trial is currently underway testing TTM compared with normothermia (NCT03114033).
2. An RCT published in 2019 compared TTM at 33°C to 37°C for patients who were not following commands after ROSC from cardiac arrest with initial nonshockable rhythm. Survival with a favorable neurological outcome (Cerebral Performance Category 1–2) was higher in the group treated with 33°C.[5] This trial included both OHCA and IHCA and is the first randomized trial on TTM after cardiac arrest to include IHCA patients. In a subgroup analysis, the benefit of TTM did not appear to differ significantly by IHCA/OHCA subgroups.
3. No RCTs of TTM have included IHCA patients with an initial shockable rhythm, and this recommendation is therefore based largely on extrapolation from OHCA studies and the study of patients with initially nonshockable rhythms that included IHCA patients. Observational studies on TTM for IHCA with any initial rhythm have reported mixed results. Two studies that included patients enrolled in the AHA Get With The Guidelines-Resuscitation registry reported either no benefit or worse outcome from TTM.[6,7] Both were limited by very low overall usage of TTM in the registry and lack of data on presence of coma, making it difficult to determine if TTM was indicated for a given IHCA patient.

This topic last received formal evidence review in 2015,[8] with an evidence update conducted for the 2020 CoSTR for ALS.[2]

Recommendations for Performance of TTM		
COR	LOE	Recommendations
1	B-R	1. We recommend selecting and maintaining a constant temperature between 32°C and 36°C during TTM.
2a	B-NR	2. It is reasonable that TTM be maintained for at least 24 h after achieving target temperature.
2b	C-LD	3. It may be reasonable to actively prevent fever in comatose patients after TTM.
3: No Benefit	A	4. We do not recommend the routine use of rapid infusion of cold IV fluids for prehospital cooling of patients after ROSC.

Recommendation-Specific Supportive Text

1. In 2013, a trial of over 900 patients compared TTM at 33°C to 36°C for patients with OHCA and any initial rhythm, excluding unwitnessed asystole, and found that 33°C was not superior to 36°C.[9] A more recent trial compared 33°C to 37°C for patients with ROSC after initial nonshockable rhythm and found improved survival with favorable neurological outcome in the group treated with 33°C.[5] There have been reports of decreasing utilization of TTM in recent years, with one hypothesis being that some clinicians interpret the inclusion of 36°C as a target temperature as being equivalent to normothermia, or no strict temperature control.[10] An updated systematic review is needed on the question of which target temperature is most beneficial. Based on the available evidence, however, TTM at a temp between 32°C and 36°C remains a Class 1 recommendation.
2. One RCT including 355 patients found no difference in outcome between TTM for 24 and 48 hours.[11] This study may have been underpowered to detect differences in clinical outcomes. The initial 2002 trials cooled patients for 12[3] and 24 hours[4] while the 2013 trial used 28 hours.[9] A larger, adaptive clinical trial is currently underway investigating multiple different durations of hypothermia ranging from 6 to 72 hours, using a target temperature of 33°C for all patients enrolled (NCT04217551). There is no clear best approach to rewarming after TTM, although a protocol of 0.5°C per hour was followed in the 2013 trial.[9] The optimal rate of rewarming, and specifically whether slower rates are beneficial, is a knowledge gap, and at least 1 trial is ongoing (NCT02555254).
3. Fever after ROSC is associated with poor neurological outcome in patients not treated with TTM, although this finding is reported less consistently in patients treated with TTM.[12–20] It has not been established whether treatment of fever is associated with an improvement in outcome, but treatment or prevention of fever appears to be a reasonable approach.
4. A 2015 systematic review found that prehospital cooling with the specific method of the rapid infusion of cold IV fluids was associated with more pulmonary edema and a higher risk of rearrest.[1] Since this review, a number of RCTs on prehospital cooling have been conducted. One trial compared the prehospital induction of hypothermia with any method (including ice packs and cold IV fluids) with no prehospital cooling, and found higher receipt of in-hospital TTM in those who had prehospital initiation. That trial found no increased adverse events in those treated with prehospital cooling.[21] Other methods of prehospital cooling, such as esophageal or nasal devices, have also been investigated; whether these affect outcomes is a knowledge gap.

This topic last received formal evidence review in 2015,[8] with an evidence update conducted for the 2020 CoSTR for ALS.[2]

REFERENCES

1. Donnino MW, Andersen LW, Berg KM, Reynolds JC, Nolan JP, Morley PT, Lang E, Cocchi MN, Xanthos T, Callaway CW, Soar J; ILCOR ALS Task Force. Temperature Management After Cardiac Arrest: An Advisory Statement by the Advanced Life Support Task Force of the International Liaison Committee on Resuscitation and the American Heart Association Emergency Cardiovascular Care Committee and the Council on Cardiopulmonary, Critical Care, Perioperative and Resuscitation. *Circulation*. 2015;132:2448–2456. doi: 10.1161/CIR.0000000000000313
2. Berg KM, Soar J, Andersen LW, Böttiger BW, Cacciola S, Callaway CW, Couper K, Cronberg T, D'Arrigo S, Deakin CD, et al; on behalf of the Adult Advanced Life Support Collaborators. Adult advanced life support: 2020 International Consensus on Cardiopulmonary Resuscitation and Emergency Cardiovascular Care Science With Treatment Recommendations. *Circulation*. 2020;142(suppl 1):S92–S139. doi: 10.1161/CIR.0000000000000893
3. Bernard SA, Gray TW, Buist MD, Jones BM, Silvester W, Gutteridge G, Smith K. Treatment of comatose survivors of out-of-hospital cardiac arrest with induced hypothermia. *N Engl J Med*. 2002;346:557–563. doi: 10.1056/NEJMoa003289
4. Hypothermia after Cardiac Arrest Study Group. Mild therapeutic hypothermia to improve the neurologic outcome after cardiac arrest. *N Engl J Med*. 2002;346:549–556. doi: 10.1056/NEJMoa012689
5. Lascarrou JB, Merdji H, Le Gouge A, Colin G, Grillet G, Girardie P, Coupez E, Dequin PF, Cariou A, Boulain T, Brule N, Frat JP, Asfar P, Pichon N, Landais M, Plantefeve G, Quenot JP, Chakarian JC, Sirodot M, Legriel S, Letheulle J, Thevenin D, Desachy A, Delahaye A, Botoc V, Vimeux S, Martino F, Giraudeau B, Reignier J; CRICS-TRIGGERSEP Group. Targeted Temperature Management for Cardiac Arrest with Nonshockable Rhythm. *N Engl J Med*. 2019;381:2327–2337. doi: 10.1056/NEJMoa1906661
6. Nichol G, Huszti E, Kim F, Fly D, Parnia S, Donnino M, Sorenson T, Callaway CW; American Heart Association Get With the Guideline-Resuscitation Investigators. Does induction of hypothermia improve outcomes after in-hospital cardiac arrest? *Resuscitation*. 2013;84:620–625. doi: 10.1016/j.resuscitation.2012.12.009
7. Chan PS, Berg RA, Tang Y, Curtis LH, Spertus JA; American Heart Association's Get With the Guidelines–Resuscitation Investigators. Association Between Therapeutic Hypothermia and Survival After In-Hospital Cardiac Arrest. *JAMA*. 2016;316:1375–1382. doi: 10.1001/jama.2016.14380

8. Callaway CW, Donnino MW, Fink EL, Geocadin RG, Golan E, Kern KB, Leary M, Meurer WJ, Peberdy MA, Thompson TM, et al. Part 8: post–cardiac arrest care: 2015 American Heart Association Guidelines Update for Cardiopulmonary Resuscitation and Emergency Cardiovascular Care. *Circulation*. 2015;132(suppl 2):S465–482. doi: 10.1161/cir.0000000000000262
9. Nielsen N, Wetterslev J, Cronberg T, Erlinge D, Gasche Y, Hassager C, Horn J, Hovdenes J, Kjaergaard J, Kuiper M, Pellis T, Stammet P, Wanscher M, Wise MP, Åneman A, Al-Subaie N, Boesgaard S, Bro-Jeppesen J, Brunetti I, Bugge JF, Hingston CD, Juffermans NP, Koopmans M, Køber L, Langørgen J, Lilja G, Møller JE, Rundgren M, Rylander C, Smid O, Werer C, Winkel P, Friberg H; TTM Trial Investigators. Targeted temperature management at 33°C versus 36°C after cardiac arrest. *N Engl J Med*. 2013;369:2197–2206. doi: 10.1056/NEJMoa1310519
10. Khera R, Humbert A, Leroux B, Nichol G, Kudenchuk P, Scales D, Baker A, Austin M, Newgard CD, Radecki R, Vilke GM, Sawyer KN, Sopko G, Idris AH, Wang H, Chan PS, Kurz MC. Hospital Variation in the Utilization and Implementation of Targeted Temperature Management in Out-of-Hospital Cardiac Arrest. *Circ Cardiovasc Qual Outcomes*. 2018;11:e004829. doi: 10.1161/CIRCOUTCOMES.118.004829
11. Kirkegaard H, Søreide E, de Haas I, Pettilä V, Taccone FS, Arus U, Storm C, Hassager C, Nielsen JF, Sørensen CA, Ilkjær S, Jeppesen AN, Grejs AM, Duez CHV, Hjort J, Larsen AI, Toome V, Tiainen M, Hästbacka J, Laitio T, Skrifvars MB. Targeted Temperature Management for 48 vs 24 Hours and Neurologic Outcome After Out-of-Hospital Cardiac Arrest: A Randomized Clinical Trial. *JAMA*. 2017;318:341–350. doi: 10.1001/jama.2017.8978
12. Nolan JP, Laver SR, Welch CA, Harrison DA, Gupta V, Rowan K. Outcome following admission to UK intensive care units after cardiac arrest: a secondary analysis of the ICNARC Case Mix Programme Database. *Anaesthesia*. 2007;62:1207–1216. doi: 10.1111/j.1365-2044.2007.05232.x
13. Langhelle A, Tyvold SS, Lexow K, Hapnes SA, Sunde K, Steen PA. In-hospital factors associated with improved outcome after out-of-hospital cardiac arrest. A comparison between four regions in Norway. *Resuscitation*. 2003;56:247–263. doi: 10.1016/s0300-9572(02)00409-4
14. Suffoletto B, Peberdy MA, van der Hoek T, Callaway C. Body temperature changes are associated with outcomes following in-hospital cardiac arrest and return of spontaneous circulation. *Resuscitation*. 2009;80:1365–1370. doi: 10.1016/j.resuscitation.2009.08.020
15. Gebhardt K, Guyette FX, Doshi AA, Callaway CW, Rittenberger JC; Post Cardiac Arrest Service. Prevalence and effect of fever on outcome following resuscitation from cardiac arrest. *Resuscitation*. 2013;84:1062–1067. doi: 10.1016/j.resuscitation.2013.03.038
16. Benz-Woerner J, Delodder F, Benz R, Cueni-Villoz N, Feihl F, Rossetti AO, Liaudet L, Oddo M. Body temperature regulation and outcome after cardiac arrest and therapeutic hypothermia. *Resuscitation*. 2012;83:338–342. doi: 10.1016/j.resuscitation.2011.10.026
17. Leary M, Grossestreuer AV, Iannacone S, Gonzalez M, Shofer FS, Povey C, Wendell G, Archer SE, Gaieski DF, Abella BS. Pyrexia and neurologic outcomes after therapeutic hypothermia for cardiac arrest. *Resuscitation*. 2013;84:1056–1061. doi: 10.1016/j.resuscitation.2012.11.003
18. Cocchi MN, Boone MD, Giberson B, Giberson T, Farrell E, Salciccioli JD, Talmor D, Williams D, Donnino MW. Fever after rewarming: incidence of pyrexia in postcardiac arrest patients who have undergone mild therapeutic hypothermia. *J Intensive Care Med*. 2014;29:365–369. doi: 10.1177/0885066613491932
19. Bro-Jeppesen J, Hassager C, Wanscher M, Søholm H, Thomsen JH, Lippert FK, Møller JE, Køber L, Kjaergaard J. Post-hypothermia fever is associated with increased mortality after out-of-hospital cardiac arrest. *Resuscitation*. 2013;84:1734–1740. doi: 10.1016/j.resuscitation.2013.07.023
20. Winters SA, Wolf KH, Kettinger SA, Seif EK, Jones JS, Bacon-Baguley T. Assessment of risk factors for post-rewarming "rebound hyperthermia" in cardiac arrest patients undergoing therapeutic hypothermia. *Resuscitation*. 2013;84:1245–1249. doi: 10.1016/j.resuscitation.2013.03.027
21. Scales DC, Cheskes S, Verbeek PR, Pinto R, Austin D, Brooks SC, Dainty KN, Goncharenko K, Mamdani M, Thorpe KE, Morrison LJ; Strategies for Post-Arrest Care SPARC Network. Prehospital cooling to improve successful targeted temperature management after cardiac arrest: A randomized controlled trial. *Resuscitation*. 2017;121:187–194. doi: 10.1016/j.resuscitation.2017.10.002

PCI After Cardiac Arrest

Recommendations for PCI After Cardiac Arrest

COR	LOE	Recommendations
1	B-NR	1. Coronary angiography should be performed emergently for all cardiac arrest patients with suspected cardiac cause of arrest and ST-segment elevation on ECG.
2a	B-NR	2. Emergent coronary angiography is reasonable for select (eg, electrically or hemodynamically unstable) adult patients who are comatose after OHCA of suspected cardiac origin but without ST-segment elevation on ECG.
2a	C-LD	3. Independent of a patient's mental status, coronary angiography is reasonable in all post–cardiac arrest patients for whom coronary angiography is otherwise indicated.

Synopsis

Coronary artery disease (CAD) is prevalent in the setting of cardiac arrest.[1–4] Patients with cardiac arrest due to shockable rhythms have demonstrated particularly high rates of severe CAD: up to 96% of patients with STEMI on their postresuscitation ECG,[2,5] up to 42% for patients without ST-segment elevation,[2,5–7] and 85% of refractory out-of-hospital VF/VT arrest patients have severe CAD.[8] The role of CAD in cardiac arrest with nonshockable rhythms is unknown.

When significant CAD is observed during post-ROSC coronary angiography, revascularization can be achieved safely in most cases.[5,7,9] Further, successful PCI is associated with improved survival in multiple observational studies.[2,6,7,10,11] Additional benefits of evaluation in the cardiac catheterization laboratory include discovery of anomalous coronary anatomy, the opportunity to assess left ventricular function and hemodynamic status, and the potential for insertion of temporary mechanical circulatory support devices.

The 2015 Guidelines Update recommended emergent coronary angiography for patients with ST-segment elevation on the post-ROSC ECG. Emergent coronary angiography and PCI have also been also associated with improved neurological outcomes in patients without STEMI on their post-ROSC resuscitation ECG.[4,12] However, a large randomized trial found no improvement in survival in patients resuscitated from OHCA with an initial shockable rhythm in whom no ST-segment elevations or signs of shock were present.[13] Multiple RCTs are underway. It remains to be tested whether patients with signs of shock benefit from emergent coronary angiography and PCI.

Recommendation-Specific Supportive Text

1. Several observational studies have demonstrated improved neurologically favorable survival when early coronary angiography is performed followed by PCI in patients with cardiac arrest who have a STEMI.[5,14–17] This led to a Class 1 recommendation in the 2015 Guidelines Update that has not been contradicted by any other recent studies. This recommendation is consistent with global recommendations for all patients with STEMI.
2. Multiple observational studies have shown an association between emergent coronary angiography and PCI and improved neurological outcomes in patients without ST-segment elevation.[5,7,14,15,18] A meta-analysis also supported the use of early coronary angiography in patients without ST-segment elevation.[19] However, a large randomized trial found no improvement in survival in patients resuscitated from OHCA with an initial shockable rhythm in whom no ST-segment elevation or signs of shock were present.[20] In addition, while coronary artery disease was found in 65% of patients who underwent coronary angiography, only 5% of patients had acute thrombotic coronary occlusions. Multiple RCTs are underway, but the role of emergent coronary angiography and PCI in patients without ST-elevation but with signs of shock remains to be tested. The use of emergent coronary angiography in patients with hemodynamic or electric instability is consistent with guidelines for non-STEMI patients.[21–23] The optimal treatment of hemodynamically and electrically stable patients without ST-segment elevation remains unclear. This area was last reviewed systematically in 2015 and requires additional systematic review after the completion of currently active trials (NCT03119571, NCT02309151, NCT02387398, NCT02641626, NCT02750462, NCT02876458).
3. Evidence suggests that patients who are comatose after ROSC benefit from invasive angiography, when indicated, as do patients who are awake.[4,14,18] Therefore, invasive coronary angiography is reasonable independent of neurological status.

This topic last received formal evidence review in 2015.[24]

REFERENCES

1. Spaulding CM, Joly LM, Rosenberg A, Monchi M, Weber SN, Dhainaut JF, Carli P. Immediate coronary angiography in survivors of out-of-hospital cardiac arrest. *N Engl J Med.* 1997;336:1629–1633. doi: 10.1056/NEJM199706053362302
2. Dumas F, Cariou A, Manzo-Silberman S, Grimaldi D, Vivien B, Rosencher J, Empana JP, Carli P, Mira JP, Jouven X, Spaulding C. Immediate percutaneous coronary intervention is associated with better survival after out-of-hospital cardiac arrest: insights from the PROCAT (Parisian Region Out of hospital Cardiac ArresT) registry. *Circ Cardiovasc Interv.* 2010;3:200–207. doi: 10.1161/CIRCINTERVENTIONS.109.913665
3. Davies MJ. Anatomic features in victims of sudden coronary death. Coronary artery pathology. *Circulation.* 1992;85(1 Suppl):I19–I24.
4. Yannopoulos D, Bartos JA, Aufderheide TP, Callaway CW, Deo R, Garcia S, Halperin HR, Kern KB, Kudenchuk PJ, Neumar RW, Raveendran G; American Heart Association Emergency Cardiovascular Care Committee. The Evolving Role of the Cardiac Catheterization Laboratory in the Management of Patients With Out-of-Hospital Cardiac Arrest: A Scientific Statement From the American Heart Association. *Circulation.* 2019;139:e530–e552. doi: 10.1161/CIR.0000000000000630
5. Kern KB, Lotun K, Patel N, Mooney MR, Hollenbeck RD, McPherson JA, McMullan PW, Unger B, Hsu CH, Seder DB; INTCAR-Cardiology Registry. Outcomes of Comatose Cardiac Arrest Survivors With and Without ST-Segment Elevation Myocardial Infarction: Importance of Coronary Angiography. *J AM COLL CARDIOL. Cardiovasc Interv.* 2015;8:1031–1040. doi: 10.1016/j.jcin.2015.02.021
6. Dumas F, Bougouin W, Geri G, Lamhaut L, Rosencher J, Pène F, Chiche JD, Varenne O, Carli P, Jouven X, Mira JP, Spaulding C, Cariou A. Emergency Percutaneous Coronary Intervention in Post-Cardiac Arrest Patients Without ST-Segment Elevation Pattern: Insights From the PROCAT II Registry. *J AM COLL CARDIOL. Cardiovasc Interv.* 2016;9:1011–1018. doi: 10.1016/j.jcin.2016.02.001
7. Garcia S, Drexel T, Bekwelem W, Raveendran G, Caldwell E, Hodgson L, Wang Q, Adabag S, Mahoney B, Frascone R, et al. Early access to the cardiac catheterization laboratory for patients resuscitated from cardiac arrest due to a shockable rhythm: the Minnesota Resuscitation Consortium Twin Cities Unified Protocol. *J Am Heart Assoc.* 2016;5:e002670. doi: 10.1161/JAHA.115.002670
8. Yannopoulos D, Bartos JA, Raveendran G, Conterato M, Frascone RJ, Trembley A, John R, Connett J, Benditt DG, Lurie KG, Wilson RF, Aufderheide TP. Coronary Artery Disease in Patients With Out-of-Hospital Refractory Ventricular Fibrillation Cardiac Arrest. *J Am Coll Cardiol.* 2017;70:1109–1117. doi: 10.1016/j.jacc.2017.06.059
9. Sideris G, Voicu S, Yannopoulos D, Dillinger JG, Adjedj J, Deye N, Gueye P, Manzo-Silberman S, Malissin I, Logeart D, Magkoutis N, Capan DD, Makhloufi S, Megarbane B, Vivien B, Cohen-Solal A, Payen D, Baud FJ, Henry P. Favourable 5-year postdischarge survival of comatose patients resuscitated from out-of-hospital cardiac arrest, managed with immediate coronary angiogram on admission. *Eur Heart J Acute Cardiovasc Care.* 2014;3:183–191. doi: 10.1177/2048872614523348
10. Geri G, Dumas F, Bougouin W, Varenne O, Daviaud F, Pene F, Lamhaut L, Chiche JD, Spaulding C, Mira JP, et al. Immediate percutaneous coronary intervention is associated with improved short- and long-term survival after out-of-hospital cardiac arrest. *Circ Cardiovasc Interv.* 2015;8 doi: 10.1161/circinterventions.114.002303
11. Zanuttini D, Armellini I, Nucifora G, Carchietti E, Trillò G, Spedicato L, Bernardi G, Proclemer A. Impact of emergency coronary angiography on in-hospital outcome of unconscious survivors after out-of-hospital cardiac arrest. *Am J Cardiol.* 2012;110:1723–1728. doi: 10.1016/j.amjcard.2012.08.006
12. Patel N, Patel NJ, Macon CJ, Thakkar B, Desai M, Rengifo-Moreno P, Alfonso CE, Myerburg RJ, Bhatt DL, Cohen MG. Trends and Outcomes of Coronary Angiography and Percutaneous Coronary Intervention After Out-of-Hospital Cardiac Arrest Associated With Ventricular Fibrillation or Pulseless Ventricular Tachycardia. *JAMA Cardiol.* 2016;1:890–899. doi: 10.1001/jamacardio.2016.2860
13. Lemkes JS, Janssens GN, van der Hoeven NW, Jewbali LSD, Dubois EA, Meuwissen M, Rijpstra TA, Bosker HA, Blans MJ, Bleeker GB, Baak R, Vlachojannis GJ, Eikemans BJW, van der Harst P, van der Horst ICC, Voskuil M, van der Heijden JJ, Beishuizen A, Stoel M, Camaro C, van der Hoeven H, Henriques JP, Vlaar APJ, Vink MA, van den Bogaard B, Heestermans TACM, de Ruijter W, Delnoij TSR, Crijns HJGM, Jessurun GAJ, Oemrawsingh PV, Gosselink MTM, Plomp K, Magro M, Elbers PWG, van de Ven PM, Oudemans-van Straaten HM, van Royen N. Coronary Angiography after Cardiac Arrest without ST-Segment Elevation. *N Engl J Med.* 2019;380:1397–1407. doi: 10.1056/NEJMoa1816897
14. Bro-Jeppesen J, Kjaergaard J, Wanscher M, Pedersen F, Holmvang L, Lippert FK, Møller JE, Køber L, Hassager C. Emergency coronary angiography in comatose cardiac arrest patients: do real-life experiences support the guidelines? *Eur Heart J Acute Cardiovasc Care.* 2012;1:291–301. doi: 10.1177/2048872612465588
15. Vyas A, Chan PS, Cram P, Nallamothu BK, McNally B, Girotra S. Early coronary angiography and survival after out-of-hospital cardiac arrest. *Circ Cardiovasc Interv.* 2015;8:e002321. doi: 10.1161/CIRCINTERVENTIONS.114.002321
16. Waldo SW, Armstrong EJ, Kulkarni A, Hoffmayer K, Kinlay S, Hsue P, Ganz P, McCabe JM. Comparison of clinical characteristics and outcomes

of cardiac arrest survivors having versus not having coronary angiography. *Am J Cardiol.* 2013;111:1253–1258. doi: 10.1016/j.amjcard.2013.01.267

17. Hosmane VR, Mustafa NG, Reddy VK, Reese CL IV, DiSabatino A, Kolm P, Hopkins JT, Weintraub WS, Rahman E. Survival and neurologic recovery in patients with ST-segment elevation myocardial infarction resuscitated from cardiac arrest. *J Am Coll Cardiol.* 2009;53:409–415. doi: 10.1016/j.jacc.2008.08.076
18. Hollenbeck RD, McPherson JA, Mooney MR, Unger BT, Patel NC, McMullan PW Jr, Hsu CH, Seder DB, Kern KB. Early cardiac catheterization is associated with improved survival in comatose survivors of cardiac arrest without STEMI. *Resuscitation.* 2014;85:88–95. doi: 10.1016/j.resuscitation.2013.07.027
19. Khan MS, Shah SMM, Mubashir A, Khan AR, Fatima K, Schenone AL, Khosa F, Samady H, Menon V. Early coronary angiography in patients resuscitated from out of hospital cardiac arrest without ST-segment elevation: A systematic review and meta-analysis. *Resuscitation.* 2017;121:127–134. doi: 10.1016/j.resuscitation.2017.10.019
20. Lemkes JS, Janssens GN, van Royen N. Coronary Angiography after Cardiac Arrest without ST-Segment Elevation. Reply. *N Engl J Med.* 2019;381:189–190. doi: 10.1056/NEJMc1906523
21. Amsterdam EA, Wenger NK, Brindis RG, Casey DE Jr, Ganiats TG, Holmes DR Jr, Jaffe AS, Jneid H, Kelly RF, Kontos MC, Levine GN, Liebson PR, Mukherjee D, Peterson ED, Sabatine MS, Smalling RW, Zieman SJ; ACC/AHA Task Force Members; Society for Cardiovascular Angiography and Interventions and the Society of Thoracic Surgeons. 2014 AHA/ACC guideline for the management of patients with non-ST-elevation acute coronary syndromes: executive summary: a report of the American College of Cardiology/American Heart Association Task Force on Practice Guidelines. *Circulation.* 2014;130:2354–2394. doi: 10.1161/CIR.0000000000000133
22. Lee L, Bates ER, Pitt B, Walton JA, Laufer N, O'Neill WW. Percutaneous transluminal coronary angioplasty improves survival in acute myocardial infarction complicated by cardiogenic shock. *Circulation.* 1988;78:1345–1351. doi: 10.1161/01.cir.78.6.1345
23. Hochman JS, Sleeper LA, Webb JG, Sanborn TA, White HD, Talley JD, Buller CE, Jacobs AK, Slater JN, Col J, McKinlay SM, LeJemtel TH. Early revascularization in acute myocardial infarction complicated by cardiogenic shock. SHOCK Investigators. Should We Emergently Revascularize Occluded Coronaries for Cardiogenic Shock. *N Engl J Med.* 1999;341:625–634. doi: 10.1056/NEJM199908263410901
24. Callaway CW, Donnino MW, Fink EL, Geocadin RG, Golan E, Kern KB, Leary M, Meurer WJ, Peberdy MA, Thompson TM, et al. Part 8: post–cardiac arrest care: 2015 American Heart Association Guidelines Update for Cardiopulmonary Resuscitation and Emergency Cardiovascular Care. *Circulation.* 2015;132(suppl 2):S465–482. doi: 10.1161/cir.0000000000000262

Neuroprognostication

General Considerations for Neuroprognostication

Introduction

Hypoxic-ischemic brain injury is the leading cause of morbidity and mortality in survivors of OHCA and accounts for a smaller but significant portion of poor outcomes after resuscitation from IHCA.[1,2] Most deaths attributable to postarrest brain injury are due to active

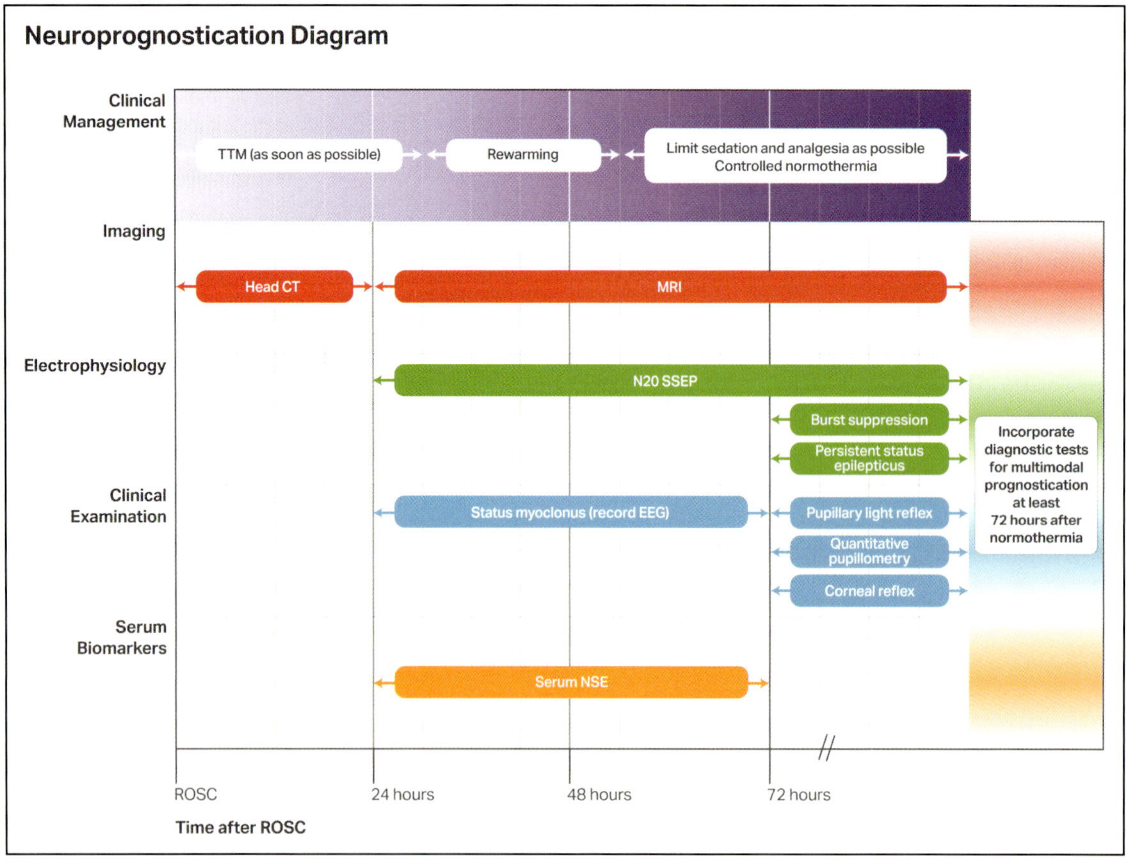

Figure 10. Recommended approach to multimodal neuroprognostication.
Neurologic prognostication incorporates multiple diagnostic tests that are synthesized into a comprehensive multimodal assessment at least 72 hours after return to normothermia and with sedation and analgesia limited as possible. Awareness and incorporation of the potential sources of error in the individual diagnostic tests is important. The suggested timing of the multimodal diagnostics is shown here. CT indicates computed tomography; EEG, electroencephalogram; MRI, magnetic resonance imaging; NSE, neuron-specific enolase; ROSC, return of spontaneous circulation; SSEP, somatosensory evoked potential; and TTM, targeted temperature management.

withdrawal of life-sustaining treatment based on a predicted poor neurological outcome. Accurate neurological prognostication is important to avoid inappropriate withdrawal of life-sustaining treatment in patients who may otherwise achieve meaningful neurological recovery and also to avoid ineffective treatment when poor outcome is inevitable (Figure 10).[3]

Recommendations for General Considerations for Neuroprognostication

COR	LOE	Recommendations
1	B-NR	1. In patients who remain comatose after cardiac arrest, we recommend that neuroprognostication involve a multimodal approach and not be based on any single finding.
1	B-NR	2. In patients who remain comatose after cardiac arrest, we recommend that neuroprognostication be delayed until adequate time has passed to ensure avoidance of confounding by medication effect or a transiently poor examination in the early postinjury period.
1	C-EO	3. We recommend that teams caring for comatose cardiac arrest survivors have regular and transparent multidisciplinary discussions with surrogates about the anticipated time course for and uncertainties around neuroprognostication.
2a	B-NR	4. In patients who remain comatose after cardiac arrest, it is reasonable to perform multimodal neuroprognostication at a minimum of 72 h after normothermia, though individual prognostic tests may be obtained earlier than this.

Synopsis

Neuroprognostication relies on interpreting the results of diagnostic tests and correlating those results with outcome. Given that a false-positive test for poor neurological outcome could lead to inappropriate withdrawal of life support from a patient who otherwise would have recovered, the most important test characteristic is specificity. Many of the tests considered are subject to error because of the effects of medications, organ dysfunction, and temperature. Furthermore, many research studies have methodological limitations including small sample sizes, single-center design, lack of blinding, the potential for self-fulfilling prophecies, and the use of outcome at hospital discharge rather than a time point associated with maximal recovery (typically 3–6 months after arrest).[3]

Because any single method of neuroprognostication has an intrinsic error rate and may be subject to confounding, multiple modalities should be used to improve decision-making accuracy.

Recommendation-Specific Supportive Text

1. The overall certainty in the evidence of neurological prognostication studies is low because of biases that limit the internal validity of the studies as well as issues of generalizability that limit their external validity. Thus, the confidence in the prognostication of the diagnostic tests studied is also low. Neuroprognostication that uses multimodal testing is felt to be better at predicting outcomes than is relying on the results of a single test to predict poor prognosis.[3,4]
2. Sedatives and neuromuscular blockers may be metabolized more slowly in post–cardiac arrest patients, and injured brains may be more sensitive to the depressant effects of various medications. Residual sedation or paralysis can confound the accuracy of clinical examinations.[5]
3. Prognostication of neurological recovery is complex and limited by uncertainty in most cases. Discordance in goals of care between clinicians and families/surrogates has been reported in more than 25% of critically ill patients.[6] Lack of adequate communication is one important factor, and regular multidisciplinary conversations may help mitigate this.
4. Operationally, the timing for prognostication is typically at least 5 days after ROSC for patients treated with TTM (which is about 72 hours after normothermia) and should be conducted under conditions that minimize the confounding effects of sedating medications. Individual test modalities may be obtained earlier and the results integrated into the multimodality assessment synthesized at least 72 hours after normothermia. In some instances, prognostication and withdrawal of life support may appropriately occur earlier because of nonneurologic disease, brain herniation, patient's goals and wishes, or clearly nonsurvivable situations.

These recommendations are supported by the 2020 CoSTR for ALS,[4] which supplements the last comprehensive review of this topic conducted in 2015.[7]

Use of the Clinical Examination in Neuroprognostication

Recommendations for Clinical Examination for Neuroprognostication		
COR	**LOE**	**Recommendations**
2b	B-NR	1. When performed with other prognostic tests, it may be reasonable to consider bilaterally absent pupillary light reflex at 72 h or more after cardiac arrest to support the prognosis of poor neurological outcome in patients who remain comatose.
2b	B-NR	2. When performed with other prognostic tests, it may be reasonable to consider quantitative pupillometry at 72 h or more after cardiac arrest to support the prognosis of poor neurological outcome in patients who remain comatose.
2b	B-NR	3. When performed with other prognostic tests, it may be reasonable to consider bilaterally absent corneal reflexes at 72 h or more after cardiac arrest to support the prognosis of poor neurological outcome in patients who remain comatose.
2b	B-NR	4. When performed with other prognostic tests, it may be reasonable to consider status myoclonus that occurs within 72 h after cardiac arrest to support the prognosis of poor neurological outcome.
2b	B-NR	5. We suggest recording EEG in the presence of myoclonus to determine if there is an associated cerebral correlate.
3: Harm	B-NR	6. The presence of undifferentiated myoclonic movements after cardiac arrest should not be used to support a poor neurological prognosis.
3: Harm	B-NR	7. We recommend that the findings of a best motor response in the upper extremities being either absent or extensor movements not be used alone for predicting a poor neurological outcome in patients who remain comatose after cardiac arrest.

Synopsis

Clinical examination findings correlate with poor outcome but are also subject to confounding by TTM and medications, and prior studies have methodological limitations. In addition to assessing level of consciousness and performing basic neurological examination, clinical examination elements may include the pupillary light reflex, pupillometry, corneal reflex, myoclonus, and status myoclonus when assessed within 1 week after cardiac arrest. The ILCOR systematic review included studies regardless of TTM status, and findings were correlated with neurological outcome at time points ranging from hospital discharge to 12 months after arrest.[4] Quantitative pupillometry is the automated assessment of pupillary reactivity, measured by the percent reduction in pupillary size and the degree of reactivity reported as the neurological pupil index. Benefits of this method are a standard and reproducible assessment. *Status myoclonus* is commonly defined as spontaneous or sound-sensitive, repetitive, irregular brief jerks in both face and limb present most of the day within 24 hours after cardiac arrest.[8] Status myoclonus differs from myoclonic status epilepticus; *myoclonic status epilepticus* is defined as status epilepticus with physical manifestation of persistent myoclonic movements and is considered a subtype of status epilepticus for these guidelines.

Recommendation-Specific Supportive Text

1. In 17 studies,[9–25] absent pupillary light reflex assessed from immediately after ROSC up to 7 days after arrest predicted poor neurological outcome with specificity ranging from 48% to 100%. The specificity varied significantly on the basis of timing, with the highest specificity seen at time points 72 hours or more after arrest.
2. Three studies evaluated quantitative pupillary light reflex[15,26,27] and 3 studies evaluated neurological pupil index[15,28,29] at time points ranging from 24 to 72 hours after arrest. Absent pupillary light reflex as assessed by quantitative pupillometry (ie, quantitative pupillary light reflex=0%) is an objective finding and, in 1 study of 271 patients, had high specificity for poor outcome when assessed at 72 hours after arrest.[15] Neurological pupil index is nonspecific and may be affected by medications; thus, an absolute neurological pupil index cutoff and a specific threshold that predicts poor prognosis is unknown.[15,28,29]
3. Eleven observational studies[9–11,14,16,17,19,21,22,30,31] evaluated absence of corneal reflexes at time points ranging from immediately after ROSC to 7 days after arrest. The specificity for poor outcome ranged from 25% to 100% and increased in the studies evaluating corneal reflexes at time points 72 hours or more after arrest (ranging from 89% to 100%). Like other examination findings, corneal reflexes are subject to confounding by medications, and few studies specifically evaluated the potential of residual medication effect.
4. In 2 studies involving 347 patients,[21,32] the presence of status myoclonus within 72 hours predicted poor neurological outcome from hospital discharge to 6 months, with specificity ranging from 97% to 100%.
5. Obtaining EEG in status myoclonus is important to rule out underlying ictal activity. In addition, status myoclonus may have an EEG correlate that is not clearly ictal but may have prognostic meaning, and additional research is needed to delineate these patterns. Some EEG-correlated patterns of status myoclonus may have poor prognosis, but there may also be more benign subtypes of status myoclonus with EEG correlates.[33,34]

6. Six observational studies[16,19,30,35–37] evaluated the presence of myoclonus within 96 hours after arrest with specificity for poor outcome ranging from 77.8% to 97.4%. There were methodological limitations in all studies, including a lack of standard definitions, lack of blinding, incomplete data about EEG correlates, and the inability to differentiate subtypes of myoclonus. The literature was so imprecise as to make it potentially harmful if undifferentiated myoclonus is used as a prognostic marker.
7. Historically, the best motor examination in the upper extremities has been used as a prognostic tool, with extensor or absent movement being correlated with poor outcome. The previous literature was limited by methodological concerns, including around inadequate control for effects of TTM and medications and self-fulfilling prophecies, and there was a lower-than-acceptable false-positive rate (10% to 15%).[7] The performance of the motor examination was not evaluated in the 2020 ILCOR systematic review. The updates made to the 2015 recommendations are based on concerns that the motor examination is subject to confounding and has an unacceptably high false-positive rate and, thus, should not be used as a prognostic tool or as a screen for subsequent testing.

These recommendations are supported by the 2020 CoSTR for ALS,[4] which supplements the last comprehensive review of this topic conducted in 2015.[7]

Use of Serum Biomarkers for Neuroprognostication

Recommendations for Serum Biomarkers for Neuroprognostication

COR	LOE	Recommendations
2b	B-NR	1. When performed in combination with other prognostic tests, it may be reasonable to consider high serum values of neuron-specific enolase (NSE) within 72 h after cardiac arrest to support the prognosis of poor neurological outcome in patients who remain comatose.
2b	C-LD	2. The usefulness of S100 calcium-binding protein (S100B), Tau, neurofilament light chain, and glial fibrillary acidic protein in neuroprognostication is uncertain.

Synopsis

Serum biomarkers are blood-based tests that measure the concentration of proteins normally found in the central nervous system (CNS). These proteins are absorbed into blood in the setting of neurological injury, and their serum levels reflect the degree of brain injury. Limitations to their prognostic utility include variability in testing methods on the basis of site and laboratory, between-laboratory inconsistency in levels, susceptibility to additional uncertainty due to hemolysis, and potential extracerebral sources of the proteins. NSE and S100B are the 2 most commonly studied markers, but others are included in this review as well. The 2020 ILCOR systematic review evaluated studies that obtained serum biomarkers within the first 7 days after arrest and correlated serum biomarker concentrations with neurological outcome. Other testing of serum biomarkers, including testing levels over serial time points after arrest, was not evaluated. A large observational cohort study investigating these and other novel serum biomarkers and their performance as prognostic biomarkers would be of high clinical significance.

Recommendation-Specific Supportive Text

1. Twelve observational studies evaluated NSE collected within 72 hours after arrest.[10,13,21,23,38–45] The maximal level that correlated with poor outcome ranged from 33 to 120 μg/L with specificity for poor outcome of 75% to 100%. The evidence is limited because of lack of blinding, laboratory inconsistencies, a broad range of thresholds needed to achieve 100% specificity, and imprecision. As such, an absolute value cutoff of NSE that predicts poor prognosis is not known, though very high levels of NSE may be used as part of multimodal prognostication. There is research interest in evaluating serial measures over the first days after arrest as a prognostic tool instead of using a single absolute value.[10,46]
2. Three observational studies[40,47,48] evaluated S100B levels within the first 72 hours after arrest. The maximal level that correlated with poor outcome ranged broadly depending on the study and the timing when it was measured after arrest. At values reported to achieve 100% specificity, test sensitivity ranged from 2.8% to 77.6%. The evidence is limited by the small number of studies and the broad range of thresholds across the studies required to achieve 100% specificity. The ILCOR review also evaluated 1 study each evaluating glial fibrillary acidic protein[44] and Tau[49] and 2 studies evaluating neurofilament light chain.[50,51] Given the low number of studies, the LOE was low, and these serum biomarkers could not be recommended for clinical practice.

These recommendations are supported by the 2020 CoSTR for ALS,[4] which supplements the last comprehensive review of this topic conducted in 2015.[7]

Use of Electrophysiological Tests for Neuroprognostication

Recommendations for Electrophysiology for Neuroprognostication		
COR	LOE	Recommendations
2b	B-NR	1. When evaluated with other prognostic tests, the prognostic value of seizures in patients who remain comatose after cardiac arrest is uncertain.
2b	B-NR	2. When performed with other prognostic tests, it may be reasonable to consider persistent status epilepticus 72 h or more after cardiac arrest to support the prognosis of poor neurological outcome.
2b	B-NR	3. When performed with other prognostic tests, it may be reasonable to consider burst suppression on EEG in the absence of sedating medications at 72 h or more after arrest to support the prognosis of poor neurological outcome.
2b	B-NR	4. When performed with other prognostic tests, it may be reasonable to consider bilaterally absent N20 somatosensory evoked potential (SSEP) waves more than 24 h after cardiac arrest to support the prognosis of poor neurological outcome.
2b	B-NR	5. When evaluated with other prognostic tests after arrest, the usefulness of rhythmic periodic discharges to support the prognosis of poor neurological outcome is uncertain.
3: No Benefit	B-NR	6. We recommend that the absence of EEG reactivity within 72 h after arrest not be used alone to support a poor neurological prognosis.

Synopsis

Electroencephalography is widely used in clinical practice to evaluate cortical brain activity and diagnose seizures. Its use as a neuroprognostic tool is promising, but the literature is limited by several factors: lack of standardized terminology and definitions, relatively small sample sizes, single center study design, lack of blinding, subjectivity in the interpretation, and lack of accounting for effects of medications. There is also inconsistency in definitions used to describe specific findings and patterns. EEG patterns that were evaluated in the 2020 ILCOR systematic review include unreactive EEG, epileptiform discharges, seizures, status epilepticus, burst suppression, and "highly malignant" EEG. Unfortunately, different studies define *highly malignant EEG* differently or imprecisely, making use of this finding unhelpful.

SSEPs are obtained by stimulating the median nerve and evaluating for the presence of a cortical N20 wave. Bilaterally absent N20 SSEP waves have been correlated with poor prognosis, but reliability of this modality is limited by requiring appropriate operator skills and care to avoid electric interference from muscle artifacts or from the ICU environment. One benefit to SSEPs is that they are subject to less interference from medications than are other modalities.

Recommendation-Specific Supportive Text

1. Five observational studies[35,52–55] evaluated the role of electrographic and/or convulsive seizures in neuroprognostication. The studies focused on electrographic seizures, though some studies also included convulsive seizures. Although the specificity of seizures in the studies included in the ILCOR systematic review was 100%, sensitivity of this finding was poor (0.6% to 26.8%), and other studies that were not included in the review found patients with postarrest seizures who had good outcomes.[36,56,57] Additional methodological concerns include selection bias for which patients underwent EEG monitoring and inconsistent definitions of seizure. The term *seizure* encompasses a broad spectrum of pathologies that likely have different prognoses, ranging from a single brief electrographic seizure to refractory status epilepticus, and this imprecision justified the more limited recommendation.
2. Six observational studies[21,55,58–61] evaluated status epilepticus within 5 days after arrest and evaluated outcomes at time points ranging from hospital discharge to 6 months after arrest. The specificity of status epilepticus for poor outcome ranged from 82.6% to 100%. Interestingly, although status epilepticus is a severe form of seizures, the specificity of status epilepticus for poor outcome was less than that which was reported in the studies examining the seizures overall (as above). Additional concerns include the inconsistent definition of *status epilepticus*, lack of blinding, and the use of status epilepticus to justify withdrawal of life-sustaining therapies leading to potential self-fulfilling prophecies.
3. Six studies[21,35,54,59,62,63] evaluated burst suppression within 120 hours after arrest. One additional study[64] subdivided burst suppression into synchronous versus heterogeneous patterns. Definitions of burst suppression varied or were not specified. Specificity ranged from 90.7% to 100%, and sensitivity was 1.1% to 51%. The lack of standardized definitions, potential for self-fulfilling prophecies, and the lack of controlling for medication effects limited the ability to make a stronger recommendation, despite the overall high specificity. Additional focus on identifying subtypes of burst suppression, such as the synchronous subtype (which appeared to be highly specific in a single study), should be investigated further. Burst suppression can

Circulation. 2020;142(suppl 2):S366–S468. DOI: 10.1161/CIR.0000000000000916

be caused by medications, so it is particularly important that providers have knowledge about the potential effects of medication on this prognostic tool.

4. Fourteen observational studies[9,13,15–17,23,59,64–70] evaluated bilaterally absent N20 SSEP waves within 96 hours after arrest and correlated the finding with outcome at time points ranging from hospital discharge to 6 months after arrest. Specificity ranged from 50% to 100%. Three studies had specificity below 100%, and additional methodological limitations included lack of blinding and potential for self-fulfilling prophecies. While the studies evaluated SSEPs obtained at any time starting immediately after arrest, there is a high likelihood of potential confounding factors early after arrest, leading to the recommendation that SSEPs should only be obtained more than 24 hours after arrest.
5. Discharges on EEG were divided into 2 types: rhythmic/periodic and nonrhythmic/periodic. Nine observational studies evaluated rhythmic/periodic discharges.[16,45,52–54,61,63,66,69] The specificity of rhythmic/periodic discharges ranged from 66.7% to 100%, with poor sensitivity (2.4%–50.8%). The studies evaluating rhythmic/periodic discharges were inconsistent in the definitions of discharges. Most did not account for effects of medications, and some studies found unacceptably low specificity. Nonetheless, as the time from the cardiac arrest increased, the specificity of rhythmic/periodic discharges for poor outcome improved. There is opportunity to develop this EEG finding as a prognostic tool. Five observational studies[52,53,64,66,69] evaluated nonrhythmic/periodic discharges. Specificity for poor outcome was low over the entire post–cardiac arrest period evaluated in the studies.
6. Ten observational studies[16,30,53–55,62,65,71–73] reported on the prognostic value of unreactive EEG. Specificity ranged from 41.7% to 100% and was below 90% in most studies. There was inconsistency in the definitions of and stimuli used for EEG reactivity. Studies also did not account for effects of temperature and medications. Thus, the overall certainty of the evidence was rated as very low.

These recommendations are supported by the 2020 CoSTR for ALS,[4] which supplements the last comprehensive review of this topic conducted in 2015.[7]

Use of Neuroimaging for Neuroprognostication

Recommendations for Neuroimaging for Neuroprognostication

COR	LOE	Recommendations
2b	B-NR	1. When performed with other prognostic tests, it may be reasonable to consider reduced gray-white ratio (GWR) on brain computed tomography (CT) after cardiac arrest to support the prognosis of poor neurological outcome in patients who remain comatose.
2b	B-NR	2. When performed with other prognostic tests, it may be reasonable to consider extensive areas of restricted diffusion on brain MRI (MRI) at 2 to 7 days after cardiac arrest to support the prognosis of poor neurological outcome in patients who remain comatose.
2b	B-NR	3. When performed with other prognostic tests, it may be reasonable to consider extensive areas of reduced apparent diffusion coefficient (ADC) on brain MRI at 2 to 7 days after cardiac arrest to support the prognosis of poor neurological outcome in patients who remain comatose.

Synopsis

Neuroimaging may be helpful after arrest to detect and quantify structural brain injury. CT and MRI are the 2 most common modalities. On CT, brain edema can be quantified as the GWR, defined as the ratio between the density (measured as Hounsfield units) of the gray matter and the white matter. Normal brain has a GWR of approximately 1.3, and this number decreases with edema. On MRI, cytotoxic injury can be measured as restricted diffusion on diffusion-weighted imaging (DWI) and can be quantified by the ADC. DWI/ADC is a sensitive measure of injury, with normal values ranging between 700 and 800×10^{-6} mm^2/s and values decreasing with injury. CT and MRI findings of brain injury evolve over the first several days after arrest, so the timing of the imaging study of interest is of particular importance as it relates to prognosis.

Recommendation-Specific Supportive Text

1. Twelve studies[23,24,31,38,66,74–79] evaluated GWR on head CT. Whole-brain GWR (GWR average) and GWR in specific regions were evaluated. The specificity was 85% to 100%, and only 1 study reported a specificity that was not 100%. Many of the studies evaluated head CTs that were obtained within the first 24 hours after arrest, though some studies included head CTs obtained up to 72 hours after arrest. There were methodological limitations, including selection bias, risk of multiple comparisons, and heterogeneity of measurement techniques, such as anatomic sites

and calculation methods. Thus, a specific GWR threshold that predicts poor prognosis with 100% specificity is unknown. Additionally, the optimal timing for obtaining head CT after arrest to optimize the GWR as a prognostic tool is unknown.

2. Five observational studies[11,23,74,80,81] investigated DWI changes on MRI within 5 days after arrest. The studies evaluated MRI qualitatively for "high signal intensity" and "positive findings," but the definitions of *positive findings* differed between studies and, in some studies, examined only specific brain regions. Specificity was 55.7% to 100%. The imprecise definition and short-term outcome in some studies led to significant uncertainty about how to use DWI MRI to predict poor prognosis. In the correct setting, a significant burden of DWI MRI findings or DWI MRI findings in specific regions of interest may be correlated with poor prognosis, but a broader recommendation could not be supported.
3. Three observational studies[82–84] investigated ADC on MRI within 7 days after arrest. The studies were designed to determine thresholds that achieved 100% specificity, though the ADC and brain volume thresholds needed to achieve that specificity varied broadly. While quantitative ADC measurements are a promising tool, their broad use is limited by feasibility concerns. Additionally, there are relatively few studies, and per other imaging features, there was heterogeneity of measurement techniques, including in sites and calculation methods. A specific ADC threshold that predicts poor prognosis is not known.

These recommendations are supported by the 2020 CoSTR for ALS,[4] which supplements the last comprehensive review of this topic conducted in 2015.[7]

REFERENCES

1. Laver S, Farrow C, Turner D, Nolan J. Mode of death after admission to an intensive care unit following cardiac arrest. *Intensive Care Med.* 2004;30:2126–2128. doi: 10.1007/s00134-004-2425-z
2. Witten L, Gardner R, Holmberg MJ, Wiberg S, Moskowitz A, Mehta S, Grossestreuer AV, Yankama T, Donnino MW, Berg KM. Reasons for death in patients successfully resuscitated from out-of-hospital and in-hospital cardiac arrest. *Resuscitation.* 2019;136:93–99. doi: 10.1016/j.resuscitation.2019.01.031
3. Geocadin RG, Callaway CW, Fink EL, Golan E, Greer DM, Ko NU, Lang E, Licht DJ, Marino BS, McNair ND, Peberdy MA, Perman SM, Sims DB, Soar J, Sandroni C; American Heart Association Emergency Cardiovascular Care Committee. Standards for Studies of Neurological Prognostication in Comatose Survivors of Cardiac Arrest: A Scientific Statement From the American Heart Association. *Circulation.* 2019;140:e517–e542. doi: 10.1161/CIR.0000000000000702
4. Berg KM, Soar J, Andersen LW, Böttiger BW, Cacciola S, Callaway CW, Couper K, Cronberg T, D'Arrigo S, Deakin CD, et al; on behalf of the Adult Advanced Life Support Collaborators. Adult advanced life support: 2020 International Consensus on Cardiopulmonary Resuscitation and Emergency Cardiovascular Care Science With Treatment Recommendations. *Circulation.* 2020;142(suppl 1):S92–S139. doi: 10.1161/CIR.0000000000000893
5. Samaniego EA, Mlynash M, Caulfield AF, Eyngorn I, Wijman CA. Sedation confounds outcome prediction in cardiac arrest survivors treated with hypothermia. *Neurocrit Care.* 2011;15:113–119. doi: 10.1007/s12028-010-9412-8
6. Wilson ME, Dobler CC, Zubek L, Gajic O, Talmor D, Curtis JR, Hinds RF, Banner-Goodspeed VM, Mueller A, Rickett DM, Elo G, Filipe M, Szucs O, Novotny PJ, Piers RD, Benoit DD. Prevalence of Disagreement About Appropriateness of Treatment Between ICU Patients/Surrogates and Clinicians. *Chest.* 2019;155:1140–1147. doi: 10.1016/j.chest.2019.02.404
7. Callaway CW, Donnino MW, Fink EL, Geocadin RG, Golan E, Kern KB, Leary M, Meurer WJ, Peberdy MA, Thompson TM, et al. Part 8: post–cardiac arrest care: 2015 American Heart Association Guidelines Update for Cardiopulmonary Resuscitation and Emergency Cardiovascular Care. *Circulation.* 2015;132(suppl 2):S465–482. doi: 10.1161/cir.0000000000000262
8. Wijdicks EF, Parisi JE, Sharbrough FW. Prognostic value of myoclonus status in comatose survivors of cardiac arrest. *Ann Neurol.* 1994;35:239–243. doi: 10.1002/ana.410350219
9. Choi SP, Park KN, Wee JH, Park JH, Youn CS, Kim HJ, Oh SH, Oh YS, Kim SH, Oh JS. Can somatosensory and visual evoked potentials predict neurological outcome during targeted temperature management in post cardiac arrest patients? *Resuscitation.* 2017;119:70–75. doi: 10.1016/j.resuscitation.2017.06.022
10. Chung-Esaki HM, Mui G, Mlynash M, Eyngorn I, Catabay K, Hirsch KG. The neuron specific enolase (NSE) ratio offers benefits over absolute value thresholds in post-cardiac arrest coma prognosis. *J Clin Neurosci.* 2018;57:99–104. doi: 10.1016/j.jocn.2018.08.020
11. Ryoo SM, Jeon SB, Sohn CH, Ahn S, Han C, Lee BK, Lee DH, Kim SH, Donnino MW, Kim WY; Korean Hypothermia Network Investigators. Predicting Outcome With Diffusion-Weighted Imaging in Cardiac Arrest Patients Receiving Hypothermia Therapy: Multicenter Retrospective Cohort Study. *Crit Care Med.* 2015;43:2370–2377. doi: 10.1097/CCM.0000000000001263
12. Javaudin F, Leclere B, Segard J, Le Bastard Q, Pes P, Penverne Y, Le Conte P, Jenvrin J, Hubert H, Escutnaire J, Batard E, Montassier E, Gr-RéAC. Prognostic performance of early absence of pupillary light reaction after recovery of out of hospital cardiac arrest. *Resuscitation.* 2018;127:8–13. doi: 10.1016/j.resuscitation.2018.03.020
13. Dhakal LP, Sen A, Stanko CM, Rawal B, Heckman MG, Hoyne JB, Dimberg EL, Freeman ML, Ng LK, Rabinstein AA, Freeman WD. Early Absent Pupillary Light Reflexes After Cardiac Arrest in Patients Treated with Therapeutic Hypothermia. *Ther Hypothermia Temp Manag.* 2016;6:116–121. doi: 10.1089/ther.2015.0035
14. Matthews EA, Magid-Bernstein J, Sobczak E, Velazquez A, Falo CM, Park S, Claassen J, Agarwal S. Prognostic Value of the Neurological Examination in Cardiac Arrest Patients After Therapeutic Hypothermia. *Neurohospitalist.* 2018;8:66–73. doi: 10.1177/1941874417733217
15. Oddo M, Sandroni C, Citerio G, Miroz JP, Horn J, Rundgren M, Cariou A, Payen JF, Storm C, Stammet P, Taccone FS. Quantitative versus standard pupillary light reflex for early prognostication in comatose cardiac arrest patients: an international prospective multicenter double-blinded study. *Intensive Care Med.* 2018;44:2102–2111. doi: 10.1007/s00134-018-5448-6
16. Fatuzzo D, Beuchat I, Alvarez V, Novy J, Oddo M, Rossetti AO. Does continuous EEG influence prognosis in patients after cardiac arrest? *Resuscitation.* 2018;132:29–32. doi: 10.1016/j.resuscitation.2018.08.023
17. Dragancea I, Horn J, Kuiper M, Friberg H, Ullén S, Wetterslev J, Cranshaw J, Hassager C, Nielsen N, Cronberg T; TTM Trial Investigators. Neurological prognostication after cardiac arrest and targeted temperature management 33°C versus 36°C: Results from a randomised controlled clinical trial. *Resuscitation.* 2015;93:164–170. doi: 10.1016/j.resuscitation.2015.04.013
18. Hofmeijer J, Beernink TM, Bosch FH, Beishuizen A, Tjepkema-Cloostermans MC, van Putten MJ. Early EEG contributes to multimodal outcome prediction of postanoxic coma. *Neurology.* 2015;85:137–143. doi: 10.1212/WNL.0000000000001742
19. Kongpolprom N, Cholkraisuwat J. Neurological Prognostications for the Therapeutic Hypothermia among Comatose Survivors of Cardiac Arrest. *Indian J Crit Care Med.* 2018;22:509–518. doi: 10.4103/ijccm.IJCCM_500_17
20. Roger C, Palmier L, Louart B, Molinari N, Claret PG, de la Coussaye JE, Lefrant JY, Muller L. Neuron specific enolase and Glasgow motor score remain useful tools for assessing neurological prognosis after out-of-hospital cardiac arrest treated with therapeutic hypothermia. *Anaesth Crit Care Pain Med.* 2015;34:231–237. doi: 10.1016/j.accpm.2015.05.004
21. Zhou SE, Maciel CB, Ormseth CH, Beekman R, Gilmore EJ, Greer DM. Distinct predictive values of current neuroprognostic guidelines in post-cardiac arrest patients. *Resuscitation.* 2019;139:343–350. doi: 10.1016/j.resuscitation.2019.03.035

22. Greer DM, Yang J, Scripko PD, Sims JR, Cash S, Wu O, Hafler JP, Schoenfeld DA, Furie KL. Clinical examination for prognostication in comatose cardiac arrest patients. *Resuscitation*. 2013;84:1546–1551. doi: 10.1016/j.resuscitation.2013.07.028
23. Kim JH, Kim MJ, You JS, Lee HS, Park YS, Park I, Chung SP. Multimodal approach for neurologic prognostication of out-of-hospital cardiac arrest patients undergoing targeted temperature management. *Resuscitation*. 2019;134:33–40. doi: 10.1016/j.resuscitation.2018.11.007
24. Lee KS, Lee SE, Choi JY, Gho YR, Chae MK, Park EJ, Choi MH, Hong JM. Useful Computed Tomography Score for Estimation of Early Neurologic Outcome in Post-Cardiac Arrest Patients With Therapeutic Hypothermia. *Circ J*. 2017;81:1628–1635. doi: 10.1253/circj.CJ-16-1327
25. Scarpino M, Carrai R, Lolli F, Lanzo G, Spalletti M, Valzania F, Lombardi M, Audenino D, Contardi S, Celani MG, et al; on behalf of the ProNeCA Study Group. Neurophysiology for predicting good and poor neurological outcome at 12 and 72 h after cardiac arrest: the ProNeCA multicentre prospective study. *Resuscitation*. 2020;147:95–103. doi: 10.1016/j.resuscitation.2019.11.014
26. Heimburger D, Durand M, Gaide-Chevronnay L, Dessertaine G, Moury PH, Bouzat P, Albaladejo P, Payen JF. Quantitative pupillometry and transcranial Doppler measurements in patients treated with hypothermia after cardiac arrest. *Resuscitation*. 2016;103:88–93. doi: 10.1016/j.resuscitation.2016.02.026
27. Solari D, Rossetti AO, Carteron L, Miroz JP, Novy J, Eckert P, Oddo M. Early prediction of coma recovery after cardiac arrest with blinded pupillometry. *Ann Neurol*. 2017;81:804–810. doi: 10.1002/ana.24943
28. Riker RR, Sawyer ME, Fischman VG, May T, Lord C, Eldridge A, Seder DB. Neurological Pupil Index and Pupillary Light Reflex by Pupillometry Predict Outcome Early After Cardiac Arrest. *Neurocrit Care*. 2020;32:152–161. doi: 10.1007/s12028-019-00717-4
29. Obling L, Hassager C, Illum C, Grand J, Wiberg S, Lindholm MG, Winther-Jensen M, Kondziella D, Kjaergaard J. Prognostic value of automated pupillometry: an unselected cohort from a cardiac intensive care unit. *Eur Heart J Acute Cardiovasc Care*. 2019:2048872619842004. doi: 10.1177/2048872619842004
30. Sivaraju A, Gilmore EJ, Wira CR, Stevens A, Rampal N, Moeller JJ, Greer DM, Hirsch LJ, Gaspard N. Prognostication of post-cardiac arrest coma: early clinical and electroencephalographic predictors of outcome. *Intensive Care Med*. 2015;41:1264–1272. doi: 10.1007/s00134-015-3834-x
31. Kim SH, Choi SP, Park KN, Youn CS, Oh SH, Choi SM. Early brain computed tomography findings are associated with outcome in patients treated with therapeutic hypothermia after out-of-hospital cardiac arrest. *Scand J Trauma*. 2013;21:57. doi: 10.1186/1757-7241-21-57
32. Ruknuddeen MI, Ramadoss R, Rajajee V, Grzeskowiak LE, Rajagopalan RE. Early clinical prediction of neurological outcome following out of hospital cardiac arrest managed with therapeutic hypothermia. *Indian J Crit Care Med*. 2015;19:304–310. doi: 10.4103/0972-5229.158256
33. Elmer J, Rittenberger JC, Faro J, Molyneaux BJ, Popescu A, Callaway CW, Baldwin M; Pittsburgh Post-Cardiac Arrest Service. Clinically distinct electroencephalographic phenotypes of early myoclonus after cardiac arrest. *Ann Neurol*. 2016;80:175–184. doi: 10.1002/ana.24697
34. Aicua RI, Rapun I, Novy J, Solari D, Oddo M, Rossetti AO. Early Lance-Adams syndrome after cardiac arrest: prevalence, time to return to awareness, and outcome in a large cohort. *Resuscitation*. 2017;115:169–172. doi: 10.1016/j.resuscitation.2017.03.020
35. Sadaka F, Doerr D, Hindia J, Lee KP, Logan W. Continuous Electroencephalogram in Comatose Postcardiac Arrest Syndrome Patients Treated With Therapeutic Hypothermia: Outcome Prediction Study. *J Intensive Care Med*. 2015;30:292–296. doi: 10.1177/0885066613517214
36. Lybeck A, Friberg H, Aneman A, Hassager C, Horn J, Kjærgaard J, Kuiper M, Nielsen N, Ullén S, Wise MP, Westhall E, Cronberg T; TTM-trial Investigators. Prognostic significance of clinical seizures after cardiac arrest and target temperature management. *Resuscitation*. 2017;114:146–151. doi: 10.1016/j.resuscitation.2017.01.017
37. Reynolds AS, Rohaut B, Holmes MG, Robinson D, Roth W, Velazquez A, Couch CK, Presciutti A, Brodie D, Moitra VK, Rabbani LE, Agarwal S, Park S, Roh DJ, Claassen J. Early myoclonus following anoxic brain injury. *Neurol Clin Pract*. 2018;8:249–256. doi: 10.1212/CPJ.0000000000000466
38. Lee BK, Jeung KW, Lee HY, Jung YH, Lee DH. Combining brain computed tomography and serum neuron specific enolase improves the prognostic performance compared to either alone in comatose cardiac arrest survivors treated with therapeutic hypothermia. *Resuscitation*. 2013;84:1387–1392. doi: 10.1016/j.resuscitation.2013.05.026
39. Vondrakova D, Kruger A, Janotka M, Malek F, Dudkova V, Neuzil P, Ostadal P. Association of neuron-specific enolase values with outcomes in cardiac arrest survivors is dependent on the time of sample collection. *Crit Care*. 2017;21:172. doi: 10.1186/s13054-017-1766-2
40. Duez CHV, Grejs AM, Jeppesen AN, Schrøder AD, Søreide E, Nielsen JF, Kirkegaard H. Neuron-specific enolase and S-100b in prolonged targeted temperature management after cardiac arrest: A randomised study. *Resuscitation*. 2018;122:79–86. doi: 10.1016/j.resuscitation.2017.11.052
41. Stammet P, Collignon O, Hassager C, Wise MP, Hovdenes J, Åneman A, Horn J, Devaux Y, Erlinge D, Kjaergaard J, Gasche Y, Wanscher M, Cronberg T, Friberg H, Wetterslev J, Pellis T, Kuiper M, Gilson G, Nielsen N; TTM-Trial Investigators. Neuron-Specific Enolase as a Predictor of Death or Poor Neurological Outcome After Out-of-Hospital Cardiac Arrest and Targeted Temperature Management at 33°C and 36°C. *J Am Coll Cardiol*. 2015;65:2104–2114. doi: 10.1016/j.jacc.2015.03.538
42. Zellner T, Gärtner R, Schopohl J, Angstwurm M. NSE and S-100B are not sufficiently predictive of neurologic outcome after therapeutic hypothermia for cardiac arrest. *Resuscitation*. 2013;84:1382–1386. doi: 10.1016/j.resuscitation.2013.03.021
43. Tsetsou S, Novy J, Pfeiffer C, Oddo M, Rossetti AO. Multimodal Outcome Prognostication After Cardiac Arrest and Targeted Temperature Management: Analysis at 36 °C. *Neurocrit Care*. 2018;28:104–109. doi: 10.1007/s12028-017-0393-8
44. Helwig K, Seeger F, Hölschermann H, Lischke V, Gerriets T, Niessner M, Foerch C. Elevated Serum Glial Fibrillary Acidic Protein (GFAP) is Associated with Poor Functional Outcome After Cardiopulmonary Resuscitation. *Neurocrit Care*. 2017;27:68–74. doi: 10.1007/s12028-016-0371-6
45. Rossetti AO, Tovar Quiroga DF, Juan E, Novy J, White RD, Ben-Hamouda N, Britton JW, Oddo M, Rabinstein AA. Electroencephalography predicts poor and good outcomes after cardiac arrest: a two-center study. *Crit Care Med*. 2017;45:e674–e682. doi: 10.1097/CCM.0000000000002337
46. Wiberg S, Hassager C, Stammet P, Winther-Jensen M, Thomsen JH, Erlinge D, Wanscher M, Nielsen N, Pellis T, Åneman A, Friberg H, Hovdenes J, Horn J, Wetterslev J, Bro-Jeppesen J, Wise MP, Kuiper M, Cronberg T, Gasche Y, Devaux Y, Kjaergaard J. Single versus Serial Measurements of Neuron-Specific Enolase and Prediction of Poor Neurological Outcome in Persistently Unconscious Patients after Out-Of-Hospital Cardiac Arrest - A TTM-Trial Substudy. *PLoS One*. 2017;12:e0168894. doi: 10.1371/journal.pone.0168894
47. Jang JH, Park WB, Lim YS, Choi JY, Cho JS, Woo JH, Choi WS, Yang HJ, Hyun SY. Combination of S100B and procalcitonin improves prognostic performance compared to either alone in patients with cardiac arrest: a prospective observational study. *Medicine (Baltimore)*. 2019;98:e14496. doi: 10.1097/MD.0000000000014496
48. Stammet P, Dankiewicz J, Nielsen N, Fays F, Collignon O, Hassager C, Wanscher M, Undèn J, Wetterslev J, Pellis T, Aneman A, Hovdenes J, Wise MP, Gilson G, Erlinge D, Horn J, Cronberg T, Kuiper M, Kjaergaard J, Gasche Y, Devaux Y, Friberg H; Target Temperature Management after Out-of-Hospital Cardiac Arrest (TTM) trial investigators. Protein S100 as outcome predictor after out-of-hospital cardiac arrest and targeted temperature management at 33 °C and 36 °C. *Crit Care*. 2017;21:153. doi: 10.1186/s13054-017-1729-7
49. Mattsson N, Zetterberg H, Nielsen N, Blennow K, Dankiewicz J, Friberg H, Lilja G, Insel PS, Rylander C, Stammet P, Aneman A, Hassager C, Kjaergaard J, Kuiper M, Pellis T, Wetterslev J, Wise M, Cronberg T. Serum tau and neurological outcome in cardiac arrest. *Ann Neurol*. 2017;82:665–675. doi: 10.1002/ana.25067
50. Moseby-Knappe M, Mattsson N, Nielsen N, Zetterberg H, Blennow K, Dankiewicz J, Dragancea I, Friberg H, Lilja G, Insel PS, Rylander C, Westhall E, Kjaergaard J, Wise MP, Hassager C, Kuiper MA, Stammet P, Wanscher MCJ, Wetterslev J, Erlinge D, Horn J, Pellis T, Cronberg T. Serum Neurofilament Light Chain for Prognosis of Outcome After Cardiac Arrest. *JAMA Neurol*. 2019;76:64–71. doi: 10.1001/jamaneurol.2018.3223
51. Rana OR, Schröder JW, Baukloh JK, Saygili E, Mischke K, Schiefer J, Weis J, Marx N, Rassaf T, Kelm M, Shin DI, Meyer C, Saygili E. Neurofilament light chain as an early and sensitive predictor of long-term neurological outcome in patients after cardiac arrest. *Int J Cardiol*. 2013;168:1322–1327. doi: 10.1016/j.ijcard.2012.12.016
52. Lamartine Monteiro M, Taccone FS, Depondt C, Lamanna I, Gaspard N, Ligot N, Mavroudakis N, Naeije G, Vincent JL, Legros B. The Prognostic Value of 48-h Continuous EEG During Therapeutic Hypothermia After Cardiac Arrest. *Neurocrit Care*. 2016;24:153–162. doi: 10.1007/s12028-015-0215-9
53. Benarous L, Gavaret M, Soda Diop M, Tobarias J, de Ghaisne de Bourmont S, Allez C, Bouzana F, Gainnier M, Trebuchon A. Sources of interrater variability

and prognostic value of standardized EEG features in post-anoxic coma after resuscitated cardiac arrest. *Clin Neurophysiol Pract.* 2019;4:20–26. doi: 10.1016/j.cnp.2018.12.001
54. Westhall E, Rossetti AO, van Rootselaar AF, Wesenberg Kjaer T, Horn J, Ullén S, Friberg H, Nielsen N, Rosén I, Åneman A, Erlinge D, Gasche Y, Hassager C, Hovdenes J, Kjaergaard J, Kuiper M, Pellis T, Stammet P, Wanscher M, Wetterslev J, Wise MP, Cronberg T; TTM-trial investigators. Standardized EEG interpretation accurately predicts prognosis after cardiac arrest. *Neurology.* 2016;86:1482–1490. doi: 10.1212/WNL.0000000000002462
55. Amorim E, Rittenberger JC, Zheng JJ, Westover MB, Baldwin ME, Callaway CW, Popescu A; Post Cardiac Arrest Service. Continuous EEG monitoring enhances multimodal outcome prediction in hypoxic-ischemic brain injury. *Resuscitation.* 2016;109:121–126. doi: 10.1016/j.resuscitation.2016.08.012
56. Rundgren M, Westhall E, Cronberg T, Rosén I, Friberg H. Continuous amplitude-integrated electroencephalogram predicts outcome in hypothermia-treated cardiac arrest patients. *Crit Care Med.* 2010;38:1838–1844. doi: 10.1097/CCM.0b013e3181eaa1e7
57. Legriel S, Hilly-Ginoux J, Resche-Rigon M, Merceron S, Pinoteau J, Henry-Lagarrigue M, Bruneel F, Nguyen A, Guezennec P, Troché G, Richard O, Pico F, Bédos JP. Prognostic value of electrographic postanoxic status epilepticus in comatose cardiac-arrest survivors in the therapeutic hypothermia era. *Resuscitation.* 2013;84:343–350. doi: 10.1016/j.resuscitation.2012.11.001
58. Oh SH, Park KN, Shon YM, Kim YM, Kim HJ, Youn CS, Kim SH, Choi SP, Kim SC. Continuous Amplitude-Integrated Electroencephalographic Monitoring Is a Useful Prognostic Tool for Hypothermia-Treated Cardiac Arrest Patients. *Circulation.* 2015;132:1094–1103. doi: 10.1161/CIRCULATIONAHA.115.015754
59. Leão RN, Ávila P, Cavaco R, Germano N, Bento L. Therapeutic hypothermia after cardiac arrest: outcome predictors. *Rev Bras Ter Intensiva.* 2015;27:322–332. doi: 10.5935/0103-507X.20150056
60. Dragancea I, Backman S, Westhall E, Rundgren M, Friberg H, Cronberg T. Outcome following postanoxic status epilepticus in patients with targeted temperature management after cardiac arrest. *Epilepsy Behav.* 2015;49:173–177. doi: 10.1016/j.yebeh.2015.04.043
61. Beretta S, Coppo A, Bianchi E, Zanchi C, Carone D, Stabile A, Padovano G, Sulmina E, Grassi A, Bogliun G, Foti G, Ferrarese C, Pesenti A, Beghi E, Avalli L. Neurological outcome of postanoxic refractory status epilepticus after aggressive treatment. *Epilepsy Behav.* 2019;101(Pt B):106374. doi: 10.1016/j.yebeh.2019.06.018
62. Alvarez V, Reinsberger C, Scirica B, O'Brien MH, Avery KR, Henderson G, Lee JW. Continuous electrodermal activity as a potential novel neurophysiological biomarker of prognosis after cardiac arrest–A pilot study. *Resuscitation.* 2015;93:128–135. doi: 10.1016/j.resuscitation.2015.06.006
63. Backman S, Cronberg T, Friberg H, Ullén S, Horn J, Kjaergaard J, Hassager C, Wanscher M, Nielsen N, Westhall E. Highly malignant routine EEG predicts poor prognosis after cardiac arrest in the Target Temperature Management trial. *Resuscitation.* 2018;131:24–28. doi: 10.1016/j.resuscitation.2018.07.024
64. Ruijter BJ, Tjepkema-Cloostermans MC, Tromp SC, van den Bergh WM, Foudraine NA, Kornips FHM, Drost G, Scholten E, Bosch FH, Beishuizen A, van Putten MJAM, Hofmeijer J. Early electroencephalography for outcome prediction of postanoxic coma: A prospective cohort study. *Ann Neurol.* 2019;86:203–214. doi: 10.1002/ana.25518
65. Grippo A, Carrai R, Scarpino M, Spalletti M, Lanzo G, Cossu C, Peris A, Valente S, Amantini A. Neurophysiological prediction of neurological good and poor outcome in post-anoxic coma. *Acta Neurol Scand.* 2017;135:641–648. doi: 10.1111/ane.12659
66. Scarpino M, Lolli F, Lanzo G, Carrai R, Spalletti M, Valzania F, Lombardi M, Audenino D, Celani MG, Marrelli A, Contardi S, Peris A, Amantini A, Sandroni C, Grippo A; ProNeCAStudy Group. Neurophysiological and neuroradiological test for early poor outcome (Cerebral Performance Categories 3-5) prediction after cardiac arrest: Prospective multicentre prognostication data. *Data Brief.* 2019;27:104755. doi: 10.1016/j.dib.2019.104755
67. De Santis P, Lamanna I, Mavroudakis N, Legros B, Vincent JL, Creteur J, Taccone FS. The potential role of auditory evoked potentials to assess prognosis in comatose survivors from cardiac arrest. *Resuscitation.* 2017;120:119–124. doi: 10.1016/j.resuscitation.2017.09.013
68. Kim SW, Oh JS, Park J, Jeong HH, Kim JH, Wee JH, Oh SH, Choi SP, Park KN; Cerebral Resuscitation and Outcome evaluation Within catholic Network (CROWN) Investigators. Short-Latency Positive Peak Following N20 Somatosensory Evoked Potential Is Superior to N20 in Predicting Neurologic Outcome After Out-of-Hospital Cardiac Arrest. *Crit Care Med.* 2018;46:e545–e551. doi: 10.1097/CCM.0000000000003083
69. Scarpino M, Carrai R, Lolli F, Lanzo G, Spalletti M, Valzania F, Lombardi M, Audenino D, Contardi S, Celani MG, Marrelli A, Mecarelli O, Minardi C, Minicucci F, Politini L, Vitelli E, Peris A, Amantini A, Sandroni C, Grippo A; ProNeCA study group. Neurophysiology for predicting good and poor neurological outcome at 12 and 72 h after cardiac arrest: The ProNeCA multicentre prospective study. *Resuscitation.* 2020;147:95–103. doi: 10.1016/j.resuscitation.2019.11.014
70. Maciel CB, Morawo AO, Tsao CY, Youn TS, Labar DR, Rubens EO, Greer DM. SSEP in Therapeutic Hypothermia Era. *J Clin Neurophysiol.* 2017;34:469–475. doi: 10.1097/WNP.0000000000000392
71. Admiraal MM, van Rootselaar AF, Hofmeijer J, Hoedemaekers CWE, van Kaam CR, Keijzer HM, van Putten MJAM, Schultz MJ, Horn J. Electroencephalographic reactivity as predictor of neurological outcome in postanoxic coma: A multicenter prospective cohort study. *Ann Neurol.* 2019;86:17–27. doi: 10.1002/ana.25507
72. Duez CHV, Johnsen B, Ebbesen MQ, Kvaløy MB, Grejs AM, Jeppesen AN, Søreide E, Nielsen JF, Kirkegaard H. Post resuscitation prognostication by EEG in 24 vs 48 h of targeted temperature management. *Resuscitation.* 2019;135:145–152. doi: 10.1016/j.resuscitation.2018.10.035
73. Liu G, Su Y, Liu Y, Jiang M, Zhang Y, Zhang Y, Gao D. Predicting Outcome in Comatose Patients: The Role of EEG Reactivity to Quantifiable Electrical Stimuli. *Evid Based Complement Alternat Med.* 2016;2016:8273716. doi: 10.1155/2016/8273716
74. Jeon CH, Park JS, Lee JH, Kim H, Kim SC, Park KH, Yi KS, Kim SM, Youn CS, Kim YM, Lee BK. Comparison of brain computed tomography and diffusion-weighted magnetic resonance imaging to predict early neurologic outcome before target temperature management comatose cardiac arrest survivors. *Resuscitation.* 2017;118:21–26. doi: 10.1016/j.resuscitation.2017.06.021
75. Kim Y, Ho LJ, Kun HC, Won CK, Hoon YJ, Ju KM, Weon KY, Yul LK, Joo KJ, Youn HS. Feasibility of optic nerve sheath diameter measured on initial brain computed tomography as an early neurologic outcome predictor after cardiac arrest *Academic Emergency Medicine* 2014;21:1121–1128.
76. Lee DH, Lee BK, Jeung KW, Jung YH, Cho YS, Cho IS, Youn CS, Kim JW, Park JS, Min YI. Relationship between ventricular characteristics on brain computed tomography and 6-month neurologic outcome in cardiac arrest survivors who underwent targeted temperature management. *Resuscitation.* 2018;129:37–42. doi: 10.1016/j.resuscitation.2018.06.008
77. Scarpino M, Lanzo G, Lolli F, Carrai R, Moretti M, Spalletti M, Cozzolino M, Peris A, Amantini A, Grippo A. Neurophysiological and neuroradiological multimodal approach for early poor outcome prediction after cardiac arrest. *Resuscitation.* 2018;129:114–120. doi: 10.1016/j.resuscitation.2018.04.016
78. Wang GN, Chen XF, Lv JR, Sun NN, Xu XQ, Zhang JS. The prognostic value of gray-white matter ratio on brain computed tomography in adult comatose cardiac arrest survivors. *J Chin Med Assoc.* 2018;81:599–604. doi: 10.1016/j.jcma.2018.03.003
79. Youn CS, Callaway CW, Rittenberger JC; Post Cardiac Arrest Service. Combination of initial neurologic examination, quantitative brain imaging and electroencephalography to predict outcome after cardiac arrest. *Resuscitation.* 2017;110:120–125. doi: 10.1016/j.resuscitation.2016.10.024
80. Greer DM, Scripko PD, Wu O, Edlow BL, Bartscher J, Sims JR, Camargo EE, Singhal AB, Furie KL. Hippocampal magnetic resonance imaging abnormalities in cardiac arrest are associated with poor outcome. *J Stroke.Cerebrovasc Dis.* 2013;22:899–905. doi: 10.1016/j.jstrokecerebrovasdis.2012.08.006
81. Jang J, Oh SH, Nam Y, Lee K, Choi HS, Jung SL, Ahn KJ, Park KN, Kim BS. Prognostic value of phase information of 2D T2*-weighted gradient echo brain imaging in cardiac arrest survivors: A preliminary study. *Resuscitation.* 2019;140:142–149. doi: 10.1016/j.resuscitation.2019.05.026
82. Moon HK, Jang J, Park KN, Kim SH, Lee BK, Oh SH, Jeung KW, Choi SP, Cho IS, Youn CS. Quantitative analysis of relative volume of low apparent diffusion coefficient value can predict neurologic outcome after cardiac arrest. *Resuscitation.* 2018;126:36–42. doi: 10.1016/j.resuscitation.2018.02.020
83. Kim J, Kim K, Hong S, Kwon B, Yun ID, Choi BS, Jung C, Lee JH, Jo YH, Kim T, et al. Low apparent diffusion coefficient cluster-based analysis of diffusion-weighted MRI for prognostication of out-of-hospital cardiac arrest survivors. *Resuscitation.* 2013;84:1393–1399. doi: 10.1016/j.resuscitation.2013.04.011
84. Hirsch KG, Fischbein N, Mlynash M, Kemp S, Bammer R, Eyngorn I, Tong J, Moseley M, Venkatasubramanian C, Caulfield AF, Albers G. Prognostic value of diffusion-weighted MRI for post-cardiac arrest coma. *Neurology.* 2020;94:e1684–e1692. doi: 10.1212/WNL.0000000000009289

RECOVERY

Recovery and Survivorship After Cardiac Arrest

Recommendations for Recovery and Survivorship After Cardiac Arrest		
COR	LOE	Recommendations
1	B-NR	1. We recommend structured assessment for anxiety, depression, posttraumatic stress, and fatigue for cardiac arrest survivors and their caregivers.
1	C-LD	2. We recommend that cardiac arrest survivors have multimodal rehabilitation assessment and treatment for physical, neurological, cardiopulmonary, and cognitive impairments before discharge from the hospital.
1	C-LD	3. We recommend that cardiac arrest survivors and their caregivers receive comprehensive, multidisciplinary discharge planning, to include medical and rehabilitative treatment recommendations and return to activity/work expectations.
2b	C-LD	4. Debriefings and referral for follow-up for emotional support for lay rescuers, EMS providers, and hospital-based healthcare workers after a cardiac arrest event may be beneficial.

Synopsis

Cardiac arrest survivors, like many survivors of critical illness, often experience a spectrum of physical, neurological, cognitive, emotional, or social issues, some of which may not become apparent until after hospital discharge. Survivorship after cardiac arrest is the journey through rehabilitation and recovery and highlights the far-reaching impact on patients, families, healthcare partners, and communities (Figure 11).[1–3]

The systems-of-care approach to cardiac arrest includes the community and healthcare response to cardiac arrest. However, with more people surviving cardiac arrest, there is a need to organize discharge planning and long-term rehabilitation care resources. Survivorship plans that address treatment, surveillance, and rehabilitation need to be provided at hospital discharge to optimize transitions of care to the outpatient setting. For many patients and families, these plans and resources may be paramount to improved quality of life after cardiac arrest. Survivorship plans help guide the patient, caregivers, and primary care providers and include a summary of the inpatient course, recommended follow-up appointments, and postdischarge recovery expectations (Figure 12).

Cardiac arrest survivors, their families, and families of nonsurvivors may be powerful advocates for community response to cardiac arrest and patient-centered outcomes. Enhancing survivorship and recovery after cardiac arrest needs to be a systematic priority, aligned with treatment recommendations for patients surviving stroke, cancer, and other critical illnesses.[3–5]

Recommendation-Specific Supportive Text

1. Approximately one third of cardiac arrest survivors experience anxiety, depression, or posttraumatic stress.[6–9] Fatigue is also common and may be due to physical, cognitive, or affective impairments.

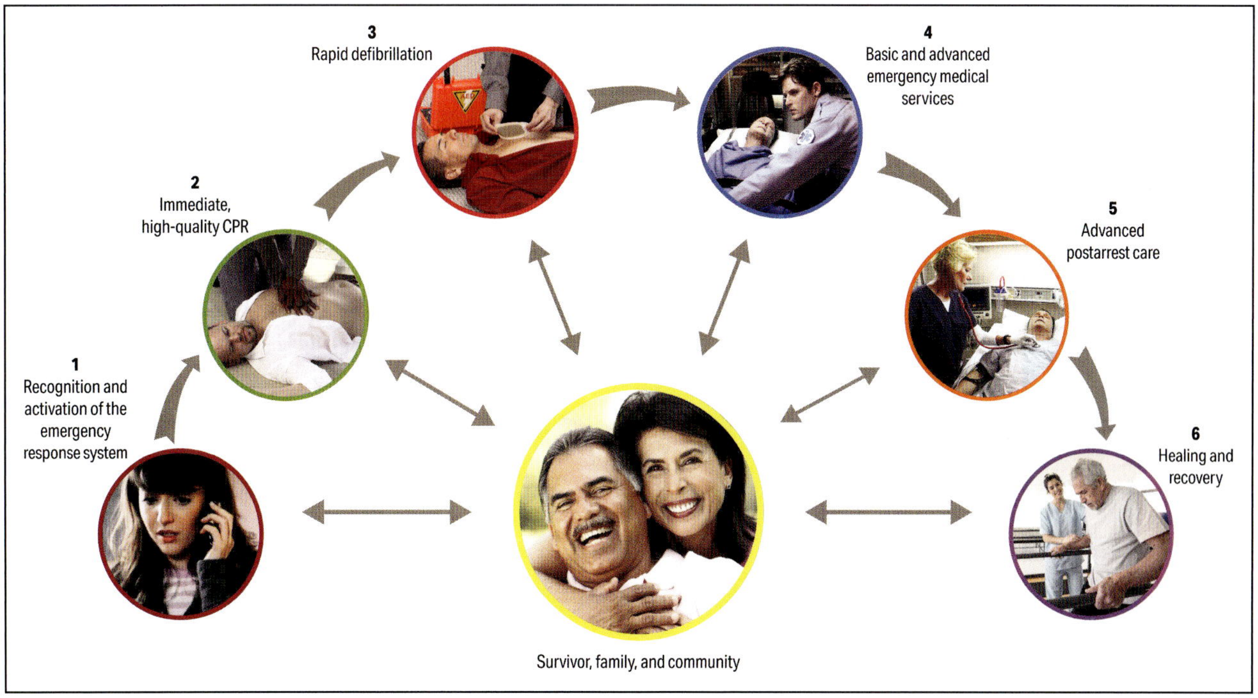

Figure 11. Centralized systems of care in cardiac arrest survivorship.[3]
CPR indicates cardiopulmonary resuscitation.

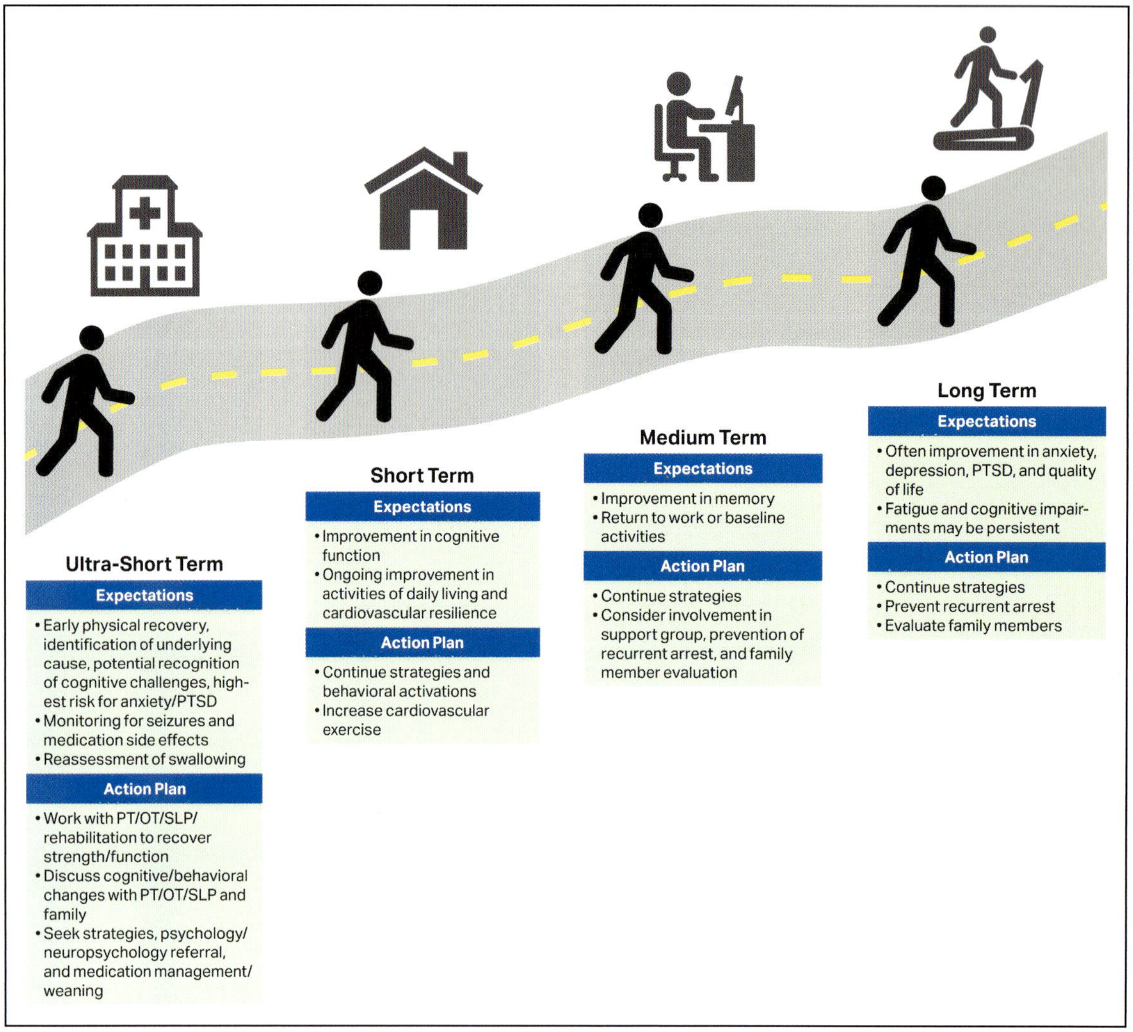

Figure 12. Roadmap to recovery in cardiac arrest survivorship.[3]
OT indicates occupational therapy; PT, physical therapy; PTSD, posttraumatic stress disorder; and SLP, speech-language pathologist.

Family or caregivers may also experience significant stress and benefit from therapy.[10–17]

2. Cognitive impairments after cardiac arrest include difficulty with memory, attention, and executive function.[18–22] Physical, neurological, and cardiopulmonary impairments are also common.[3] Early evaluation for cardiac rehabilitation and physical, occupational, and speech language therapy may be helpful to develop strategies to recover from, overcome, or adapt to impairments.[3,23–25]
3. Community reintegration and return to work or other activities may be slow and depend on social support and relationships.[26–29] Patients need direction about when to begin driving and when to return to intimacy.[30,31]
4. Rescuers may experience anxiety or posttraumatic stress about providing or not providing BLS.[23,32] Hospital-based care providers may also experience emotional or psychological effects of caring for a patient with cardiac arrest.[34] Team debriefings may allow a review of team performance (education, quality improvement) as well as recognition of the natural stressors associated with caring for a patient near death.[35]

These recommendations are supported by "Sudden Cardiac Arrest Survivorship: a Scientific Statement From the AHA."[3]

REFERENCES

1. Iwashyna TJ. Survivorship will be the defining challenge of critical care in the 21st century. *Ann Intern Med.* 2010;153:204–205. doi: 10.7326/0003-4819-153-3-201008030-00013
2. Hope AA, Munro CL. Understanding and Improving Critical Care Survivorship. *Am J Crit Care.* 2019;28:410–412. doi: 10.4037/ajcc2019442
3. Sawyer KN, Camp-Rogers TR, Kotini-Shah P, Del Rios M, Gossip MR, Moitra VK, Haywood KL, Dougherty CM, Lubitz SA, Rabinstein AA, Rittenberger JC, Callaway CW, Abella BS, Geocadin RG, Kurz MC; American Heart Association Emergency Cardiovascular Care Committee; Council on Cardiovascular and Stroke Nursing; Council on Genomic and Precision Medicine; Council on Quality of Care and Outcomes Research; and Stroke Council. Sudden Cardiac Arrest Survivorship: A Scientific Statement From the American Heart Association. *Circulation.* 2020;141:e654–e685. doi: 10.1161/CIR.0000000000000747

4. Nekhlyudov L, O'Malley D M, Hudson SV. Integrating primary care providers in the care of cancer survivors: gaps in evidence and future opportunities. *Lancet Oncol.* 2017;18:e30–e38. doi: 10.1016/S1470-2045(16)30570-8
5. Committee on Cancer Survivorship: Improving Care and Quality of life. *From Cancer Patient to Cancer Survivor—Lost in Transition.* Washington, DC: Institute of Medicine and National Research Council of the National Academies of Sciences; 2006.
6. Wilder Schaaf KP, Artman LK, Peberdy MA, Walker WC, Ornato JP, Gossip MR, Kreutzer JS; Virginia Commonwealth University ARCTIC Investigators. Anxiety, depression, and PTSD following cardiac arrest: a systematic review of the literature. *Resuscitation.* 2013;84:873–877. doi: 10.1016/j.resuscitation.2012.11.021
7. Presciutti A, Verma J, Pavol M, Anbarasan D, Falo C, Brodie D, Rabbani LE, Roh DJ, Park S, Claassen J, Agarwal S. Posttraumatic stress and depressive symptoms characterize cardiac arrest survivors' perceived recovery at hospital discharge. *Gen Hosp Psychiatry.* 2018;53:108–113. doi: 10.1016/j.genhosppsych.2018.02.006
8. Presciutti A, Sobczak E, Sumner JA, Roh DJ, Park S, Claassen J, Kronish I, Agarwal S. The impact of psychological distress on long-term recovery perceptions in survivors of cardiac arrest. *J Crit Care.* 2019;50:227–233. doi: 10.1016/j.jcrc.2018.12.011
9. Lilja G, Nilsson G, Nielsen N, Friberg H, Hassager C, Koopmans M, Kuiper M, Martini A, Mellinghoff J, Pelosi P, Wanscher M, Wise MP, Östman I, Cronberg T. Anxiety and depression among out-of-hospital cardiac arrest survivors. *Resuscitation.* 2015;97:68–75. doi: 10.1016/j.resuscitation.2015.09.389
10. Doolittle ND, Sauvé MJ. Impact of aborted sudden cardiac death on survivors and their spouses: the phenomenon of different reference points. *Am J Crit Care.* 1995;4:389–396.
11. Pusswald G, Fertl E, Faltl M, Auff E. Neurological rehabilitation of severely disabled cardiac arrest survivors. Part II. Life situation of patients and families after treatment. *Resuscitation.* 2000;47:241–248. doi: 10.1016/s0300-9572(00)00240-9
12. Löf S, Sandström A, Engström A. Patients treated with therapeutic hypothermia after cardiac arrest: relatives' experiences. *J Adv Nurs.* 2010;66:1760–1768. doi: 10.1111/j.1365-2648.2010.05352.x
13. Weslien M, Nilstun T, Lundqvist A, Fridlund B. When the unreal becomes real: family members' experiences of cardiac arrest. *Nurs Crit Care.* 2005;10:15–22. doi: 10.1111/j.1362-1017.2005.00094.x
14. Wallin E, Larsson IM, Rubertsson S, Kristoferzon ML. Relatives' experiences of everyday life six months after hypothermia treatment of a significant other's cardiac arrest. *J Clin Nurs.* 2013;22:1639–1646. doi: 10.1111/jocn.12112
15. Larsson IM, Wallin E, Rubertsson S, Kristoferzon ML. Relatives' experiences during the next of kin's hospital stay after surviving cardiac arrest and therapeutic hypothermia. *Eur J Cardiovasc Nurs.* 2013;12:353–359. doi: 10.1177/1474515112459618
16. Dougherty CM. Longitudinal recovery following sudden cardiac arrest and internal cardioverter defibrillator implantation: survivors and their families. *Am J Crit Care.* 1994;3:145–154.
17. Dougherty CM. Family-focused interventions for survivors of sudden cardiac arrest. *J Cardiovasc Nurs.* 1997;12:45–58. doi: 10.1097/00005082-199710000-00006
18. Lilja G, Nielsen N, Friberg H, Horn J, Kjaergaard J, Nilsson F, Pellis T, Wetterslev J, Wise MP, Bosch F, Bro-Jeppesen J, Brunetti I, Buratti AF, Hassager C, Hofgren C, Insorsi A, Kuiper M, Martini A, Palmer N, Rundgren M, Rylander C, van der Veen A, Wanscher M, Watkins H, Cronberg T. Cognitive function in survivors of out-of-hospital cardiac arrest after target temperature management at 33°C versus 36°C. *Circulation.* 2015;131:1340–1349. doi: 10.1161/CIRCULATIONAHA.114.014414
19. Tiainen M, Poutiainen E, Oksanen T, Kaukonen KM, Pettilä V, Skrifvars M, Varpula T, Castrén M. Functional outcome, cognition and quality of life after out-of-hospital cardiac arrest and therapeutic hypothermia: data from a randomized controlled trial. *Scand J Trauma Resusc Emerg Med.* 2015;23:12. doi: 10.1186/s13049-014-0084-9
20. Buanes EA, Gramstad A, Søvig KK, Hufthammer KO, Flaatten H, Husby T, Langørgen J, Heltne JK. Cognitive function and health-related quality of life four years after cardiac arrest. *Resuscitation.* 2015;89:13–18. doi: 10.1016/j.resuscitation.2014.12.021
21. Mateen FJ, Josephs KA, Trenerry MR, Felmlee-Devine MD, Weaver AL, Carone M, White RD. Long-term cognitive outcomes following out-of-hospital cardiac arrest: a population-based study. *Neurology.* 2011;77:1438–1445. doi: 10.1212/WNL.0b013e318232ab33
22. Steinbusch CVM, van Heugten CM, Rasquin SMC, Verbunt JA, Moulaert VRM. Cognitive impairments and subjective cognitive complaints after survival of cardiac arrest: A prospective longitudinal cohort study. *Resuscitation.* 2017;120:132–137. doi: 10.1016/j.resuscitation.2017.08.007
23. Nolan JP, Soar J, Cariou A, Cronberg T, Moulaert VR, Deakin CD, Bottiger BW, Friberg H, Sunde K, Sandroni C. European Resuscitation Council and European Society of Intensive Care Medicine 2015 guidelines for post-resuscitation care. *Intensive Care Med.* 2015;41:2039–2056. doi: 10.1007/s00134-015-4051-3
24. Moulaert VR, Verbunt JA, Bakx WG, Gorgels AP, de Krom MC, Heuts PH, Wade DT, van Heugten CM. 'Stand still., and move on', a new early intervention service for cardiac arrest survivors and their caregivers: rationale and description of the intervention. *Clin Rehabil.* 2011;25:867–879. doi: 10.1177/0269215511399937
25. Cowan MJ, Pike KC, Budzynski HK. Psychosocial nursing therapy following sudden cardiac arrest: impact on two-year survival. *Nurs Res.* 2001;50:68–76. doi: 10.1097/00006199-200103000-00002
26. Lundgren-Nilsson A, Rosén H, Hofgren C, Sunnerhagen KS. The first year after successful cardiac resuscitation: function, activity, participation and quality of life. *Resuscitation.* 2005;66:285–289. doi: 10.1016/j.resuscitation.2005.04.001
27. Middelkamp W, Moulaert VR, Verbunt JA, van Heugten CM, Bakx WG, Wade DT. Life after survival: long-term daily life functioning and quality of life of patients with hypoxic brain injury as a result of a cardiac arrest. *Clin Rehabil.* 2007;21:425–431. doi: 10.1177/0269215507075307
28. Kragholm K, Wissenberg M, Mortensen RN, Fonager K, Jensen SE, Rajan S, Lippert FK, Christensen EF, Hansen PA, Lang-Jensen T, Hendriksen OM, Kober L, Gislason G, Torp-Pedersen C, Rasmussen BS. Return to Work in Out-of-Hospital Cardiac Arrest Survivors: A Nationwide Register-Based Follow-Up Study. *Circulation.* 2015;131:1682–1690. doi: 10.1161/CIRCULATIONAHA.114.011366
29. Lilja G, Nielsen N, Bro-Jeppesen J, Dunford H, Friberg H, Hofgren C, Horn J, Insorsi A, Kjaergaard J, Nilsson F, Pelosi P, Winters T, Wise MP, Cronberg T. Return to Work and Participation in Society After Out-of-Hospital Cardiac Arrest. *Circ Cardiovasc Qual Outcomes.* 2018;11:e003566. doi: 10.1161/CIRCOUTCOMES.117.003566
30. Dougherty CM, Benoliel JQ, Bellin C. Domains of nursing intervention after sudden cardiac arrest and automatic internal cardioverter defibrillator implantation. *Heart Lung.* 2000;29:79–86.
31. Forslund AS, Lundblad D, Jansson JH, Zingmark K, Söderberg S. Risk factors among people surviving out-of-hospital cardiac arrest and their thoughts about what lifestyle means to them: a mixed methods study. *BMC Cardiovasc Disord.* 2013;13:62. doi: 10.1186/1471-2261-13-62
32. Møller TP, Hansen CM, Fjordholt M, Pedersen BD, Østergaard D, Lippert FK. Debriefing bystanders of out-of-hospital cardiac arrest is valuable. *Resuscitation.* 2014;85:1504–1511. doi: 10.1016/j.resuscitation.2014.08.006
33. Deleted in proof.
34. Clark R, McLean C. The professional and personal debriefing needs of ward based nurses after involvement in a cardiac arrest: An explorative qualitative pilot study. *Intensive Crit Care Nurs.* 2018;47:78–84. doi: 10.1016/j.iccn.2018.03.009
35. Ireland S, Gilchrist J, Maconochie I. Debriefing after failed paediatric resuscitation: a survey of current UK practice. *Emerg Med J.* 2008;25:328–330. doi: 10.1136/emj.2007.048942

SPECIAL CIRCUMSTANCES OF RESUSCITATION

Accidental Hypothermia

Recommendations for Accidental Hypothermia		
COR	**LOE**	**Recommendations**
1	C-LD	1. Full resuscitative measures, including extracorporeal rewarming when available, are recommended for all victims of accidental hypothermia without characteristics that deem them unlikely to survive and without any obviously lethal traumatic injury.
1	C-EO	2. Victims of accidental hypothermia should not be considered dead before rewarming has been provided unless there are signs of obvious death.
2b	C-LD	3. It may be reasonable to perform defibrillation attempts according to the standard BLS algorithm concurrent with rewarming strategies.
2b	C-LD	4. It may be reasonable to consider administration of epinephrine during cardiac arrest according to the standard ACLS algorithm concurrent with rewarming strategies.

Synopsis

Severe accidental environmental hypothermia (body temperature less than 30°C [86°F]) causes marked decrease in both heart rate and respiratory rate and may make it difficult to determine if a patient is truly in cardiac arrest. A victim may also appear clinically dead because of the effects of very low body temperature. Lifesaving procedures, including standard BLS and ACLS, are therefore important to continue until a patient is rewarmed unless the victim is obviously dead (eg, rigor mortis or nonsurvivable traumatic injury). Aggressive rewarming, possibly including invasive techniques, may be required and may necessitate transport to the hospital sooner than would be done in other OHCA circumstances.[1] The specific care of patients who are victims of an avalanche are not included in these guidelines but can be found elsewhere.[2]

Recommendation-Specific Supportive Text

1. Patients with accidental hypothermia often present with marked CNS and cardiovascular depression and the appearance of death or near death, necessitating the need for prompt full resuscitative measures unless there are signs of obvious death. Along with providing standard BLS and ALS treatment, next steps include preventing additional evaporative heat loss by removing wet garments and insulating the victim from further environmental exposures. For patients with severe hypothermia (less than 30°C [86°F]) with a perfusing rhythm, core rewarming is often used. Techniques include administration of warm humidified oxygen, warm IV fluids, and intrathoracic or intraperitoneal warm-water lavage.[3–5]For patients with severe hypothermia and cardiac arrest, extracorporeal rewarming allows for most rapid rewarming when available.[6–11] Severe hyperkalemia and very low core temperatures may also predict resuscitation futility.[12,13]
2. When the victim is hypothermic, pulse and respiratory rates may be slow or difficult to detect,[13,14] and the ECG may even show asystole, making it important to perform lifesaving interventions until the victim is warmed and/or obviously dead. Because severe hypothermia is frequently preceded by other disorders (eg, drug overdose, alcohol use, trauma), it is advisable to look for and treat these underlying conditions while simultaneously treating hypothermia.
3. The hypothermic heart may be unresponsive to cardiovascular drugs, pacemaker stimulation, and defibrillation; however, the data to support this are essentially theoretical.[15] If VT or VF persists after a single shock, the value of deferring subsequent defibrillations until a target temperature is achieved is uncertain. There is no evidence to suggest a benefit from deviating from standard BLS protocol for defibrillation.
4. Evidence in humans of the effect of vasopressors or other medications during cardiac arrest in the setting of hypothermia consists of case reports only.[11,16,17] A systematic review of several animal studies concluded that use of vasopressors during hypothermic cardiac arrest did increase ROSC.[18] No evidence was identified at the time of prior review for harm from following standard ACLS, including vasopressor medications, during hypothermic cardiac arrest.

This topic last received formal evidence review in 2010.[1]

REFERENCES

1. Vanden Hoek TL, Morrison LJ, Shuster M, Donnino M, Sinz E, Lavonas EJ, Jeejeebhoy FM, Gabrielli A. Part 12: cardiac arrest in special situations: 2010 American Heart Association Guidelines for Cardiopulmonary Resuscitation and Emergency Cardiovascular Care. *Circulation.* 2010;122(suppl 3):S829–S861. doi: 10.1161/CIRCULATIONAHA.110.971069
2. Brugger H, Durrer B, Elsensohn F, Paal P, Strapazzon G, Winterberger E, Zafren K, Boyd J. Resuscitation of avalanche victims: Evidence-based guidelines of the international commission for mountain emergency medicine (ICAR MEDCOM): intended for physicians and other advanced life support personnel. *Resuscitation.* 2013;84:539–546. doi: 10.1016/j.resuscitation.2012.10.020
3. Kangas E, Niemelä H, Kojo N. Treatment of hypothermic circulatory arrest with thoracotomy and pleural lavage. *Ann Chir Gynaecol.* 1994;83:258–260.
4. Walters DT. Closed thoracic cavity lavage for hypothermia with cardiac arrest. *Ann Emerg Med.* 1991;20:439–440. doi: 10.1016/s0196-0644(05)81687-7
5. Plaisier BR. Thoracic lavage in accidental hypothermia with cardiac arrest–report of a case and review of the literature. *Resuscitation.* 2005;66:99–104. doi: 10.1016/j.resuscitation.2004.12.024

6. Farstad M, Andersen KS, Koller ME, Grong K, Segadal L, Husby P. Rewarming from accidental hypothermia by extracorporeal circulation. A retrospective study. *Eur J Cardiothorac Surg*. 2001;20:58–64. doi: 10.1016/s1010-7940(01)00713-8
7. Sheridan RL, Goldstein MA, Stoddard FJ Jr, Walker TG. Case records of the Massachusetts General Hospital. Case 41-2009. A 16-year-old boy with hypothermia and frostbite. *N Engl J Med*. 2009;361:2654–2662. doi: 10.1056/NEJMcpc0910088
8. Gilbert M, Busund R, Skagseth A, Nilsen PA, Solbø JP. Resuscitation from accidental hypothermia of 13.7 degrees C with circulatory arrest. *Lancet*. 2000;355:375–376. doi: 10.1016/S0140-6736(00)01021-7
9. Coleman E, Doddakula K, Meeke R, Marshall C, Jahangir S, Hinchion J. An atypical case of successful resuscitation of an accidental profound hypothermia patient, occurring in a temperate climate. *Perfusion*. 2010;25:103–106. doi: 10.1177/0267659110366066
10. Althaus U, Aeberhard P, Schüpbach P, Nachbur BH, Mühlemann W. Management of profound accidental hypothermia with cardiorespiratory arrest. *Ann Surg*. 1982;195:492–495. doi: 10.1097/00000658-198204000-00018
11. Dobson JA, Burgess JJ. Resuscitation of severe hypothermia by extracorporeal rewarming in a child. *J Trauma*. 1996;40:483–485. doi: 10.1097/00005373-199603000-00032
12. Brugger H, Bouzat P, Pasquier M, Mair P, Fieler J, Darocha T, Blancher M, de Riedmatten M, Falk M, Paal P, Strapazzon G, Zafren K, Brodmann Maeder M. Cut-off values of serum potassium and core temperature at hospital admission for extracorporeal rewarming of avalanche victims in cardiac arrest: A retrospective multi-centre study. *Resuscitation*. 2019;139:222–229. doi: 10.1016/j.resuscitation.2019.04.025
13. Paal P, Gordon L, Strapazzon G, Brodmann Maeder M, Putzer G, Walpoth B, Wanscher M, Brown D, Holzer M, Broessner G, Brugger H. Accidental hypothermia-an update: The content of this review is endorsed by the International Commission for Mountain Emergency Medicine (ICAR MEDCOM). *Scand J Trauma Resusc Emerg Med*. 2016;24:111. doi: 10.1186/s13049-016-0303-7
14. Danzl DF, Pozos RS. Accidental hypothermia. *N Engl J Med*. 1994;331:1756–1760. doi: 10.1056/NEJM199412293312607
15. Clift J, Munro-Davies L. Best evidence topic report. Is defibrillation effective in accidental severe hypothermia in adults? *Emerg Med J*. 2007;24:50–51. doi: 10.1136/emj.2006.044404
16. Winegard C. Successful treatment of severe hypothermia and prolonged cardiac arrest with closed thoracic cavity lavage. *J Emerg Med*. 1997;15:629–632. doi: 10.1016/s0736-4679(97)00139-x
17. Lienhart HG, John W, Wenzel V. Cardiopulmonary resuscitation of a near-drowned child with a combination of epinephrine and vasopressin. *Pediatr Crit Care Med*. 2005;6:486–488. doi: 10.1097/01.PCC.0000163673.40424.E7
18. Wira CR, Becker JU, Martin G, Donnino MW. Anti-arrhythmic and vasopressor medications for the treatment of ventricular fibrillation in severe hypothermia: a systematic review of the literature. *Resuscitation*. 2008;78:21–29. doi: 10.1016/j.resuscitation.2008.01.025

Anaphylaxis

Introduction

Between 1.6% and 5.1% of US adults have suffered anaphylaxis.[1] Approximately 200 Americans die from anaphylaxis annually, mostly from adverse reactions to medication.[2] Although anaphylaxis is a multisystem disease, life-threatening manifestations most often involve the respiratory tract (edema, bronchospasm) and/or the circulatory system (vasodilatory shock). Epinephrine is the cornerstone of treatment for anaphylaxis.[3–5]

Recommendation for Cardiac Arrest From Anaphylaxis

COR	LOE	Recommendation
1	C-LD	1. In cardiac arrest secondary to anaphylaxis, standard resuscitative measures and immediate administration of epinephrine should take priority.

Recommendation-Specific Supportive Text

1. There are no RCTs evaluating alternative treatment algorithms for cardiac arrest due to anaphylaxis. Evidence is limited to case reports and extrapolations from nonfatal cases, interpretation of pathophysiology, and consensus opinion. Urgent support of airway, breathing, and circulation is essential in suspected anaphylactic reactions. Because of limited evidence, the cornerstone of management of cardiac arrest secondary to anaphylaxis is standard BLS and ACLS, including airway management and early epinephrine. There is no proven benefit from the use of antihistamines, inhaled beta agonists, and IV corticosteroids during anaphylaxis-induced cardiac arrest.

Recommendations for Anaphylaxis Without Cardiac Arrest

COR	LOE	Recommendations
1	C-LD	1. Epinephrine should be administered early by intramuscular injection (or autoinjector) to all patients with signs of a systemic allergic reaction, especially hypotension, airway swelling, or difficulty breathing.
1	C-LD	2. The recommended dose of epinephrine in anaphylaxis is 0.2 to 0.5 mg (1:1000) intramuscularly, to be repeated every 5 to 15 min as needed.
1	C-LD	3. In patients with anaphylactic shock, close hemodynamic monitoring is recommended.
1	C-LD	4. Given the potential for the rapid development of oropharyngeal or laryngeal edema, immediate referral to a health professional with expertise in advanced airway placement, including surgical airway management, is recommended.
2a	C-LD	5. When an IV line is in place, it is reasonable to consider the IV route for epinephrine in anaphylactic shock, at a dose of 0.05 to 0.1 mg (0.1 mg/mL, aka 1:10 000).
2a	C-LD	6. IV infusion of epinephrine is a reasonable alternative to IV boluses for treatment of anaphylaxis in patients not in cardiac arrest.
2b	C-LD	7. IV infusion of epinephrine may be considered for postarrest shock in patients with anaphylaxis.

Recommendation-Specific Supportive Text

1. All patients with evidence of anaphylaxis require early treatment with epinephrine. Severe anaphylaxis may cause complete obstruction of the airway and/or cardiovascular collapse from vasogenic shock. Administration of epinephrine may be lifesaving.[6] Intramuscular is the preferred initial route because of ease of administration, effectiveness, and safety.[7]
2. Injection of epinephrine into the lateral aspect of the thigh produces rapid peak plasma epinephrine concentrations.[7] The adult epinephrine intramuscular

autoinjector will deliver 0.3 mg of epinephrine, and the pediatric epinephrine intramuscular autoinjector will deliver 0.15 mg of epinephrine. Many patients will require additional doses, with recurrence of symptoms after 5 to 15 minutes reported.[8]

3. Patients in anaphylactic shock are critically ill, and cardiovascular and respiratory status can change quickly, making close monitoring imperative.[9]
4. When anaphylaxis produces obstructive airway edema, rapid advanced airway management is critical. In some cases, emergency cricothyroidotomy or tracheostomy may be required.[10,11]
5. IV epinephrine is an appropriate alternative to intramuscular administration in anaphylactic shock when an IV is in place. An IV dose of 0.05 to 0.1 mg (5% to 10% of the epinephrine dose used routinely in cardiac arrest) has been used successfully for anaphylactic shock.[9] Although not specifically studied by this route in anaphylaxis, IO epinephrine is also likely to be effective at comparable doses.
6. In a canine model of anaphylactic shock, a continuous infusion of epinephrine was more effective at treating hypotension than no treatment or bolus epinephrine treatment were.[12] If shock recurs after initial treatment, IV infusion (5–15 μg/min) may also better allow for careful titration and avoidance of overdosing epinephrine.
7. Although data specific to patients with ROSC after cardiac arrest from anaphylaxis was not identified, an observational study of anaphylactic shock suggests that IV infusion of epinephrine (5–15 μg/min), along with other resuscitative measures such as volume resuscitation, can be successful in the treatment of anaphylactic shock.[13] Because of its role in the treatment of anaphylaxis, epinephrine is a logical choice for the treatment of postarrest shock in this setting.

This topic last received formal evidence review in 2010.[14]

REFERENCES

1. Wood RA, Camargo CA Jr, Lieberman P, Sampson HA, Schwartz LB, Zitt M, Collins C, Tringale M, Wilkinson M, Boyle J, et al. Anaphylaxis in America: the prevalence and characteristics of anaphylaxis in the United States. *J Allergy Clin Immunol.* 2014;133:461–467. doi: 10.1016/j.jaci.2013.08.016
2. Jerschow E, Lin RY, Scaperotti MM, McGinn AP. Fatal anaphylaxis in the United States, 1999-2010: temporal patterns and demographic associations. *J Allergy Clin Immunol.* 2014;134:1318.e7–1328.e7. doi: 10.1016/j.jaci.2014.08.018
3. Dhami S, Panesar SS, Roberts G, Muraro A, Worm M, Bilò MB, Cardona V, Dubois AE, DunnGalvin A, Eigenmann P, Fernandez-Rivas M, Halken S, Lack G, Niggemann B, Rueff F, Santos AF, Vlieg-Boerstra B, Zolkipli ZQ, Sheikh A; EAACI Food Allergy and Anaphylaxis Guidelines Group. Management of anaphylaxis: a systematic review. *Allergy.* 2014;69:168–175. doi: 10.1111/all.12318
4. Sheikh A, Simons FE, Barbour V, Worth A. Adrenaline auto-injectors for the treatment of anaphylaxis with and without cardiovascular collapse in the community. *Cochrane Database Syst Rev.* 2012:CD008935. doi: 10.1002/14651858.CD008935.pub2
5. Shaker MS, Wallace DV, Golden DBK, Oppenheimer J, Bernstein JA, Campbell RL, Dinakar C, Ellis A, Greenhawt M, Khan DA, Lang DM, Lang ES, Lieberman JA, Portnoy J, Rank MA, Stukus DR, Wang J, Riblet N, Bobrownicki AMP, Bontrager T, Dusin J, Foley J, Frederick B, Fregene E, Hellerstedt S, Hassan F, Hess K, Horner C, Huntington K, Kasireddy P, Keeler D, Kim B, Lieberman P, Lindhorst E, McEnany F, Milbank J, Murphy H, Pando O, Patel AK, Ratliff N, Rhodes R, Robertson K, Scott H, Snell A, Sullivan R, Trivedi V, Wickham A, Shaker MS, Wallace DV, Shaker MS, Wallace DV, Bernstein JA, Campbell RL, Dinakar C, Ellis A, Golden DBK, Greenhawt M, Lieberman JA, Rank MA, Stukus DR, Wang J, Shaker MS, Wallace DV, Golden DBK, Bernstein JA, Dinakar C, Ellis A, Greenhawt M, Horner C, Khan DA, Lieberman JA, Oppenheimer J, Rank MA, Shaker MS, Stukus DR, Wang J; Collaborators; Chief Editors; Workgroup Contributors; Joint Task Force on Practice Parameters Reviewers. Anaphylaxis-a 2020 practice parameter update, systematic review, and Grading of Recommendations, Assessment, Development and Evaluation (GRADE) analysis. *J Allergy Clin Immunol.* 2020;145:1082–1123. doi: 10.1016/j.jaci.2020.01.017
6. Sheikh A, Shehata YA, Brown SG, Simons FE. Adrenaline (epinephrine) for the treatment of anaphylaxis with and without shock. *Cochrane Database Syst Rev.* 2008:CD006312. doi: 10.1002/14651858.CD006312.pub2
7. Simons FE, Gu X, Simons KJ. Epinephrine absorption in adults: intramuscular versus subcutaneous injection. *J Allergy Clin Immunol.* 2001;108:871–873. doi: 10.1067/mai.2001.119409
8. Korenblat P, Lundie MJ, Dankner RE, Day JH. A retrospective study of epinephrine administration for anaphylaxis: how many doses are needed? *Allergy Asthma Proc.* 1999;20:383–386. doi: 10.2500/108854199778251834
9. Bochner BS, Lichtenstein LM. Anaphylaxis. *N Engl J Med.* 1991;324:1785–1790. doi: 10.1056/NEJM199106203242506
10. Yilmaz R, Yuksekbas O, Erkol Z, Bulut ER, Arslan MN. Postmortem findings after anaphylactic reactions to drugs in Turkey. *Am J Forensic Med Pathol.* 2009;30:346–349. doi: 10.1097/PAF.0b013e3181c0e7bb
11. Yunginger JW, Sweeney KG, Sturner WQ, Giannandrea LA, Teigland JD, Bray M, Benson PA, York JA, Biedrzycki L, Squillace DL. Fatal food-induced anaphylaxis. *JAMA.* 1988;260:1450–1452.
12. Mink SN, Simons FE, Simons KJ, Becker AB, Duke K. Constant infusion of epinephrine, but not bolus treatment, improves haemodynamic recovery in anaphylactic shock in dogs. *Clin Exp Allergy.* 2004;34:1776–1783. doi: 10.1111/j.1365-2222.2004.02106.x
13. Brown SG, Blackman KE, Stenlake V, Heddle RJ. Insect sting anaphylaxis; prospective evaluation of treatment with intravenous adrenaline and volume resuscitation. *Emerg Med J.* 2004;21:149–154. doi: 10.1136/emj.2003.009449
14. Vanden Hoek TL, Morrison LJ, Shuster M, Donnino M, Sinz E, Lavonas EJ, Jeejeebhoy FM, Gabrielli A. Part 12: cardiac arrest in special situations: 2010 American Heart Association Guidelines for Cardiopulmonary Resuscitation and Emergency Cardiovascular Care. *Circulation.* 2010;122(suppl 3):S829–S861. doi: 10.1161/CIRCULATIONAHA.110.971069

Cardiac Arrest Due to Asthma

Recommendations for Management of Cardiac Arrest Due to Asthma

COR	LOE	Recommendations
1	C-LD	1. For asthmatic patients with cardiac arrest, sudden elevation in peak inspiratory pressures or difficulty ventilating should prompt evaluation for tension pneumothorax.
2a	C-LD	2. Due to the potential effects of intrinsic positive end-expiratory pressure (auto-PEEP) and risk of barotrauma in an asthmatic patient with cardiac arrest, a ventilation strategy of low respiratory rate and tidal volume is reasonable.
2a	C-LD	3. If increased auto-PEEP or sudden decrease in blood pressure is noted in asthmatics receiving assisted ventilation in a periarrest state, a brief disconnection from the bag mask or ventilator with compression of the chest wall to relieve air-trapping can be effective.

Synopsis

Severe exacerbations of asthma can lead to profound respiratory distress, retention of carbon dioxide, and air trapping, resulting in acute respiratory acidosis and high intrathoracic pressure. Deaths from acute asthma have decreased in the United States, but asthma continues to be the acute cause of death for over 3500 adults per year.[1,2] Patients with respiratory arrest from asthma develop life-threatening acute respiratory acidosis.[3] Both the profound acidemia and the decreased venous return to the heart from elevated intrathoracic pressure are likely causes of cardiac arrest in asthma.

Care of any patient with cardiac arrest in the setting of acute exacerbation of asthma begins with standard BLS. There are also no specific alterations to ACLS for patients with cardiac arrest from asthma, although airway management and ventilation increase in importance given the likelihood of an underlying respiratory cause of arrest. Acute asthma management was reviewed in detail in the 2010 Guidelines.[4] For 2020, the writing group focused attention on additional ACLS considerations specific to asthma patients in the immediate periarrest period.

Recommendation-Specific Supportive Text

1. Tension pneumothorax is a rare life-threatening complication of asthma and a potentially reversible cause of arrest.[5] Although usually occurring in patients receiving mechanical ventilation, cases in spontaneously breathing patients have been reported.[5–7] High peak airway pressures resulting from positive-pressure ventilation can lead to pneumothorax. While difficulty ventilating an asthmatic patient in extremis is more likely due to hyperinflation and high intrathoracic pressure, evaluation for tension pneumothorax remains important.
2. The acute respiratory failure that can precipitate cardiac arrest in asthma patients is characterized by severe obstruction leading to air trapping. Because of the limitation in exhalational air flow, delivery of large tidal volumes at a higher respiratory rate can lead to progressive worsening of air trapping and a decrease in effective ventilation. An approach using lower tidal volumes, lower respiratory rate, and increased expiratory time may minimize the risk of auto-PEEP and barotrauma.[8]
3. Breath stacking in an asthma patient with limited ability to exhale can lead to increases in intrathoracic pressure, decreases in venous return and coronary perfusion pressure, and cardiac arrest.[9–11] This can manifest as increased difficulty ventilating a patient, high airway pressure alarms on a ventilator, or sudden decreases in blood pressure. Brief disconnection from the ventilator or a pause in bag-mask ventilation and compression of the thorax to aid exhalation may relieve hyperinflation.

This topic last received formal evidence review in 2010.[4]

REFERENCES

1. Moorman JE, Akinbami LJ, Bailey CM, Zahran HS, King ME, Johnson CA, Liu X. National surveillance of asthma: United States, 2001-2010. *Vital Health Stat 3*. 2012:1–58.
2. Centers for Disease Control and Prevention. AsthmaStats: asthma as the underlying cause of death. 2016. https://www.cdc.gov/asthma/asthma_stats/documents/AsthmStat_Mortality_2001-2016-H.pdf. Accessed April 20, 2020.
3. Molfino NA, Nannini LJ, Martelli AN, Slutsky AS. Respiratory arrest in near-fatal asthma. *N Engl J Med*. 1991;324:285–288. doi: 10.1056/NEJM199101313240502
4. Vanden Hoek TL, Morrison LJ, Shuster M, Donnino M, Sinz E, Lavonas EJ, Jeejeebhoy FM, Gabrielli A. Part 12: cardiac arrest in special situations: 2010 American Heart Association Guidelines for Cardiopulmonary Resuscitation and Emergency Cardiovascular Care. *Circulation*. 2010;122(suppl 3):S829–S861. doi: 10.1161/CIRCULATIONAHA.110.971069
5. Leigh-Smith S, Christey G. Tension pneumothorax in asthma. *Resuscitation*. 2006;69:525–527. doi: 10.1016/j.resuscitation.2005.10.011
6. Metry AA. Acute severe asthma complicated with tension pneumothorax and hemopneumothorax. *Int J Crit Illn Inj Sci*. 2019;9:91–95. doi: 10.4103/IJCIIS.IJCIIS_83_18
7. Karakaya Z, Demir S, Sagay SS, Karakaya O, Ozdinç S. Bilateral spontaneous pneumothorax, pneumomediastinum, and subcutaneous emphysema: rare and fatal complications of asthma. *Case Rep Emerg Med*. 2012;2012:242579. doi: 10.1155/2012/242579
8. Leatherman J. Mechanical ventilation for severe asthma. *Chest*. 2015;147:1671–1680. doi: 10.1378/chest.14-1733
9. Myles PS, Madder H, Morgan EB. Intraoperative cardiac arrest after unrecognized dynamic hyperinflation. *Br J Anaesth*. 1995;74:340–342. doi: 10.1093/bja/74.3.340
10. Mercer M. Cardiac arrest after unrecognized dynamic inflation. *Br J Anaesth*. 1995;75:252. doi: 10.1093/bja/75.2.252
11. Berlin D. Hemodynamic consequences of auto-PEEP. *J Intensive Care Med*. 2014;29:81–86. doi: 10.1177/0885066612445712

Cardiac Arrest After Cardiac Surgery

Recommendations for Cardiac Arrest After Cardiac Surgery

COR	LOE	Recommendations
1	B-NR	1. External chest compressions should be performed if emergency resternotomy is not immediately available.
1	C-LD	2. In a trained provider-witnessed arrest of a post–cardiac surgery patient, immediate defibrillation for VF/VT should be performed. CPR should be initiated if defibrillation is not successful within 1 min.
1	C-EO	3. In a trained provider-witnessed arrest of a post–cardiac surgery patient where pacer wires are already in place, we recommend immediate pacing in an asystolic or bradycardic arrest. CPR should be initiated if pacing is not successful within 1 min.
2a	B-NR	4. For patients with cardiac arrest after cardiac surgery, it is reasonable to perform resternotomy early in an appropriately staffed and equipped ICU.
2a	C-LD	5. Open-chest CPR can be useful if cardiac arrest develops during surgery when the chest or abdomen is already open, or in the early postoperative period after cardiothoracic surgery.
2b	C-LD	6. In post–cardiac surgery patients who are refractory to standard resuscitation procedures, mechanical circulatory support may be effective in improving outcome.

Synopsis

Cardiac arrest occurs after 1% to 8% of cardiac surgery cases.[1–8] Etiologies include tachyarrhythmias such as VT or VF, bradyarrhythmias such as heart block or asystole, obstructive causes such as tamponade or pneumothorax, technical factors such as dysfunction of a new valve, occlusion of a grafted artery, or bleeding. Like all patients with cardiac arrest, the immediate goal is restoration of perfusion with CPR, initiation of ACLS, and rapid identification and correction of the cause of cardiac arrest. Unlike most other cardiac arrests, these patients typically develop cardiac arrest in a highly monitored setting such as an ICU, with highly trained staff available to perform rescue therapies.

These guidelines are not meant to be comprehensive. A recent consensus statement on this topic has been published by the Society of Thoracic Surgeons.[9]

Recommendation-Specific Supportive Text

1. Case reports have rarely described damage to the heart due to external chest compressions.[10–14] However, other case series have not reported such damage,[8] and external chest compressions remain the only means of providing perfusion in some circumstances. In this case, the risk of external chest compressions is far outweighed by the certain death in the absence of perfusion.
2. VF is the presenting rhythm in 25% to 50% of cases of cardiac arrest after cardiac surgery. Immediate defibrillation by a trained provider presents distinct advantages in these patients, whereas the morbidity associated with external chest compressions or resternotomy may substantially impact recovery. Sparse data have been published addressing this question. Limited data are available from defibrillator threshold testing with backup transthoracic defibrillation, using variable waveforms and energy doses.[15–17] First shock success over 90% was observed in most of these studies, though pooled results from 15 studies found a defibrillation success rate of 78% for the first shock, 35% for the second, and 14% for the third shock.[18] The Society of Thoracic Surgeons Task Force on Resuscitation After Cardiac Surgery[9] and the European Association for Cardio-Thoracic Surgery[18] recommend 3 stacked defibrillations within 1 minute, before initiation of CPR. This departure from standard ACLS is likely warranted in the post–cardiac surgery setting because of the highly monitored setting and unique risks of compressions and resternotomy.
3. In post–cardiac surgery patients with asystole or bradycardic arrest in the ICU with pacing leads in place, pacing can be initiated immediately by trained providers. Available hemodynamic monitoring modalities in conjunction with manual pulse detection provide an opportunity to confirm myocardial capture and adequate cardiac function. When pacing attempts are not immediately successful, standard ACLS including CPR is indicated. This protocol is supported by the surgical societies,[9,18] though no data are available to support its use.
4. No RCTs of resternotomy timing have been performed. However, good outcomes have been observed with rapid resternotomy protocols when performed by experienced providers in an appropriately equipped ICU.[1,4,8,19–25] Other studies are neutral or show no benefit of resternotomy compared with standard therapy.[3,6,26,27] Resternotomy performed outside of the ICU results in poor outcomes.[1,3] The Society of Thoracic Surgeons recommends that resternotomy be a standard part of the resuscitation protocols for at least 10 days after surgery.[9]
5. No randomized RCTs have been performed comparing open-chest with external CPR. Two small studies have demonstrated improved hemodynamic effects of open-chest CPR when compared with external chest compressions in cardiac surgery patients.[3,4]
6. Multiple case series have demonstrated potential benefit from mechanical circulatory support including ECMO and cardiopulmonary bypass in patients who are refractory to standard resuscitation procedures.[24,28–34] No RCT has been performed to date.

This topic last received formal evidence review in 2010.[35] These recommendations were supplemented by a 2017 review published by the Society of Thoracic Surgeons.[9]

REFERENCES

1. Mackay JH, Powell SJ, Osgathorp J, Rozario CJ. Six-year prospective audit of chest reopening after cardiac arrest. *Eur J Cardiothorac Surg.* 2002;22:421–425. doi: 10.1016/s1010-7940(02)00294-4
2. Birdi I, Chaudhuri N, Lenthall K, Reddy S, Nashef SA. Emergency reinstitution of cardiopulmonary bypass following cardiac surgery: outcome justifies the cost. *Eur J Cardiothorac Surg.* 2000;17:743–746. doi: 10.1016/s1010-7940(00)00453-x
3. Pottle A, Bullock I, Thomas J, Scott L. Survival to discharge following open chest cardiac compression (OCCC). A 4-year retrospective audit in a cardiothoracic specialist centre–Royal Brompton and Harefield NHS Trust, United Kingdom. *Resuscitation.* 2002;52:269–272. doi: 10.1016/s0300-9572(01)00479-8
4. Anthi A, Tzelepis GE, Alivizatos P, Michalis A, Palatianos GM, Geroulanos S. Unexpected cardiac arrest after cardiac surgery: incidence, predisposing causes, and outcome of open chest cardiopulmonary resuscitation. *Chest.* 1998;113:15–19. doi: 10.1378/chest.113.1.15
5. Charalambous CP, Zipitis CS, Keenan DJ. Chest reexploration in the intensive care unit after cardiac surgery: a safe alternative to returning to the operating theater. *Ann Thorac Surg.* 2006;81:191–194. doi: 10.1016/j.athoracsur.2005.06.024
6. Wahba A, Götz W, Birnbaum DE. Outcome of cardiopulmonary resuscitation following open heart surgery. *Scand Cardiovasc J.* 1997;31:147–149. doi: 10.3109/14017439709058084
7. LaPar DJ, Ghanta RK, Kern JA, Crosby IK, Rich JB, Speir AM, Kron IL, Ailawadi G; and the Investigators for the Virginia Cardiac Surgery Quality

Initiative. Hospital variation in mortality from cardiac arrest after cardiac surgery: an opportunity for improvement? *Ann Thorac Surg.* 2014;98:534–539. doi: 10.1016/j.athoracsur.2014.03.030
8. el-Banayosy A, Brehm C, Kizner L, Hartmann D, Körtke H, Körner MM, Minami K, Reichelt W, Körfer R. Cardiopulmonary resuscitation after cardiac surgery: a two-year study. *J Cardiothorac Vasc Anesth.* 1998;12:390–392. doi: 10.1016/s1053-0770(98)90189-6
9. Society of Thoracic Surgeons Task Force on Resuscitation After Cardiac Surgery. The Society of Thoracic Surgeons expert consensus for the resuscitation of patients who arrest after cardiac surgery. *Ann Thorac Surg.* 2017;103:1005–1020. doi: 10.1016/j.athoracsur.2016.10.033
10. Böhrer H, Gust R, Böttiger BW. Cardiopulmonary resuscitation after cardiac surgery. *J Cardiothorac Vasc Anesth.* 1995;9:352. doi: 10.1016/s1053-0770(05)80355-6
11. Ricci M, Karamanoukian HL, D'Ancona G, Jajkowski MR, Bergsland J, Salerno TA. Avulsion of an H graft during closed-chest cardiopulmonary resuscitation after minimally invasive coronary artery bypass graft surgery. *J Cardiothorac Vasc Anesth.* 2000;14:586–587. doi: 10.1053/jcan.2000.9440
12. Kempen PM, Allgood R. Right ventricular rupture during closed-chest cardiopulmonary resuscitation after pneumonectomy with pericardiotomy: a case report. *Crit Care Med.* 1999;27:1378–1379. doi: 10.1097/00003246-199907000-00033
13. Sokolove PE, Willis-Shore J, Panacek EA. Exsanguination due to right ventricular rupture during closed-chest cardiopulmonary resuscitation. *J Emerg Med.* 2002;23:161–164. doi: 10.1016/s0736-4679(02)00504-8
14. Fosse E, Lindberg H. Left ventricular rupture following external chest compression. *Acta Anaesthesiol Scand.* 1996;40:502–504. doi: 10.1111/j.1399-6576.1996.tb04476.x
15. Szili-Torok T, Theuns D, Verblaauw T, Scholten M, Kimman GJ, Res J, Jordaens L. Transthoracic defibrillation of short-lasting ventricular fibrillation: a randomised trial for comparison of the efficacy of low-energy biphasic rectilinear and monophasic damped sine shocks. *Acta Cardiol.* 2002;57:329–334. doi: 10.2143/AC.57.5.2005448
16. Higgins SL, O'Grady SG, Banville I, Chapman FW, Schmitt PW, Lank P, Walker RG, Ilina M. Efficacy of lower-energy biphasic shocks for transthoracic defibrillation: a follow-up clinical study. *Prehosp Emerg Care.* 2004;8:262–267. doi: 10.1016/j.prehos.2004.02.002
17. Bardy GH, Marchlinski FE, Sharma AD, Worley SJ, Luceri RM, Yee R, Halperin BD, Fellows CL, Ahern TS, Chilson DA, Packer DL, Wilber DJ, Mattioni TA, Reddy R, Kronmal RA, Lazzara R. Multicenter comparison of truncated biphasic shocks and standard damped sine wave monophasic shocks for transthoracic ventricular defibrillation. Transthoracic Investigators. *Circulation.* 1996;94:2507–2514. doi: 10.1161/01.cir.94.10.2507
18. Dunning J, Fabbri A, Kolh PH, Levine A, Lockowandt U, Mackay J, Pavie AJ, Strang T, Versteegh MI, Nashef SA; EACTS Clinical Guidelines Committee. Guideline for resuscitation in cardiac arrest after cardiac surgery. *Eur J Cardiothorac Surg.* 2009;36:3–28. doi: 10.1016/j.ejcts.2009.01.033
19. Mackay JH, Powell SJ, Charman SC, Rozario C. Resuscitation after cardiac surgery: are we ageist? *Eur J Anaesthesiol.* 2004;21:66–71. doi: 10.1017/s0265021504001115
20. Raman J, Saldanha RF, Branch JM, Esmore DS, Spratt PM, Farnsworth AE, Harrison GA, Chang VP, Shanahan MX. Open cardiac compression in the postoperative cardiac intensive care unit. *Anaesth Intensive Care.* 1989;17:129–135. doi: 10.1177/0310057X8901700202
21. Karhunen JP, Sihvo EI, Suojaranta-Ylinen RT, Rämö OJ, Salminen US. Predictive factors of hemodynamic collapse after coronary artery bypass grafting: a case-control study. *J Cardiothorac Vasc Anesth.* 2006;20:143–148. doi: 10.1053/j.jvca.2005.11.005
22. Fairman RM, Edmunds LH Jr. Emergency thoracotomy in the surgical intensive care unit after open cardiac operation. *Ann Thorac Surg.* 1981;32:386–391. doi: 10.1016/s0003-4975(10)61761-4
23. Ngaage DL, Cowen ME. Survival of cardiorespiratory arrest after coronary artery bypass grafting or aortic valve surgery. *Ann Thorac Surg.* 2009;88:64–68. doi: 10.1016/j.athoracsur.2009.03.042
24. Rousou JA, Engelman RM, Flack JE III, Deaton DW, Owen SG. Emergency cardiopulmonary bypass in the cardiac surgical unit can be a lifesaving measure in postoperative cardiac arrest. *Circulation.* 1994;90(5 Pt 2):II280–II284.
25. Dimopoulou I, Anthi A, Michalis A, Tzelepis GE. Functional status and quality of life in long-term survivors of cardiac arrest after cardiac surgery. *Crit Care Med.* 2001;29:1408–1411. doi: 10.1097/00003246-200107000-00018
26. Feng WC, Bert AA, Browning RA, Singh AK. Open cardiac massage and periresuscitative cardiopulmonary bypass for cardiac arrest following cardiac surgery. *J Cardiovasc Surg (Torino).* 1995;36:319–321.
27. Kaiser GC, Naunheim KS, Fiore AC, Harris HH, McBride LR, Pennington DG, Barner HB, Willman VL. Reoperation in the intensive care unit. *Ann Thorac Surg.* 1990;49:903–7; discussion 908. doi: 10.1016/0003-4975(90)90863-2
28. Chen YS, Chao A, Yu HY, Ko WJ, Wu IH, Chen RJ, Huang SC, Lin FY, Wang SS. Analysis and results of prolonged resuscitation in cardiac arrest patients rescued by extracorporeal membrane oxygenation. *J Am Coll Cardiol.* 2003;41:197–203. doi: 10.1016/s0735-1097(02)02716-x
29. Dalton HJ, Siewers RD, Fuhrman BP, Del Nido P, Thompson AE, Shaver MG, Dowhy M. Extracorporeal membrane oxygenation for cardiac rescue in children with severe myocardial dysfunction. *Crit Care Med.* 1993;21:1020–1028. doi: 10.1097/00003246-199307000-00016
30. Ghez O, Feier H, Ughetto F, Fraisse A, Kreitmann B, Metras D. Postoperative extracorporeal life support in pediatric cardiac surgery: recent results. *ASAIO J.* 2005;51:513–516. doi: 10.1097/01.mat.0000178039.53714.57
31. Duncan BW, Ibrahim AE, Hraska V, del Nido PJ, Laussen PC, Wessel DL, Mayer JE Jr, Bower LK, Jonas RA. Use of rapid-deployment extracorporeal membrane oxygenation for the resuscitation of pediatric patients with heart disease after cardiac arrest. *J Thorac Cardiovasc Surg.* 1998;116:305–311. doi: 10.1016/s0022-5223(98)70131-x
32. Newsome LR, Ponganis P, Reichman R, Nakaji N, Jaski B, Hartley M. Portable percutaneous cardiopulmonary bypass: use in supported coronary angioplasty, aortic valvuloplasty, and cardiac arrest. *J Cardiothorac Vasc Anesth.* 1992;6:328–331. doi: 10.1016/1053-0770(92)90151-v
33. Parra DA, Totapally BR, Zahn E, Jacobs J, Aldousany A, Burke RP, Chang AC. Outcome of cardiopulmonary resuscitation in a pediatric cardiac intensive care unit. *Crit Care Med.* 2000;28:3296–3300. doi: 10.1097/00003246-200009000-00030
34. Overlie PA. Emergency use of cardiopulmonary bypass. *J Interv Cardiol.* 1995;8:239–247. doi: 10.1111/j.1540-8183.1995.tb00541.x
35. Vanden Hoek TL, Morrison LJ, Shuster M, Donnino M, Sinz E, Lavonas EJ, Jeejeebhoy FM, Gabrielli A. Part 12: cardiac arrest in special situations: 2010 American Heart Association Guidelines for Cardiopulmonary Resuscitation and Emergency Cardiovascular Care. *Circulation.* 2010;122(suppl 3):S829–S861. doi: 10.1161/CIRCULATIONAHA.110.971069

Drowning

Recommendations for Drowning

COR	LOE	Recommendations
1	C-LD	1. Rescuers should provide CPR, including rescue breathing, as soon as an unresponsive submersion victim is removed from the water.
1	C-LD	2. All victims of drowning who require any form of resuscitation (including rescue breathing alone) should be transported to the hospital for evaluation and monitoring, even if they appear to be alert and demonstrate effective cardiorespiratory function at the scene.
2b	C-LD	3. Mouth-to-mouth ventilation in the water may be helpful when administered by a trained rescuer if it does not compromise safety.
3: No Benefit	B-NR	4. Routine stabilization of the cervical spine in the absence of circumstances that suggest a spinal injury is not recommended.

Synopsis

Each year, drowning is responsible for approximately 0.7% of deaths worldwide, or more than 500 000 deaths per year.[1,2] A recent study using data from the United States reported a survival rate of 13% after cardiac arrest associated with drowning.[3] People at increased risk for drowning include children, those with seizure disorders, and those intoxicated with alcohol or other drugs.[1] Although survival is uncommon after prolonged submersion, successful resuscitations have been reported.[4–9] For this reason, scene resuscitation should be initiated and the victim transported to the hospital unless there are obvious signs of death. Standard BLS and ACLS are the cornerstones of treatment, with airway management and ventilation being of particular importance because of the respiratory cause of arrest. The evidence for these recommendations was last reviewed thoroughly in 2010.

Recommendation-Specific Supportive Text

1. The duration and severity of hypoxia sustained as a result of drowning is the single most important determinant of outcome.[10,11] With outcome in mind, as soon as an unresponsive submersion victim is removed from the water, rescuers should provide CPR, with rescue breathing, if appropriately trained. Prompt initiation of rescue breathing increases the victim's chance of survival.[12]
2. Multiple observational evaluations, primarily in pediatric patients, have demonstrated that decompensation after fresh or salt-water drowning can occur in the first 4 to 6 hours after the event.[13,14] This supports transporting all victims to a medical facility for monitoring for at least 4 to 6 hours if feasible.
3. The immediate cause of death in drowning is hypoxemia. Based on the training of the rescuers, and only if scene safety can be maintained for the rescuer, sometimes ventilation can be provided in the water ("in-water resuscitation"), which may lead to improved patient outcomes compared with delaying ventilation until the victim is out of the water.[8]
4. The reported incidence of cervical spine injury in drowning victims is low (0.009%).[15,16] Routine stabilization of the cervical spine in the absence of circumstances that suggest a spinal injury is unlikely to benefit the patient and may delay needed resuscitation.[16,17]

These recommendations incorporate the results of a 2020 ILCOR CoSTR, which focused on prognostic factors in drowning.[18] Otherwise, this topic last received formal evidence review in 2010.[19] These guidelines were supplemented by "Wilderness Medical Society Clinical Practice Guidelines for the Treatment and Prevention of Drowning: 2019 Update."[20]

REFERENCES

1. Szpilman D, Bierens JJ, Handley AJ, Orlowski JP. Drowning. *N Engl J Med.* 2012;366:2102–2110. doi: 10.1056/NEJMra1013317
2. Peden MM, McGee K. The epidemiology of drowning worldwide. *Inj Control Saf Promot.* 2003;10:195–199. doi: 10.1076/icsp.10.4.195.16772
3. Reynolds JC, Hartley T, Michiels EA, Quan L. Long-Term Survival After Drowning-Related Cardiac Arrest. *J Emerg Med.* 2019;57:129–139. doi: 10.1016/j.jemermed.2019.05.029
4. Southwick FS, Dalglish PH Jr. Recovery after prolonged asystolic cardiac arrest in profound hypothermia. A case report and literature review. *JAMA.* 1980;243:1250–1253.
5. Siebke H, Rod T, Breivik H, Link B. Survival after 40 minutes; submersion without cerebral sequeae. *Lancet.* 1975;1:1275–1277. doi: 10.1016/s0140-6736(75)92554-4
6. Bolte RG, Black PG, Bowers RS, Thorne JK, Corneli HM. The use of extracorporeal rewarming in a child submerged for 66 minutes. *JAMA.* 1988;260:377–379.
7. Gilbert M, Busund R, Skagseth A, Nilsen PA, Solbø JP. Resuscitation from accidental hypothermia of 13.7 degrees C with circulatory arrest. *Lancet.* 2000;355:375–376. doi: 10.1016/S0140-6736(00)01021-7
8. Szpilman D, Soares M. In-water resuscitation–is it worthwhile? *Resuscitation.* 2004;63:25–31. doi: 10.1016/j.resuscitation.2004.03.017
9. Allman FD, Nelson WB, Pacentine GA, McComb G. Outcome following cardiopulmonary resuscitation in severe pediatric near-drowning. *Am J Dis Child.* 1986;140:571–575. doi: 10.1001/archpedi.1986.02140200081033
10. Youn CS, Choi SP, Yim HW, Park KN. Out-of-hospital cardiac arrest due to drowning: An Utstein Style report of 10 years of experience from St. Mary's Hospital. *Resuscitation.* 2009;80:778–783. doi: 10.1016/j.resuscitation.2009.04.007
11. Suominen P, Baillie C, Korpela R, Rautanen S, Ranta S, Olkkola KT. Impact of age, submersion time and water temperature on outcome in near-drowning. *Resuscitation.* 2002;52:247–254. doi: 10.1016/s0300-9572(01)00478-6
12. Kyriacou DN, Arcinue EL, Peek C, Kraus JF. Effect of immediate resuscitation on children with submersion injury. *Pediatrics.* 1994;94(2 Pt 1):137–142.
13. Causey AL, Tilelli JA, Swanson ME. Predicting discharge in uncomplicated near-drowning. *Am J Emerg Med.* 2000;18:9–11. doi: 10.1016/s0735-6757(00)90039-1
14. Noonan L, Howrey R, Ginsburg CM. Freshwater submersion injuries in children: a retrospective review of seventy-five hospitalized patients. *Pediatrics.* 1996;98(3 Pt 1):368–371.
15. Weinstein MD, Krieger BP. Near-drowning: epidemiology, pathophysiology, and initial treatment. *J Emerg Med.* 1996;14:461–467. doi: 10.1016/0736-4679(96)00097-2
16. Watson RS, Cummings P, Quan L, Bratton S, Weiss NS. Cervical spine injuries among submersion victims. *J Trauma.* 2001;51:658–662. doi: 10.1097/00005373-200110000-00006
17. Hwang V, Shofer FS, Durbin DR, Baren JM. Prevalence of traumatic injuries in drowning and near drowning in children and adolescents. *Arch Pediatr Adolesc Med.* 2003;157:50–53. doi: 10.1001/archpedi.157.1.50
18. Olasveengen TM, Mancini ME, Perkins GD, Avis S, Brooks S, Castrén M, Chung SP, Considine J, Couper K, Escalante R, et al; on behalf of the Adult Basic Life Support Collaborators. Adult basic life support: 2020 International Consensus on Cardiopulmonary Resuscitation and Emergency Cardiovascular Care Science With Treatment Recommendations. *Circulation.* 2020;142(suppl 1):S41–S91. doi: 10.1161/CIR.0000000000000892
19. Vanden Hoek TL, Morrison LJ, Shuster M, Donnino M, Sinz E, Lavonas EJ, Jeejeebhoy FM, Gabrielli A. Part 12: cardiac arrest in special situations: 2010 American Heart Association Guidelines for Cardiopulmonary Resuscitation and Emergency Cardiovascular Care. *Circulation.* 2010;122(suppl 3):S829–S861. doi: 10.1161/CIRCULATIONAHA.110.971069
20. Schmidt AC, Sempsrott JR, Hawkins SC, Arastu AS, Cushing TA, Auerbach PS. Wilderness Medical Society Clinical Practice Guidelines for the Treatment and Prevention of Drowning: 2019 Update. *Wilderness Environ Med.* 2019;30(4S):S70–S86. doi: 10.1016/j.wem.2019.06.007

Electrolyte Abnormalities

Recommendations for Electrolyte Abnormalities in Cardiac Arrest		
COR	**LOE**	**Recommendations**
1	C-LD	1. For cardiac arrest with known or suspected hyperkalemia, in addition to standard ACLS care, IV calcium should be administered.
1	C-LD	2. For cardiotoxicity and cardiac arrest from severe hypomagnesemia, in addition to standard ACLS care, IV magnesium is recommended.
2b	C-EO	3. For cardiac arrest with known or suspected hypermagnesemia, in addition to standard ACLS care, it may be reasonable to administer empirical IV calcium.
3: Harm	C-LD	4. IV bolus administration of potassium for cardiac arrest in suspected hypokalemia is not recommended.

Synopsis

Electrolyte abnormalities may cause or contribute to cardiac arrest, hinder resuscitative efforts, and affect hemodynamic recovery after cardiac arrest. In addition to standard ACLS, specific interventions may be lifesaving for cases of hyperkalemia and hypermagnesemia.

Hyperkalemia is commonly caused by renal failure and can precipitate cardiac arrhythmias and cardiac arrest. The clinical signs associated with severe hyperkalemia (more than 6.5 mmol/L) include flaccid paralysis, paresthesia, depressed deep tendon reflexes, or shortness of breath.[1–3] The early electrocardiographic signs include peaked T waves on the ECG followed by flattened or absent T waves, prolonged PR interval, widened QRS complex, deepened S waves, and merging of S and T waves.[4,5] As hyperkalemia progresses, the ECG can develop idioventricular rhythms, form a sine-wave pattern, and develop into an asystolic cardiac arrest.[4,5] Severe hypokalemia is less common but can occur in the setting of gastrointestinal or renal losses and can lead to life-threatening ventricular arrhythmias.[6–8] Severe hypermagnesemia is most likely to occur in the obstetric setting in patients being treated with IV magnesium for preeclampsia or eclampsia. At very elevated levels, hypermagnesemia can lead to altered consciousness, bradycardia or ventricular arrhythmias, and cardiac arrest.[9,10] Hypomagnesemia can occur in the setting of gastrointestinal illness or malnutrition, among other causes, and, when significant, can lead to both atrial and ventricular arrhythmias.[11]

Recommendation-Specific Supportive Text

1. In addition to standard ACLS, several therapies have long been recommended to treat life-threatening hyperkalemia.[12] These include IV administration of calcium and/or bicarbonate, insulin with glucose, and/or inhaled albuterol. Parenteral calcium may stabilize the myocardial cell membrane and is therefore the most likely to be useful during cardiac arrest and can be given by the IV or IO route. A typical dose is 5 to 10 mL of 10% calcium chloride solution, or 15 to 30 mL of 10% calcium gluconate solution, administered via IV or IO line over 2 to 5 minutes.[12] Standard use of sodium polystyrene (Kayexalate) is now discouraged because of poor efficacy and the risk of bowel complications. Emergent hemodialysis in the hospital setting remains a definitive treatment for life-threatening hyperkalemia.
2. Although the administration of IV magnesium has not been found to be beneficial for VF/VT in the absence of prolonged QT, consideration of its use for cardiac arrest in patients with prolonged QT is advised.[13] Hypomagnesemia can cause or aggravate prolonged QT, is associated with multiple arrhythmias, and may precipitate cardiac arrest.[11] This provides physiological rationale for the restoration of normal levels, although standard ACLS remains the cornerstone of treatment. Recommendations for treatment of torsades de pointes are provided in the Wide Complex Tachycardia section.
3. Administration of IV or IO calcium, in the doses suggested for hyperkalemia, may improve hemodynamics in severe magnesium toxicity, supporting its use in cardiac arrest although direct evidence is lacking.[14]
4. The controlled administration of IV potassium for ventricular arrhythmias due to severe hypokalemia may be useful, but case reports have generally included infusion of potassium and not bolus dosing.[15] Bolus dosing without adverse cardiac effects was reported in at least 1 small case series of cardiac surgery patients where it was administered in a highly monitored setting by an anesthesiologist, but the efficacy of this for cardiac arrest is not known, and safety concerns remain.[16]

This topic last received formal evidence review in 2010.[12]

REFERENCES

1. Weiner ID, Wingo CS. Hyperkalemia: a potential silent killer. *J Am Soc Nephrol.* 1998;9:1535–1543.
2. Weiner M, Epstein FH. Signs and symptoms of electrolyte disorders. *Yale J Biol Med.* 1970;43:76–109.
3. Rastegar A, Soleimani M, Rastergar A. Hypokalaemia and hyperkalaemia. *Postgrad Med J.* 2001;77:759–764. doi: 10.1136/pmj.77.914.759
4. Mattu A, Brady WJ, Robinson DA. Electrocardiographic manifestations of hyperkalemia. *Am J Emerg Med.* 2000;18:721–729. doi: 10.1053/ajem.2000.7344
5. Frohnert PP, Giuliani ER, Friedberg M, Johnson WJ, Tauxe WN. Statistical investigation of correlations between serum potassium levels and electrocardiographic findings in patients on intermittent hemodialysis therapy. *Circulation.* 1970;41:667–676. doi: 10.1161/01.cir.41.4.667
6. Gennari FJ. Hypokalemia. *N Engl J Med.* 1998;339:451–458. doi: 10.1056/NEJM199808133390707
7. Clausen TG, Brocks K, Ibsen H. Hypokalemia and ventricular arrhythmias in acute myocardial infarction. *Acta Med Scand.* 1988;224:531–537. doi: 10.1111/j.0954-6820.1988.tb19623.x
8. Slovis C, Jenkins R. ABC of clinical electrocardiography: Conditions not primarily affecting the heart. *BMJ.* 2002;324:1320–1323. doi: 10.1136/bmj.324.7349.1320

9. McDonnell NJ, Muchatuta NA, Paech MJ. Acute magnesium toxicity in an obstetric patient undergoing general anaesthesia for caesarean delivery. *Int J Obstet Anesth*. 2010;19:226–231. doi: 10.1016/j.ijoa.2009.09.009
10. McDonnell NJ. Cardiopulmonary arrest in pregnancy: two case reports of successful outcomes in association with perimortem Caesarean delivery. *Br J Anaesth*. 2009;103:406–409. doi: 10.1093/bja/aep176
11. Hansen BA, Bruserud Ø. Hypomagnesemia in critically ill patients. *J Intensive Care*. 2018;6:21. doi: 10.1186/s40560-018-0291-y
12. Vanden Hoek TL, Morrison LJ, Shuster M, Donnino M, Sinz E, Lavonas EJ, Jeejeebhoy FM, Gabrielli A. Part 12: cardiac arrest in special situations: 2010 American Heart Association Guidelines for Cardiopulmonary Resuscitation and Emergency Cardiovascular Care. *Circulation*. 2010;122(suppl 3):S829–S861. doi: 10.1161/CIRCULATIONAHA.110.971069
13. Panchal AR, Berg KM, Kudenchuk PJ, Del Rios M, Hirsch KG, Link MS, Kurz MC, Chan PS, Cabañas JG, Morley PT, Hazinski MF, Donnino MW. 2018 American Heart Association Focused Update on Advanced Cardiovascular Life Support Use of Antiarrhythmic Drugs During and Immediately After Cardiac Arrest: An Update to the American Heart Association Guidelines for Cardiopulmonary Resuscitation and Emergency Cardiovascular Care. *Circulation*. 2018;138:e740–e749. doi: 10.1161/CIR.0000000000000613
14. Van Hook JW. Endocrine crises. Hypermagnesemia. *Crit Care Clin*. 1991;7:215–223.
15. Curry P, Fitchett D, Stubbs W, Krikler D. Ventricular arrhythmias and hypokalaemia. *Lancet*. 1976;2:231–233. doi: 10.1016/s0140-6736(76)91029-1
16. McCall BB, Mazzei WJ, Scheller MS, Thomas TC. Effects of central bolus injections of potassium chloride on arterial potassium concentration in patients undergoing cardiopulmonary bypass. *J Cardiothorac Anesth*. 1990;4:571–576. doi: 10.1016/0888-6296(90)90406-6

Opioid Overdose

Introduction

The ongoing opioid epidemic has resulted in an increase in opioid-associated OHCA, leading to approximately 115 deaths per day in the United States and predominantly impacting patients from 25 to 65 years old.[1–3] Initially, isolated opioid toxicity is associated with CNS and respiratory depression that progresses to respiratory arrest followed by cardiac arrest. Most opioid-associated deaths also involve the coingestion of multiple drugs or medical and mental health comorbidities.[4–7]

In creating these recommendations, the writing group considered the difficulty in accurately differentiating opioid-associated resuscitative emergencies from other causes of cardiac and respiratory arrest. Opioid-associated resuscitative emergencies are defined by the presence of cardiac arrest, respiratory arrest, or severe life-threatening instability (such as severe CNS or respiratory depression, hypotension, or cardiac arrhythmia) that is suspected to be due to opioid toxicity. In these situations, the mainstay of care remains the early recognition of an emergency followed by the activation of the emergency response systems (Figures 13 and 14). Opioid overdoses deteriorate to cardiopulmonary arrest because of loss of airway patency and lack of breathing; therefore, addressing the airway and ventilation in a periarrest patient is of the highest priority. The next steps in care, including the performance of CPR and the administration of naloxone, are discussed in detail below.

Additional recommendations about opioid overdose response education are provided in "Part 6: Resuscitation Education Science."

Recommendations for Acute Management of Opioid Overdose

COR	LOE	Recommendations
1	C-LD	1. For patients in respiratory arrest, rescue breathing or bag-mask ventilation should be maintained until spontaneous breathing returns, and standard BLS and/or ACLS measures should continue if return of spontaneous breathing does not occur.
1	C-EO	2. For patients known or suspected to be in cardiac arrest, in the absence of a proven benefit from the use of naloxone, standard resuscitative measures should take priority over naloxone administration, with a focus on high-quality CPR (compressions plus ventilation).
1	C-EO	3. Lay and trained responders should not delay activating emergency response systems while awaiting the patient's response to naloxone or other interventions.
2a	B-NR	4. For a patient with suspected opioid overdose who has a definite pulse but no normal breathing or only gasping (ie, a respiratory arrest), in addition to providing standard BLS and/or ACLS care, it is reasonable for responders to administer naloxone.

Recommendation-Specific Supportive Text

1. Initial management should focus on support of the patient's airway and breathing. This begins with opening the airway followed by delivery of rescue breaths, ideally with the use of a bag-mask or barrier device.[8–10] Provision of ACLS should continue if return of spontaneous breathing does not occur.
2. Because there are no studies demonstrating improvement in patient outcomes from administration of naloxone during cardiac arrest, provision of CPR should be the focus of initial care.[3] Naloxone can be administered along with standard ACLS care if it does not delay components of high-quality CPR.
3. Early activation of the emergency response system is critical for patients with suspected opioid overdose. Rescuers cannot be certain that the person's clinical condition is due to opioid-induced respiratory depression alone. This is particularly true in first aid and BLS, where determination of the presence of a pulse is unreliable.[11,12] Naloxone is ineffective in other medical conditions, including overdose involving nonopioids and cardiac arrest from any cause. Second, patients who respond to naloxone administration may develop recurrent CNS and/or respiratory depression and require longer periods of observation before safe discharge.[13–16]
4. Twelve studies examined the use of naloxone in respiratory arrest, of which 5 compared

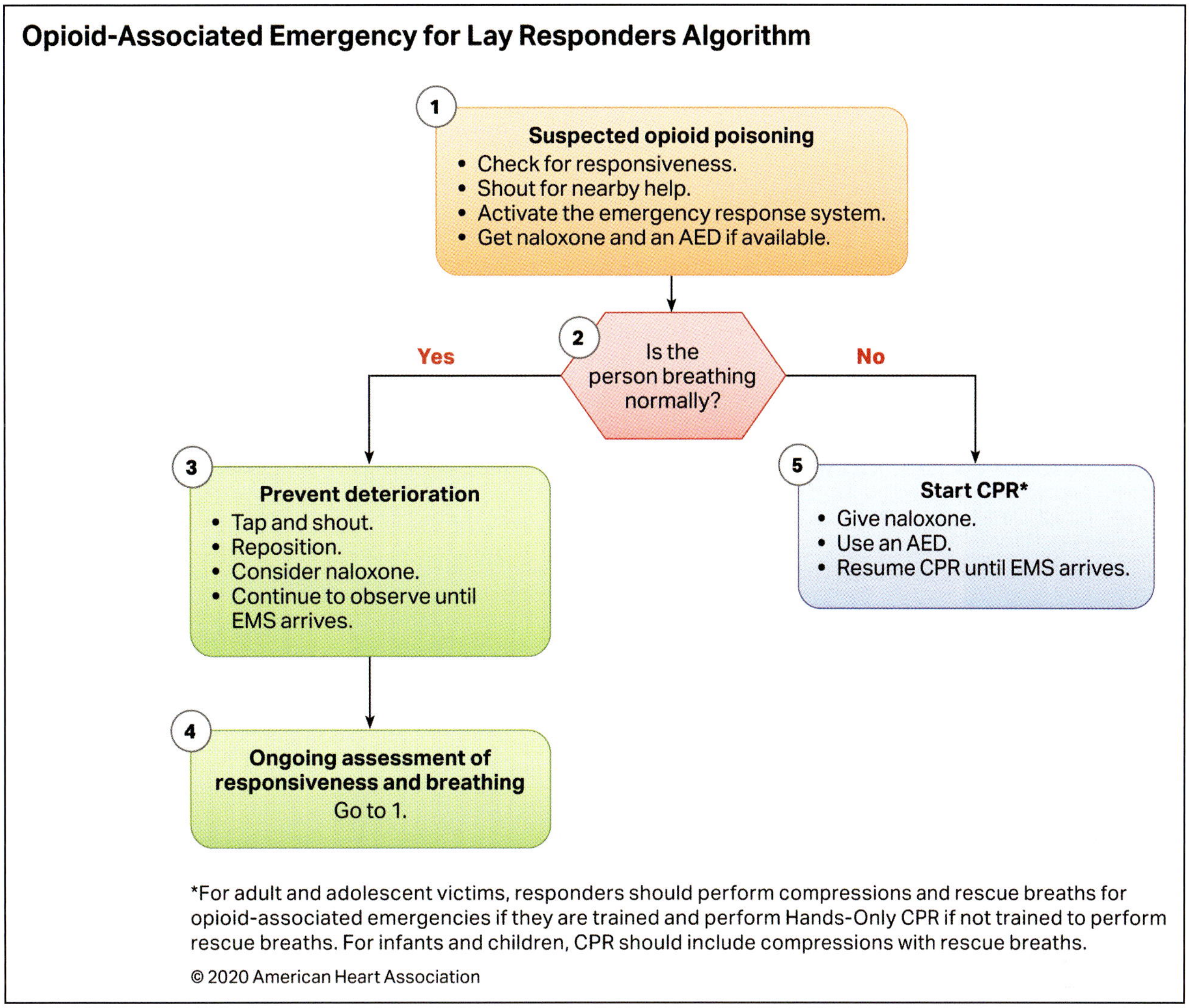
Opioid-Associated Emergency for Lay Responders Algorithm
1
Suspected opioid poisoning
• Check for responsiveness.
• Shout for nearby help.
• Activate the emergency response system.
• Get naloxone and an AED if available.
2
Is the person breathing normally?
Yes
No
3
Prevent deterioration
• Tap and shout.
• Reposition.
• Consider naloxone.
• Continue to observe until EMS arrives.
4
Ongoing assessment of responsiveness and breathing
Go to 1.
5
Start CPR*
• Give naloxone.
• Use an AED.
• Resume CPR until EMS arrives.
*For adult and adolescent victims, responders should perform compressions and rescue breaths for opioid-associated emergencies if they are trained and perform Hands-Only CPR if not trained to perform rescue breaths. For infants and children, CPR should include compressions with rescue breaths.
© 2020 American Heart Association

Figure 13. Opioid-Associated Emergency for Lay Responders Algorithm.
AED indicates automated external defibrillator; CPR, cardiopulmonary resuscitation; and EMS, emergency medical services.

intramuscular, intravenous, and/or intranasal routes of naloxone administration (2 RCT,[17,18] 3 non-RCT[19–21]) and 9 assessed the safety of naloxone use or were observational studies of naloxone use.[22–30] These studies report that naloxone is safe and effective in treatment of opioid-induced respiratory depression and that complications are rare and dose related.

Recommendations for Postresuscitation Management of Opioid Overdose

COR	LOE	Recommendations
1	C-LD	1. After return of spontaneous breathing, patients should be observed in a healthcare setting until the risk of recurrent opioid toxicity is low and the patient's level of consciousness and vital signs have normalized.
2a	C-LD	2. If recurrent opioid toxicity develops, repeated small doses or an infusion of naloxone can be beneficial.

Recommendation-Specific Supportive Text

1. Patients who respond to naloxone administration may develop recurrent CNS and/or respiratory depression. Although abbreviated observation periods may be adequate for patients with fentanyl, morphine, or heroin overdose,[28,30–34] longer periods of observation may be required to safely discharge a patient with life-threatening overdose of a long-acting or sustained-release opioid.[13–15] Prehospital providers who are faced with the challenge of a patient refusing transport after treatment for a life-threatening overdose are advised to follow local protocols and practices for determination of patient capacity to refuse care.
2. Because the duration of action of naloxone may be shorter than the respiratory depressive effect of the opioid, particularly long-acting formulations, repeat doses of naloxone, or a naloxone infusion may be required.[13–15]

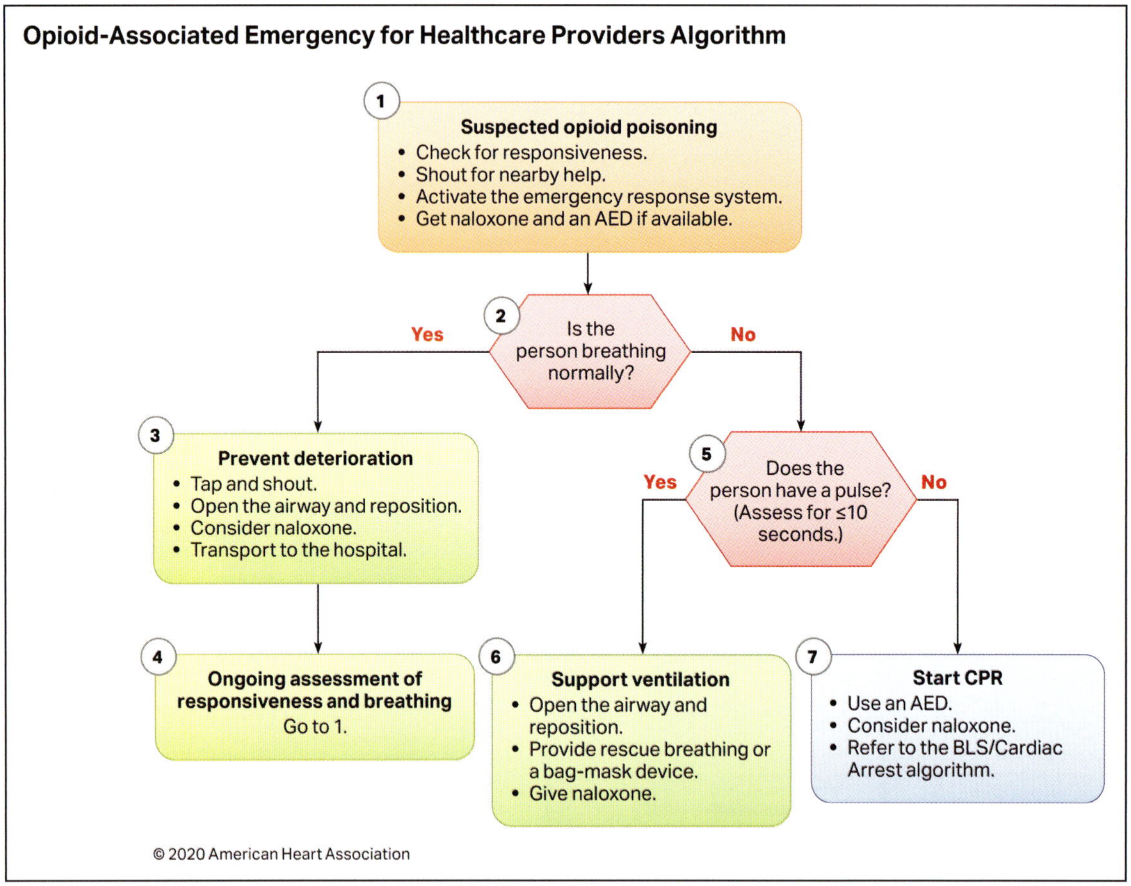

Figure 14. Opioid-Associated Emergency for Healthcare Providers Algorithm.
AED indicates automated external defibrillator; and BLS, basic life support.

These recommendations are supported by the 2020 AHA scientific statement on opioid-associated OHCA.[3]

REFERENCES

1. Scholl L, Seth P, Kariisa M, Wilson N, Baldwin G. Drug and opioid-involved overdose deaths—United States, 2013-2017. *MMWR Morb Mortal Wkly Rep*. 2018;67:1419–1427. doi: 10.15585/mmwr.mm675152e1
2. Jones CM, Einstein EB, Compton WM. Changes in synthetic opioid involvement in drug overdose deaths in the United States, 2010-2016. *JAMA*. 2018;319:1819–1821. doi: 10.1001/jama.2018.2844
3. Dezfulian C, Orkin AM, Maron BA, Elmer J, Girota S, Gladwin MT, Merchant RM, Panchal AR, Perman SM, Starks M, et al; on behalf of the American Heart Association Council on Cardiopulmonary, Critical Care, Perioperative and Resuscitation; Council on Arteriosclerosis, Thrombosis and Vascular Biology; Council on Cardiovascular and Stroke Nursing; and Council on Clinical Cardiology. Opioid-associated out-of-hospital cardiac arrest: distinctive clinical features and implications for healthcare and public responses: a scientific statement from the American Heart Association. *Circulation*. In press.
4. Jones CM, Paulozzi LJ, Mack KA; Centers for Disease Control and Prevention (CDC). Alcohol involvement in opioid pain reliever and benzodiazepine drug abuse-related emergency department visits and drug-related deaths - United States, 2010. *MMWR Morb Mortal Wkly Rep*. 2014;63:881–885.
5. Madadi P, Hildebrandt D, Lauwers AE, Koren G. Characteristics of opioid-users whose death was related to opioid-toxicity: a population-based study in Ontario, Canada. *PLoS One*. 2013;8:e60600. doi: 10.1371/journal.pone.0060600
6. Paulozzi LJ, Logan JE, Hall AJ, McKinstry E, Kaplan JA, Crosby AE. A comparison of drug overdose deaths involving methadone and other opioid analgesics in West Virginia. *Addiction*. 2009;104:1541–1548. doi: 10.1111/j.1360-0443.2009.02650.x
7. Webster LR, Cochella S, Dasgupta N, Fakata KL, Fine PG, Fishman SM, Grey T, Johnson EM, Lee LK, Passik SD, Peppin J, Porucznik CA, Ray A, Schnoll SH, Stieg RL, Wakeland W. An analysis of the root causes for opioid-related overdose deaths in the United States. *Pain Med*. 2011;12 Suppl 2:S26–S35. doi: 10.1111/j.1526-4637.2011.01134.x
8. Kleinman ME, Brennan EE, Goldberger ZD, Swor RA, Terry M, Bobrow BJ, Gazmuri RJ, Travers AH, Rea T. Part 5: adult basic life support and cardiopulmonary resuscitation quality: 2015 American Heart Association Guidelines Update for Cardiopulmonary Resuscitation and Emergency Cardiovascular Care. *Circulation*. 2015;132(suppl 2):S414–S435. doi: 10.1161/CIR.0000000000000259
9. Guildner CW. Resuscitation—opening the airway: a comparative study of techniques for opening an airway obstructed by the tongue. *JACEP*. 1976;5:588–590. doi: 10.1016/s0361-1124(76)80217-1
10. Wenzel V, Keller C, Idris AH, Dörges V, Lindner KH, Brimacombe JR. Effects of smaller tidal volumes during basic life support ventilation in patients with respiratory arrest: good ventilation, less risk? *Resuscitation*. 1999;43:25–29. doi: 10.1016/s0300-9572(99)00118-5
11. Bahr J, Klingler H, Panzer W, Rode H, Kettler D. Skills of lay people in checking the carotid pulse. *Resuscitation*. 1997;35:23–26. doi: 10.1016/s0300-9572(96)01092-1
12. Eberle B, Dick WF, Schneider T, Wisser G, Doetsch S, Tzanova I. Checking the carotid pulse check: diagnostic accuracy of first responders in patients with and without a pulse. *Resuscitation*. 1996;33:107–116. doi: 10.1016/s0300-9572(96)01016-7
13. Clarke SF, Dargan PI, Jones AL. Naloxone in opioid poisoning: walking the tightrope. *Emerg Med J*. 2005;22:612–616. doi: 10.1136/emj.2003.009613
14. Etherington J, Christenson J, Innes G, Grafstein E, Pennington S, Spinelli JJ, Gao M, Lahiffe B, Wanger K, Fernandes C. Is early discharge safe after naloxone reversal of presumed opioid overdose? *CJEM*. 2000;2:156–162. doi: 10.1017/s1481803500004863

15. Zuckerman M, Weisberg SN, Boyer EW. Pitfalls of intranasal naloxone. *Prehosp Emerg Care.* 2014;18:550–554. doi: 10.3109/10903127.2014.896961
16. Heaton JD, Bhandari B, Faryar KA, Huecker MR. Retrospective Review of Need for Delayed Naloxone or Oxygen in Emergency Department Patients Receiving Naloxone for Heroin Reversal. *J Emerg Med.* 2019;56:642–651. doi: 10.1016/j.jemermed.2019.02.015
17. Kelly AM, Kerr D, Dietze P, Patrick I, Walker T, Koutsogiannis Z. Randomised trial of intranasal versus intramuscular naloxone in prehospital treatment for suspected opioid overdose. *Med J Aust.* 2005;182:24–27.
18. Kerr D, Kelly AM, Dietze P, Jolley D, Barger B. Randomized controlled trial comparing the effectiveness and safety of intranasal and intramuscular naloxone for the treatment of suspected heroin overdose. *Addiction.* 2009;104:2067–2074. doi: 10.1111/j.1360-0443.2009.02724.x
19. Wanger K, Brough L, Macmillan I, Goulding J, MacPhail I, Christenson JM. Intravenous vs subcutaneous naloxone for out-of-hospital management of presumed opioid overdose. *Acad Emerg Med.* 1998;5:293–299. doi: 10.1111/j.1553-2712.1998.tb02707.x
20. Barton ED, Colwell CB, Wolfe T, Fosnocht D, Gravitz C, Bryan T, Dunn W, Benson J, Bailey J. Efficacy of intranasal naloxone as a needleless alternative for treatment of opioid overdose in the prehospital setting. *J Emerg Med.* 2005;29:265–271. doi: 10.1016/j.jemermed.2005.03.007
21. Robertson TM, Hendey GW, Stroh G, Shalit M. Intranasal naloxone is a viable alternative to intravenous naloxone for prehospital narcotic overdose. *Prehosp Emerg Care.* 2009;13:512–515. doi: 10.1080/10903120903144866
22. Cetrullo C, Di Nino GF, Melloni C, Pieri C, Zanoni A. [Naloxone antagonism toward opiate analgesic drugs. Clinical experimental study]. *Minerva Anestesiol.* 1983;49:199–204.
23. Osterwalder JJ. Naloxone–for intoxications with intravenous heroin and heroin mixtures–harmless or hazardous? A prospective clinical study. *J Toxicol Clin Toxicol.* 1996;34:409–416. doi: 10.3109/15563659609013811
24. Sporer KA, Firestone J, Isaacs SM. Out-of-hospital treatment of opioid overdoses in an urban setting. *Acad Emerg Med.* 1996;3:660–667. doi: 10.1111/j.1553-2712.1996.tb03487.x
25. Stokland O, Hansen TB, Nilsen JE. [Prehospital treatment of heroin intoxication in Oslo in 1996]. *Tidsskr Nor Laegeforen.* 1998;118:3144–3146.
26. Buajordet I, Naess AC, Jacobsen D, Brørs O. Adverse events after naloxone treatment of episodes of suspected acute opioid overdose. *Eur J Emerg Med.* 2004;11:19–23. doi: 10.1097/00063110-200402000-00004
27. Cantwell K, Dietze P, Flander L. The relationship between naloxone dose and key patient variables in the treatment of non-fatal heroin overdose in the prehospital setting. *Resuscitation.* 2005;65:315–319. doi: 10.1016/j.resuscitation.2004.12.012
28. Boyd JJ, Kuisma MJ, Alaspää AO, Vuori E, Repo JV, Randell TT. Recurrent opioid toxicity after pre-hospital care of presumed heroin overdose patients. *Acta Anaesthesiol Scand.* 2006;50:1266–1270. doi: 10.1111/j.1399-6576.2006.01172.x
29. Nielsen K, Nielsen SL, Siersma V, Rasmussen LS. Treatment of opioid overdose in a physician-based prehospital EMS: frequency and long-term prognosis. *Resuscitation.* 2011;82:1410–1413. doi: 10.1016/j.resuscitation.2011.05.027
30. Wampler DA, Molina DK, McManus J, Laws P, Manifold CA. No deaths associated with patient refusal of transport after naloxone-reversed opioid overdose. *Prehosp Emerg Care.* 2011;15:320–324. doi: 10.3109/10903127.2011.569854
31. Vilke GM, Sloane C, Smith AM, Chan TC. Assessment for deaths in out-of-hospital heroin overdose patients treated with naloxone who refuse transport. *Acad Emerg Med.* 2003;10:893–896. doi: 10.1111/j.1553-2712.2003.tb00636.x
32. Rudolph SS, Jehu G, Nielsen SL, Nielsen K, Siersma V, Rasmussen LS. Prehospital treatment of opioid overdose in Copenhagen–is it safe to discharge on-scene? *Resuscitation.* 2011;82:1414–1418. doi: 10.1016/j.resuscitation.2011.06.027
33. Moss ST, Chan TC, Buchanan J, Dunford JV, Vilke GM. Outcome study of prehospital patients signed out against medical advice by field paramedics. *Ann Emerg Med.* 1998;31:247–250. doi: 10.1016/s0196-0644(98)70315-4
34. Christenson J, Etherington J, Grafstein E, Innes G, Pennington S, Wanger K, Fernandes C, Spinelli JJ, Gao M. Early discharge of patients with presumed opioid overdose: development of a clinical prediction rule. *Acad Emerg Med.* 2000;7:1110–1118. doi: 10.1111/j.1553-2712.2000.tb01260.x

Cardiac Arrest in Pregnancy

Introduction

Approximately 1 in 12 000 admissions for delivery in the United States results in a maternal cardiac arrest.[1] Although it remains a rare event, the incidence has been increasing.[2] Reported maternal and fetal/neonatal survival rates vary widely.[3–8] Invariably, the best outcomes for both mother and fetus are through successful maternal resuscitation. Common causes of maternal cardiac arrest are hemorrhage, heart failure, amniotic fluid embolism, sepsis, aspiration pneumonitis, venous thromboembolism, preeclampsia/eclampsia, and complications of anesthesia.[1,4,6]

Current literature is largely observational, and some treatment decisions are based primarily on the physiology of pregnancy and extrapolations from nonarrest pregnancy states.[9] High-quality resuscitative and therapeutic interventions that target the most likely cause of cardiac arrest are paramount in this population. Perimortem cesarean delivery (PMCD) at or greater than 20 weeks uterine size, sometimes referred to as *resuscitative hysterotomy*, appears to improve outcomes of maternal cardiac arrest when resuscitation does not rapidly result in ROSC (Figure 15).[10–14] Further, shorter time intervals from arrest to delivery appear to lead to improved maternal and neonatal outcomes.[15] However, the clinical decision to perform PMCD—and its timing with respect to maternal cardiac arrest—is complex because of the variability in level of practitioner and team training, patient factors (eg, etiology of arrest, gestational age), and system resources. Finally, case reports and case series using ECMO in maternal cardiac arrest patients report good maternal survival.[16] The treatment of cardiac arrest in late pregnancy represents a major scientific gap.

Recommendations for Planning and Preparation for Cardiac Arrest in Pregnancy

COR	LOE	Recommendations
1	C-LD	1. Team planning for cardiac arrest in pregnancy should be done in collaboration with the obstetric, neonatal, emergency, anesthesiology, intensive care, and cardiac arrest services.
1	C-LD	2. Because immediate ROSC cannot always be achieved, local resources for a perimortem cesarean delivery should be summoned as soon as cardiac arrest in a woman in the second half of pregnancy is recognized.
1	C-EO	3. Protocols for management of OHCA in pregnancy should be developed to facilitate timely transport to a center with capacity to immediately perform perimortem cesarean delivery while providing ongoing resuscitation.

Recommendation-Specific Supportive Text

1. To assure successful maternal resuscitation, all potential stakeholders need to be engaged in the

planning and training for cardiac arrest in pregnancy, including the possible need for PMCD. Based on similarly rare but time-critical interventions, planning, simulation training and mock emergencies will assist in facility preparedness.[17–21]

2. Since initial efforts for maternal resuscitation may not be successful, preparation for PMCD should begin early in the resuscitation, since decreased time to PMCD is associated with better maternal and fetal outcomes.[8]
3. In cases of prehospital maternal arrest, rapid transport directly to a facility capable of PMCD and neonatal resuscitation, with early activation of the receiving facility's adult resuscitation, obstetric, and neonatal resuscitation teams, provides the best chance for a successful outcome.

Recommendations for Resuscitation of Cardiac Arrest in Pregnancy

COR	LOE	Recommendations
1	C-LD	1. Priorities for the pregnant woman in cardiac arrest should include provision of high-quality CPR and relief of aortocaval compression through left lateral uterine displacement.
1	C-LD	2. Because pregnant patients are more prone to hypoxia, oxygenation and airway management should be prioritized during resuscitation from cardiac arrest in pregnancy.
1	C-EO	3. Because of potential interference with maternal resuscitation, fetal monitoring should not be undertaken during cardiac arrest in pregnancy.
1	C-EO	4. We recommend targeted temperature management for pregnant women who remain comatose after resuscitation from cardiac arrest.
1	C-EO	5. During targeted temperature management of the pregnant patient, it is recommended that the fetus be continuously monitored for bradycardia as a potential complication, and obstetric and neonatal consultation should be sought.

Recommendation-Specific Supportive Text

1. The gravid uterus can compress the inferior vena cava, impeding venous return, thereby reducing stroke volume and cardiac output. In the supine position, aortocaval compression can occur for singleton pregnancies starting at approximately 20 weeks of gestational age or when the fundal height is at or above the level of the umbilicus.[22] Manual left lateral uterine displacement effectively relieves aortocaval pressure in patients with hypotension (Figure 16).[23,23a,23b]
2. Airway, ventilation, and oxygenation are particularly important in the setting of pregnancy because of increased maternal metabolism and decreased functional reserve capacity due to the gravid uterus, making pregnant patients more prone to hypoxia. Furthermore, fetal hypoxia has known detrimental effects. Both of these considerations support earlier advanced airway management for the pregnant patient.
3. Resuscitation of the pregnant woman, including PMCD when indicated, is the first priority because it may lead to increased survival of both the woman and the fetus.[9] Fetal monitoring does not achieve this goal and may distract from maternal resuscitation efforts, particularly defibrillation and preparation of the abdomen for PMCD.
4. There are no randomized trials of the use of TTM in pregnancy. However, there are several case reports of good maternal and fetal outcome with the use of TTM after cardiac arrest.[24,25]
5. After successful maternal resuscitation, the undelivered fetus remains susceptible to the effects of hypothermia, acidosis, hypoxemia, and hypotension, all of which can occur in the setting of post-ROSC care with TTM. In addition, deterioration of fetal status may be an early warning sign of maternal decompensation.

Recommendations for Cardiac Arrest and PMCD

COR	LOE	Recommendations
1	C-LD	1. During cardiac arrest, if the pregnant woman with a fundus height at or above the umbilicus has not achieved ROSC with usual resuscitation measures plus manual left lateral uterine displacement, it is advisable to prepare to evacuate the uterus while resuscitation continues.
1	C-LD	2. In situations such as nonsurvivable maternal trauma or prolonged pulselessness, in which maternal resuscitative efforts are considered futile, there is no reason to delay performing perimortem cesarean delivery in appropriate patients.
2a	C-EO	3. To accomplish delivery early, ideally within 5 min after the time of arrest, it is reasonable to immediately prepare for perimortem cesarean delivery while initial BLS and ACLS interventions are being performed.

Recommendation-Specific Supportive Text

1. Evacuation of the gravid uterus relieves aortocaval compression and may increase the likelihood of ROSC.[10–14] In the latter half of pregnancy, PMCD may be considered part of maternal resuscitation, regardless of fetal viability.[26]
2. Early delivery is associated with better maternal and neonatal survival.[15] In situations incompatible with maternal survival, early delivery of the fetus may also improve neonatal survival.[26]
3. The optimal timing for the performance of PMCD is not well established and must logically vary on the basis of provider skill set and available resources as well as patient and/or cardiac arrest

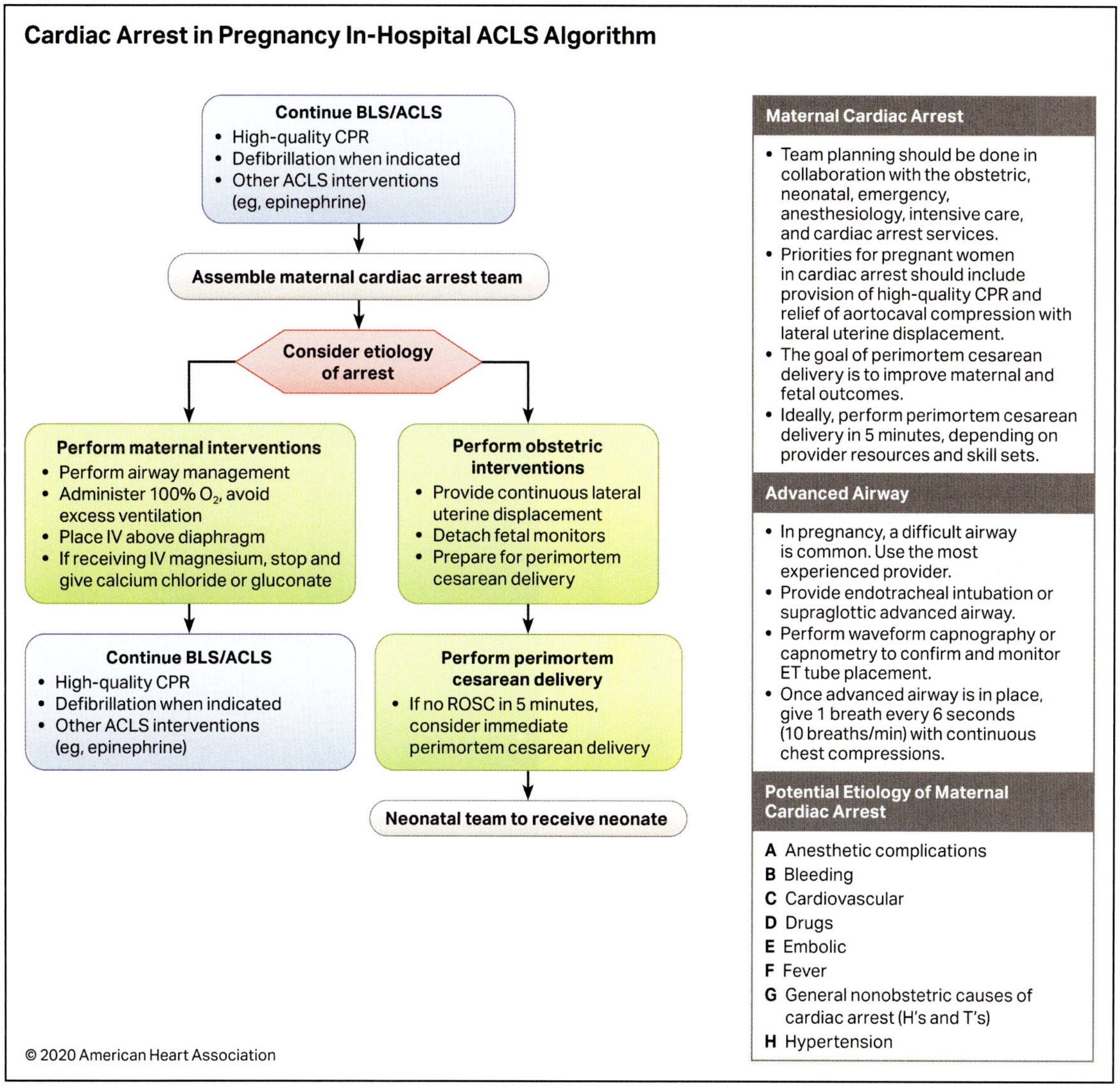
Cardiac Arrest in Pregnancy In-Hospital ACLS Algorithm
Continue BLS/ACLS
• High-quality CPR
• Defibrillation when indicated
• Other ACLS interventions (eg, epinephrine)
Assemble maternal cardiac arrest team
Consider etiology of arrest
Perform maternal interventions
• Perform airway management
• Administer 100% O_2, avoid excess ventilation
• Place IV above diaphragm
• If receiving IV magnesium, stop and give calcium chloride or gluconate
Perform obstetric interventions
• Provide continuous lateral uterine displacement
• Detach fetal monitors
• Prepare for perimortem cesarean delivery
Continue BLS/ACLS
• High-quality CPR
• Defibrillation when indicated
• Other ACLS interventions (eg, epinephrine)
Perform perimortem cesarean delivery
• If no ROSC in 5 minutes, consider immediate perimortem cesarean delivery
Neonatal team to receive neonate
Maternal Cardiac Arrest
• Team planning should be done in collaboration with the obstetric, neonatal, emergency, anesthesiology, intensive care, and cardiac arrest services.
• Priorities for pregnant women in cardiac arrest should include provision of high-quality CPR and relief of aortocaval compression with lateral uterine displacement.
• The goal of perimortem cesarean delivery is to improve maternal and fetal outcomes.
• Ideally, perform perimortem cesarean delivery in 5 minutes, depending on provider resources and skill sets.
Advanced Airway
• In pregnancy, a difficult airway is common. Use the most experienced provider.
• Provide endotracheal intubation or supraglottic advanced airway.
• Perform waveform capnography or capnometry to confirm and monitor ET tube placement.
• Once advanced airway is in place, give 1 breath every 6 seconds (10 breaths/min) with continuous chest compressions.
Potential Etiology of Maternal Cardiac Arrest
A Anesthetic complications
B Bleeding
C Cardiovascular
D Drugs
E Embolic
F Fever
G General nonobstetric causes of cardiac arrest (H's and T's)
H Hypertension
© 2020 American Heart Association

Figure 15. Cardiac Arrest in Pregnancy In-Hospital ACLS Algorithm.
ACLS indicates advanced cardiovascular life support; BLS, basic life support; CPR, cardiopulmonary resuscitation; ET, endotracheal; IV, intravenous; and ROSC, return of spontaneous circulation.

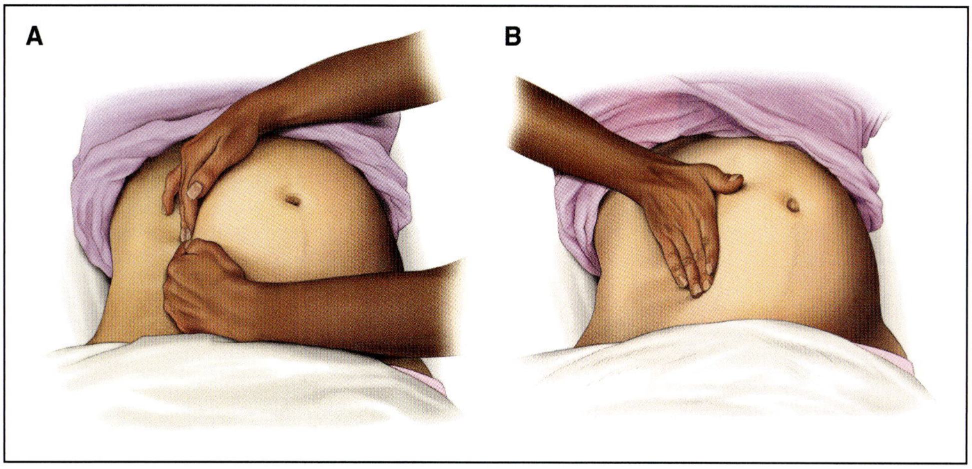

Figure 16. A, Manual left lateral uterine displacement, performed with 2-handed technique. B, 1-handed technique during resuscitation.

characteristics. A systematic review of the literature evaluated all case reports of cardiac arrest in pregnancy about the timing of PMCD, but the wide range of case heterogeneity and reporting bias does not allow for conclusions.[15] Survival of the mother has been reported up to 39 minutes after the onset of maternal cardiac arrest.[4,10,27–29] In a systematic review of literature published 1980 to 2010, the median time from maternal cardiac arrest to delivery was 9 minutes in surviving mothers and 20 minutes in nonsurviving mothers.[15] In the same study, the median time to PMCD was 10 minutes in surviving and 20 minutes in nonsurviving neonates. The time to delivery was within 4 minutes in only 4/57 (7%) reported cases.[15] In a UK cohort study,[4] the median time from collapse to PMCD was 3 minutes in women who survived compared with 12 minutes in nonsurvivors. In this study, 24/25 infants survived when PMCD occurred within 5 minutes after maternal cardiac arrest compared with 7/10 infants when PMCD occurred more than 5 minutes after cardiac arrest. Neonatal survival has been documented with PMCD performed up to 30 minutes after the onset of maternal cardiac arrest.[10] The expert recommendation for timing for PMCD in cardiac arrest at less than 5 minutes remains an important goal, though rarely achieved.[9] There is no evidence for a specific survival threshold at 4 minutes.[8]

These recommendations are supported by "Cardiac Arrest in Pregnancy: a Scientific Statement From the AHA"[9] and a 2020 evidence update.[30]

REFERENCES

1. Mhyre JM, Tsen LC, Einav S, Kuklina EV, Leffert LR, Bateman BT. Cardiac arrest during hospitalization for delivery in the United States, 1998-2011. *Anesthesiology.* 2014;120:810–818. doi: 10.1097/ALN.0000000000000159
2. Centers for Disease Control and Prevention. Pregnancy-related deaths: data from 14 U.S. maternal mortality review committees, 2008-2017. https://www.cdc.gov/reproductivehealth/maternal-mortality/erase-mm/mmr-data-brief.html. Accessed April 22, 2020.
3. Kobori S, Toshimitsu M, Nagaoka S, Yaegashi N, Murotsuki J. Utility and limitations of perimortem cesarean section: A nationwide survey in Japan. *J Obstet Gynaecol Res.* 2019;45:325–330. doi: 10.1111/jog.13819
4. Beckett VA, Knight M, Sharpe P. The CAPS Study: incidence, management and outcomes of cardiac arrest in pregnancy in the UK: a prospective, descriptive study. *BJOG.* 2017;124:1374–1381. doi: 10.1111/1471-0528.14521
5. Maurin O, Lemoine S, Jost D, Lanoë V, Renard A, Travers S, The Paris Fire Brigade Cardiac Arrest Work Group, Lapostolle F, Tourtier JP. Maternal out-of-hospital cardiac arrest: A retrospective observational study. *Resuscitation.* 2019;135:205–211. doi: 10.1016/j.resuscitation.2018.11.001
6. Schaap TP, Overtoom E, van den Akker T, Zwart JJ, van Roosmalen J, Bloemenkamp KWM. Maternal cardiac arrest in the Netherlands: A nationwide surveillance study. *Eur J Obstet Gynecol Reprod Biol.* 2019;237:145–150. doi: 10.1016/j.ejogrb.2019.04.028
7. Lipowicz AA, Cheskes S, Gray SH, Jeejeebhoy F, Lee J, Scales DC, Zhan C, Morrison LJ; Rescu Investigators. Incidence, outcomes and guideline compliance of out-of-hospital maternal cardiac arrest resuscitations: A population-based cohort study. *Resuscitation.* 2018;132:127–132. doi: 10.1016/j.resuscitation.2018.09.003
8. Benson MD, Padovano A, Bourjeily G, Zhou Y. Maternal collapse: Challenging the four-minute rule. *EBioMedicine.* 2016;6:253–257. doi: 10.1016/j.ebiom.2016.02.042
9. Jeejeebhoy FM, Zelop CM, Lipman S, Carvalho B, Joglar J, Mhyre JM, Katz VL, Lapinsky SE, Einav S, Warnes CA, Page RL, Griffin RE, Jain A, Dainty KN, Arafeh J, Windrim R, Koren G, Callaway CW; American Heart Association Emergency Cardiovascular Care Committee, Council on Cardiopulmonary, Critical Care, Perioperative and Resuscitation, Council on Cardiovascular Diseases in the Young, and Council on Clinical Cardiology. Cardiac Arrest in Pregnancy: A Scientific Statement From the American Heart Association. *Circulation.* 2015;132:1747–1773. doi: 10.1161/CIR.0000000000000300
10. Dijkman A, Huisman CM, Smit M, Schutte JM, Zwart JJ, van Roosmalen JJ, Oepkes D. Cardiac arrest in pregnancy: increasing use of perimortem caesarean section due to emergency skills training? *BJOG.* 2010;117:282–287. doi: 10.1111/j.1471-0528.2009.02461.x
11. Page-Rodriguez A, Gonzalez-Sanchez JA. Perimortem cesarean section of twin pregnancy: case report and review of the literature. *Acad Emerg Med.* 1999;6:1072–1074. doi: 10.1111/j.1553-2712.1999.tb01199.x
12. Cardosi RJ, Porter KB. Cesarean delivery of twins during maternal cardiopulmonary arrest. *Obstet Gynecol.* 1998;92(4 Pt 2):695–697. doi: 10.1016/s0029-7844(98)00127-6
13. Rose CH, Faksh A, Traynor KD, Cabrera D, Arendt KW, Brost BC. Challenging the 4- to 5-minute rule: from perimortem cesarean to resuscitative hysterotomy. *Am J Obstetr Gynecol.* 2015;213:653–656. doi: 10.1016/j.ajog.2015.07.019
14. Tambawala ZY, Cherawala M, Maqbool S, Hamza LK. Resuscitative hysterotomy for maternal collapse in a triplet pregnancy. *BMJ Case Rep.* 2020;13:e235328. doi: 10.1136/bcr-2020-235328
15. Einav S, Kaufman N, Sela HY. Maternal cardiac arrest and perimortem caesarean delivery: evidence or expert-based? *Resuscitation.* 2012;83:1191–1200. doi: 10.1016/j.resuscitation.2012.05.005
16. Biderman P, Carmi U, Setton E, Fainblut M, Bachar O, Einav S. Maternal Salvage With Extracorporeal Life Support: Lessons Learned in a Single Center. *Anesth Analg.* 2017;125:1275–1280. doi: 10.1213/ANE.0000000000002262
17. Lipman SS, Daniels KI, Arafeh J, Halamek LP. The case for OBLS: a simulation-based obstetric life support program. *Semin Perinatol.* 2011;35:74–79. doi: 10.1053/j.semperi.2011.01.006
18. Petrone P, Talving P, Browder T, Teixeira PG, Fisher O, Lozornio A, Chan LS. Abdominal injuries in pregnancy: a 155-month study at two level 1 trauma centers. *Injury.* 2011;42:47–49. doi: 10.1016/j.injury.2010.06.026
19. Al-Foudri H, Kevelighan E, Catling S. CEMACH 2003–5 *Saving Mothers' Lives*: lessons for anaesthetists. *Continuing Education in Anaesthesia Critical Care & Pain.* 2010;10:81–87. doi: 10.1093/bjaceaccp/mkq009
20. The Joint Commission. TJC Sentinel Event Alert 44: preventing maternal death. https://www.jointcommission.org/resources/patient-safety-topics/sentinel-event/sentinel-event-alert-newsletters/sentinel-event-alert-issue-44-preventing-maternal-death/. Accessed May 11, 2020.
21. The Joint Commission. Sentinel Event Alert: Preventing infant death and injury during delivery. 2004. https://www.jointcommission.org/resources/patient-safety-topics/sentinel-event/sentinel-event-alert-newsletters/sentinel-event-alert-issue-30-preventing-infant-death-and-injury-during-delivery/. Accessed February 28, 2020.
22. Goodwin AP, Pearce AJ. The human wedge. A manoeuvre to relieve aortocaval compression during resuscitation in late pregnancy. *Anaesthesia.* 1992;47:433–434. doi: 10.1111/j.1365-2044.1992.tb02228.x
23. Cyna AM, Andrew M, Emmett RS, Middleton P, Simmons SW. Techniques for preventing hypotension during spinal anaesthesia for caesarean section. *Cochrane Database Syst Rev.* 2006:CD002251. doi: 10.1002/14651858.CD002251.pub2

23a. Rees SG, Thurlow JA, Gardner IC, Scrutton MJ, Kinsella SM. Maternal cardiovascular consequences of positioning after spinal anaesthesia for Caesarean section: left 15 degree table tilt vs. left lateral. *Anaesthesia.* 2002;57:15–20. doi: 10.1046/j.1365-2044.2002.02325.x

23b. Mendonca C, Griffiths J, Ateleanu B, Collis RE. Hypotension following combined spinal-epidural anaesthesia for Caesarean section. Left lateral position vs. tilted supine position. *Anaesthesia.* 2003;58:428–431. doi: 10.1046/j.1365-2044.2003.03090.x

24. Rittenberger JC, Kelly E, Jang D, Greer K, Heffner A. Successful outcome utilizing hypothermia after cardiac arrest in pregnancy: a case report. *Crit Care Med.* 2008;36:1354–1356. doi: 10.1097/CCM.0b013e318169ee99

25. Chauhan A, Musunuru H, Donnino M, McCurdy MT, Chauhan V, Walsh M. The use of therapeutic hypothermia after cardiac arrest in a pregnant patient. *Ann Emerg Med.* 2012;60:786–789. doi: 10.1016/j.annemergmed.2012.06.004
26. Svinos H. Towards evidence based emergency medicine: best BETs from the Manchester Royal Infirmary. BET 1. Emergency caesarean section in cardiac arrest before the third trimester. *Emerg Med J.* 2008;25:764–765. doi: 10.1136/emj.2008.066860
27. Kam CW. Perimortem caesarean sections (PMCS). *J Accid Emerg Med.* 1994;11:57–58. doi: 10.1136/emj.11.1.57-b
28. Kupas DF, Harter SC, Vosk A. Out-of-hospital perimortem cesarean section. *Prehosp Emerg Care.* 1998;2:206–208. doi: 10.1080/10903129808958874
29. Oates S, Williams GL, Rees GA. Cardiopulmonary resuscitation in late pregnancy. *BMJ.* 1988;297:404–405. doi: 10.1136/bmj.297.6645.404
30. Berg KM, Soar J, Andersen LW, Böttiger BW, Cacciola S, Callaway CW, Couper K, Cronberg T, D'Arrigo S, Deakin CD, et al; on behalf of the Adult Advanced Life Support Collaborators. Adult advanced life support: 2020 International Consensus on Cardiopulmonary Resuscitation and Emergency Cardiovascular Care Science With Treatment Recommendations. *Circulation.* 2020;142(suppl 1):S92–S139. doi: 10.1161/CIR.0000000000000893

Pulmonary Embolism

Recommendations for Pulmonary Embolism

COR	LOE	Recommendations
2a	C-LD	1. In patients with confirmed pulmonary embolism as the precipitant of cardiac arrest, thrombolysis, surgical embolectomy, and mechanical embolectomy are reasonable emergency treatment options.
2b	C-LD	2. Thrombolysis may be considered when cardiac arrest is suspected to be caused by pulmonary embolism.

Synopsis

This topic was reviewed in an ILCOR systematic review for 2020.[1] PE is a potentially reversible cause of shock and cardiac arrest. Acute increase in right ventricular pressure due to pulmonary artery obstruction and release of vasoactive mediators produces cardiogenic shock that may rapidly progress to cardiovascular collapse. Management of acute PE is determined by disease severity.[2] Fulminant PE, characterized by cardiac arrest or severe hemodynamic instability, defines the subset of massive PE that is the focus of these recommendations. Pulseless electrical activity is the presenting rhythm in 36% to 53% of PE-related cardiac arrests, while primary shockable rhythms are uncommon.[3–5]

Prompt systemic anticoagulation is generally indicated for patients with massive and submassive PE to prevent clot propagation and support endogenous clot dissolution over weeks. Anticoagulation alone is inadequate for patients with fulminant PE. Pharmacological and mechanical therapies to rapidly reverse pulmonary artery occlusion and restore adequate pulmonary and systemic circulation have emerged as primary therapies for massive PE, including fulminant PE.[2,6] Current advanced treatment options include systemic thrombolysis, surgical or percutaneous mechanical embolectomy, and ECPR.

Recommendation-Specific Supportive Text

1. In the 2020 ILCOR systematic review, no randomized trials were identified addressing the treatment of cardiac arrest caused by confirmed PE. Observational studies of fibrinolytic therapy for suspected PE were found to have substantial bias and showed mixed results in terms of improvement in outcomes.[3,7–10] Two case series totaling 21 patients with PE undergoing CPR who underwent surgical embolectomy reported 30-day survival rates of 12.5% and 71.4%, respectively.[11,12] A case series of patients with PE-related cardiac arrest reported ROSC in 6 of 7 patients (86%) treated with percutaneous mechanical thrombectomy.[13] In terms of potential adverse effects, a clinical trial and several observational studies show that the risk of major bleeding in patients receiving thrombolysis and CPR is relatively low.[7–9] In spite of the uncertainty of benefit, the risk of death from cardiac arrest outweighs the risk of bleeding from thrombolysis and/or the risks of mechanical or surgical interventions. Because there is no clear benefit to one approach over the other, choice of thrombolysis or surgical or mechanical thrombectomy will depend on timing and available expertise.
2. The approach to cardiac arrest when PE is suspected but not confirmed is less clear, given that a misdiagnosis could place the patient at risk for bleeding without benefit. Recent evidence, however, suggests that the risk of major bleeding is not significantly higher in cardiac arrest patients receiving thrombolysis.[8] PE is difficult to diagnose in the intra-arrest setting, and when ROSC is not obtained and PE is strongly suspected, the evidence supports consideration of thrombolysis.[1]

These recommendations are supported by a 2020 ILCOR systematic review.[1]

REFERENCES

1. Berg KM, Soar J, Andersen LW, Böttiger BW, Cacciola S, Callaway CW, Couper K, Cronberg T, D'Arrigo S, Deakin CD, et al; on behalf of the Adult Advanced Life Support Collaborators. Adult advanced life support: 2020 International Consensus on Cardiopulmonary Resuscitation and Emergency Cardiovascular Care Science With Treatment Recommendations. *Circulation.* 2020;142(suppl 1):S92–S139. doi: 10.1161/CIR.0000000000000893
2. Jaff MR, McMurtry MS, Archer SL, Cushman M, Goldenberg N, Goldhaber SZ, Jenkins JS, Kline JA, Michaels AD, Thistlethwaite P, Vedantham S, White RJ, Zierler BK; American Heart Association Council on Cardiopulmonary, Critical Care, Perioperative and Resuscitation; American Heart Association Council on Peripheral Vascular Disease; American Heart Association Council on Arteriosclerosis, Thrombosis and Vascular Biology. Management of massive and submassive pulmonary embolism, iliofemoral deep vein thrombosis, and chronic thromboembolic pulmonary hypertension: a scientific statement from the American Heart Association. *Circulation.* 2011;123:1788–1830. doi: 10.1161/CIR.0b013e318214914f

3. Kürkciyan I, Meron G, Sterz F, Janata K, Domanovits H, Holzer M, Berzlanovich A, Bankl HC, Laggner AN. Pulmonary embolism as a cause of cardiac arrest: presentation and outcome. *Arch Intern Med.* 2000;160:1529–1535. doi: 10.1001/archinte.160.10.1529
4. Courtney DM, Kline JA. Prospective use of a clinical decision rule to identify pulmonary embolism as likely cause of outpatient cardiac arrest. *Resuscitation.* 2005;65:57–64. doi: 10.1016/j.resuscitation.2004.07.018
5. Comess KA, DeRook FA, Russell ML, Tognazzi-Evans TA, Beach KW. The incidence of pulmonary embolism in unexplained sudden cardiac arrest with pulseless electrical activity. *Am J Med.* 2000;109:351–356. doi: 10.1016/s0002-9343(00)00511-8
6. Wood KE. Major pulmonary embolism: review of a pathophysiologic approach to the golden hour of hemodynamically significant pulmonary embolism. *Chest.* 2002;121:877–905. doi: 10.1378/chest.121.3.877
7. Böttiger BW, Arntz HR, Chamberlain DA, Bluhmki E, Belmans A, Danays T, Carli PA, Adgey JA, Bode C, Wenzel V; TROICA Trial Investigators; European Resuscitation Council Study Group. Thrombolysis during resuscitation for out-of-hospital cardiac arrest. *N Engl J Med.* 2008;359:2651–2662. doi: 10.1056/NEJMoa070570
8. Javaudin F, Lascarrou JB, Le Bastard Q, Bourry Q, Latour C, De Carvalho H, Le Conte P, Escutnaire J, Hubert H, Montassier E, Leclère B; Research Group of the French National Out-of-Hospital Cardiac Arrest Registry (GR-RéAC). Thrombolysis During Resuscitation for Out-of-Hospital Cardiac Arrest Caused by Pulmonary Embolism Increases 30-Day Survival: Findings From the French National Cardiac Arrest Registry. *Chest.* 2019;156:1167–1175. doi: 10.1016/j.chest.2019.07.015
9. Yousuf T, Brinton T, Ahmed K, Iskander J, Woznicka D, Kramer J, Kopiec A, Chadaga AR, Ortiz K. Tissue Plasminogen Activator Use in Cardiac Arrest Secondary to Fulminant Pulmonary Embolism. *J Clin Med Res.* 2016;8:190–195. doi: 10.14740/jocmr2452w
10. Janata K, Holzer M, Kürkciyan I, Losert H, Riedmüller E, Pikula B, Laggner AN, Laczika K. Major bleeding complications in cardiopulmonary resuscitation: the place of thrombolytic therapy in cardiac arrest due to massive pulmonary embolism. *Resuscitation.* 2003;57:49–55. doi: 10.1016/s0300-9572(02)00430-6
11. Doerge HC, Schoendube FA, Loeser H, Walter M, Messmer BJ. Pulmonary embolectomy: review of a 15-year experience and role in the age of thrombolytic therapy. *Eur J Cardiothorac Surg.* 1996;10:952–957. doi: 10.1016/s1010-7940(96)80396-4
12. Konstantinov IE, Saxena P, Koniuszko MD, Alvarez J, Newman MA. Acute massive pulmonary embolism with cardiopulmonary resuscitation: management and results. *Tex Heart Inst J.* 2007;34:41–5; discussion 45.
13. Fava M, Loyola S, Bertoni H, Dougnac A. Massive pulmonary embolism: percutaneous mechanical thrombectomy during cardiopulmonary resuscitation. *J Vasc Interv Radiol.* 2005;16:119–123. doi: 10.1097/01.RVI.0000146173.85401.BA

Toxicity: Benzodiazepines

Recommendation for Benzodiazepine Overdose		
COR	**LOE**	**Recommendation**
3: Harm	B-R	1. The administration of flumazenil to patients with undifferentiated coma confers risk and is not recommended.

Synopsis

Benzodiazepine overdose causes CNS and respiratory depression and, particularly when taken with other sedatives (eg, opioids), can cause respiratory arrest and cardiac arrest. Flumazenil, a specific benzodiazepine antagonist, restores consciousness, protective airway reflexes, and respiratory drive but can have significant side effects including seizures and arrhythmia.[1] These risks are increased in patients with benzodiazepine dependence and with coingestion of cyclic antidepressant medications. The half-life of flumazenil is shorter than many benzodiazepines, necessitating close monitoring after flumazenil administration.[2] An alternative to flumazenil administration is respiratory support with bag-mask ventilation followed by ETI and mechanical ventilation until the benzodiazepine has been metabolized.

Recommendation-Specific Supportive Text

1. A recent meta-analysis of 13 RCTs (990 evaluable patients) found that adverse events and serious adverse events were more common in patients who were randomized to receive flumazenil than placebo (number needed to harm: 5.5 for all adverse events and 50 for serious adverse events).[1] The most commonly encountered adverse events were psychiatric (anxiety, agitation, aggressive behavior); serious adverse events reported included tachycardia, supraventricular arrhythmia, premature ventricular complexes, seizures, and hypotension. Although no patient died in these clinical trials, rare cases of death associated with flumazenil administration have been reported.[3,4] Administration of flumazenil to a patient with undifferentiated overdose may confer an unnecessary risk to the patient, making a focus on providing supportive care the best approach.

This topic last received formal evidence review in 2010.[5]

REFERENCES

1. Penninga EI, Graudal N, Ladekarl MB, Jürgens G. Adverse Events Associated with Flumazenil Treatment for the Management of Suspected Benzodiazepine Intoxication–A Systematic Review with Meta-Analyses of Randomised Trials. *Basic Clin Pharmacol Toxicol.* 2016;118:37–44. doi: 10.1111/bcpt.12434
2. Bowden CA, Krenzelok EP. Clinical applications of commonly used contemporary antidotes. A US perspective. *Drug Saf.* 1997;16:9–47. doi: 10.2165/00002018-199716010-00002
3. Katz Y, Boulos M, Singer P, Rosenberg B. Cardiac arrest associated with flumazenil. *BMJ.* 1992;304:1415. doi: 10.1136/bmj.304.6839.1415-b
4. Burr W, Sandham P, Judd A. Death after flumazepil. *BMJ.* 1989;298:1713. doi: 10.1136/bmj.298.6689.1713-a
5. Vanden Hoek TL, Morrison LJ, Shuster M, Donnino M, Sinz E, Lavonas EJ, Jeejeebhoy FM, Gabrielli A. Part 12: cardiac arrest in special situations: 2010 American Heart Association Guidelines for Cardiopulmonary Resuscitation and Emergency Cardiovascular Care. *Circulation.* 2010;122(suppl 3):S829–S861. doi: 10.1161/CIRCULATIONAHA.110.971069

Toxicity: β-Adrenergic Blockers and Calcium Channel Blockers

Introduction

β-Adrenergic receptor antagonists ("β-adrenergic blockers") and L-type calcium channel antagonists ("calcium channel blockers") are common antihypertensive and cardiac rate control medications. Because the β-adrenergic receptor regulates the activity of the L-type calcium channel,[1] overdose of these medications presents similarly, causing life-threatening hypotension and/or bradycardia that may be refractory to standard treatments such as vasopressor infusions.[2,3] For patients with refractory hemodynamic instability, therapeutic options include administration of high-dose insulin, IV calcium, or glucagon, and consultation with a medical toxicologist or regional poison center can help determine the optimal therapy. Resuscitation from cardiac arrest caused by β-adrenergic blocker or calcium channel blocker overdose follows standard resuscitation guidelines.

Recommendations for β-Adrenergic Blocker Overdose

COR	LOE	Recommendations
2a	C-LD	1. In patients with β-adrenergic blocker overdose who are in refractory shock, administration of high-dose insulin with glucose is reasonable.
2a	C-LD	2. In patients with β-adrenergic blocker overdose who are in refractory shock, administration of IV glucagon is reasonable.
2b	C-LD	3. In patients with β-adrenergic blocker overdose who are in refractory shock, administration of calcium may be considered.
2b	C-LD	4. In patients with β-adrenergic blocker overdose who are in shock refractory to pharmacological therapy, ECMO might be considered.

Recommendation-Specific Supportive Text

1. Animal studies, case reports, and case series have reported increased heart rate and improved hemodynamics after high-dose insulin administration for β-adrenergic blocker toxicity.[4–6] The typical insulin dose used in these studies is a bolus of 1 U/kg, followed by an infusion of 1 U/kg per hour titrated to clinical effect; dextrose and potassium infusions are coadministered.[2,7] No controlled studies on this topic have been identified.
2. Although there are no controlled studies, several case reports and small case series have reported improvement in bradycardia and hypotension after glucagon administration.[8–10]
3. Limited animal data and rare case reports suggest possible utility of calcium to improve heart rate and hypotension in β-adrenergic blocker toxicity.[11–13]
4. Case reports and at least 1 retrospective observational study have been published on survival after ECMO in patients presenting with refractory shock from β-adrenergic blocker overdose.[14,15] The evidence for ECMO for any cardiac arrest is very limited, but refractory shock from a reversible cause such as drug toxicity may be a situation when ECMO could convey a benefit.

These recommendations are supported by the 2018 American College of Cardiology, AHA, and Heart Rhythm Society guideline on the evaluation and management of patients with bradycardia and cardiac conduction delay.[16]

Recommendations for Calcium Channel Blocker Overdose

COR	LOE	Recommendations
2a	C-LD	1. In patients with calcium channel blocker overdose who are in refractory shock, administration of calcium is reasonable.
2a	C-LD	2. In patients with calcium channel blocker overdose who are in refractory shock, administration of high-dose insulin with glucose is reasonable.
2b	C-LD	3. In patients with calcium channel blocker overdose who are in refractory shock, administration of IV glucagon may be considered.
2b	C-LD	4. In patients with calcium channel blocker overdose who are in shock refractory to pharmacological therapy, ECMO might be considered.

Recommendation-Specific Supportive Text

1. No controlled studies examine the effect of IV calcium for calcium channel blocker toxicity.[16] Case series and case reports have reported variable efficacy with low incidence of adverse effects. A systematic review noted consistent benefit in animal studies but inconsistent results in human reports.[17–21] A 2017 expert consensus statement recommended calcium as first-line treatment for catecholamine-refractory shock from calcium channel blockers, acknowledging a very low certainty of evidence for this intervention.[22]
2. Two systematic reviews have identified animal studies, case reports, and human observational studies that have reported increased heart rate and improved hemodynamics after high-dose insulin administration for calcium channel blocker toxicity.[4,16,21,23,24] As with β-adrenergic blocker overdose, the typical insulin dose used in these studies is a bolus of 1 U/kg, followed by an infusion of 1 U/kg per hour titrated to clinical effect; dextrose and potassium infusions are coadministered.[2,4,7,21]
3. Findings in both animal studies and human case reports/case series on the effect of glucagon in calcium channel blocker toxicity have been inconsistent, with some reporting increase in heart rate and some reporting no effect.[21]
4. At least 1 retrospective study on ECMO use for patients with cardiac arrest or refractory shock in the setting of drug toxicity has reported improved outcomes.[14] As with all retrospective studies, the risk of bias is high because of other considerations in deciding which patients will be treated with ECMO. A recent consensus statement supports the use of ECMO for refractory shock from a reversible causes such as drug toxicity.[22]

These recommendations are supported by the 2018 American College of Cardiology, AHA, and Heart Rhythm Society guideline on the evaluation and management of patients with bradycardia and cardiac conduction delay.[16]

REFERENCES

1. van der Heyden MA, Wijnhoven TJ, Opthof T. Molecular aspects of adrenergic modulation of cardiac L-type Ca2+ channels. *Cardiovasc Res.* 2005;65:28–39. doi: 10.1016/j.cardiores.2004.09.028
2. Graudins A, Lee HM, Druda D. Calcium channel antagonist and beta-blocker overdose: antidotes and adjunct therapies. *Br J Clin Pharmacol.* 2016;81:453–461. doi: 10.1111/bcp.12763
3. Levine M, Curry SC, Padilla-Jones A, Ruha AM. Critical care management of verapamil and diltiazem overdose with a focus on vasopressors: a 25-year experience at a single center. *Ann Emerg Med.* 2013;62:252–258. doi: 10.1016/j.annemergmed.2013.03.018
4. Engebretsen KM, Kaczmarek KM, Morgan J, Holger JS. High-dose insulin therapy in beta-blocker and calcium channel-blocker poisoning. *Clin Toxicol (Phila).* 2011;49:277–283. doi: 10.3109/15563650.2011.582471
5. Seegobin K, Maharaj S, Deosaran A, Reddy P. Severe beta blocker and calcium channel blocker overdose: Role of high dose insulin. *Am J Emerg Med.* 2018;36:736.e5–736.e6. doi: 10.1016/j.ajem.2018.01.038
6. Doepker B, Healy W, Cortez E, Adkins EJ. High-dose insulin and intravenous lipid emulsion therapy for cardiogenic shock induced by intentional calcium-channel blocker and Beta-blocker overdose: a case series. *J Emerg Med.* 2014;46:486–490. doi: 10.1016/j.jemermed.2013.08.135
7. Holger JS, Stellpflug SJ, Cole JB, Harris CR, Engebretsen KM. High-dose insulin: a consecutive case series in toxin-induced cardiogenic shock. *Clin Toxicol (Phila).* 2011;49:653–658. doi: 10.3109/15563650.2011.593522
8. Love JN, Sachdeva DK, Bessman ES, Curtis LA, Howell JM. A potential role for glucagon in the treatment of drug-induced symptomatic bradycardia. *Chest.* 1998;114:323–326. doi: 10.1378/chest.114.1.323
9. Bailey B. Glucagon in beta-blocker and calcium channel blocker overdoses: a systematic review. *J Toxicol Clin Toxicol.* 2003;41:595–602. doi: 10.1081/clt-120023761
10. Peterson CD, Leeder JS, Sterner S. Glucagon therapy for beta-blocker overdose. *Drug Intell Clin Pharm.* 1984;18:394–398. doi: 10.1177/106002808401800507
11. Pertoldi F, D'Orlando L, Mercante WP. Electromechanical dissociation 48 hours after atenolol overdose: usefulness of calcium chloride. *Ann Emerg Med.* 1998;31:777–781. doi: 10.1016/s0196-0644(98)70241-0
12. Love JN, Hanfling D, Howell JM. Hemodynamic effects of calcium chloride in a canine model of acute propranolol intoxication. *Ann Emerg Med.* 1996;28:1–6. doi: 10.1016/s0196-0644(96)70129-4
13. Teo LK, Tham DJW, Chong CP. A case of massive atenolol overdose successfully managed with intravenous calcium chloride. *East J Med.* 2018;21:213–215.
14. Masson R, Colas V, Parienti JJ, Lehoux P, Massetti M, Charbonneau P, Saulnier F, Daubin C. A comparison of survival with and without extracorporeal life support treatment for severe poisoning due to drug intoxication. *Resuscitation.* 2012;83:1413–1417. doi: 10.1016/j.resuscitation.2012.03.028
15. Rotella JA, Greene SL, Koutsogiannis Z, Graudins A, Hung Leang Y, Kuan K, Baxter H, Bourke E, Wong A. Treatment for beta-blocker poisoning: a systematic review. *Clin Toxicol (Phila).* 2020:1–41. doi: 10.1080/15563650.2020.1752918
16. Kusumoto FM, Schoenfeld MH, Barrett C, Edgerton JR, Ellenbogen KA, Gold MR, Goldschlager NF, Hamilton RM, Joglar JA, Kim RJ, Lee R, Marine JE, McLeod CJ, Oken KR, Patton KK, Pellegrini CN, Selzman KA, Thompson A, Varosy PD. 2018 ACC/AHA/HRS Guideline on the Evaluation and Management of Patients With Bradycardia and Cardiac Conduction Delay: A Report of the American College of Cardiology/American Heart Association Task Force on Clinical Practice Guidelines and the Heart Rhythm Society. *Circulation.* 2019;140:e382–e482. doi: 10.1161/CIR.0000000000000628
17. Howarth DM, Dawson AH, Smith AJ, Buckley N, Whyte IM. Calcium channel blocking drug overdose: an Australian series. *Hum Exp Toxicol.* 1994;13:161–166. doi: 10.1177/096032719401300304
18. Crump BJ, Holt DW, Vale JA. Lack of response to intravenous calcium in severe verapamil poisoning. *Lancet.* 1982;2:939–940. doi: 10.1016/s0140-6736(82)90912-6
19. Ghosh S, Sircar M. Calcium channel blocker overdose: experience with amlodipine. *Indian J Crit Care Med.* 2008;12:190–193. doi: 10.4103/0972-5229.45080
20. Henry M, Kay MM, Viccellio P. Cardiogenic shock associated with calcium-channel and beta blockers: reversal with intravenous calcium chloride. *Am J Emerg Med.* 1985;3:334–336. doi: 10.1016/0735-6757(85)90060-9
21. St-Onge M, Dubé PA, Gosselin S, Guimont C, Godwin J, Archambault PM, Chauny JM, Frenette AJ, Darveau M, Le Sage N, Poitras J, Provencher J, Juurlink DN, Blais R. Treatment for calcium channel blocker poisoning: a systematic review. *Clin Toxicol (Phila).* 2014;52:926–944. doi: 10.3109/15563650.2014.965827
22. St-Onge M, Anseeuw K, Cantrell FL, Gilchrist IC, Hantson P, Bailey B, Lavergne V, Gosselin S, Kerns W II, Laliberté M, Lavonas EJ, Juurlink DN, Muscedere J, Yang CC, Sinuff T, Rieder M, Mégarbane B. Experts Consensus Recommendations for the Management of Calcium Channel Blocker Poisoning in Adults. *Crit Care Med.* 2017;45:e306–e315. doi: 10.1097/CCM.0000000000002087
23. Greene SL, Gawarammana I, Wood DM, Jones AL, Dargan PI. Relative safety of hyperinsulinaemia/euglycaemia therapy in the management of calcium channel blocker overdose: a prospective observational study. *Intensive Care Med.* 2007;33:2019–2024. doi: 10.1007/s00134-007-0768-y
24. Espinoza TR, Bryant SM, Aks SE. Hyperinsulin therapy for calcium channel antagonist poisoning: a seven-year retrospective study. *Am J Ther.* 2013;20:29–31. doi: 10.1097/MJT.0b013e31824d5fbd

Toxicity: Cocaine

Recommendations for Cocaine Toxicity

COR	LOE	Recommendations
2a	B-NR	1. For patients with cocaine-induced hypertension, tachycardia, agitation, or chest discomfort, benzodiazepines, alpha blockers, calcium channel blockers, nitroglycerin, and/or morphine can be beneficial.
2b	C-LD	2. Although contradictory evidence exists, it may be reasonable to avoid the use of pure β-adrenergic blocker medications in the setting of cocaine toxicity.

Synopsis

Cocaine toxicity can cause adverse effects on the cardiovascular system, including dysrhythmia, hypertension, tachycardia and coronary artery vasospasm, and cardiac conduction delays. These effects can also precipitate acute coronary syndrome and stroke. Human experimental data suggest that benzodiazepines (diazepam, lorazepam), alpha blockers (phentolamine), calcium channel blockers (verapamil), morphine, and nitroglycerine are all safe and potentially beneficial in the cocaine-intoxicated patient; no data are available comparing these approaches.[1–5] Contradictory data surround the use of β-adrenergic blockers.[6–8] Patients suffering from cocaine toxicity can deteriorate quickly depending on the amount and timing of ingestion. If cardiac arrest develops as the result of cocaine toxicity, there is no evidence to suggest deviation from standard BLS and ALS guidelines, with specific treatment strategies used in the post–cardiac arrest phase as needed if there is evidence of severe cardiotoxicity or neurotoxicity. Once ROSC is achieved, urgent consultation with a medical toxicologist or regional poison center is suggested.

Recommendation-Specific Supportive Text

1. No large RCT evaluating different treatment strategies for patients suffering from acute cocaine toxicity exists. A systematic review of the

literature identified 5 small prospective trials, 3 retrospective studies, and multiple case reports and case series with contradictory results. Some literature reports good favorable outcomes while others report significant adverse events.[9]

2. A well-conducted human trial showed that administration of propranolol reduces coronary blood flow in patients with cocaine exposure.[8] Although recent systematic reviews suggest that β-adrenergic blocker use may not be harmful,[6,7] safe alternatives are available.

This topic last received formal evidence review in 2010.[10]

REFERENCES

1. Baumann BM, Perrone J, Hornig SE, Shofer FS, Hollander JE. Randomized, double-blind, placebo-controlled trial of diazepam, nitroglycerin, or both for treatment of patients with potential cocaine-associated acute coronary syndromes. *Acad Emerg Med.* 2000;7:878–885. doi: 10.1111/j.1553-2712.2000.tb02065.x
2. Negus BH, Willard JE, Hillis LD, Glamann DB, Landau C, Snyder RW, Lange RA. Alleviation of cocaine-induced coronary vasoconstriction with intravenous verapamil. *Am J Cardiol.* 1994;73:510–513. doi: 10.1016/0002-9149(94)90684-x
3. Saland KE, Hillis LD, Lange RA, Cigarroa JE. Influence of morphine sulfate on cocaine-induced coronary vasoconstriction. *Am J Cardiol.* 2002;90:810–811. doi: 10.1016/s0002-9149(02)02622-x
4. Hollander JE, Hoffman RS, Gennis P, Fairweather P, DiSano MJ, Schumb DA, Feldman JA, Fish SS, Dyer S, Wax P. Nitroglycerin in the treatment of cocaine associated chest pain–clinical safety and efficacy. *J Toxicol Clin Toxicol.* 1994;32:243–256. doi: 10.3109/15563659409017957
5. Honderick T, Williams D, Seaberg D, Wears R. A prospective, randomized, controlled trial of benzodiazepines and nitroglycerine or nitroglycerine alone in the treatment of cocaine-associated acute coronary syndromes. *Am J Emerg Med.* 2003;21:39–42. doi: 10.1053/ajem.2003.50010
6. Pham D, Addison D, Kayani W, Misra A, Jneid H, Resar J, Lakkis N, Alam M. Outcomes of beta blocker use in cocaine-associated chest pain: a meta-analysis. *Emerg Med J.* 2018;35:559–563. doi: 10.1136/emermed-2017-207065
7. Shin D, Lee ES, Bohra C, Kongpakpaisarn K. In-Hospital and Long-Term Outcomes of Beta-Blocker Treatment in Cocaine Users: A Systematic Review and Meta-analysis. *Cardiol Res.* 2019;10:40–47. doi: 10.14740/cr831
8. Lange RA, Cigarroa RG, Flores ED, McBride W, Kim AS, Wells PJ, Bedotto JB, Danziger RS, Hillis LD. Potentiation of cocaine-induced coronary vasoconstriction by beta-adrenergic blockade. *Ann Intern Med.* 1990;112:897–903. doi: 10.7326/0003-4819-112-12-897
9. Richards JR, Garber D, Laurin EG, Albertson TE, Derlet RW, Amsterdam EA, Olson KR, Ramoska EA, Lange RA. Treatment of cocaine cardiovascular toxicity: a systematic review. *Clin Toxicol (Phila).* 2016;54:345–364. doi: 10.3109/15563650.2016.1142090
10. Vanden Hoek TL, Morrison LJ, Shuster M, Donnino M, Sinz E, Lavonas EJ, Jeejeebhoy FM, Gabrielli A. Part 12: cardiac arrest in special situations: 2010 American Heart Association Guidelines for Cardiopulmonary Resuscitation and Emergency Cardiovascular Care. *Circulation.* 2010;122(suppl 3):S829–S861. doi: 10.1161/CIRCULATIONAHA.110.971069

Toxicity: Local Anesthetics

Recommendation for Local Anesthetic Overdose

COR	LOE	Recommendation
2b	C-LD	1. It may be reasonable to administer IV lipid emulsion, concomitant with standard resuscitative care, to patients with local anesthetic systemic toxicity (LAST), and particularly to patients who have premonitory neurotoxicity or cardiac arrest due to bupivacaine toxicity.

Synopsis

Local anesthetic overdose (also known as *local anesthetic systemic toxicity*, or LAST) is a life-threatening emergency that can present with neurotoxicity or fulminant cardiovascular collapse.[1,2] The most commonly reported agents associated with LAST are bupivacaine, lidocaine, and ropivacaine.[2]

By definition, LAST is a special circumstance in which alternative approaches should be considered in addition to standard BLS and ALS. Case reports and animal data have suggested that IV lipid emulsion may be of benefit.[2–5] LAST results in profound inhibition of voltage-gated channels (especially sodium transduction) in the cell membrane. The potential mechanisms of action of IV lipid emulsion include active shuttling of the local anesthetic drug away from the heart and brain, increased cardiac contractility, vasoconstriction, and cardioprotective effects.[1]

The reported incidence of LAST ranges from 0 to 2 per 1000 nerve blocks[2] but appears to be decreasing as a result of increasing awareness of toxicity and improved techniques.[1]

Recommendation-Specific Supportive Text

1. Since the last time these recommendations were formally reviewed,[6] several detailed systematic reviews of the literature and a practice advisory from the American Society of Regional Anesthesia and Pain Medicine have been published.[1–5] There are still no published RCTs or studies with a comparison with standard resuscitative care. Human data come from approximately 100 case reports published until 2014,[6] with an additional 47 separate cases in 35 articles between 2014 and November 2016, although patients in only 10 of these 47 cases received any CPR.[2] In the identified cases, the results cannot easily be interpreted or attributed to IV lipid emulsion given the lack of a comparative group. The administration of IV lipid emulsion is thought to be relatively benign, although pancreatitis and acute respiratory distress syndrome have been associated with its use.[7]

This topic last received formal evidence review in 2015.[6]

REFERENCES

1. Neal JM, Barrington MJ, Fettiplace MR, Gitman M, Memtsoudis SG, Morwald EE, Rubin DS, Weinberg G. The Third American Society of Regional Anesthesia and Pain Medicine Practice advisory on local anesthetic systemic toxicity: executive summary 2017. *Reg Anesth Pain Med.* 2018;43:113–123. doi: 10.1097/AAP.0000000000000720
2. Gitman M, Barrington MJ. Local Anesthetic Systemic Toxicity: A Review of Recent Case Reports and Registries. *Reg Anesth Pain Med.* 2018;43:124–130. doi: 10.1097/AAP.0000000000000721
3. Cao D, Heard K, Foran M, Koyfman A. Intravenous lipid emulsion in the emergency department: a systematic review of recent literature. *J Emerg Med.* 2015;48:387–397. doi: 10.1016/j.jemermed.2014.10.009
4. Gosselin S, Hoegberg LC, Hoffman RS, Graudins A, Stork CM, Thomas SH, Stellpflug SJ, Hayes BD, Levine M, Morris M, Nesbitt-Miller A, Turgeon AF, Bailey B, Calello DP, Chuang R, Bania TC, Mégarbane B, Bhalla A, Lavergne V. Evidence-based recommendations on the use of intravenous

lipid emulsion therapy in poisoning. *Clin Toxicol (Phila).* 2016;54:899–923. doi: 10.1080/15563650.2016.1214275
5. Hoegberg LC, Bania TC, Lavergne V, Bailey B, Turgeon AF, Thomas SH, Morris M, Miller-Nesbitt A, Mégarbane B, Magder S, Gosselin S; Lipid Emulsion Workgroup. Systematic review of the effect of intravenous lipid emulsion therapy for local anesthetic toxicity. *Clin Toxicol (Phila).* 2016;54:167–193. doi: 10.3109/15563650.2015.1121270
6. Lavonas EJ, Drennan IR, Gabrielli A, Heffner AC, Hoyte CO, Orkin AM, Sawyer KN, Donnino MW. Part 10: special circumstances of resuscitation: 2015 American Heart Association Guidelines Update for Cardiopulmonary Resuscitation and Emergency Cardiovascular Care. *Circulation.* 2015;132(suppl 2):S501–S518. doi: 10.1161/CIR.0000000000000264
7. Levine M, Skolnik AB, Ruha AM, Bosak A, Menke N, Pizon AF. Complications following antidotal use of intravenous lipid emulsion therapy. *J Med Toxicol.* 2014;10:10–14. doi: 10.1007/s13181-013-0356-1

Toxicity: Sodium Channel Blockers, Including Tricyclic Antidepressants

Recommendations for Cardiac Arrest Due to Sodium Channel Blockers, Including Tricyclic Antidepressants

COR	LOE	Recommendation
2a	C-LD	1. Administration of sodium bicarbonate for cardiac arrest or life-threatening cardiac conduction delays (ie, QRS prolongation more than 120 ms) due to sodium channel blocker/tricyclic antidepressant (TCA) overdose can be beneficial.
2b	C-LD	2. The use of ECMO for cardiac arrest or refractory shock due to sodium channel blocker/TCA toxicity may be considered.

Synopsis

Overdose of sodium channel–blocking medications, such as TCAs and other drugs (eg, cocaine, flecainide, citalopram), can cause hypotension, dysrhythmia, and death by blockade of cardiac sodium channels, among other mechanisms. Characteristic ECG findings include tachycardia and QRS prolongation with a right bundle branch pattern.[1,2] TCA toxicity can mimic a Brugada type 1 ECG pattern.[3]

The standard therapy for hypotension or cardiotoxicity from sodium channel blocker poisoning consists of sodium boluses and serum alkalization, typically achieved through administration of sodium bicarbonate boluses. This approach is supported by animal studies and human case reports and has recently been systematically reviewed.[4]

A clinical trial studied administration of magnesium in addition to sodium bicarbonate for patients with TCA-induced hypotension, acidosis, and/or QRS prolongation.[5] Although overall outcomes were better in the magnesium group, no statistically significant effect was found in mortality, the magnesium patients were significantly less ill than controls at study entry, and methodologic flaws render this work preliminary.

Although case reports describe good outcomes after the use of ECMO[6] and IV lipid emulsion therapy[7–10] for severe sodium channel blocker cardiotoxicity, no controlled human studies could be found, and limited animal data do not support lipid emulsion efficacy.[11]

No human controlled studies were found evaluating treatment of cardiac arrest due to TCA toxicity, although 1 study demonstrated termination of amitriptyline-induced VT in dogs.[12]

Recommendation-Specific Supportive Text

1. The administration of hypertonic (8.4%, 1 mEq/mL) sodium bicarbonate solution for treatment of sodium channel blockade due to TCAs and other toxicants is supported by human observational studies[13,14] and animal experiments.[12,15–22] This literature has recently been systematically reviewed.[4] Although dose-finding studies are not available, an initial dose of 1 to 2 mEq/kg (1–2 mL/kg of 1 mEq/mL [8.4%]) sodium bicarbonate, repeated as needed to achieve clinical stability while avoiding extreme hypernatremia or alkalemia) has historically been recommended and appears effective.
2. Case reports support the use of ECMO for patients with refractory shock due to TCA toxicity.[23,24] Although the overall evidence for ECPR to improve outcomes is limited, because TCA toxicity is a reversible cause of cardiogenic shock/cardiac arrest, use of ECPR/ECMO in patients with life-threatening toxicity refractory to other therapy is logical.

This topic last received formal evidence review in 2010.[25]

REFERENCES

1. Harrigan RA, Brady WJ. ECG abnormalities in tricyclic antidepressant ingestion. *Am J Emerg Med.* 1999;17:387–393. doi: 10.1016/s0735-6757(99)90094-3
2. Thanacoody HK, Thomas SH. Tricyclic antidepressant poisoning: cardiovascular toxicity. *Toxicol Rev.* 2005;24:205–214. doi: 10.2165/00139709-200524030-00013
3. Bebarta VS, Phillips S, Eberhardt A, Calihan KJ, Waksman JC, Heard K. Incidence of Brugada electrocardiographic pattern and outcomes of these patients after intentional tricyclic antidepressant ingestion. *Am J Cardiol.* 2007;100:656–660. doi: 10.1016/j.amjcard.2007.03.077
4. Bruccoleri RE, Burns MM. A Literature Review of the Use of Sodium Bicarbonate for the Treatment of QRS Widening. *J Med Toxicol.* 2016;12:121–129. doi: 10.1007/s13181-015-0483-y
5. Emamhadi M, Mostafazadeh B, Hassanijirdehi M. Tricyclic antidepressant poisoning treated by magnesium sulfate: a randomized, clinical trial. *Drug Chem Toxicol.* 2012;35:300–303. doi: 10.3109/01480545.2011.614249
6. Koschny R, Lutz M, Seckinger J, Schwenger V, Stremmel W, Eisenbach C. Extracorporeal life support and plasmapheresis in a case of severe polyintoxication. *J Emerg Med.* 2014;47:527–531. doi: 10.1016/j.jemermed.2014.04.044
7. Kiberd MB, Minor SF. Lipid therapy for the treatment of a refractory amitriptyline overdose. *CJEM.* 2012;14:193–197. doi: 10.2310/8000.2011.110486
8. Agarwala R, Ahmed SZ, Wiegand TJ. Prolonged use of intravenous lipid emulsion in a severe tricyclic antidepressant overdose. *J Med Toxicol.* 2014;10:210–214. doi: 10.1007/s13181-013-0353-4
9. Cao D, Heard K, Foran M, Koyfman A. Intravenous lipid emulsion in the emergency department: a systematic review of recent literature. *J Emerg Med.* 2015;48:387–397. doi: 10.1016/j.jemermed.2014.10.009
10. Odigwe CC, Tariq M, Kotecha T, Mustafa U, Senussi N, Ikwu I, Bhattacharya A, Ngene JI, Ojiako K, Iroegbu N. Tricyclic antidepressant overdose treated with adjunctive lipid rescue and plasmapheresis. *Proc (Bayl Univ Med Cent).* 2016;29:284–287. doi: 10.1080/08998280.2016.11929437
11. Varney SM, Bebarta VS, Vargas TE, Boudreau S, Castaneda M. Intravenous lipid emulsion therapy does not improve hypotension compared to sodium bicarbonate for tricyclic antidepressant toxicity: a randomized, controlled pilot study in a swine model. *Acad Emerg Med.* 2014;21:1212–1219. doi: 10.1111/acem.12513

12. Sasyniuk BI, Jhamandas V, Valois M. Experimental amitriptyline intoxication: treatment of cardiac toxicity with sodium bicarbonate. *Ann Emerg Med.* 1986;15:1052–1059. doi: 10.1016/s0196-0644(86)80128-7
13. Köppel C, Wiegreffe A, Tenczer J. Clinical course, therapy, outcome and analytical data in amitriptyline and combined amitriptyline/chlordiazepoxide overdose. *Hum Exp Toxicol.* 1992;11:458–465. doi: 10.1177/096032719201100604
14. Hoffman JR, Votey SR, Bayer M, Silver L. Effect of hypertonic sodium bicarbonate in the treatment of moderate-to-severe cyclic antidepressant overdose. *Am J Emerg Med.* 1993;11:336–341. doi: 10.1016/0735-6757(93)90163-6
15. Brown TC. Tricyclic antidepressant overdosage: experimental studies on the management of circulatory complications. *Clin Toxicol.* 1976;9:255–272. doi: 10.3109/15563657608988129
16. Nattel S, Mittleman M. Treatment of ventricular tachyarrhythmias resulting from amitriptyline toxicity in dogs. *J Pharmacol Exp Ther.* 1984;231:430–435.
17. Pentel P, Benowitz N. Efficacy and mechanism of action of sodium bicarbonate in the treatment of desipramine toxicity in rats. *J Pharmacol Exp Ther.* 1984;230:12–19.
18. Hedges JR, Baker PB, Tasset JJ, Otten EJ, Dalsey WC, Syverud SA. Bicarbonate therapy for the cardiovascular toxicity of amitriptyline in an animal model. *J Emerg Med.* 1985;3:253–260. doi: 10.1016/0736-4679(85)90427-5
19. Knudsen K, Abrahamsson J. Epinephrine and sodium bicarbonate independently and additively increase survival in experimental amitriptyline poisoning. *Crit Care Med.* 1997;25:669–674. doi: 10.1097/00003246-199704000-00019
20. Tobis JM, Aronow WS. Effect of amitriptyline antidotes on repetitive extrasystole threshold. *Clin Pharmacol Ther.* 1980;27:602–606. doi: 10.1038/clpt.1980.85
21. McCabe JL, Cobaugh DJ, Menegazzi JJ, Fata J. Experimental tricyclic antidepressant toxicity: a randomized, controlled comparison of hypertonic saline solution, sodium bicarbonate, and hyperventilation. *Ann Emerg Med.* 1998;32(3 Pt 1):329–333. doi: 10.1016/s0196-0644(98)70009-5
22. Bou-Abboud E, Nattel S. Relative role of alkalosis and sodium ions in reversal of class I antiarrhythmic drug-induced sodium channel blockade by sodium bicarbonate. *Circulation.* 1996;94:1954–1961. doi: 10.1161/01.cir.94.8.1954
23. Goodwin DA, Lally KP, Null DM Jr. Extracorporeal membrane oxygenation support for cardiac dysfunction from tricyclic antidepressant overdose. *Crit Care Med.* 1993;21:625–627. doi: 10.1097/00003246-199304000-00025
24. de Lange DW, Sikma MA, Meulenbelt J. Extracorporeal membrane oxygenation in the treatment of poisoned patients. *Clin Toxicol (Phila).* 2013;51:385–393. doi: 10.3109/15563650.2013.800876
25. Vanden Hoek TL, Morrison LJ, Shuster M, Donnino M, Sinz E, Lavonas EJ, Jeejeebhoy FM, Gabrielli A. Part 12: cardiac arrest in special situations: 2010 American Heart Association Guidelines for Cardiopulmonary Resuscitation and Emergency Cardiovascular Care. *Circulation.* 2010;122(suppl 3):S829–S861. doi: 10.1161/CIRCULATIONAHA.110.971069

Toxicity: Carbon Monoxide, Digoxin, and Cyanide

Recommendations for Carbon Monoxide, Digoxin, and Cyanide Poisoning

COR	LOE	Recommendations
1	B-R	1. Antidigoxin Fab antibodies should be administered to patients with severe cardiac glycoside toxicity.
2b	B-R	2. Hyperbaric oxygen therapy may be helpful in the treatment of acute carbon monoxide poisoning in patients with severe toxicity.
2a	C-LD	3. Hydroxocobalamin and 100% oxygen, with or without sodium thiosulfate, can be beneficial for cyanide poisoning.

Synopsis

Digoxin poisoning can cause severe bradycardia, AV nodal blockade, and life-threatening ventricular arrhythmias. Poisoning from other cardiac glycosides, such as oleander, foxglove, and digitoxin, have similar effects. Prompt treatment of cardiac glycoside toxicity is imperative to prevent or treat life-threatening arrhythmias.

Carbon monoxide poisoning reduces the ability of hemoglobin to deliver oxygen and also causes direct cellular damage to the brain and myocardium, leading to death or long-term risk of neurological and myocardial injury. Although cardiac arrest due to carbon monoxide poisoning is almost always fatal, studies about neurological sequelae from less-severe carbon monoxide poisoning may be relevant.

The toxicity of cyanide is predominantly due to the cessation of aerobic cell metabolism. Cyanide reversibly binds to the ferric ion cytochrome oxidase in the mitochondria and stops cellular respiration and adenosine triphosphate production. Cyanide poisoning may result from smoke inhalation, industrial exposures, self-poisoning, terrorism, or the administration of sodium nitroprusside. Symptoms typically occur within minutes, and findings may include arrhythmias, apnea, hypotension with bradycardia, seizures, and cardiovascular collapse.[1] Lactic acidosis is a sensitive and specific finding.[2,3] Immediate antidotes include hydroxocobalamin and nitrites; however, the former has a much better safety profile. Sodium thiosulfate enhances the effectiveness of nitrites by enhancing the detoxification of cyanide, though its role in patients treated with hydroxocobalamin is less certain.[4] Novel antidotes are in development.

Recommendation-Specific Supportive Text

1. There are no data evaluating the use of antidotes to digoxin overdose specifically in the setting of cardiac arrest. Data from 1 RCT[5] and 4 case series[6–9] concluded that antidigoxin Fab fragments are safe and effective for the treatment of serious cardiac arrhythmias induced by digitalis and other cardiac glycoside overdose.
2. Few patients who develop cardiac arrest from carbon monoxide poisoning survive to hospital discharge, regardless of the treatment administered after ROSC, though rare good outcomes have been described.[10–12] Clinical trials of hyperbaric oxygen therapy to prevent neurological injury from carbon monoxide poisoning yield conflicting results; patients with cardiac arrest were excluded from all trials.[13,14] Hyperbaric oxygen therapy has a low incidence of side effects.
3. Several studies demonstrate that patients with known or suspected cyanide toxicity presenting with cardiovascular instability or cardiac arrest who undergo prompt treatment with IV hydroxocobalamin, a cyanide scavenger,[2,15–19] can have reversal of life-threatening toxicity. Whether the addition of sodium thiosulfate, a cofactor for cyanide metabolism, enhances the antidotal effect of

hydroxocobalamin is controversial. Four studies in animals[20–23] and 2 studies in humans[2,24] demonstrated enhanced effectiveness of hydroxocobalamin when sodium thiosulfate was coadministered, though this is not the case in other models.[4]

This topic last received formal evidence review in 2010.[25]

REFERENCES

1. Parker-Cote JL, Rizer J, Vakkalanka JP, Rege SV, Holstege CP. Challenges in the diagnosis of acute cyanide poisoning. *Clin Toxicol (Phila).* 2018;56:609–617. doi: 10.1080/15563650.2018.1435886
2. Baud FJ, Barriot P, Toffis V, Riou B, Vicaut E, Lecarpentier Y, Bourdon R, Astier A, Bismuth C. Elevated blood cyanide concentrations in victims of smoke inhalation. *N Engl J Med.* 1991;325:1761–1766. doi: 10.1056/NEJM199112193252502
3. Baud FJ, Borron SW, Bavoux E, Astier A, Hoffman JR. Relation between plasma lactate and blood cyanide concentrations in acute cyanide poisoning. *BMJ.* 1996;312:26–27. doi: 10.1136/bmj.312.7022.26
4. Bebarta VS, Pitotti RL, Dixon P, Lairet JR, Bush A, Tanen DA. Hydroxocobalamin versus sodium thiosulfate for the treatment of acute cyanide toxicity in a swine (Sus scrofa) model. *Ann Emerg Med.* 2012;59:532–539. doi: 10.1016/j.annemergmed.2012.01.022
5. Eddleston M, Rajapakse S, Rajakanthan, Jayalath S, Sjöström L, Santharaj W, Thenabadu PN, Sheriff MH, Warrell DA. Anti-digoxin Fab fragments in cardiotoxicity induced by ingestion of yellow oleander: a randomised controlled trial. *Lancet.* 2000;355:967–972. doi: 10.1016/s0140-6736(00)90014-x
6. Smith TW, Butler VP Jr, Haber E, Fozzard H, Marcus FI, Bremner WF, Schulman IC, Phillips A. Treatment of life-threatening digitalis intoxication with digoxin-specific Fab antibody fragments: experience in 26 cases. *N Engl J Med.* 1982;307:1357–1362. doi: 10.1056/NEJM198211253072201
7. Antman EM, Wenger TL, Butler VP Jr, Haber E, Smith TW. Treatment of 150 cases of life-threatening digitalis intoxication with digoxin-specific Fab antibody fragments. Final report of a multicenter study. *Circulation.* 1990;81:1744–1752. doi: 10.1161/01.cir.81.6.1744
8. Wenger TL, Butler VP Jr, Haber E, Smith TW. Treatment of 63 severely digitalis-toxic patients with digoxin-specific antibody fragments. *J Am Coll Cardiol.* 1985;5(suppl A):118A–123A. doi: 10.1016/s0735-1097(85)80471-x
9. Hickey AR, Wenger TL, Carpenter VP, Tilson HH, Hlatky MA, Furberg CD, Kirkpatrick CH, Strauss HC, Smith TW. Digoxin Immune Fab therapy in the management of digitalis intoxication: safety and efficacy results of an observational surveillance study. *J Am Coll Cardiol.* 1991;17:590–598. doi: 10.1016/s0735-1097(10)80170-6
10. Hampson NB, Zmaeff JL. Outcome of patients experiencing cardiac arrest with carbon monoxide poisoning treated with hyperbaric oxygen. *Ann Emerg Med.* 2001;38:36–41. doi: 10.1067/mem.2001.115532
11. Sloan EP, Murphy DG, Hart R, Cooper MA, Turnbull T, Barreca RS, Ellerson B. Complications and protocol considerations in carbon monoxide-poisoned patients who require hyperbaric oxygen therapy: report from a ten-year experience. *Ann Emerg Med.* 1989;18:629–634. doi: 10.1016/s0196-0644(89)80516-5
12. Mumma BE, Shellenbarger D, Callaway CW, Katz KD, Guyette FX, Rittenberger JC. Neurologic recovery following cardiac arrest due to carbon monoxide poisoning. *Resuscitation.* 2009;80:835. doi: 10.1016/j.resuscitation.2009.03.027
13. Buckley NA, Juurlink DN, Isbister G, Bennett MH, Lavonas EJ. Hyperbaric oxygen for carbon monoxide poisoning. *Cochrane Database Syst Rev.* 2011:CD002041. doi: 10.1002/14651858.CD002041.pub3
14. American College of Emergency Physicians Clinical Policies Subcommittee on Carbon Monoxide Poisoning, Wolf SJ, Maloney GE, Shih RD, Shy BD, Brown MD. Clinical policy: critical issues in the evaluation and management of adult patients presenting to the emergency department with acute carbon monoxide poisoning. *Ann Emerg Med.* 2017;69:98.e6–107.e6. doi: 10.1016/j.annemergmed.2016.11.003
15. Borron SW, Baud FJ, Barriot P, Imbert M, Bismuth C. Prospective study of hydroxocobalamin for acute cyanide poisoning in smoke inhalation. *Ann Emerg Med.* 2007;49:794–801, 801.e1. doi: 10.1016/j.annemergmed.2007.01.026
16. Fortin JL, Giocanti JP, Ruttimann M, Kowalski JJ. Prehospital administration of hydroxocobalamin for smoke inhalation-associated cyanide poisoning: 8 years of experience in the Paris Fire Brigade. *Clin Toxicol (Phila).* 2006;44(suppl 1):37–44. doi: 10.1080/15563650600811870
17. Borron SW, Baud FJ, Mégarbane B, Bismuth C. Hydroxocobalamin for severe acute cyanide poisoning by ingestion or inhalation. *Am J Emerg Med.* 2007;25:551–558. doi: 10.1016/j.ajem.2006.10.010
18. Houeto P, Hoffman JR, Imbert M, Levillain P, Baud FJ. Relation of blood cyanide to plasma cyanocobalamin concentration after a fixed dose of hydroxocobalamin in cyanide poisoning. *Lancet.* 1995;346:605–608. doi: 10.1016/s0140-6736(95)91437-4
19. Espinoza OB, Perez M, Ramirez MS. Bitter cassava poisoning in eight children: a case report. *Vet Hum Toxicol.* 1992;34:65.
20. Hall AH, Rumack BH. Hydroxycobalamin/sodium thiosulfate as a cyanide antidote. *J Emerg Med.* 1987;5:115–121. doi: 10.1016/0736-4679(87)90074-6
21. Höbel M, Engeser P, Nemeth L, Pill J. The antidote effect of thiosulphate and hydroxocobalamin in formation of nitroprusside intoxication of rabbits. *Arch Toxicol.* 1980;46:207–213. doi: 10.1007/BF00310436
22. Mengel K, Krämer W, Isert B, Friedberg KD. Thiosulphate and hydroxocobalamin prophylaxis in progressive cyanide poisoning in guinea-pigs. *Toxicology.* 1989;54:335–342. doi: 10.1016/0300-483x(89)90068-1
23. Friedberg KD, Shukla UR. The efficiency of aquocobalamine as an antidote in cyanide poisoning when given alone or combined with sodium thiosulfate. *Arch Toxicol.* 1975;33:103–113. doi: 10.1007/BF00353235
24. Forsyth JC, Mueller PD, Becker CE, Osterloh J, Benowitz NL, Rumack BH, Hall AH. Hydroxocobalamin as a cyanide antidote: safety, efficacy and pharmacokinetics in heavily smoking normal volunteers. *J Toxicol Clin Toxicol.* 1993;31:277–294. doi: 10.3109/15563659309000395
25. Vanden Hoek TL, Morrison LJ, Shuster M, Donnino M, Sinz E, Lavonas EJ, Jeejeebhoy FM, Gabrielli A. Part 12: cardiac arrest in special situations: 2010 American Heart Association Guidelines for Cardiopulmonary Resuscitation and Emergency Cardiovascular Care. *Circulation.* 2010;122(suppl 3):S829–S861. doi: 10.1161/CIRCULATIONAHA.110.971069

KNOWLEDGE GAPS AND PRIORITIES OF RESEARCH

As part of the overall work for development of these guidelines, the writing group was able to review a large amount of literature concerning the management of adult cardiac arrest. One expected challenge faced through this process was the lack of data in many areas of cardiac arrest research. This challenge was faced in both the 2010 Guidelines and 2015 Guidelines Update processes, where only a small percent of guideline recommendations (1%) were based on high-grade LOE (A) and nearly three quarters were based on low-grade LOE (C).[1]

Similar challenges were faced in the 2020 Guidelines process, where a number of critical knowledge gaps were identified in adult cardiac arrest management. These topics were identified as not only areas where no information was identified but also where the results of ongoing research could impact the recommendation directly. Throughout the recommendation-specific text, the need for specific research is identified to facilitate the next steps in the evolution of these questions.

Critical knowledge gaps are summarized in Table 4.

REFERENCES

1. Morrison LJ, Gent LM, Lang E, Nunnally ME, Parker MJ, Callaway CW, Nadkarni VM, Fernandez AR, Billi JE, Egan JR, et al. Part 2: evidence evaluation and management of conflicts of interest: 2015 American Heart Association Guidelines Update for Cardiopulmonary Resuscitation and Emergency Cardiovascular Care. *Circulation.* 2015;132(suppl 2):S368–S382. doi: 10.1161/CIR.0000000000000253

Table 4. 2020 Adult Guidelines Critical Knowledge Gaps

Sequence of Resuscitation	
Initiation of resuscitation	What are optimal strategies to enhance lay rescuer performance of CPR?
Metrics for high-quality CPR	What is optimal for the CPR duty cycle (the proportion of time spent in compression relative to the total time of the compression-plus-decompression cycle)?
Metrics for high-quality CPR	What is the validity and reliability of $ETCO_2$ in nonintubated patients?
Metrics for high-quality CPR	For patients with an arterial line in place, does targeting CPR to a particular blood pressure improve outcomes?
Metrics for high-quality CPR	How does integrated team performance, as opposed to performance on individual resuscitation skills, affect resuscitation outcomes?
Defibrillation	Is there an ideal time in the CPR cycle for defibrillator charging?
Defibrillation	Can artifact-filtering algorithms for analysis of ECG rhythms during CPR in a real-time clinical setting decrease pauses in chest compressions and improve outcomes?
Defibrillation	Does preshock waveform analysis lead to improved outcome?
Defibrillation	Do double sequential defibrillation and/or alternative defibrillator pad positioning affect outcome in cardiac arrest with shockable rhythm?
Vascular access	Is the IO route of drug administration safe and efficacious in cardiac arrest, and does efficacy vary by IO site?
Vasopressor medications during cardiac arrest	Does epinephrine, when administered early after cardiac arrest, improve survival with favorable neurological outcome?
Nonvasopressor medications during cardiac arrest	Do antiarrhythmic drugs, when given in combination for cardiac arrest, improve outcomes from cardiac arrest with shockable rhythm?
Nonvasopressor medications during cardiac arrest	Do prophylactic antiarrhythmic medications on ROSC after successful defibrillation decrease arrhythmia recurrence and improve outcome?
Nonvasopressor medications during cardiac arrest	Do steroids improve shock or other outcomes in patients who remain hypotensive after ROSC?
Adjuncts to CPR	Does the use of point-of-care cardiac ultrasound during cardiac arrest improve outcomes?
Adjuncts to CPR	Is targeting a specific $ETCO_2$ value during CPR beneficial, and what degree of rise in $ETCO_2$ indicates ROSC?
Termination of resuscitation	Can $ETCO_2$ be used for intra-arrest prognostication, in combination with other metrics?
Termination of resuscitation	Can point-of-care cardiac ultrasound, in conjunction with other factors, inform termination of resuscitation?
Advanced Techniques and Devices for Resuscitation	
Advanced airway placement	What is the optimal approach to advanced airway management for IHCA?
Advanced airway placement	There is a need for further research specifically on the interface between patient factors and the experience, training, tools, and skills of the provider when choosing an approach to airway management.
Advanced airway placement	What is the specific type, amount, and interval between airway management training experiences to maintain proficiency?
Alternative CPR techniques and devices	Which populations are most likely to benefit from ECPR?
Specific Arrhythmia Management	
Atrial fibrillation or flutter with rapid ventricular response	What is the optimal energy needed for cardioversion of atrial fibrillation and atrial flutter?
Bradycardia	What is the optimal approach, vasopressor or transcutaneous pacing, in managing symptomatic bradycardia?
Care After ROSC	
Postresuscitation care	Does avoidance of hyperoxia in the postarrest period lead to improved outcomes?
Postresuscitation care	What is the effect of hypocarbia or hypercarbia on outcome after cardiac arrest?
Postresuscitation care	Does the treatment of nonconvulsive seizures, common in postarrest patients, improve patient outcomes?
Postresuscitation care	What are the optimal pharmacological treatment regimens for the management of postarrest seizures?
Postresuscitation care	Do neuroprotective agents improve favorable neurological outcome after arrest?
Postresuscitation care	What is the most efficacious management approach for postarrest cardiogenic shock, including pharmacological, catheter intervention, or implantable device?
Postresuscitation care	Is there a role for prophylactic antiarrhythmics after ROSC?
Targeted temperature management	Does targeted temperature management, compared to strict normothermia, improve outcomes?
Targeted temperature management	What is the optimal temperature goal for targeted temperature management?

(Continued)

Table 4. Continued

Targeted temperature management	What is the optimal duration for targeted temperature management before rewarming?
Targeted temperature management	What is the best approach to rewarming postarrest patients after treatment with targeted temperature management?
PCI after cardiac arrest	Does emergent PCI for patients with ROSC after VF/VT cardiac arrest and no STEMI but with signs of shock or electric instability improve outcomes?
Neuroprognostication	What is the interrater agreement for physical examination findings such as pupillary light reflex, corneal reflex, and myoclonus/status myoclonus?
Neuroprognostication	Can we identify consistent NSE and S100B thresholds for predicting poor neurological outcome after cardiac arrest?
Neuroprognostication	Are NSE and S100B helpful when checked later than 72 h after ROSC?
Neuroprognostication	Are glial fibrillary acidic protein, serum tau protein, and neurofilament light chain valuable for neuroprognostication?
Neuroprognostication	More uniform definitions for *status epilepticus*, *malignant EEG patterns,* and other EEG patterns are needed to be able to compare prognostic values across studies.
Neuroprognostication	What is the optimal timing for head CT for prognostication?
Neuroprognostication	Is there a consistent threshold value for prognostication for GWR or ADC?
Neuroprognostication	Standardization of methods for quantifying GWR and ADC would be useful.
Recovery	
Recovery and survivorship after cardiac arrest	What do survivor-derived outcome measures of the impact of cardiac arrest survival look like, and how do they differ from current generic or clinician-derived measures?
Recovery and survivorship after cardiac arrest	Are there in-hospital interventions that can reduce or prevent physical impairment after cardiac arrest?
Recovery and survivorship after cardiac arrest	Which patients develop affective/psychological disorders of well-being after cardiac arrest, and are they treatable/preventable/recoverable?
Recovery and survivorship after cardiac arrest	Does hospital-based protocolized discharge planning for cardiac arrest survivors improve access to/ referral to rehabilitation services or patient outcomes?
Special Circumstances of Resuscitation	
Accidental hypothermia	What combination of features can identify patients with no chance of survival, even if rewarmed?
Accidental hypothermia	Should severely hypothermic patients receive intubation and mechanical ventilation or simply warm humidified oxygen?
Accidental hypothermia	Should severely hypothermic patients in VF who fail an initial defibrillation attempt receive additional defibrillation?
Accidental hypothermia	Should severely hypothermic patients in cardiac arrest receive epinephrine or other resuscitation medications? If so, what dose and schedule should be used?
Drowning	In what situations is attempted resuscitation of the drowning victim futile?
Drowning	How long after mild drowning events should patients be observed for late-onset respiratory effects?
Electrolyte abnormalities	What is the optimal treatment for hyperkalemia with life-threatening arrhythmia or cardiac arrest?
Opioid overdose	What is the minimum safe observation period after reversal of respiratory depression from opioid overdose with naloxone? Does this vary based on the opioid involved?
Opioid overdose	Is there benefit to naloxone administration in patients with opioid-associated cardiac arrest who are receiving CPR with ventilation?
Opioid overdose	What is the ideal initial dose of naloxone in a setting where fentanyl and fentanyl analogues are responsible for a large proportion of opioid overdose?
Opioid overdose	In cases of suspected opioid overdose managed by a non–healthcare provider who is not capable of reliably checking a pulse, is initiation of CPR beneficial?
Pregnancy	What is the ideal timing of PMCD for a pregnant woman in cardiac arrest?
Pulmonary embolism	Which patients with cardiac arrest due to "suspected" pulmonary embolism benefit from emergency thrombolysis during resuscitation?
Toxicity: β-adrenergic blockers and calcium channel blockers	What is the ideal sequencing of modalities (traditional vasopressors, calcium, glucagon, high-dose insulin) for refractory shock due to β-adrenergic blocker or calcium channel blocker overdose?
Toxicity: local anesthetics	What are the ideal dose and formulation of IV lipid emulsion therapy?
Toxicity: carbon monoxide, digoxin, and cyanide	Which patients with cyanide poisoning benefit from antidotal therapy?
Toxicity: carbon monoxide, digoxin, and cyanide	Does sodium thiosulfate provide additional benefit to patients with cyanide poisoning who are treated with hydroxocobalamin?

ADC indicates apparent diffusion coefficient; CPR, cardiopulmonary resuscitation; CT, computed tomography; ECG, electrocardiogram; ECPR, extracorporeal cardiopulmonary resuscitation; EEG, electroencephalogram; $ETCO_2$, end-tidal carbon dioxide; GWR, gray-white ratio; IHCA, in-hospital cardiac arrest; IO, intraosseous; IV, intravenous; NSE, neuron-specific enolase; PCI, percutaneous coronary intervention; PMCD, perimortem cesarean delivery; ROSC, return of spontaneous circulation; S100B, S100 calcium binding protein; STEMI, ST-segment elevation myocardial infarction; and VF, ventricular fibrillation.

ARTICLE INFORMATION

The American Heart Association requests that this document be cited as follows: Panchal AR, Bartos JA, Cabañas JG, Donnino MW, Drennan IR, Hirsch KG, Kudenchuk PJ, Kurz MC, Lavonas EJ, Morley PT, O'Neil BJ, Peberdy MA, Rittenberger JC, Rodriguez AJ, Sawyer KN, Berg KM; on behalf of the Adult Basic and Advanced Life Support Writing Group. Part 3: adult basic and advanced life support: 2020 American Heart Association Guidelines for Cardiopulmonary Resuscitation and Emergency Cardiovascular Care. *Circulation*. 2020;142(suppl 2):S366–S468. doi: 10.1161/CIR.0000000000000916

Acknowledgments

The writing group acknowledges the following contributors: Julie Arafeh, RN, MSN; Justin L. Benoit, MD, MS; Maureen Chase; MD, MPH; Antonio Fernandez; Edison Ferreira de Paiva, MD, PhD; Bryan L. Fischberg, NRP; Gustavo E. Flores, MD, EMT-P; Peter Fromm, MPH, RN; Raul Gazmuri, MD, PhD; Blayke Courtney Gibson, MD; Theresa Hoadley, MD, PhD; Cindy H. Hsu, MD, PhD; Mahmoud Issa, MD; Adam Kessler, DO; Mark S. Link, MD; David J. Magid, MD, MPH; Keith Marrill, MD; Tonia Nicholson, MBBS; Joseph P. Ornato, MD; Garrett Pacheco, MD; Michael Parr, MB; Rahul Pawar, MBBS, MD; James Jaxton, MD; Sarah M. Perman, MD, MSCE; James Pribble, MD; Derek Robinett, MD; Daniel Rolston, MD; Comilla Sasson, MD, PhD; Sree Veena Satyapriya, MD; Travis Sharkey, MD, PhD; Jasmeet Soar, MA, MB, BChir; Deb Torman, MBA, MEd, AT, ATC, EMT-P; Benjamin Von Schweinitz; Anezi Uzendu, MD; and Carolyn M. Zelop, MD.

The writing group would also like to acknowledge the outstanding contributions of David J. Magid, MD, MPH.

Disclosures

Appendix 1. Writing Group Disclosures

Writing Group Member	Employment	Research Grant	Other Research Support	Speakers' Bureau/ Honoraria	Expert Witness	Ownership Interest	Consultant/ Advisory Board	Other
Ashish R. Panchal	The Ohio State University	None	None	None	None	None	None	None
Katherine M. Berg	Beth Israel Deaconess Medical Center	NHLBI Grant K23 HL128814†	None	None	None	None	None	None
Jason A. Bartos	University of Minnesota	None	None	None	None	None	None	Abbott Labs*; Biotronik Inc*; Edwards Lifesciences Corp*; Inari Medical, Inc*; Maquet Cardiovascular US Sales, LLC*; Stryker Corp*; Zoll Circulation, Inc*
José G. Cabañas	Wake County Emergency Medical Services	None	None	None	None	None	None	None
Michael W. Donnino	Beth Israel Deaconess Med Center	NIH†; General Electric*; Kaneka (Investigator-initiated)*	None	Speaking engagements with respect to cardiac arrest topics*	None	None	None	None
Ian R. Drennan	Sunnybrook Health Sciences Center (Canada)	None	None	None	None	None	None	None
Karen G. Hirsch	Stanford University	NIH (Salary support for research activities in cardiac arrest)*; AHA (Salary support for research related to cardiac arrest)*	None	None	None	None	None	None
Peter J. Kudenchuk	University of Washington	NIH (PI at my institution for the SIREN Network)†	None	None	None	None	None	None
Michael C. Kurz	University of Alabama at Birmingham	DOD (DSMB member for PACT trial)*; NIH (CO-I for R21 examining mast cell degranulation in OHCA)*	None	Zoll Medical Corp*	None	None	Zoll Circulation, Inc†	Zoll Circulation, Inc†
Eric J. Lavonas	Denver Health Emergency Medicine	BTG Pharmaceuticals (Denver Health (Dr Lavonas' employer) has research, call center, consulting, and teaching agreements with BTG Pharmaceuticals. BTG manufactures the digoxin antidote, DigiFab. Dr Lavonas does not receive bonus or incentive compensation, and these agreements involve an unrelated product. When these guidelines were developed, Dr Lavonas recused from discussions related to digoxin poisoning.)†	None	None	None	None	None	American Heart Association (Senior Science Editor)†

(*Continued*)

Appendix 1. Continued

Writing Group Member	Employment	Research Grant	Other Research Support	Speakers' Bureau/ Honoraria	Expert Witness	Ownership Interest	Consultant/ Advisory Board	Other
Peter T. Morley	University of Melbourne, Royal Melbourne Hospital (Australia)	None	None	None	None	None	None	None
Brian J. O'Neil	Wayne State University	SIREN Network (Clinical trial network through NHLBI)*	None	Zoll circulation*; Genentech*	None	None	None	None
Mary Ann Peberdy	Virginia Commonwealth University	None	None	None	None	None	None	None
Jon C. Rittenberger	Guthrie Medical Center	NIH- SIREN (ICECAP Trial)*; AHA (Grant In Aid)*	None	None	Bailey Glasser*	None	Hibernaid, LLC*	None
Amber J. Rodriguez	American Heart Association	None	None	None	None	None	None	None
Kelly N. Sawyer	University of Pittsburgh	None	None	None	None	None	None	None

This table represents the relationships of writing group members that may be perceived as actual or reasonably perceived conflicts of interest as reported on the Disclosure Questionnaire, which all members of the writing group are required to complete and submit. A relationship is considered to be "significant" if (a) the person receives $10 000 or more during any 12-month period, or 5% or more of the person's gross income; or (b) the person owns 5% or more of the voting stock or share of the entity, or owns $10 000 or more of the fair market value of the entity. A relationship is considered to be "modest" if it is less than "significant" under the preceding definition.

*Modest.

†Significant.

Appendix 2. Reviewer Disclosures

Reviewer	Employment	Research Grant	Other Research Support	Speakers' Bureau/ Honoraria	Expert Witness	Ownership Interest	Consultant/ Advisory Board	Other
Clifton Callaway	University of Pittsburgh	NIH (Grants to study emergency care, including treatment of cardiac arrest and cardiac emergencies)†	None	None	None	None	None	None
Alix Carter	Dalhousie University (Canada)	Maritime Heart (descriptive factors survival ohca)*	None	None	None	None	None	None
Henry Halperin	Johns Hopkins University	Zoll Circulation (CPR research)†; NIH (CPR research)†	None	None	None	None	None	None
Timothy Henry	The Christ Hospital	None	None	None	None	None	None	None
Jonathan Jui	Oregon Health and Science University	NIH (HL 126938)*	None	None	None	None	None	None
Tommaso Pellis	AAS 5 Friuli Occidentale (Italy)	None	None	None	None	None	None	None
Fred Severyn	Denver Health and Hospital Authority; University of Colorado Anschutz Medical Campus; University of Arkansas for Medical Sciences	None	None	None	None	None	None	None
Andrew H. Travers	Emergency Health Services, Nova Scotia (Canada)	None	None	None	None	None	None	None

This table represents the relationships of reviewers that may be perceived as actual or reasonably perceived conflicts of interest as reported on the Disclosure Questionnaire, which all reviewers are required to complete and submit. A relationship is considered to be "significant" if (a) the person receives $10 000 or more during any 12-month period, or 5% or more of the person's gross income; or (b) the person owns 5% or more of the voting stock or share of the entity, or owns $10 000 or more of the fair market value of the entity. A relationship is considered to be "modest" if it is less than "significant" under the preceding definition.

*Modest.

†Significant.

Circulation

Part 4: Pediatric Basic and Advanced Life Support

2020 American Heart Association Guidelines for Cardiopulmonary Resuscitation and Emergency Cardiovascular Care

Alexis A. Topjian, MD, MSCE, Chair
Tia T. Raymond, MD, Vice-Chair
Dianne Atkins, MD
Melissa Chan, MD
Jonathan P. Duff, MD, MEd
Benny L. Joyner Jr, MD, MPH
Javier J. Lasa, MD
Eric J. Lavonas, MD, MS
Arielle Levy, MD, MEd
Melissa Mahgoub, PhD
Garth D. Meckler, MD, MSHS
Kathryn E. Roberts, MSN, RN
Robert M. Sutton, MD, MSCE
Stephen M. Schexnayder, MD
On behalf of the Pediatric Basic and Advanced Life Support Collaborators

TOP 10 TAKE-HOME MESSAGES

1. High-quality cardiopulmonary resuscitation (CPR) is the foundation of resuscitation. New data reaffirm the key components of high-quality CPR: providing adequate chest compression rate and depth, minimizing interruptions in CPR, allowing full chest recoil between compressions, and avoiding excessive ventilation.
2. A respiratory rate of 20 to 30 breaths per minute is new for infants and children who are (a) receiving CPR with an advanced airway in place or (b) receiving rescue breathing and have a pulse.
3. For patients with nonshockable rhythms, the earlier epinephrine is administered after CPR initiation, the more likely the patient is to survive.
4. Using a cuffed endotracheal tube decreases the need for endotracheal tube changes.
5. The routine use of cricoid pressure does not reduce the risk of regurgitation during bag-mask ventilation and may impede intubation success.
6. For out-of-hospital cardiac arrest, bag-mask ventilation results in the same resuscitation outcomes as advanced airway interventions such as endotracheal intubation.
7. Resuscitation does not end with return of spontaneous circulation (ROSC). Excellent post–cardiac arrest care is critically important to achieving the best patient outcomes. For children who do not regain consciousness after ROSC, this care includes targeted temperature management and continuous electroencephalography monitoring. The prevention and/or treatment of hypotension, hyperoxia or hypoxia, and hypercapnia or hypocapnia is important.
8. After discharge from the hospital, cardiac arrest survivors can have physical, cognitive, and emotional challenges and may need ongoing therapies and interventions.
9. Naloxone can reverse respiratory arrest due to opioid overdose, but there is no evidence that it benefits patients in cardiac arrest.
10. Fluid resuscitation in sepsis is based on patient response and requires frequent reassessment. Balanced crystalloid, unbalanced crystalloid, and colloid fluids are all acceptable for sepsis resuscitation. Epinephrine or norepinephrine infusions are used for fluid-refractory septic shock.

PREAMBLE

More than 20 000 infants and children have a cardiac arrest per year in the United States.[1–4] In 2015, emergency medical service–documented out-of-hospital cardiac arrest (OHCA) occurred in more than 7000 infants and children.[4]

Key Words: AHA Scientific Statements ■ arrhythmia ■ cardiopulmonary resuscitation ■ defibrillation ■ heart arrest ■ pediatrics ■ post–cardiac arrest care

https://www.ahajournals.org/journal/circ

Approximately 11.4% of pediatric OHCA patients survived to hospital discharge, but outcomes varied by age, with survival rates of 17.1% in adolescents, 13.2% in children, and 4.9% in infants. In the same year, pediatric in-hospital cardiac arrest (IHCA) incidence was 12.66 events per 1000 infant and child hospital admissions, with an overall survival to hospital discharge rate of 41.1%.[4] Neurological outcomes remain difficult to assess across the pediatric age spectrum, with variability in reporting metrics and time to follow-up across studies of both OHCA and IHCA. Favorable neurological outcome has been reported in up to 47% of survivors to discharge.[5] Despite increases in survival from IHCA, there is more to be done to improve both survival and neurological outcomes.[6]

The International Liaison Committee on Resuscitation (ILCOR) Formula for Survival emphasizes 3 essential components for good resuscitation outcomes: guidelines based on sound resuscitation science, effective education of the lay public and resuscitation providers, and implementation of a well-functioning Chain of Survival.[7]

These guidelines contain recommendations for pediatric basic and advanced life support, excluding the newborn period, and are based on the best available resuscitation science. The Chain of Survival (Section 2), which is now expanded to include recovery from cardiac arrest, requires coordinated efforts from medical professionals in a variety of disciplines and, in the case of OHCA, from bystanders, emergency dispatchers, and first responders. In addition, specific recommendations about the training of resuscitation providers are provided in Part 6: Resuscitation Education Science, and recommendations about systems of care are provided in Part 7.

INTRODUCTION

Scope of Guidelines

These guidelines are intended to be a resource for lay rescuers and healthcare providers to identify and treat infants and children in the prearrest, intra-arrest, and postarrest states. These apply to infants and children in multiple settings; the community, prehospital, and the hospital environment. Prearrest, intra-arrest, and postarrest topics are reviewed, including cardiac arrest in special circumstances, such as in patients with congenital heart disease.

For the purposes of the pediatric advanced life support guidelines, pediatric patients are infants, children, and adolescents up to 18 years of age, excluding newborns. For pediatric basic life support (BLS), guidelines apply as follows:

- Infant guidelines apply to infants younger than approximately 1 year of age.
- Child guidelines apply to children approximately 1 year of age until puberty. For teaching purposes, puberty is defined as breast development in females and the presence of axillary hair in males.
- For those with signs of puberty and beyond, adult basic life support guidelines should be followed.

Resuscitation of the neonate is addressed in "Part 5: Neonatal Resuscitation" and applies to the newborn typically only during the first hospitalization following birth. Pediatric basic and advanced life support guidelines apply to neonates (less than 30 days old) after hospital discharge.

Coronavirus Disease 2019 Guidance

Together with other professional societies, the American Heart Association (AHA) has provided interim guidance for basic and advanced life support in adults, children, and neonates with suspected or confirmed coronavirus disease 2019 (COVID-19). Because evidence and guidance are evolving with the COVID-19 situation, this interim guidance is maintained separately from the emergency cardiovascular care (ECC) guidelines. Readers are directed to the AHA website for the most recent guidance.[8]

Organization of the Pediatric Writing Committee

The Pediatric Writing Group consisted of pediatric clinicians including intensivists, cardiac intensivists, cardiologists, emergency medicine physicians, medical toxicologists, and nurses. Volunteers with recognized expertise in resuscitation are nominated by the writing group chair and selected by the AHA ECC Committee. The AHA has rigorous conflict of interest policies and procedures to minimize the risk of bias or improper influence during development of the guidelines.[9] Prior to appointment, writing group members and peer reviewers disclosed all commercial relationships and other potential (including intellectual) conflicts. Writing group members whose research led to changes in guidelines were required to declare those conflicts during discussions and abstain from voting on those specific recommendations. This process is described more fully in "Part 2: Evidence Evaluation and Guidelines Development." Disclosure information for writing group members is listed in Appendix 1.

Methodology and Evidence Review

These pediatric guidelines are based on the extensive evidence evaluation performed in conjunction with the ILCOR and affiliated ILCOR member councils. Three different types of evidence reviews (systematic reviews, scoping reviews, and evidence updates) were used in

Table 1. Applying Class of Recommendation and Level of Evidence to Clinical Strategies, Interventions, Treatments, or Diagnostic Testing in Patient Care (Updated May 2019)*

CLASS (STRENGTH) OF RECOMMENDATION

CLASS 1 (STRONG) — **Benefit >>> Risk**

Suggested phrases for writing recommendations:
- Is recommended
- Is indicated/useful/effective/beneficial
- Should be performed/administered/other
- Comparative-Effectiveness Phrases†:
  - Treatment/strategy A is recommended/indicated in preference to treatment B
  - Treatment A should be chosen over treatment B

CLASS 2a (MODERATE) — **Benefit >> Risk**

Suggested phrases for writing recommendations:
- Is reasonable
- Can be useful/effective/beneficial
- Comparative-Effectiveness Phrases†:
  - Treatment/strategy A is probably recommended/indicated in preference to treatment B
  - It is reasonable to choose treatment A over treatment B

CLASS 2b (WEAK) — **Benefit ≥ Risk**

Suggested phrases for writing recommendations:
- May/might be reasonable
- May/might be considered
- Usefulness/effectiveness is unknown/unclear/uncertain or not well-established

CLASS 3: No Benefit (MODERATE) (Generally, LOE A or B use only) — **Benefit = Risk**

Suggested phrases for writing recommendations:
- Is not recommended
- Is not indicated/useful/effective/beneficial
- Should not be performed/administered/other

Class 3: Harm (STRONG) — **Risk > Benefit**

Suggested phrases for writing recommendations:
- Potentially harmful
- Causes harm
- Associated with excess morbidity/mortality
- Should not be performed/administered/other

LEVEL (QUALITY) OF EVIDENCE‡

LEVEL A
- High-quality evidence‡ from more than 1 RCT
- Meta-analyses of high-quality RCTs
- One or more RCTs corroborated by high-quality registry studies

LEVEL B-R — **(Randomized)**
- Moderate-quality evidence‡ from 1 or more RCTs
- Meta-analyses of moderate-quality RCTs

LEVEL B-NR — **(Nonrandomized)**
- Moderate-quality evidence‡ from 1 or more well-designed, well-executed nonrandomized studies, observational studies, or registry studies
- Meta-analyses of such studies

LEVEL C-LD — **(Limited Data)**
- Randomized or nonrandomized observational or registry studies with limitations of design or execution
- Meta-analyses of such studies
- Physiological or mechanistic studies in human subjects

LEVEL C-EO — **(Expert Opinion)**
- Consensus of expert opinion based on clinical experience

COR and LOE are determined independently (any COR may be paired with any LOE).

A recommendation with LOE C does not imply that the recommendation is weak. Many important clinical questions addressed in guidelines do not lend themselves to clinical trials. Although RCTs are unavailable, there may be a very clear clinical consensus that a particular test or therapy is useful or effective.

* The outcome or result of the intervention should be specified (an improved clinical outcome or increased diagnostic accuracy or incremental prognostic information).

† For comparative-effectiveness recommendations (COR 1 and 2a; LOE A and B only), studies that support the use of comparator verbs should involve direct comparisons of the treatments or strategies being evaluated.

‡ The method of assessing quality is evolving, including the application of standardized, widely-used, and preferably validated evidence grading tools; and for systematic reviews, the incorporation of an Evidence Review Committee.

COR indicates Class of Recommendation; EO, expert opinion; LD, limited data; LOE, Level of Evidence; NR, nonrandomized; R, randomized; and RCT, randomized controlled trial.

the 2020 process.[10,11] After review by the ILCOR Science Advisory Committee Chair, the evidence update worksheets were included in Appendix C of the *2020 ILCOR Consensus on CPR and ECC Science With Treatment Recommendations*.[11a] Each of these resulted in a description of the literature that facilitated guideline development. This process is described more fully in "Part 2: Evidence Evaluation and Guidelines Development."[12]

Class of Recommendation and Level of Evidence

The writing group reviewed all relevant and current AHA Guidelines for Cardiopulmonary Resuscitation (CPR) and ECC and all relevant *2020 ILCOR Consensus on CPR and ECC Science With Treatment Recommendations* evidence and recommendations to determine if current guidelines should be reaffirmed, revised, or retired or if new recommendations were needed. The writing group then drafted, reviewed, and approved recommendations, assigning to each a Class of Recommendation (COR; ie, strength) and Level of Evidence (LOE; ie, quality, certainty). Criteria for each COR and LOE are described in Table 1.

Guideline Structure

The 2020 Guidelines are organized in discrete modules of information on specific topics or management issues.[13] Each modular "knowledge chunk" includes a table of recommendations using standard AHA nomenclature of

COR and LOE. Recommendations are presented in order of COR: most potential benefit (Class 1), followed by lesser certainty of benefit (Class 2), and finally potential for harm or no benefit (Class 3). Following the COR, recommendations are ordered by the certainty of supporting LOE: Level A (high-quality randomized controlled trials) to Level C-EO (expert opinion). This order does not reflect the order in which care should be provided.

A brief introduction or short synopsis is provided to contextualize the recommendations with important background information and overarching management or treatment concepts. Recommendation-specific supportive text clarifies the rationale and key study data supporting the recommendations. When appropriate, flow diagrams or additional tables are included. Hyperlinked references are provided to facilitate quick access and review.

Document Review and Approval

The guideline was submitted for blinded peer review to 5 subject matter experts nominated by the AHA. Peer reviewer feedback was provided for guidelines in draft format and again in final format. The guideline was also reviewed and approved for publication by the AHA Science Advisory and Coordinating Committee and AHA Executive Committee. Disclosure information for peer reviewers is listed in Appendix 2.

Abbreviations

Abbreviation	Meaning/Phrase
ACLS	advanced cardiovascular life support
AED	automated external defibrillator
ALS	advanced life support
AHA	American Heart Association
BLS	basic life support
COI	conflict of interest
COR	Class of Recommendation
CPR	cardiopulmonary resuscitation
ECC	emergency cardiovascular care
ECLS	extracorporeal life support
ECMO	extracorporeal membrane oxygenation
ECPR	extracorporeal cardiopulmonary resuscitation
EO	Expert Opinion
ETI	endotracheal intubation
FBAO	foreign body airway obstruction
IHCA	in-hospital cardiac arrest
ILCOR	International Liaison Committee on Resuscitation
LD	limited data
LOE	Level of Evidence
MCS	mechanical circulatory support
NR	nonrandomized
OHCA	out-of-hospital cardiac arrest
PALS	pediatric advanced life support
PICO	population, intervention, comparator, outcome
pVT	pulseless ventricular tachycardia
RCT	randomized clinical trial
ROSC	return of spontaneous circulation
SGA	supraglottic airway
TTM	targeted temperature management
VF	ventricular fibrillation

REFERENCES

1. Holmberg MJ, Ross CE, Fitzmaurice GM, Chan PS, Duval-Arnould J, Grossestreuer AV, Yankama T, Donnino MW, Andersen LW; American Heart Association's Get With The Guidelines–Resuscitation Investigators. Annual Incidence of Adult and Pediatric In-Hospital Cardiac Arrest in the United States. *Circ Cardiovasc Qual Outcomes.* 2019;12:e005580.
2. Atkins DL, Everson-Stewart S, Sears GK, Daya M, Osmond MH, Warden CR, Berg RA; Resuscitation Outcomes Consortium Investigators. Epidemiology and outcomes from out-of-hospital cardiac arrest in children: the Resuscitation Outcomes Consortium Epistry-Cardiac Arrest. *Circulation.* 2009;119:1484–1491. doi: 10.1161/CIRCULATIONAHA.108.802678
3. Knudson JD, Neish SR, Cabrera AG, Lowry AW, Shamszad P, Morales DL, Graves DE, Williams EA, Rossano JW. Prevalence and outcomes of pediatric in-hospital cardiopulmonary resuscitation in the United States: an analysis of the Kids' Inpatient Database*. *Crit Care Med.* 2012;40:2940–2944. doi: 10.1097/CCM.0b013e31825feb3f
4. Virani SS, Alonso A, Benjamin EJ, Bittencourt MS, Callaway CW, Carson AP, Chamberlain AM, Chang AR, Cheng S, Delling FN, et al: on behalf of the American Heart Association Council on Epidemiology and Prevention Statistics Committee and Stroke Statistics Subcommittee. Heart disease and stroke statistics—2020 update: a report from the American Heart Association. *Circulation.* 2020;141:e139–e596. doi: 10.1161/CIR.0000000000000757
5. Matos RI, Watson RS, Nadkarni VM, Huang HH, Berg RA, Meaney PA, Carroll CL, Berens RJ, Praestgaard A, Weissfeld L, Spinella PC; American Heart Association's Get With The Guidelines–Resuscitation (Formerly the National Registry of Cardiopulmonary Resuscitation) Investigators. Duration of cardiopulmonary resuscitation and illness category impact survival and neurologic outcomes for in-hospital pediatric cardiac arrests. *Circulation.* 2013;127:442–451. doi: 10.1161/CIRCULATIONAHA.112.125625
6. Girotra S, Spertus JA, Li Y, Berg RA, Nadkarni VM, Chan PS; American Heart Association Get With the Guidelines–Resuscitation Investigators. Survival trends in pediatric in-hospital cardiac arrests: an analysis from Get With the Guidelines-Resuscitation. *Circ Cardiovasc Qual Outcomes.* 2013;6:42–49. doi: 10.1161/CIRCOUTCOMES.112.967968
7. Søreide E, Morrison L, Hillman K, Monsieurs K, Sunde K, Zideman D, Eisenberg M, Sterz F, Nadkarni VM, Soar J, Nolan JP; Utstein Formula for Survival Collaborators. The formula for survival in resuscitation. *Resuscitation.* 2013;84:1487–1493. doi: 10.1016/j.resuscitation.2013.07.020
8. American Heart Association. CPR & ECC. https://cpr.heart.org/. Accessed June 19, 2020.
9. American Heart Association. Conflict of interest policy. https://www.heart.org/en/about-us/statements-and-policies/conflict-of-interest-policy. Accessed December 31, 2019.
10. International Liaison Committee on Resuscitation (ILCOR). Continuous evidence evaluation guidance and templates: 2020 evidence update process final. https://www.ilcor.org/documents/continuous-evidence-evaluation-guidance-and-templates. Accessed December 31, 2019.
11. Institute of Medicine (US) Committee of Standards for Systematic Reviews of Comparative Effectiveness Research. *Finding What Works in Health Care: Standards for Systematic Reviews.* Eden J, Levit L, Berg A, Morton S, eds. Washington, DC: The National Academies Press; 2011.

11a. Maconochie IK, Aickin R, Hazinski MF, Atkins DL, Bingham R, Couto TB, Guerguerian A-M, Nadkarni VM, Ng K-C, Nuthall GA, et al; on behalf of the Pediatric Life Support Collaborators. Pediatric life support: 2020 International Consensus on Cardiopulmonary Resuscitation and Emergency Cardiovascular Care Science With Treatment Recommendations. *Circulation.* 2020;142(suppl 1):S140–S184. doi: 10.1161/CIR.0000000000000894

12. Magid DJ, Aziz K, Cheng A, Hazinski MF, Hoover AV, Mahgoub M, Panchal AR, Sasson C, Topjian AA, Rodriguez AJ, et al. Part 2: evidence evaluation and guidelines development: 2020 American Heart Association Guidelines for Cardiopulmonary Resuscitation and Emergency Cardiovascular Care. *Circulation.* 2020;142(suppl 2):S358–S365. doi: 10.1161/CIR.0000000000000898
13. Levine GN, O'Gara PT, Beckman JA, Al-Khatib SM, Birtcher KK, Cigarroa JE, de Las Fuentes L, Deswal A, Fleisher LA, Gentile F, Goldberger ZD, Hlatky MA, Joglar JA, Piano MR, Wijeysundera DN. Recent Innovations, Modifications, and Evolution of ACC/AHA Clinical Practice Guidelines: An Update for Our Constituencies: A Report of the American College of Cardiology/American Heart Association Task Force on Clinical Practice Guidelines. *Circulation.* 2019;139:e879–e886. doi: 10.1161/CIR.0000000000000651

MAJOR CONCEPTS

The epidemiology, pathophysiology, and common etiologies of pediatric cardiac arrest are distinct from adult and neonatal cardiac arrest. Cardiac arrest in infants and children does not usually result from a primary cardiac cause; rather, it is the end result of progressive respiratory failure or shock. In these patients, cardiac arrest is preceded by a variable period of deterioration, which eventually results in cardiopulmonary failure, bradycardia, and cardiac arrest. In children with congenital heart disease, cardiac arrest is often due to a primary cardiac cause, although the etiology is distinct from adults.

Outcomes for pediatric IHCA have improved over the past 20 years, in part because of early recognition, high-quality CPR, postarrest care, and extracorporeal cardiopulmonary resuscitation (ECPR).[1,2] In a recent analysis of the Get With The Guidelines Resuscitation Registry, a large multicenter, hospital-based cardiac arrest registry, pediatric cardiac arrest survival to hospital discharge was 19% in 2000 and 38% in 2018.[2] Survival has increased on average by 0.67% per year, though that increase has plateaued since 2010.[2] New directions of research and therapy may be required to improve cardiac arrest survival. More cardiac arrest events now occur in an intensive care unit (ICU) setting, suggesting that patients at risk for cardiac arrest are being identified sooner and transferred to a higher level of care.[3]

Survival rates from OHCA remain less encouraging. In a recent analysis of the Resuscitation Outcomes Consortium Epidemiological Registry, a multicenter OHCA registry, annual survival to hospital discharge of pediatric OHCA between 2007 and 2012 ranged from 6.7% to 10.2% depending on region and patient age.[4] There was no significant change in these rates over time, consistent with other national registries from Japan and from Australia and New Zealand.[5,6] In the Resuscitation Outcomes Consortium Epidemiological Registry, survival of OHCA was higher in regions with more arrests that were witnessed by emergency medical services and with higher bystander CPR rates, stressing the importance of early recognition and treatment of these patients.[4]

As survival rates from pediatric cardiac arrest increase, there has been a shift with more focus on neurodevelopmental, physical, and emotional outcomes of survivors. Recent studies demonstrate that a quarter of patients with favorable outcomes have global cognitive impairment and that 85% of older children who were reported to have favorable outcomes have selective neuropsychological deficits.[7]

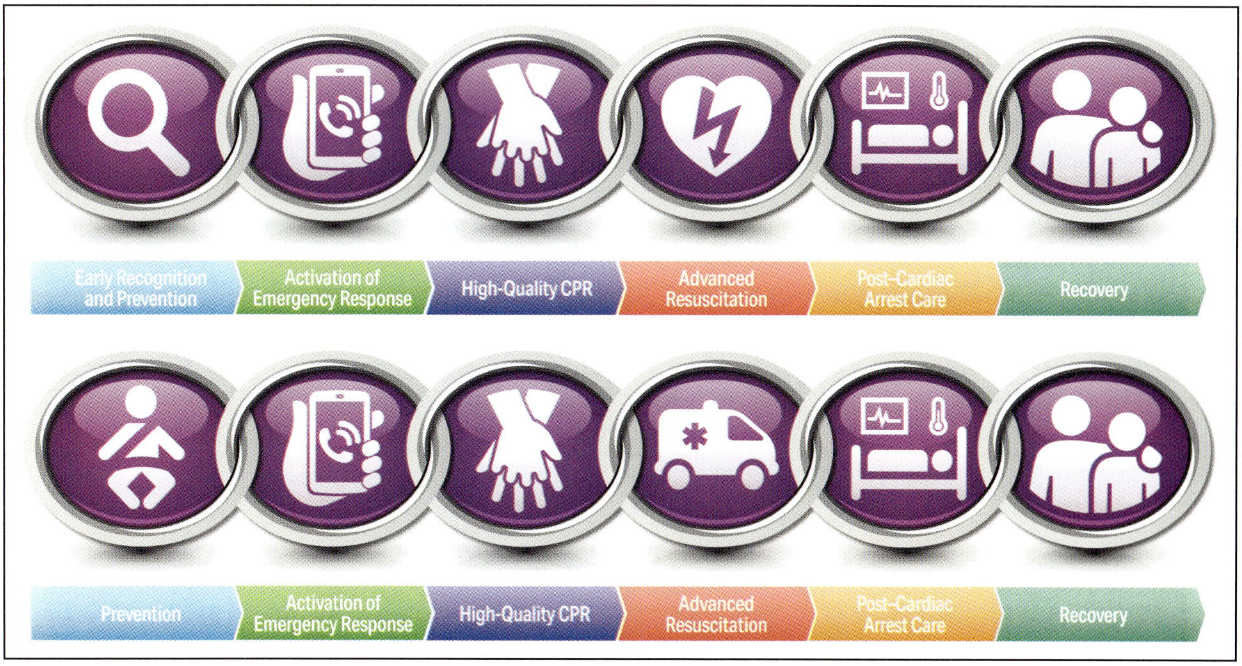

Figure 1. Pediatric Chains of Survival for in-hospital (top) and out-of-hospital (bottom) cardiac arrest.
CPR indicates cardiopulmonary resuscitation.

The Pediatric Chain of Survival

Historically, cardiac arrest care has largely focused on the management of the cardiac arrest itself, highlighting high-quality CPR, early defibrillation, and effective teamwork. However, there are aspects of prearrest and postarrest care that are critical to improve outcomes. As pediatric cardiac arrest survival rates have plateaued, the prevention of cardiac arrest becomes even more important. In the out-of-hospital environment, this includes safety initiatives (eg, bike helmet laws), sudden infant death syndrome prevention, lay rescuer CPR training, and early access to emergency care. When OHCA occurs, early bystander CPR is critical in improving outcomes. In the in-hospital environment, cardiac arrest prevention includes early recognition and treatment of patients at risk for cardiac arrest such as neonates undergoing cardiac surgical procedures, patients presenting with acute fulminant myocarditis, acute decompensated heart failure, or pulmonary hypertension.

Following resuscitation from cardiac arrest, management of the post–cardiac arrest syndrome (which may include brain dysfunction, myocardial dysfunction with low cardiac output, and ischemia or reperfusion injury) is important to avoid known contributors to secondary injury, such as hypotension.[8,9] Accurate neuroprognostication is important to guide caregiver discussions and decision-making. Finally, given the high risk of neurodevelopmental impairment in cardiac arrest survivors, early referral for rehabilitation assessment and intervention is key.

To highlight these different aspects of cardiac arrest management, the Pediatric Chain of Survival has been updated (Figure 1). A separate OHCA Chain of Survival has been created to distinguish the differences between OHCA and IHCA. In both the OHCA and IHCA chains, a sixth link has been added to stress the importance of recovery, which focuses on short- and long-term treatment evaluation, and support for survivors and their families. For both chains of survival, activating the emergency response is followed immediately by the initiation of high-quality CPR. If help is nearby or a cell phone is available, activating the emergency response and starting CPR can be nearly simultaneous. However, in the out-of-hospital setting, a single rescuer who does not have access to a cell phone should begin CPR (compressions-airway-breathing) for infants and children before calling for help because respiratory arrest is the most common cause of cardiac arrest and help may not be nearby. In the event of sudden witnessed collapse, rescuers should use an available automatic external defibrillator (AED), because early defibrillation can be lifesaving.

REFERENCES

1. Girotra S, Spertus JA, Li Y, Berg RA, Nadkarni VM, Chan PS; American Heart Association Get With the Guidelines–Resuscitation Investigators. Survival trends in pediatric in-hospital cardiac arrests: an analysis from Get With the Guidelines-Resuscitation. *Circ Cardiovasc Qual Outcomes.* 2013;6:42–49. doi: 10.1161/CIRCOUTCOMES.112.967968
2. Holmberg MJ, Wiberg S, Ross CE, Kleinman M, Hoeyer-Nielsen AK, Donnino MW, Andersen LW. Trends in Survival After Pediatric In-Hospital Cardiac Arrest in the United States. *Circulation.* 2019;140:1398–1408. doi: 10.1161/CIRCULATIONAHA.119.041667
3. Berg RA, Sutton RM, Holubkov R, Nicholson CE, Dean JM, Harrison R, Heidemann S, Meert K, Newth C, Moler F, Pollack M, Dalton H, Doctor A, Wessel D, Berger J, Shanley T, Carcillo J, Nadkarni VM; Eunice Kennedy Shriver National Institute of Child Health and Human Development Collaborative Pediatric Critical Care Research Network and for the American Heart Association's Get With the Guidelines-Resuscitation (formerly the National Registry of Cardiopulmonary Resuscitation) Investigators. Ratio of PICU versus ward cardiopulmonary resuscitation events is increasing. *Crit Care Med.* 2013;41:2292–2297. doi: 10.1097/CCM.0b013e31828cf0c0
4. Fink EL, Prince DK, Kaltman JR, Atkins DL, Austin M, Warden C, Hutchison J, Daya M, Goldberg S, Herren H, Tijssen JA, Christenson J, Vaillancourt C, Miller R, Schmicker RH, Callaway CW; Resuscitation Outcomes Consortium. Unchanged pediatric out-of-hospital cardiac arrest incidence and survival rates with regional variation in North America. *Resuscitation.* 2016;107:121–128. doi: 10.1016/j.resuscitation.2016.07.244
5. Kitamura T, Iwami T, Kawamura T, Nitta M, Nagao K, Nonogi H, Yonemoto N, Kimura T; Japanese Circulation Society Resuscitation Science Study Group. Nationwide improvements in survival from out-of-hospital cardiac arrest in Japan. *Circulation.* 2012;126:2834–2843. doi: 10.1161/CIRCULATIONAHA.112.109496
6. Straney LD, Schlapbach LJ, Yong G, Bray JE, Millar J, Slater A, Alexander J, Finn J; Australian and New Zealand Intensive Care Society Paediatric Study Group. Trends in PICU Admission and Survival Rates in Children in Australia and New Zealand Following Cardiac Arrest. *Pediatr Crit Care Med.* 2015;16:613–620. doi: 10.1097/PCC.0000000000000425
7. Slomine BS, Silverstein FS, Christensen JR, Page K, Holubkov R, Dean JM, Moler FW. Neuropsychological Outcomes of Children 1 Year After Pediatric Cardiac Arrest: Secondary Analysis of 2 Randomized Clinical Trials. *JAMA Neurol.* 2018;75:1502–1510. doi: 10.1001/jamaneurol.2018.2628
8. Topjian AA, de Caen A, Wainwright MS, Abella BS, Abend NS, Atkins DL, Bembea MM, Fink EL, Guerguerian AM, Haskell SE, Kilgannon JH, Lasa JJ, Hazinski MF. Pediatric Post-Cardiac Arrest Care: A Scientific Statement From the American Heart Association. *Circulation.* 2019;140:e194–e233. doi: 10.1161/CIR.0000000000000697
9. Laverriere EK, Polansky M, French B, Nadkarni VM, Berg RA, Topjian AA. Association of Duration of Hypotension With Survival After Pediatric Cardiac Arrest. *Pediatr Crit Care Med.* 2020;21:143–149. doi: 10.1097/PCC.0000000000002119

SEQUENCE OF RESUSCITATION

Rapid recognition of cardiac arrest, immediate initiation of high-quality chest compressions, and delivery of effective ventilations are critical to improve outcomes from cardiac arrest. Lay rescuers should not delay starting CPR in a child with no "signs of life." Healthcare providers may consider assessing the presence of a pulse as long as the initiation of CPR is not delayed more than 10 seconds. Palpation for the presence or absence of a pulse is not reliable as the sole determinant of cardiac arrest and the need for chest compressions. In infants and children, asphyxial cardiac arrest is more common than cardiac arrest from a primary cardiac event; therefore, effective ventilation is important during resuscitation of children. When CPR is initiated, the sequence is compressions-airway-breathing.

High-quality CPR generates blood flow to vital organs and increases the likelihood of return of spontaneous circulation (ROSC). The 5 main components of high-quality CPR are (1) adequate chest compression depth, (2) optimal chest compression rate, (3) minimizing interruptions in CPR (ie, maximizing chest compression fraction or the proportion of time that chest compressions are provided for cardiac arrest), (4) allowing full chest recoil between compressions, and (5) avoiding excessive ventilation. Compressions of inadequate depth and rate,[1,2] incomplete chest recoil,[3] and high ventilation rates[4,5] are common during pediatric resuscitation.

Initiation of CPR

Recommendations for Initiation of CPR

COR	LOE	Recommendations
1	C-LD	1. Lay rescuers should begin CPR for any victim who is unresponsive, not breathing normally, and does not have signs of life; do not check for a pulse.[6–20]
2a	C-LD	2. In infants and children with no signs of life, it is reasonable for healthcare providers to check for a pulse for up to 10 s and begin compressions unless a definite pulse is felt.[21–23]
2b	C-EO	3. It may be reasonable to initiate CPR with compressions-airway-breathing over airway-breathing-compressions.[24]

Recommendation-Specific Supportive Text

1. Lay rescuers are unable to reliably determine the presence or absence of a pulse.[6–20]
2. No clinical trials have compared manual pulse checks with observations of "signs of life." However, adult and pediatric studies have identified a high error rate and harmful CPR pauses during manual pulse checks by trained rescuers.[21–23] In 1 study, healthcare provider pulse palpation accuracy was 78%[21] compared with lay rescuer pulse palpation accuracy of 47% at 5 seconds and 73% at 10 seconds.[6]
3. One pediatric study demonstrated only a small delay (5.74 seconds) in commencement of rescue breathing with compressions-airway-breathing compared with airway-breathing-compressions.[24] Although the evidence is of low certainty, continuing to recommend compressions-airway-breathing likely results in minimal delays in rescue breathing and allows for a consistent approach to cardiac arrest treatment in adults and children.

Components of High-Quality CPR

Recommendations for Components of High-Quality CPR

COR	LOE	Recommendations
1	B-NR	1. CPR using chest compressions with rescue breaths should be provided to infants and children in cardiac arrest.[25–29]
1	B-NR	2. For infants and children, if bystanders are unwilling or unable to deliver rescue breaths, it is recommended that rescuers should provide chest compressions only.[27,28]
1	C-EO	3. After each compression, rescuers should allow the chest to recoil completely.[2,3,30]
2a	C-LD	4. It is reasonable to use a chest compression rate of ≈100–120/min for infants and children.[31,32]
2a	C-LD	5. For infants and children, it is reasonable for rescuers to provide chest compressions that depress the chest at least one third the anterior-posterior diameter of the chest, which equates to approximately 1.5 inches (4 cm) in infants to 2 inches (5 cm) in children. Once children have reached puberty, it is reasonable to use the adult compression depth of at least 5 cm but no more than 6 cm.[33–36]
2a	C-EO	6. For healthcare providers, it is reasonable to perform a rhythm check, lasting no more than 10 s, approximately every 2 min.
2a	C-EO	7. It is reasonable to ventilate with 100% oxygen during CPR.
2a	C-EO	8. When performing CPR without an advanced airway, it is reasonable for single rescuers to provide a compression-to-ventilation ratio of 30:2 and for 2 rescuers to provide a compression-to-ventilation ratio of 15:2.[25]
2b	C-LD	9. When performing CPR in infants and children with an advanced airway, it may be reasonable to target a respiratory rate range of 1 breath every 2–3 s (20–30 breaths/min), accounting for age and clinical condition. Rates exceeding these recommendations may compromise hemodynamics.[5]

Recommendation-Specific Supportive Text

1. Large observational studies of children with OHCA show the best outcomes with compression-ventilation CPR, though outcomes for infants with OHCA are often poor regardless of resuscitation strategy.[25–29]
2. Large observational studies of children with OHCA show that compression-only CPR is superior to no bystander CPR, though outcomes for infants with OHCA are often poor.[27,28]
3. Allowing complete chest re-expansion improves the flow of blood returning to the heart and thereby blood flow to the body during CPR. There are no pediatric studies evaluating the effect of residual leaning during CPR, although

leaning during pediatric CPR is common.[2,3] In 1 observational study of invasively monitored and anesthetized children, leaning was associated with elevated cardiac filling pressures, leading to decreased coronary perfusion pressures during sinus rhythm.[30]

4. A small observational study found that a compression rate of at least 100/min was associated with improved systolic and diastolic blood pressures during CPR for pediatric IHCA.[31] One multicenter, observational study of pediatric IHCA demonstrated increased systolic blood pressures with chest compression rates between 100 and 120/min when compared with rates exceeding 120/min.[32] Rates less than 100/min were associated with improved survival compared to rates of 100 to 120/min; however, the median rate in this slower category was approximately 95/min (ie, very close to 100/min).[32]
5. Three anthropometric studies have shown that the pediatric chest can be compressed to one third of the anterior-posterior chest diameter without damaging intrathoracic organs.[33–35] An observational study found an improvement in rates of ROSC and 24-hour survival, when at least 60% of 30-second epochs of CPR achieve an average chest compression depth greater than 5 cm for pediatric IHCA.[36]
6. Current recommendations include a brief rhythm check every 2 minutes when a monitor or AED is available.
7. There are no human studies addressing the effect of varying inhaled oxygen concentrations during CPR on outcomes in infants and children.
8. The optimum compression-to-ventilation ratio is uncertain. Large observational studies of children with OHCA demonstrated better outcomes with compression-ventilation CPR with ratios of either 15:2 or 30:2 compared with compression-only CPR.[25]
9. One small, multicenter observational study of intubated pediatric patients found that ventilation rates (at least 30 breaths/min in children less than 1 year of age, at least 25 breaths/min in older children) were associated with improved rates of ROSC and survival.[5] However, increasing ventilation rates are associated with decreased systolic blood pressure in children. The optimum ventilation rate during continuous chest compressions in children with an advanced airway is based on limited data and requires further study.

Recommendations 1 and 2 were reviewed in the "2017 American Heart Association Focused Update on Pediatric Basic Life Support and Cardiopulmonary Resuscitation Quality: An Update to the American Heart Association Guidelines for Cardiopulmonary Resuscitation and Emergency Cardiovascular Care."[37]

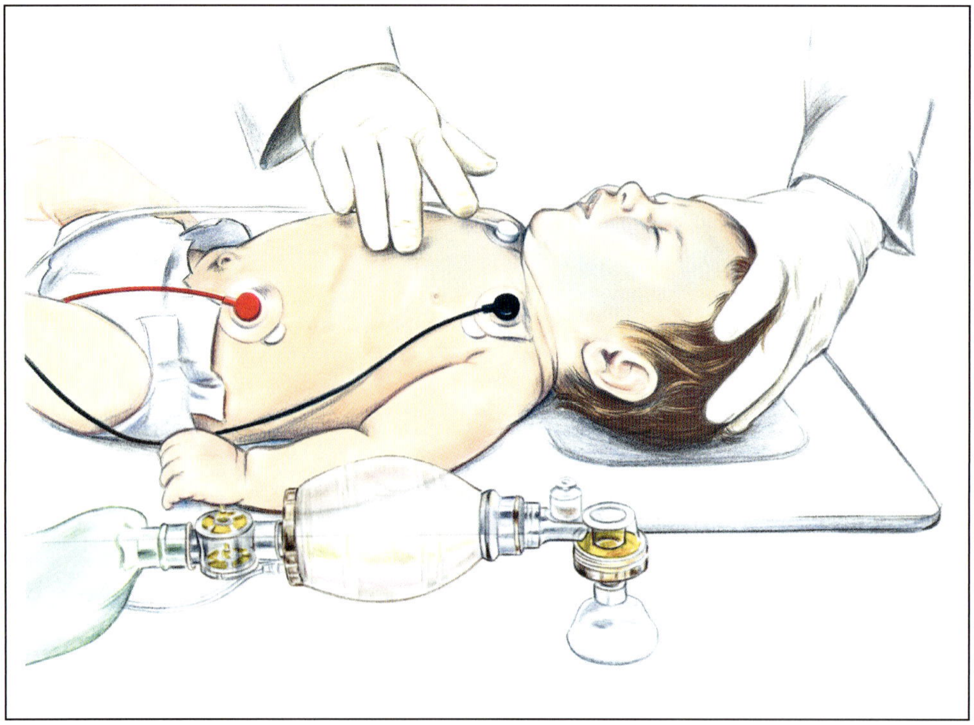

Figure 2. 2-Finger compressions.

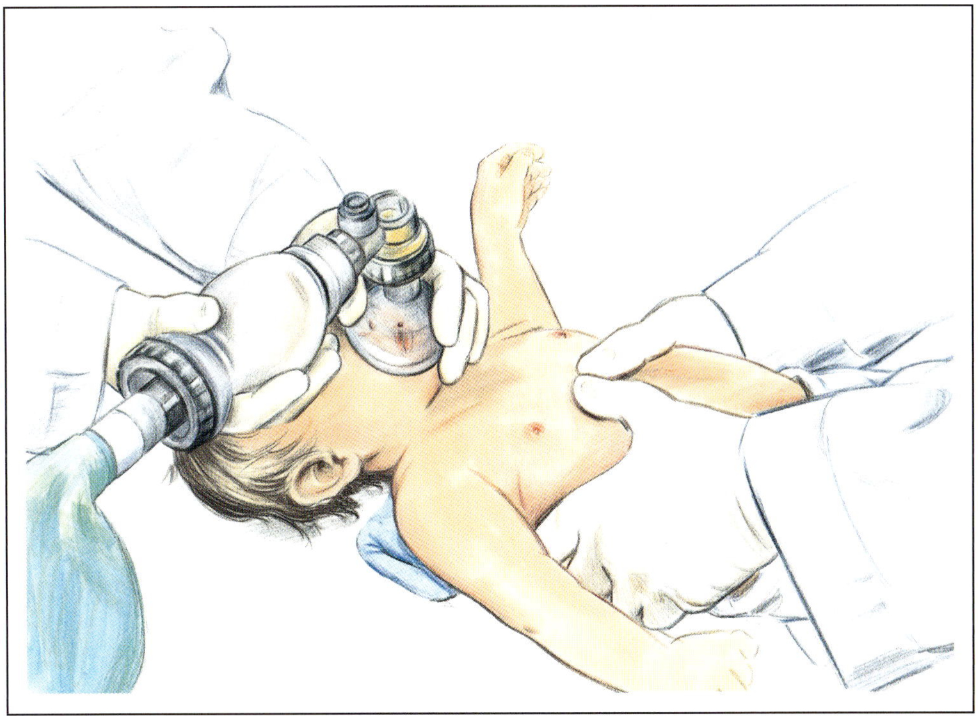

Figure 3. **2-Thumb–encircling hands compressions.**

CPR Technique

Recommendations for CPR Technique		
COR	**LOE**	**Recommendations**
1	C-LD	1. For infants, single rescuers (whether lay rescuers or healthcare providers) should compress the sternum with 2 fingers (Figure 2) or 2 thumbs placed just below the intermammary line.[38–41]
1	C-LD	2. For infants, the 2-thumb–encircling hands technique (Figure 3) is recommended when CPR is provided by 2 rescuers. If the rescuer cannot physically encircle the victim's chest, compress the chest with 2 fingers.[42–46]
2b	C-LD	3. For children, it may be reasonable to use either a 1- or 2-hand technique to perform chest compressions.[47–49]
2b	C-EO	4. For infants, if the rescuer is unable to achieve guideline recommended depths (at least one third the anterior-posterior diameter of the chest), it may be reasonable to use the heel of 1 hand.

Recommendation-Specific Supportive Text

1. One anthropometric[38] and 3 radiological studies[39–41] found that optimal cardiac compressions occur when fingers are placed just below the intermammary line. One observational pediatric study found that blood pressure was higher when compressions were performed over the lower third of the sternum compared to the midsternum.[41] See Figure 2 for the 2-finger technique.
2. Systematic reviews suggest that the 2-thumb–encircling hands technique may improve CPR quality when compared with 2-finger compressions, particularly for depth.[42,43] However, recent manikin studies suggest that the 2-thumb–encircling hands technique may be associated with lower chest compression fractions (percent of cardiac arrest time that chest compression are provided)[44] and incomplete chest recoil,[45,46] especially when performed by single rescuers. See Figure 3 for the 2-thumb–encircling hands technique.
3. There are no pediatric-specific clinical data to determine if the 1-hand or 2-hand technique produces better outcomes for children receiving CPR. In manikin studies, the 2-hand technique has been associated with improved compression depth,[47] compression force,[48] and less rescuer fatigue.[49]
4. There were no human studies comparing the 1-hand compression versus the 2-thumb–encircling hands technique in infants.

Support Surfaces for CPR

Recommendations for Support Surfaces for CPR		
COR	**LOE**	**Recommendations**
1	C-LD	1. During IHCA, when available, activate the bed's "CPR mode" to increase mattress stiffness.[50–53]
2a	C-LD	2. It is reasonable to perform chest compressions on a firm surface.[53–59]
2a	C-LD	3. During IHCA, it is reasonable to use a backboard to improve chest compression depth.[53,55,56,60–63]

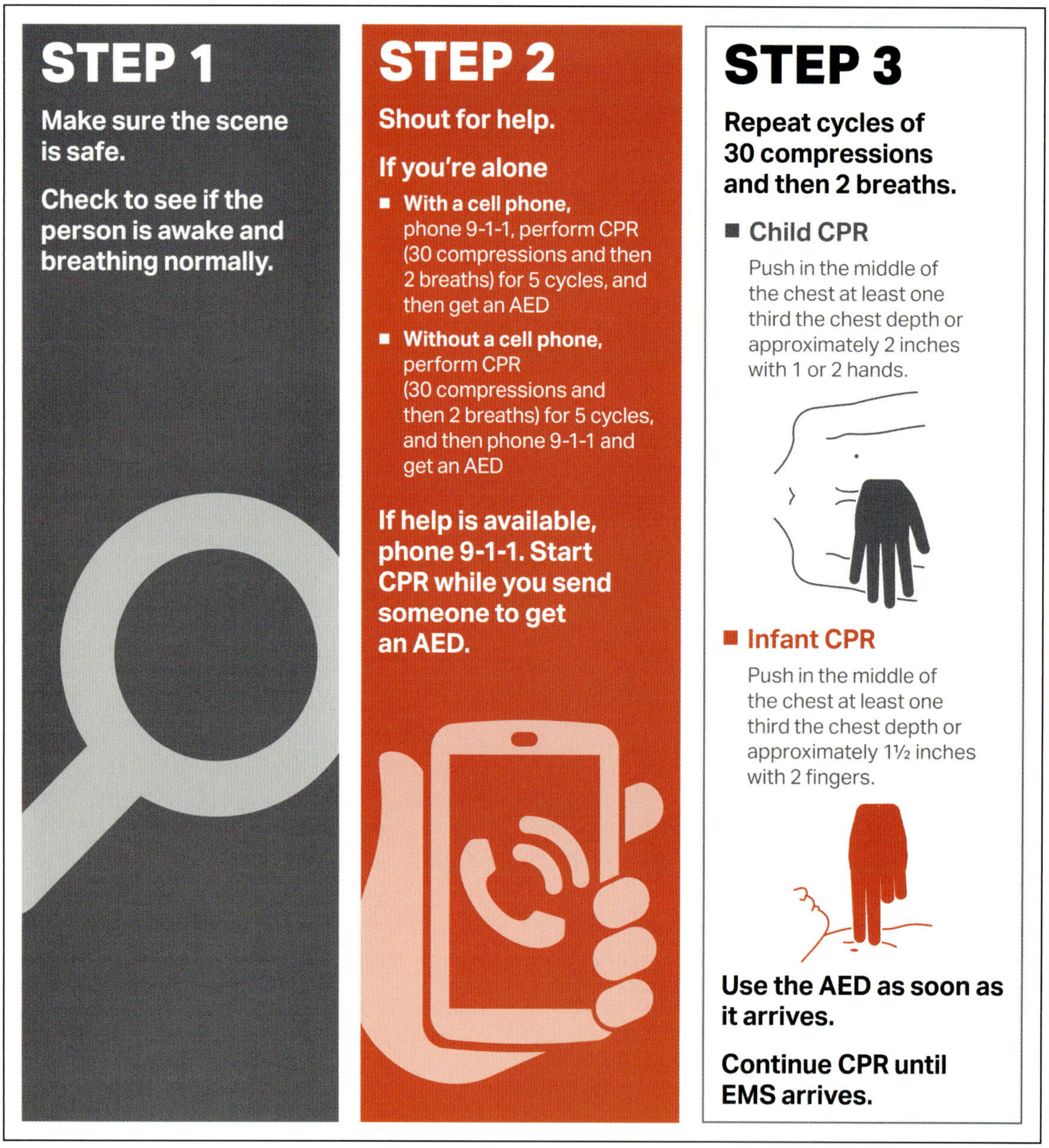

Figure 4. Pediatric BLS for lay rescuers.
AED indicates automated external defibrillator; BLS, basic life support; CPR, cardiopulmonary resuscitation; and EMS, emergency medical services.

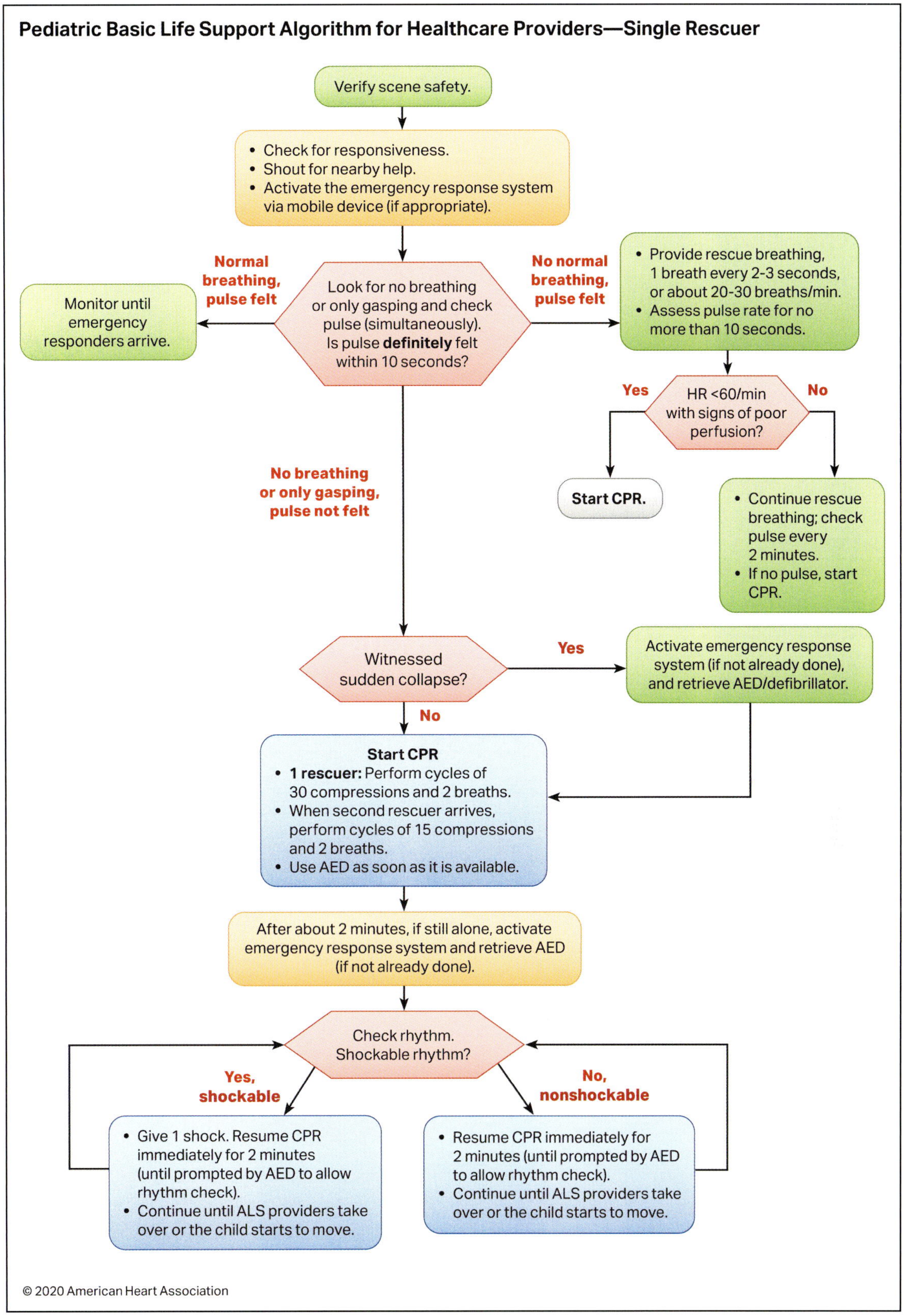
Pediatric Basic Life Support Algorithm for Healthcare Providers—Single Rescuer
Verify scene safety.
• Check for responsiveness.
• Shout for nearby help.
• Activate the emergency response system via mobile device (if appropriate).
Look for no breathing or only gasping and check pulse (simultaneously). Is pulse definitely felt within 10 seconds?
Normal breathing, pulse felt
Monitor until emergency responders arrive.
No normal breathing, pulse felt
• Provide rescue breathing, 1 breath every 2-3 seconds, or about 20-30 breaths/min.
• Assess pulse rate for no more than 10 seconds.
HR <60/min with signs of poor perfusion?
Yes
Start CPR.
No
• Continue rescue breathing; check pulse every 2 minutes.
• If no pulse, start CPR.
No breathing or only gasping, pulse not felt
Witnessed sudden collapse?
Yes
Activate emergency response system (if not already done), and retrieve AED/defibrillator.
No
Start CPR
• 1 rescuer: Perform cycles of 30 compressions and 2 breaths.
• When second rescuer arrives, perform cycles of 15 compressions and 2 breaths.
• Use AED as soon as it is available.
After about 2 minutes, if still alone, activate emergency response system and retrieve AED (if not already done).
Check rhythm. Shockable rhythm?
Yes, shockable
• Give 1 shock. Resume CPR immediately for 2 minutes (until prompted by AED to allow rhythm check).
• Continue until ALS providers take over or the child starts to move.
No, nonshockable
• Resume CPR immediately for 2 minutes (until prompted by AED to allow rhythm check).
• Continue until ALS providers take over or the child starts to move.
© 2020 American Heart Association

Figure 5. Pediatric Basic Life Support Algorithm for Healthcare Providers—Single Rescuer.
AED indicates automated external defibrillator; ALS, advanced life support; CPR, cardiopulmonary resuscitation; and HR, heart rate.

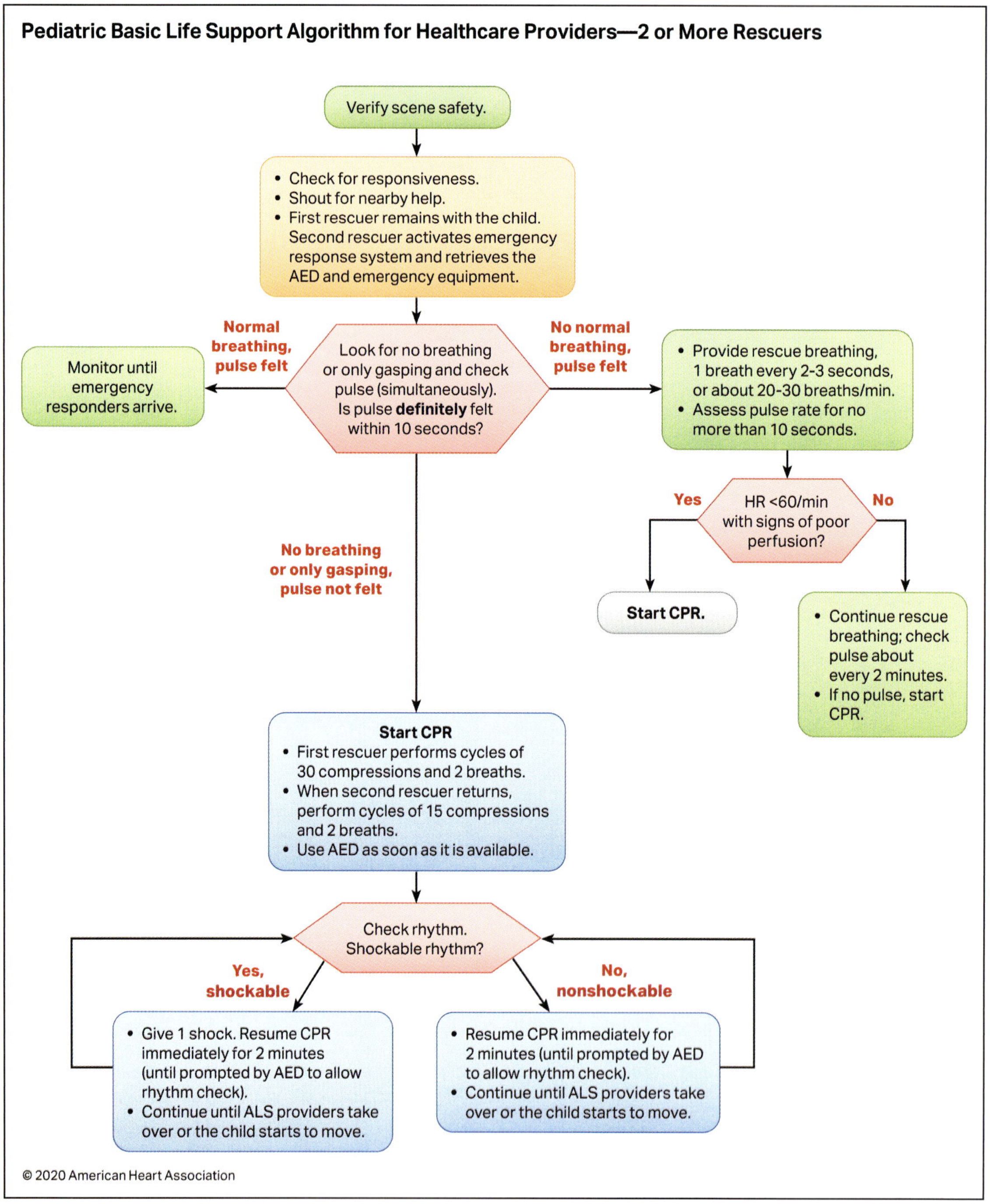
Pediatric Basic Life Support Algorithm for Healthcare Providers—2 or More Rescuers
Verify scene safety.
• Check for responsiveness.
• Shout for nearby help.
• First rescuer remains with the child. Second rescuer activates emergency response system and retrieves the AED and emergency equipment.
Normal breathing, pulse felt
Monitor until emergency responders arrive.
Look for no breathing or only gasping and check pulse (simultaneously). Is pulse definitely felt within 10 seconds?
No normal breathing, pulse felt
• Provide rescue breathing, 1 breath every 2-3 seconds, or about 20-30 breaths/min.
• Assess pulse rate for no more than 10 seconds.
Yes
HR <60/min with signs of poor perfusion?
No
Start CPR.
• Continue rescue breathing; check pulse about every 2 minutes.
• If no pulse, start CPR.
No breathing or only gasping, pulse not felt
Start CPR
• First rescuer performs cycles of 30 compressions and 2 breaths.
• When second rescuer returns, perform cycles of 15 compressions and 2 breaths.
• Use AED as soon as it is available.
Check rhythm. Shockable rhythm?
Yes, shockable
No, nonshockable
• Give 1 shock. Resume CPR immediately for 2 minutes (until prompted by AED to allow rhythm check).
• Continue until ALS providers take over or the child starts to move.
• Resume CPR immediately for 2 minutes (until prompted by AED to allow rhythm check).
• Continue until ALS providers take over or the child starts to move.
© 2020 American Heart Association

Figure 6. Pediatric Basic Life Support Algorithm for Healthcare Providers—2 or More Rescuers.
AED indicates automated external defibrillator; ALS, advanced life support; CPR, cardiopulmonary resuscitation; and HR, heart rate.

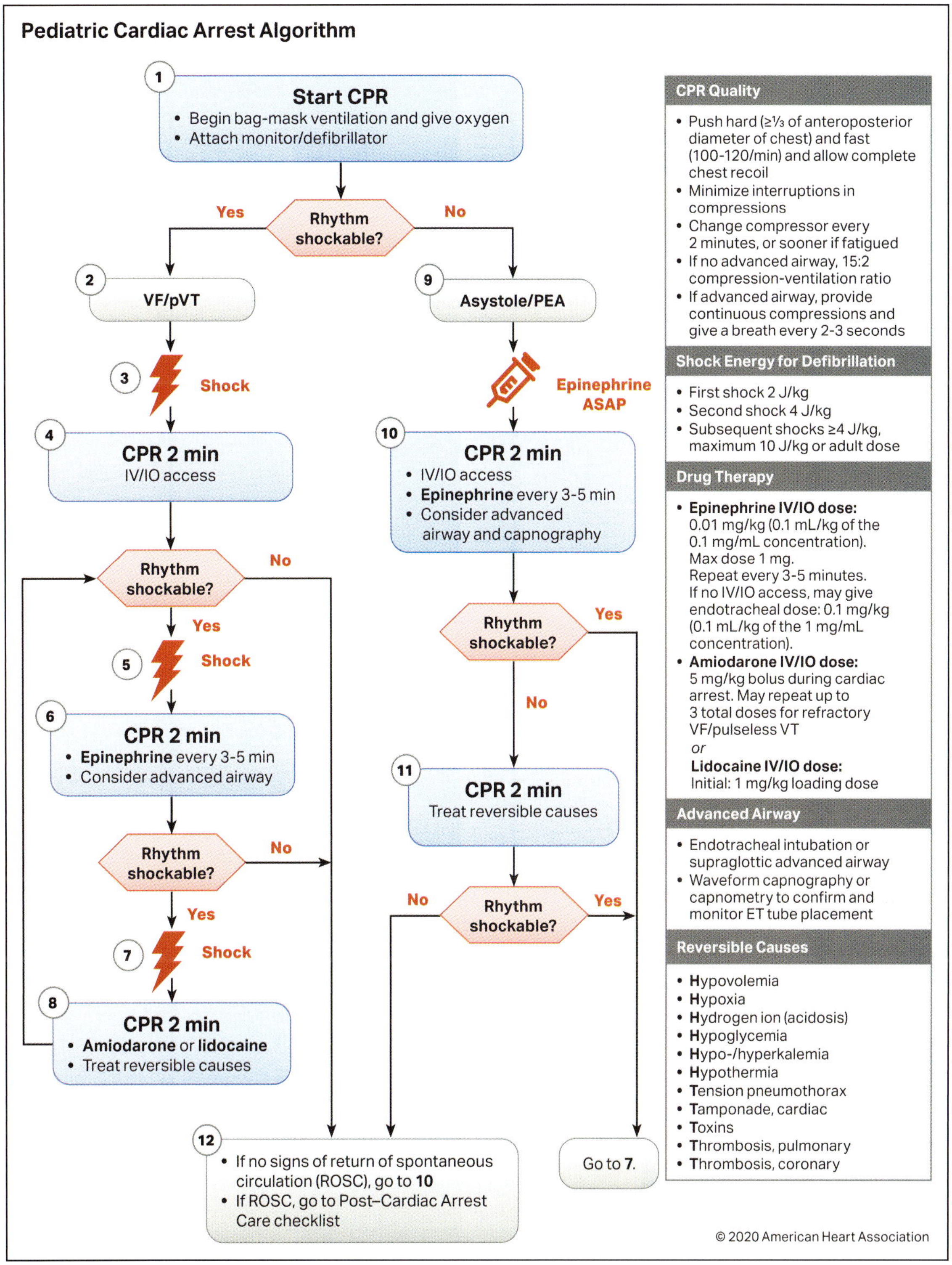

Figure 7. Pediatric Cardiac Arrest Algorithm.
ASAP indicates as soon as possible; CPR, cardiopulmonary resuscitation; ET, endotracheal; HR, heart rate; IO, intraosseous; IV, intravenous; PEA, pulseless electrical activity; and VF/pVT, ventricular fibrillation/pulseless ventricular tachycardia.

Recommendation-Specific Supportive Text

1. "CPR mode" is available on some hospital beds to stiffen the mattress during CPR. Manikin models indicate that mattress compression ranges between 12% and 57% of total compression depth, with softer mattresses being compressed the most.[50–53] This can lead to reduced sternal displacement and a reduction in effective chest compression depth.
2. Manikin studies and 1 pediatric case series show that effective compression depth can be achieved even on a soft surface, providing the CPR provider increases overall compression depth to compensate for mattress compression.[53–59]
3. Meta-analysis of 6 studies[53,56,60–63] showed a 3-mm (95% CI 1–4 mm) improvement in chest compression depth associated with backboard use when CPR was performed on a manikin placed on a mattress or bed.

Opening the Airway

Recommendations for Opening the Airway

COR	LOE	Recommendations
1	C-LD	1. Unless a cervical spine injury is suspected, use a head tilt–chin lift maneuver to open the airway.[64]
1	C-EO	2. For the trauma patient with suspected cervical spinal injury, use a jaw thrust without head tilt to open the airway.
1	C-EO	3. For the trauma patient with suspected cervical spinal injury, if the jaw thrust does not open the airway, use a head tilt–chin lift maneuver.

Recommendation-Specific Supportive Text

1. No data directly address the ideal method to open or maintain airway patency. One retrospective cohort study evaluated various head-tilt angles in neonates and young infants undergoing diagnostic MRI and found that the highest proportion of patent airways was at a head-tilt angle of 144 to 150 degrees based on a regression analysis.[64]
2. While no pediatric studies evaluate jaw thrust versus head tilt–chin lift to open the airway, the jaw thrust is widely accepted as an effective way to open the airway, and this maneuver theoretically limits cervical motion compared with the head tilt–chin lift.
3. There are no pediatric studies evaluating the impact of a head tilt–chin lift maneuver to open the airway in a trauma patient with suspected cervical spine injury. However, if providers are unable to open the airway and deliver effective ventilations using a jaw thrust, given the importance of a patent airway, using a head tilt–chin lift maneuver is recommended.

Figures 4, 5, 6, and 7 show, respectively, an infographic for pediatric BLS for lay rescuers, the current pediatric BLS algorithms for healthcare provider, single-rescuer CPR and 2-rescuer CPR, and the current algorithm for pediatric cardiac arrest.

REFERENCES

1. Niles DE, Duval-Arnould J, Skellett S, Knight L, Su F, Raymond TT, Sweberg T, Sen AI, Atkins DL, Friess SH, de Caen AR, Kurosawa H, Sutton RM, Wolfe H, Berg RA, Silver A, Hunt EA, Nadkarni VM; pediatric Resuscitation Quality (pediRES-Q) Collaborative Investigators. Characterization of Pediatric In-Hospital Cardiopulmonary Resuscitation Quality Metrics Across an International Resuscitation Collaborative. *Pediatr Crit Care Med.* 2018;19:421–432. doi: 10.1097/PCC.0000000000001520
2. Sutton RM, Niles D, Nysaether J, Abella BS, Arbogast KB, Nishisaki A, Maltese MR, Donoghue A, Bishnoi R, Helfaer MA, Myklebust H, Nadkarni V. Quantitative analysis of CPR quality during in-hospital resuscitation of older children and adolescents. *Pediatrics.* 2009;124:494–499. doi: 10.1542/peds.2008-1930
3. Niles D, Nysaether J, Sutton R, Nishisaki A, Abella BS, Arbogast K, Maltese MR, Berg RA, Helfaer M, Nadkarni V. Leaning is common during in-hospital pediatric CPR, and decreased with automated corrective feedback. *Resuscitation.* 2009;80:553–557. doi: 10.1016/j.resuscitation.2009.02.012
4. McInnes AD, Sutton RM, Orioles A, Nishisaki A, Niles D, Abella BS, Maltese MR, Berg RA, Nadkarni V. The first quantitative report of ventilation rate during in-hospital resuscitation of older children and adolescents. *Resuscitation.* 2011;82:1025–1029. doi: 10.1016/j.resuscitation.2011.03.020
5. Sutton RM, Reeder RW, Landis WP, Meert KL, Yates AR, Morgan RW, Berger JT, Newth CJ, Carcillo JA, McQuillen PS, Harrison RE, Moler FW, Pollack MM, Carpenter TC, Notterman DA, Holubkov R, Dean JM, Nadkarni VM, Berg RA; Eunice Kennedy Shriver National Institute of Child Health and Human Development Collaborative Pediatric Critical Care Research Network (CPCCRN). Ventilation Rates and Pediatric In-Hospital Cardiac Arrest Survival Outcomes. *Crit Care Med.* 2019;47:1627–1636. doi: 10.1097/CCM.0000000000003898
6. Bahr J, Klingler H, Panzer W, Rode H, Kettler D. Skills of lay people in checking the carotid pulse. *Resuscitation.* 1997;35:23–26. doi: 10.1016/s0300-9572(96)01092-1
7. Brearley S, Shearman CP, Simms MH. Peripheral pulse palpation: an unreliable physical sign. *Ann R Coll Surg Engl.* 1992;74:169–171.
8. Cavallaro DL, Melker RJ. Comparison of two techniques for detecting cardiac activity in infants. *Crit Care Med.* 1983;11:189–190. doi: 10.1097/00003246-198303000-00009
9. Inagawa G, Morimura N, Miwa T, Okuda K, Hirata M, Hiroki K. A comparison of five techniques for detecting cardiac activity in infants. *Paediatr Anaesth.* 2003;13:141–146. doi: 10.1046/j.1460-9592.2003.00970.x
10. Kamlin CO, O'Donnell CP, Everest NJ, Davis PG, Morley CJ. Accuracy of clinical assessment of infant heart rate in the delivery room. *Resuscitation.* 2006;71:319–321. doi: 10.1016/j.resuscitation.2006.04.015
11. Lee CJ, Bullock LJ. Determining the pulse for infant CPR: time for a change? *Mil Med.* 1991;156:190–193.
12. Mather C, O'Kelly S. The palpation of pulses. *Anaesthesia.* 1996;51:189–191. doi: 10.1111/j.1365-2044.1996.tb07713.x
13. Ochoa FJ, Ramalle-Gómara E, Carpintero JM, García A, Saralegui I. Competence of health professionals to check the carotid pulse. *Resuscitation.* 1998;37:173–175. doi: 10.1016/s0300-9572(98)00055-0
14. Owen CJ, Wyllie JP. Determination of heart rate in the baby at birth. *Resuscitation.* 2004;60:213–217. doi: 10.1016/j.resuscitation.2003.10.002
15. Sarti A, Savron F, Casotto V, Cuttini M. Heartbeat assessment in infants: a comparison of four clinical methods. *Pediatr Crit Care Med.* 2005;6:212–215. doi: 10.1097/01.PCC.0000154952.59176.E0
16. Sarti A, Savron F, Ronfani L, Pelizzo G, Barbi E. Comparison of three sites to check the pulse and count heart rate in hypotensive infants. *Paediatr Anaesth.* 2006;16:394–398. doi: 10.1111/j.1460-9592.2005.01803.x
17. Tanner M, Nagy S, Peat JK. Detection of infant's heart beat/pulse by caregivers: a comparison of 4 methods. *J Pediatr.* 2000;137:429–430. doi: 10.1067/mpd.2000.107188
18. Whitelaw CC, Goldsmith LJ. Comparison of two techniques for determining the presence of a pulse in an infant. *Acad Emerg Med.* 1997;4:153–154. doi: 10.1111/j.1553-2712.1997.tb03725.x

19. Dick WF, Eberle B, Wisser G, Schneider T. The carotid pulse check revisited: what if there is no pulse? *Crit Care Med*. 2000;28(suppl):N183–N185. doi: 10.1097/00003246-200011001-00002
20. Eberle B, Dick WF, Schneider T, Wisser G, Doetsch S, Tzanova I. Checking the carotid pulse check: diagnostic accuracy of first responders in patients with and without a pulse. *Resuscitation*. 1996;33:107–116. doi: 10.1016/s0300-9572(96)01016-7
21. Tibballs J, Russell P. Reliability of pulse palpation by healthcare personnel to diagnose paediatric cardiac arrest. *Resuscitation*. 2009;80:61–64. doi: 10.1016/j.resuscitation.2008.10.002
22. Tibballs J, Weeranatna C. The influence of time on the accuracy of healthcare personnel to diagnose paediatric cardiac arrest by pulse palpation. *Resuscitation*. 2010;81:671–675. doi: 10.1016/j.resuscitation.2010.01.030
23. O'Connell KJ, Keane RR, Cochrane NH, Sandler AB, Donoghue AJ, Kerrey BT, Myers SR, Vazifedan T, Mullan PC. Pauses in compressions during pediatric CPR: Opportunities for improving CPR quality. *Resuscitation*. 2019;145:158–165. doi: 10.1016/j.resuscitation.2019.08.015
24. Lubrano R, Cecchetti C, Bellelli E, Gentile I, Loayza Levano H, Orsini F, Bertazzoni G, Messi G, Rugolotto S, Pirozzi N, Elli M. Comparison of times of intervention during pediatric CPR maneuvers using ABC and CAB sequences: a randomized trial. *Resuscitation*. 2012;83:1473–1477. doi: 10.1016/j.resuscitation.2012.04.011
25. Kitamura T, Iwami T, Kawamura T, Nagao K, Tanaka H, Nadkarni VM, Berg RA, Hiraide A; implementation working group for All-Japan Utstein Registry of the Fire and Disaster Management Agency. Conventional and chest-compression-only cardiopulmonary resuscitation by bystanders for children who have out-of-hospital cardiac arrests: a prospective, nationwide, population-based cohort study. *Lancet*. 2010;375:1347–1354. doi: 10.1016/S0140-6736(10)60064-5
26. Goto Y, Maeda T, Goto Y. Impact of dispatcher-assisted bystander cardiopulmonary resuscitation on neurological outcomes in children with out-of-hospital cardiac arrests: a prospective, nationwide, population-based cohort study. *J Am Heart Assoc*. 2014;3:e000499. doi: 10.1161/JAHA.113.000499
27. Naim MY, Burke RV, McNally BF, Song L, Griffis HM, Berg RA, Vellano K, Markenson D, Bradley RN, Rossano JW. Association of Bystander Cardiopulmonary Resuscitation With Overall and Neurologically Favorable Survival After Pediatric Out-of-Hospital Cardiac Arrest in the United States: A Report From the Cardiac Arrest Registry to Enhance Survival Surveillance Registry. *JAMA Pediatr*. 2017;171:133–141. doi: 10.1001/jamapediatrics.2016.3643
28. Fukuda T, Ohashi-Fukuda N, Kobayashi H, Gunshin M, Sera T, Kondo Y, Yahagi N. Conventional Versus Compression-Only Versus No-Bystander Cardiopulmonary Resuscitation for Pediatric Out-of-Hospital Cardiac Arrest. *Circulation*. 2016;134:2060–2070. doi: 10.1161/CIRCULATIONAHA.116.023831
29. Ashoor HM, Lillie E, Zarin W, Pham B, Khan PA, Nincic V, Yazdi F, Ghassemi M, Ivory J, Cardoso R, Perkins GD, de Caen AR, Tricco AC; ILCOR Basic Life Support Task Force. Effectiveness of different compression-to-ventilation methods for cardiopulmonary resuscitation: A systematic review. *Resuscitation*. 2017;118:112–125. doi: 10.1016/j.resuscitation.2017.05.032
30. Glatz AC, Nishisaki A, Niles DE, Hanna BD, Eilevstjonn J, Diaz LK, Gillespie MJ, Rome JJ, Sutton RM, Berg RA, Nadkarni VM. Sternal wall pressure comparable to leaning during CPR impacts intrathoracic pressure and haemodynamics in anaesthetized children during cardiac catheterization. *Resuscitation*. 2013;84:1674–1679. doi: 10.1016/j.resuscitation.2013.07.010
31. Sutton RM, French B, Nishisaki A, Niles DE, Maltese MR, Boyle L, Stavland M, Eilevstjønn J, Arbogast KB, Berg RA, et al. American Heart Association cardiopulmonary resuscitation quality targets are associated with improved arterial blood pressure during pediatric cardiac arrest. *Resuscitation*. 2013;84:168–172. doi: 10.1016/j.resuscitation.2012.08.335
32. Sutton RM, Reeder RW, Landis W, Meert KL, Yates AR, Berger JT, Newth CJ, Carcillo JA, McQuillen PS, Harrison RE, Moler FW, Pollack MM, Carpenter TC, Notterman DA, Holubkov R, Dean JM, Nadkarni VM, Berg RA; Eunice Kennedy Shriver National Institute of Child Health and Human Development Collaborative Pediatric Critical Care Research Network (CPCCRN) Investigators. Chest compression rates and pediatric in-hospital cardiac arrest survival outcomes. *Resuscitation*. 2018;130:159–166. doi: 10.1016/j.resuscitation.2018.07.015
33. Kao PC, Chiang WC, Yang CW, Chen SJ, Liu YP, Lee CC, Hsidh MJ, Ko PC, Chen SC, Ma MH. What is the correct depth of chest compression for infants and children? A radiological study. *Pediatrics*. 2009;124:49–55. doi: 10.1542/peds.2008-2536
34. Sutton RM, Niles D, Nysaether J, Arbogast KB, Nishisaki A, Maltese MR, Bishnoi R, Helfaer MA, Nadkarni V, Donoghue A. Pediatric CPR quality monitoring: analysis of thoracic anthropometric data. *Resuscitation*. 2009;80:1137–1141. doi: 10.1016/j.resuscitation.2009.06.031
35. Braga MS, Dominguez TE, Pollock AN, Niles D, Meyer A, Myklebust H, Nysaether J, Nadkarni V. Estimation of optimal CPR chest compression depth in children by using computer tomography. *Pediatrics*. 2009;124:e69–e74. doi: 10.1542/peds.2009-0153
36. Sutton RM, French B, Niles DE, Donoghue A, Topjian AA, Nishisaki A, Leffelman J, Wolfe H, Berg RA, Nadkarni VM, et al. 2010 American Heart Association recommended compression depths during pediatric in-hospital resuscitations are associated with survival. *Resuscitation*. 2014;85:1179–1184. doi: 10.1016/j.resuscitation.2014.05.007
37. Atkins DL, de Caen AR, Berger S, Samson RA, Schexnayder SM, Joyner BL Jr, Bigham BL, Niles DE, Duff JP, Hunt EA, Meaney PA. 2017 American Heart Association Focused Update on Pediatric Basic Life Support and Cardiopulmonary Resuscitation Quality: An Update to the American Heart Association Guidelines for Cardiopulmonary Resuscitation and Emergency Cardiovascular Care. *Circulation*. 2018;137:e1–e6. doi: 10.1161/CIR.0000000000000540
38. Clements F, McGowan J. Finger position for chest compressions in cardiac arrest in infants. *Resuscitation*. 2000;44:43–46. doi: 10.1016/s0300-9572(99)00165-3
39. Finholt DA, Kettrick RG, Wagner HR, Swedlow DB. The heart is under the lower third of the sternum. Implications for external cardiac massage. *Am J Dis Child*. 1986;140:646–649. doi: 10.1001/archpedi.1986.02140210044022
40. Phillips GW, Zideman DA. Relation of infant heart to sternum: its significance in cardiopulmonary resuscitation. *Lancet*. 1986;1:1024–1025. doi: 10.1016/s0140-6736(86)91284-5
41. Orlowski JP. Optimum position for external cardiac compression in infants and young children. *Ann Emerg Med*. 1986;15:667–673. doi: 10.1016/s0196-0644(86)80423-1
42. Douvanas A, Koulouglioti C, Kalafati M. A comparison between the two methods of chest compression in infant and neonatal resuscitation: a review according to 2010 CPR guidelines. *J Matern Fetal Neonatal Med*. 2018;31:805–816. doi: 10.1080/14767058.2017.1295953
43. Lee JE, Lee J, Oh J, Park CH, Kang H, Lim TH, Yoo KH. Comparison of two-thumb encircling and two-finger technique during infant cardiopulmonary resuscitation with single rescuer in simulation studies: a systematic review and meta-analysis. *Medicine (Baltimore)*. 2019;98:e17853. doi: 10.1097/MD.0000000000017853
44. Lee SY, Hong JY, Oh JH, Son SH. The superiority of the two-thumb over the two-finger technique for single-rescuer infant cardiopulmonary resuscitation. *Eur J Emerg Med*. 2018;25:372–376. doi: 10.1097/MEJ.0000000000000461
45. Tsou JY, Kao CL, Chang CJ, Tu YF, Su FC, Chi CH. Biomechanics of two-thumb versus two-finger chest compression for cardiopulmonary resuscitation in an infant manikin model. *Eur J Emerg Med*. 2020;27:132–136. doi: 10.1097/MEJ.0000000000000631
46. Pellegrino JL, Bogumil D, Epstein JL, Burke RV. Two-thumb-encircling advantageous for lay responder infant CPR: a randomised manikin study. *Arch Dis Child*. 2019;104:530–534. doi: 10.1136/archdischild-2018-314893
47. Kim MJ, Lee HS, Kim S, Park YS. Optimal chest compression technique for paediatric cardiac arrest victims. *Scand J Trauma Resusc Emerg Med*. 2015;23:36. doi: 10.1186/s13049-015-0118-y
48. Stevenson AG, McGowan J, Evans AL, Graham CA. CPR for children: one hand or two? *Resuscitation*. 2005;64:205–208. doi: 10.1016/j.resuscitation.2004.07.012
49. Peska E, Kelly AM, Kerr D, Green D. One-handed versus two-handed chest compressions in paediatric cardio-pulmonary resuscitation. *Resuscitation*. 2006;71:65–69. doi: 10.1016/j.resuscitation.2006.02.007
50. Lin Y, Wan B, Belanger C, Hecker K, Gilfoyle E, Davidson J, Cheng A. Reducing the impact of intensive care unit mattress compressibility during CPR: a simulation-based study. *Adv Simul (Lond)*. 2017;2:22. doi: 10.1186/s41077-017-0057-y
51. Noordergraaf GJ, Paulussen IW, Venema A, van Berkom PF, Woerlee PH, Scheffer GJ, Noordergraaf A. The impact of compliant surfaces on in-hospital chest compressions: effects of common mattresses and a backboard. *Resuscitation*. 2009;80:546–552. doi: 10.1016/j.resuscitation.2009.03.023
52. Oh J, Chee Y, Song Y, Lim T, Kang H, Cho Y. A novel method to decrease mattress compression during CPR using a mattress compression cover and a vacuum pump. *Resuscitation*. 2013;84:987–991. doi: 10.1016/j.resuscitation.2012.12.027

53. Song Y, Oh J, Lim T, Chee Y. A new method to increase the quality of cardiopulmonary resuscitation in hospital. *Conf Proc IEEE Eng Med Biol Soc.* 2013;2013:469–472. doi: 10.1109/EMBC.2013.6609538
54. Beesems SG, Koster RW. Accurate feedback of chest compression depth on a manikin on a soft surface with correction for total body displacement. *Resuscitation.* 2014;85:1439–1443. doi: 10.1016/j.resuscitation.2014.08.005
55. Nishisaki A, Maltese MR, Niles DE, Sutton RM, Urbano J, Berg RA, Nadkarni VM. Backboards are important when chest compressions are provided on a soft mattress. *Resuscitation.* 2012;83:1013–1020. doi: 10.1016/j.resuscitation.2012.01.016
56. Sato H, Komasawa N, Ueki R, Yamamoto N, Fujii A, Nishi S, Kaminoh Y. Backboard insertion in the operating table increases chest compression depth: a manikin study. *J Anesth.* 2011;25:770–772. doi: 10.1007/s00540-011-1196-2
57. Lee S, Oh J, Kang H, Lim T, Kim W, Chee Y, Song Y, Ahn C, Cho JH. Proper target depth of an accelerometer-based feedback device during CPR performed on a hospital bed: a randomized simulation study. *Am J Emerg Med.* 2015;33:1425–1429. doi: 10.1016/j.ajem.2015.07.010
58. Oh J, Song Y, Kang B, Kang H, Lim T, Suh Y, Chee Y. The use of dual accelerometers improves measurement of chest compression depth. *Resuscitation.* 2012;83:500–504. doi: 10.1016/j.resuscitation.2011.09.028
59. Ruiz de Gauna S, González-Otero DM, Ruiz J, Gutiérrez JJ, Russell JK. A feasibility study for measuring accurate chest compression depth and rate on soft surfaces using two accelerometers and spectral analysis. *Biomed Res Int.* 2016;2016:6596040. doi: 10.1155/2016/6596040
60. Andersen LØ, Isbye DL, Rasmussen LS. Increasing compression depth during manikin CPR using a simple backboard. *Acta Anaesthesiol Scand.* 2007;51:747–750. doi: 10.1111/j.1399-6576.2007.01304.x
61. Fischer EJ, Mayrand K, Ten Eyck RP. Effect of a backboard on compression depth during cardiac arrest in the ED: a simulation study. *Am J Emerg Med.* 2016;34:274–277. doi: 10.1016/j.ajem.2015.10.035
62. Perkins GD, Smith CM, Augre C, Allan M, Rogers H, Stephenson B, Thickett DR. Effects of a backboard, bed height, and operator position on compression depth during simulated resuscitation. *Intensive Care Med.* 2006;32:1632–1635. doi: 10.1007/s00134-006-0273-8
63. Sanri E, Karacabey S. The Impact of Backboard Placement on Chest Compression Quality: A Mannequin Study. *Prehosp Disaster Med.* 2019;34:182–187. doi: 10.1017/S1049023X19000153
64. Bhalala US, Hemani M, Shah M, Kim B, Gu B, Cruz A, Arunachalam P, Tian E, Yu C, Punnoose J, Chen S, Petrillo C, Brown A, Munoz K, Kitchen G, Lam T, Bosemani T, Huisman TA, Allen RH, Acharya S. Defining Optimal Head-Tilt Position of Resuscitation in Neonates and Young Infants Using Magnetic Resonance Imaging Data. *PLoS One.* 2016;11:e0151789. doi: 10.1371/journal.pone.0151789

ADVANCED AIRWAY INTERVENTIONS DURING CPR

Most pediatric cardiac arrests are triggered by respiratory deterioration. Airway management and effective ventilation are fundamental to pediatric resuscitation. Although the majority of patients can be successfully ventilated with bag-mask ventilation, this method requires interruptions in chest compressions and is associated with risk of aspiration and barotrauma.

Advanced airway interventions, such as supraglottic airway (SGA) placement or endotracheal intubation (ETI), may improve ventilation, reduce the risk of aspiration, and enable uninterrupted compression delivery. However, airway placement may interrupt the delivery of compressions or result in a malpositioned device. Advanced airway placement requires specialized equipment and skilled providers, and it may be difficult for professionals who do not routinely intubate children.

Recommendation for Advanced Airway Interventions During CPR

COR	LOE	Recommendation
2a	C-LD	1. Bag-mask ventilation is reasonable compared with advanced airway interventions (SGA and ETI) in the management of children during cardiac arrest in the out-of-hospital setting.[1–4]

Recommendation-Specific Supportive Text

1. A clinical trial and 2 propensity-matched retrospective studies show that ETI and bag-mask ventilation achieve similar rates of survival with good neurological function and survival to hospital discharge in pediatric patients with OHCA.[1–3] Propensity-matched retrospective studies also show similar rates of survival with good neurological function and survival to discharge when comparing SGA with bag-mask ventilation in pediatric OHCA.[2,3] No difference was observed in outcomes between SGA and ETI.[2,3] There are limited data to compare outcomes between bag-mask ventilation versus ETI in the management of IHCA,[4] and there are no hospital-based studies of SGA. The data are not sufficient to support a recommendation for advanced airway use in IHCA. There may be specific circumstances or populations in which early advanced airway interventions are beneficial.

This recommendation was reviewed in the "2019 American Heart Association Focused Update on Pediatric Advanced Life Support: An Update to the American Heart Association Guidelines for Cardiopulmonary Resuscitation and Emergency Cardiovascular Care."[5]

REFERENCES

1. Gausche M, Lewis RJ, Stratton SJ, Haynes BE, Gunter CS, Goodrich SM, Poore PD, McCollough MD, Henderson DP, Pratt FD, et al. Effect of out-of-hospital pediatric endotracheal intubation on survival and neurological outcome: a controlled clinical trial. *JAMA.* 2000;283:783–790.
2. Hansen ML, Lin A, Eriksson C, Daya M, McNally B, Fu R, Yanez D, Zive D, Newgard C; CARES surveillance group. A comparison of pediatric airway management techniques during out-of-hospital cardiac arrest using the CARES database. *Resuscitation.* 2017;120:51–56. doi: 10.1016/j.resuscitation.2017.08.015
3. Ohashi-Fukuda N, Fukuda T, Doi K, Morimura N. Effect of prehospital advanced airway management for pediatric out-of-hospital cardiac arrest. *Resuscitation.* 2017;114:66–72. doi: 10.1016/j.resuscitation.2017.03.002
4. Andersen LW, Raymond TT, Berg RA, Nadkarni VM, Grossestreuer AV, Kurth T, Donnino MW; American Heart Association's Get With The Guidelines–Resuscitation Investigators. Association Between Tracheal Intubation During Pediatric In-Hospital Cardiac Arrest and Survival. *JAMA.* 2016;316:1786–1797. doi: 10.1001/jama.2016.14486
5. Duff JP, Topjian AA, Berg MD, Chan M, Haskell SE, Joyner BL Jr, Lasa JJ, Ley SJ, Raymond TT, Sutton RM, Hazinski MF, Atkins DL. 2019 American Heart Association Focused Update on Pediatric Advanced Life Support: An Update to the American Heart Association Guidelines for Cardiopulmonary Resuscitation and Emergency Cardiovascular Care. *Circulation.* 2019;140:e904–e914. doi: 10.1161/CIR.0000000000000731

DRUG ADMINISTRATION DURING CPR

Vasoactive agents, such as epinephrine, are used during cardiac arrest to restore spontaneous circulation by optimizing coronary perfusion and maintaining cerebral perfusion, but the benefit and optimal timing of administration remain unclear.[1,2] Antiarrhythmics reduce the risk of recurrent ventricular fibrillation (VF) and pulseless ventricular tachycardia (pVT) following defibrillation and may improve defibrillation success. Routine use of sodium bicarbonate and calcium is not supported by current data.[3–7] However, there are specific circumstances when their administration is indicated, such as electrolyte imbalances and certain drug toxicities.

Medication dosing for children is based on weight, which is often difficult to obtain in an emergency setting. There are numerous approaches to estimating weight when an actual weight cannot be obtained.[8]

Drug Administration During Cardiac Arrest

Recommendations for Drug Administration During Cardiac Arrest

COR	LOE	Recommendations
2a	C-LD	1. For pediatric patients in any setting, it is reasonable to administer epinephrine. IV/IO is preferable to endotracheal tube (ETT) administration.[2,9–11]
2a	C-LD	2. For pediatric patients in any setting, it is reasonable to administer the initial dose of epinephrine within 5 min from the start of chest compressions.[12–16]
2a	C-LD	3. For pediatric patients in any setting, it is reasonable to administer epinephrine every 3–5 min until ROSC is achieved.[17,18]
2b	C-LD	4. For shock-refractory VF/pVT, either amiodarone or lidocaine may be used.[19,20]
3: Harm	B-NR	5. Routine administration of sodium bicarbonate is not recommended in pediatric cardiac arrest in the absence of hyperkalemia or sodium channel blocker (eg, tricyclic antidepressant) toxicity.[5–7,21–25]
3: Harm	B-NR	6. Routine calcium administration is not recommended for pediatric cardiac arrest in the absence of documented hypocalcemia, calcium channel blocker overdose, hypermagnesemia, or hyperkalemia.[3,4,23]

Recommendation-Specific Supportive Text

1. There are limited data in pediatrics comparing epinephrine administration to no epinephrine administration in any setting. In an OHCA study of 65 children, 12 patients did not receive epinephrine due to lack of a route of administration, and only 1 child had ROSC.[2] An OHCA study of 9 children who had cardiac arrest during sport or exertion noted a survival rate of 67%, of whom 83% did not receive epinephrine. All survivors received early chest compressions (within 5 minutes) and early defibrillation (within 10 minutes), and the initial cardiac arrest rhythm was a shockable rhythm.[9] Intravenous/intraosseous (IV/IO) administration of epinephrine is preferred over ETT administration when possible.[10,11]
2. One retrospective observational study of children with IHCA who received epinephrine for an initial nonshockable rhythm demonstrated that, for every minute delay in administration of epinephrine, there was a significant decrease in ROSC, survival at 24 hours, survival to discharge, and survival with favorable neurological outcome.[12] Patients who received epinephrine within 5 minutes of CPR compared to those who received epinephrine more than 5 minutes after CPR initiation were more likely to survive to discharge.[12] Four observational studies of pediatric OHCA demonstrated that earlier epinephrine administration increased rates of ROSC,[13,14] survival to ICU admission,[14] survival to discharge,[14,16] and 30-day survival.[15]
3. One observational study demonstrated an increased survival rate at 1 year in the group that was administered epinephrine at an interval of less than 5 minutes.[17] One observational study of pediatric IHCA demonstrated that an average epinephrine administration interval of 5 to 8 minutes and of 8 to 10 minutes was associated with increased odds of survival compared with an epinephrine interval of 1 to 5 minutes.[18] Both studies[17,18] calculated the average interval of epinephrine doses by averaging all doses over total arrest time, which does not account for potential differences in dosing intervals throughout resuscitations of varying duration. No studies of pediatric OHCA on frequency of epinephrine dosing were identified.
4. Two studies examined drug therapy of VF/pVT in infants and children.[19,20] In Valdes et al, administration of lidocaine, but not amiodarone, was associated with higher rates of ROSC and survival to hospital admission.[19] Neither lidocaine nor amiodarone significantly affected the odds of survival to hospital discharge; neurological outcome was not assessed. A propensity-matched study of an IHCA registry demonstrated no difference in outcomes for patients receiving lidocaine compared with amiodarone.[20]
5. A recent evidence review identified 8 observational studies of sodium bicarbonate administration during cardiac arrest.[5–7,21–25] Bicarbonate administration was associated with worse survival outcomes for both IHCA and OHCA. There are special circumstances in which bicarbonate is used, such as the treatment of hyperkalemia and

sodium channel blocker toxicity, including from tricyclic antidepressants.

6. Two observational studies examining the administration of calcium during cardiac arrest demonstrated worse survival and ROSC with calcium administration.[4,23] There are special circumstances in which calcium administration is used, such as hypocalcemia, calcium channel blocker overdose, hypermagnesemia, and hyperkalemia.[3]

Recommendation 4 was reviewed in "2018 American Heart Association Focused Update on Pediatric Advanced Life Support: An Update to the American Heart Association Guidelines for Cardiopulmonary Resuscitation and Emergency Cardiovascular Care."[26]

Weight-Based Dosing of Resuscitation Medications

Recommendations for Weight-Based Dosing of Resuscitation Medications

COR	LOE	Recommendations
1	C-EO	1. For resuscitation medication dosing, it is recommended to use the child's body weight to calculate resuscitation drug doses while not exceeding the recommended dose for adults.[27–31]
2b	B-NR	2. When possible, inclusion of body habitus or anthropomorphic measurements may improve the accuracy of length-based estimated weight.[8]
2b	C-LD	3. If the child's weight is unknown, a body length tape for estimating weight and other cognitive aids to calculate resuscitation drug dosing and administration may be considered.[29,32,33]

Recommendation-Specific Supportive Text

1. There are many theoretical concerns about the use of actual body weight (especially in overweight or obese patients).[27–29] However, there are no data about the safety and efficacy of adjusting medication dosing in obese patients. Such adjustments could result in inaccurate dosing of medications.[30,31]
2. Several studies suggest that inclusion of body habitus or anthropometric measurements further refines and improves weight estimations using length-based measures.[8] However, there is considerable variation in these methods, and the training required to use these measures may not be practical in every context.
3. Cognitive aids can assist in the accurate approximation of body weight (described as being within 10% to 20% of measured total body weight). Several recent studies demonstrated high variability of weight estimates, with a tendency toward underestimation of total body weight yet closely approximating ideal body weight.[29,32,33]

REFERENCES

1. Campbell ME, Byrne PJ. Cardiopulmonary resuscitation and epinephrine infusion in extremely low birth weight infants in the neonatal intensive care unit. *J Perinatol*. 2004;24:691–695. doi: 10.1038/sj.jp.7211174
2. Dieckmann RA, Vardis R. High-dose epinephrine in pediatric out-of-hospital cardiopulmonary arrest. *Pediatrics*. 1995;95:901–913.
3. Kette F, Ghuman J, Parr M. Calcium administration during cardiac arrest: a systematic review. *Eur J Emerg Med*. 2013;20:72–78. doi: 10.1097/MEJ.0b013e328358e336
4. Lasa JJ, Alali A, Minard CG, Parekh D, Kutty S, Gaies M, Raymond TT, Guerguerian AM, Atkins D, Foglia E, et al; on behalf of the American Heart Association's Get With the Guidelines-Resuscitation Investigators. Cardiopulmonary resuscitation in the pediatric cardiac catheterization laboratory: A report from the American Heart Association's Get With the Guidelines-Resuscitation Registry. *Pediatr Crit Care Med*. 2019;20:1040–1047. doi: 10.1097/PCC.0000000000002038
5. Matamoros M, Rodriguez R, Callejas A, Carranza D, Zeron H, Sánchez C, Del Castillo J, López-Herce J; Iberoamerican Pediatric Cardiac Arrest Study Network (RIBEPCI). In-hospital pediatric cardiac arrest in Honduras. *Pediatr Emerg Care*. 2015;31:31–35. doi: 10.1097/PEC.0000000000000323
6. Nehme Z, Namachivayam S, Forrest A, Butt W, Bernard S, Smith K. Trends in the incidence and outcome of paediatric out-of-hospital cardiac arrest: A 17-year observational study. *Resuscitation*. 2018;128:43–50. doi: 10.1016/j.resuscitation.2018.04.030
7. Raymond TT, Stromberg D, Stigall W, Burton G, Zaritsky A; American Heart Association's Get With The Guidelines-Resuscitation Investigators. Sodium bicarbonate use during in-hospital pediatric pulseless cardiac arrest - a report from the American Heart Association Get With The Guidelines®-Resuscitation. *Resuscitation*. 2015;89:106–113. doi: 10.1016/j.resuscitation.2015.01.007
8. Young KD, Korotzer NC. Weight Estimation Methods in Children: A Systematic Review. *Ann Emerg Med*. 2016;68:441–451.e10. doi: 10.1016/j.annemergmed.2016.02.043
9. Enright K, Turner C, Roberts P, Cheng N, Browne G. Primary cardiac arrest following sport or exertion in children presenting to an emergency department: chest compressions and early defibrillation can save lives, but is intravenous epinephrine always appropriate? *Pediatr Emerg Care*. 2012;28:336–339. doi: 10.1097/PEC.0b013e31824d8c78
10. Niemann JT, Stratton SJ, Cruz B, Lewis RJ. Endotracheal drug administration during out-of-hospital resuscitation: where are the survivors? *Resuscitation*. 2002;53:153–157. doi: 10.1016/s0300-9572(02)00004-7
11. Niemann JT, Stratton SJ. Endotracheal versus intravenous epinephrine and atropine in out-of-hospital "primary" and postcountershock asystole. *Crit Care Med*. 2000;28:1815–1819. doi: 10.1097/00003246-200006000-00022
12. Andersen LW, Berg KM, Saindon BZ, Massaro JM, Raymond TT, Berg RA, Nadkarni VM, Donnino MW; American Heart Association Get With the Guidelines–Resuscitation Investigators. Time to Epinephrine and Survival After Pediatric In-Hospital Cardiac Arrest. *JAMA*. 2015;314:802–810. doi: 10.1001/jama.2015.9678
13. Lin YR, Wu MH, Chen TY, Syue YJ, Yang MC, Lee TH, Lin CM, Chou CC, Chang CF, Li CJ. Time to epinephrine treatment is associated with the risk of mortality in children who achieve sustained ROSC after traumatic out-of-hospital cardiac arrest. *Crit Care*. 2019;23:101. doi: 10.1186/s13054-019-2391-z
14. Lin YR, Li CJ, Huang CC, Lee TH, Chen TY, Yang MC, Chou CC, Chang CF, Huang HW, Hsu HY, Chen WL. Early Epinephrine Improves the Stabilization of Initial Post-resuscitation Hemodynamics in Children With Nonshockable Out-of-Hospital Cardiac Arrest. *Front Pediatr*. 2019;7:220. doi: 10.3389/fped.2019.00220
15. Fukuda T, Kondo Y, Hayashida K, Sekiguchi H, Kukita I. Time to epinephrine and survival after paediatric out-of-hospital cardiac arrest. *Eur Heart J Cardiovasc Pharmacother*. 2018;4:144–151. doi: 10.1093/ehjcvp/pvx023
16. Hansen M, Schmicker RH, Newgard CD, Grunau B, Scheuermeyer F, Cheskes S, Vithalani V, Alnaji F, Rea T, Idris AH, Herren H, Hutchison J, Austin M, Egan D, Daya M; Resuscitation Outcomes Consortium Investigators. Time to Epinephrine Administration and Survival From Nonshockable Out-of-Hospital Cardiac Arrest Among Children and Adults. *Circulation*. 2018;137:2032–2040. doi: 10.1161/CIRCULATIONAHA.117.033067

17. Meert K, Telford R, Holubkov R, Slomine BS, Christensen JR, Berger J, Ofori-Amanfo G, Newth CJL, Dean JM, Moler FW. Paediatric in-hospital cardiac arrest: factors associated with survival and neurobehavioural outcome one year later. *Resuscitation*. 2018;124:96–105. doi: 10.1016/j.resuscitation.2018.01.013
18. Hoyme DB, Patel SS, Samson RA, Raymond TT, Nadkarni VM, Gaies MG, Atkins DL; American Heart Association Get With The Guidelines–Resuscitation Investigators. Epinephrine dosing interval and survival outcomes during pediatric in-hospital cardiac arrest. *Resuscitation*. 2017;117:18–23. doi: 10.1016/j.resuscitation.2017.05.023
19. Valdes SO, Donoghue AJ, Hoyme DB, Hammond R, Berg MD, Berg RA, Samson RA; American Heart Association Get With The Guidelines-Resuscitation Investigators. Outcomes associated with amiodarone and lidocaine in the treatment of in-hospital pediatric cardiac arrest with pulseless ventricular tachycardia or ventricular fibrillation. *Resuscitation*. 2014;85:381–386. doi: 10.1016/j.resuscitation.2013.12.008
20. Holmberg MJ, Ross CE, Atkins DL, Valdes SO, Donnino MW, Andersen LW; on behalf of the American Heart Association's Get With The Guidelines-Resuscitation Pediatric Research Task Force. Lidocaine versus amiodarone for pediatric in-hospital cardiac arrest: an observational study. *Resuscitation*. 2020:Epub ahead of print. doi: 10.1016/j.resuscitation.2019.12.033
21. López-Herce J, del Castillo J, Cañadas S, Rodríguez-Núñez A, Carrillo A; Spanish Study Group of Cardiopulmonary Arrest in Children. In-hospital pediatric cardiac arrest in Spain. *Rev Esp Cardiol (Engl Ed)*. 2014;67:189–195. doi: 10.1016/j.rec.2013.07.017
22. Wolfe HA, Sutton RM, Reeder RW, Meert KL, Pollack MM, Yates AR, Berger JT, Newth CJ, Carcillo JA, McQuillen PS, Harrison RE, Moler FW, Carpenter TC, Notterman DA, Holubkov R, Dean JM, Nadkarni VM, Berg RA; Eunice Kennedy Shriver National Institute of Child Health; Human Development Collaborative Pediatric Critical Care Research Network; Pediatric Intensive Care Quality of Cardiopulmonary Resuscitation Investigators. Functional outcomes among survivors of pediatric in-hospital cardiac arrest are associated with baseline neurologic and functional status, but not with diastolic blood pressure during CPR. *Resuscitation*. 2019;143:57–65. doi: 10.1016/j.resuscitation.2019.08.006
23. Mok YH, Loke AP, Loh TF, Lee JH. Characteristics and Risk Factors for Mortality in Paediatric In-Hospital Cardiac Events in Singapore: Retrospective Single Centre Experience. *Ann Acad Med Singapore*. 2016;45:534–541.
24. Del Castillo J, López-Herce J, Cañadas S, Matamoros M, Rodríguez-Núnez A, Rodríguez-Calvo A, Carrillo A; Iberoamerican Pediatric Cardiac Arrest Study Network RIBEPCI. Cardiac arrest and resuscitation in the pediatric intensive care unit: a prospective multicenter multinational study. *Resuscitation*. 2014;85:1380–1386. doi: 10.1016/j.resuscitation.2014.06.024
25. Wu ET, Li MJ, Huang SC, Wang CC, Liu YP, Lu FL, Ko WJ, Wang MJ, Wang JK, Wu MH. Survey of outcome of CPR in pediatric in-hospital cardiac arrest in a medical center in Taiwan. *Resuscitation*. 2009;80:443–448. doi: 10.1016/j.resuscitation.2009.01.006
26. Duff JP, Topjian A, Berg MD, Chan M, Haskell SE, Joyner BL Jr, Lasa JJ, Ley SJ, Raymond TT, Sutton RM, Hazinski MF, Atkins DL. 2018 American Heart Association Focused Update on Pediatric Advanced Life Support: An Update to the American Heart Association Guidelines for Cardiopulmonary Resuscitation and Emergency Cardiovascular Care. *Circulation*. 2018;138:e731–e739. doi: 10.1161/CIR.0000000000000612
27. Wells M, Goldstein LN, Bentley A. It is time to abandon age-based emergency weight estimation in children! A failed validation of 20 different age-based formulas. *Resuscitation*. 2017;116:73–83. doi: 10.1016/j.resuscitation.2017.05.018
28. Tanner D, Negaard A, Huang R, Evans N, Hennes H. A Prospective Evaluation of the Accuracy of Weight Estimation Using the Broselow Tape in Overweight and Obese Pediatric Patients in the Emergency Department. *Pediatr Emerg Care*. 2017;33:675–678. doi: 10.1097/PEC.0000000000000894
29. Waseem M, Chen J, Leber M, Giambrone AE, Gerber LM. A reexamination of the accuracy of the Broselow tape as an instrument for weight estimation. *Pediatr Emerg Care*. 2019;35:112–116. doi: 10.1097/PEC.0000000000000982
30. van Rongen A, Brill MJE, Vaughns JD, Välitalo PAJ, van Dongen EPA, van Ramshorst B, Barrett JS, van den Anker JN, Knibbe CAJ. Higher midazolam clearance in obese adolescents compared with morbidly obese adults. *Clin Pharmacokinet*. 2018;57:601–611. doi: 10.1007/s40262-017-0579-4
31. Vaughns JD, Ziesenitz VC, Williams EF, Mushtaq A, Bachmann R, Skopp G, Weiss J, Mikus G, van den Anker JN. Use of fentanyl in adolescents with clinically severe obesity undergoing bariatric surgery: a pilot study. *Paediatr Drugs*. 2017;19:251–257. doi: 10.1007/s40272-017-0216-6
32. Shrestha K, Subedi P, Pandey O, Shakya L, Chhetri K, House DR. Estimating the weight of children in Nepal by Broselow, PAWPER XL and Mercy method. *World J Emerg Med*. 2018;9:276–281. doi: 10.5847/wjem.j.1920-8642.2018.04.007
33. Wells M, Goldstein LN, Bentley A. The accuracy of paediatric weight estimation during simulated emergencies: the effects of patient position, patient cooperation, and human errors. *Afr J Emerg Med*. 2018;8:43–50. doi: 10.1016/j.afjem.2017.12.003

MANAGEMENT OF VF/pVT

The risk of VF/pVT steadily increases throughout childhood and adolescence but remains less frequent than in adults. Cardiac arrest due to an initial rhythm of VF/pVT has better rates of survival to hospital discharge with favorable neurological function than cardiac arrests due to an initial nonshockable rhythm. Shockable rhythms may be the initial rhythm of the cardiac arrest (primary VF/pVT) or may develop during the resuscitation (secondary VF/pVT). Defibrillation is the definitive treatment for VF/pVT. The shorter the duration of VF/pVT, the more likely that the shock will result in a perfusing rhythm. Both manual defibrillators and AEDs can be used to treat VF/pVT in children. Manual defibrillators are preferred when a shockable rhythm is identified by a healthcare provider because the energy dose can be titrated to the patient's weight. AEDs have high specificity in recognizing pediatric shockable rhythms. Biphasic, instead of monophasic, defibrillators are recommended because less energy is required to achieve termination of VF/pVT, with fewer side effects. Many AEDs are equipped to attenuate (reduce) the energy dose to make them suitable for infants and children younger than 8 years of age.

Energy Dose

Recommendations for Energy Dose

COR	LOE	Recommendations
2a	C-LD	1. It is reasonable to use an initial dose of 2–4 J/kg of monophasic or biphasic energy for defibrillation, but, for ease of teaching, an initial dose of 2 J/kg may be considered.[1–7]
2b	C-LD	2. For refractory VF, it may be reasonable to increase the defibrillation dose to 4 J/kg.[1–7]
2b	C-LD	3. For subsequent energy levels, a dose of 4 J/kg may be reasonable, and higher energy levels may be considered, though not to exceed 10 J/kg or the adult maximum dose.[1–7]

Recommendation-Specific Supportive Text

1. 1, 2, and 3. A systematic review[1] demonstrated no relationship between energy dose and any outcome. No randomized controlled trials were available, and most studies only evaluated the first shock. An IHCA case series of 71 shocks in 27 patients concluded that 2 J/kg terminated VF, but neither the subsequent rhythm nor the outcome of

the resuscitation was reported.[2] A small case series of prolonged OHCA observed that 2 to 4 J/kg shock terminated VF 14 times in 11 patients, resulting in asystole or pulseless electric activity, with no survivors to hospital discharge.[3] In 1 observational study of IHCA,[4] a higher initial energy dose of more than 3 to 5 J/kg was less effective than 1 to 3 J/kg in achieving ROSC. Three small, observational studies of pediatric IHCA[3,5] and OHCA[6] found no specific initial energy dose that was associated with successful defibrillation. One study suggested that 2 J/kg was an ineffective dose, especially for secondary VF.[7]

Coordination of Shock and CPR

Recommendations for Coordination of Shock and CPR		
COR	**LOE**	**Recommendations**
1	C-EO	1. Perform CPR until the device is ready to deliver a shock.[8–12]
1	C-EO	2. A single shock followed by immediate chest compressions is recommended for children with VF/pVT.[13,14]
1	C-EO	3. Minimize interruptions of chest compressions.[13,15]

Recommendation-Specific Supportive Text

1. There are currently no pediatric data available regarding the optimal timing of CPR prior to defibrillation. Adult studies demonstrate no benefit of a prolonged period of CPR prior to initial defibrillation.[8–12]
2. There are currently no pediatric data concerning the best sequence for coordination of shocks and CPR. Adult studies comparing a 1-shock protocol versus a 3-shock protocol for treatment of VF suggest significant survival benefit with the single-shock protocol.[13,14]
3. Prolonged pauses in chest compressions decrease blood flow and oxygen delivery to vital organs, such as the brain and heart, and are associated with lower survival.[13,15]

Defibrillator Paddle Size, Type, and Position

Recommendations for Defibrillator Paddle Size, Type, and Position		
COR	**LOE**	**Recommendations**
1	C-EO	1. Use the largest paddles or self-adhering electrodes that will fit on the child's chest while still maintaining good separation between the pads/paddles.[16–18]
2b	C-LD	2. When affixing self-adhering pads, either anterior-lateral placement or anterior-posterior placement may be reasonable.[7,19]
2b	C-LD	3. Paddles and self-adhering pads may be considered equally effective in delivering electricity.[20]

Recommendation-Specific Supportive Text

1. Larger pad or paddle size decreases transthoracic impedance, which is a major determinant of current delivery.[16–18]
2. One human and 1 porcine study demonstrated no significant difference in shock success or ROSC when comparing anterior-lateral with anterior-posterior position.[7,19]
3. One study demonstrated no significant difference in median time to shock with paddles compared with self-adhesive pads.[20]

Type of Defibrillator

Recommendations for Type of Defibrillator		
COR	**LOE**	**Recommendations**
1	C-LD	1. When using an AED on infants and children <8 y old, use of a pediatric attenuator is recommended.[21–32]
1	C-EO	2. For infants under the care of a trained healthcare provider, a manual defibrillator is recommended when a shockable rhythm is identified.[33,34]
2b	C-EO	3. If neither a manual defibrillator nor an AED equipped with a pediatric attenuator is available, an AED without a dose attenuator may be used.[26–28,30,35]

Recommendation-Specific Supportive Text

1. Shockable rhythms are infrequent in infants.[21,22] Studies of rhythm identification algorithms have demonstrated high specificity for shockable rhythms in infants and children.[23–25] Although there are no direct comparisons between pediatric attenuator and nonattenuator AED-delivered shocks, multiple case reports and case series document shock success with survival when a pediatric attenuator was used.[26–32]
2. There are no specific studies comparing manual defibrillators with AEDs in infants or children. Manual defibrillators are preferred for in-hospital use because the energy dose can be titrated to the patient's weight. In adults, use of an AED in hospitals did not improve survival,[33] and the peri-shock pauses needed for rhythm analysis were prolonged.[34]
3. AEDs without pediatric modifications deliver 120 to 360 Joules, exceeding the recommended dose for children weighing less than 25 kg. However, there are reports of safe and effective AED use in infants and young children when the dose exceeded 2 to 4 J/kg.[26–28,30,35] Because defibrillation is the only effective therapy for VF, an AED without a dose attenuator may be lifesaving.

Circulation. 2020;142(suppl 2):S469–S523. DOI: 10.1161/CIR.0000000000000901

REFERENCES

1. Mercier E, Laroche E, Beck B, Le Sage N, Cameron PA, Émond M, Berthelot S, Mitra B, Ouellet-Pelletier J. Defibrillation energy dose during pediatric cardiac arrest: Systematic review of human and animal model studies. *Resuscitation.* 2019;139:241–252. doi: 10.1016/j.resuscitation.2019.04.028
2. Gutgesell HP, Tacker WA, Geddes LA, Davis S, Lie JT, McNamara DG. Energy dose for ventricular defibrillation of children. *Pediatrics.* 1976;58:898–901.
3. Berg MD, Samson RA, Meyer RJ, Clark LL, Valenzuela TD, Berg RA. Pediatric defibrillation doses often fail to terminate prolonged out-of-hospital ventricular fibrillation in children. *Resuscitation.* 2005;67:63–67. doi: 10.1016/j.resuscitation.2005.04.018
4. Meaney PA, Nadkarni VM, Atkins DL, Berg MD, Samson RA, Hazinski MF, Berg RA; American Heart Association National Registry of Cardiopulmonary Resuscitation Investigators. Effect of defibrillation energy dose during in-hospital pediatric cardiac arrest. *Pediatrics.* 2011;127:e16–e23. doi: 10.1542/peds.2010-1617
5. Rodríguez-Núñez A, López-Herce J, del Castillo J, Bellón JM; and the Iberian-American Paediatric Cardiac Arrest Study Network RIBEPCI. Shockable rhythms and defibrillation during in-hospital pediatric cardiac arrest. *Resuscitation.* 2014;85:387–391. doi: 10.1016/j.resuscitation.2013.11.015
6. Rossano JW, Quan L, Kenney MA, Rea TD, Atkins DL. Energy doses for treatment of out-of-hospital pediatric ventricular fibrillation. *Resuscitation.* 2006;70:80–89. doi: 10.1016/j.resuscitation.2005.10.031
7. Tibballs J, Carter B, Kiraly NJ, Ragg P, Clifford M. External and internal biphasic direct current shock doses for pediatric ventricular fibrillation and pulseless ventricular tachycardia. *Pediatr Crit Care Med.* 2011;12:14–20. doi: 10.1097/PCC.0b013e3181dbb4fc
8. Baker PW, Conway J, Cotton C, Ashby DT, Smyth J, Woodman RJ, Grantham H; Clinical Investigators. Defibrillation or cardiopulmonary resuscitation first for patients with out-of-hospital cardiac arrests found by paramedics to be in ventricular fibrillation? A randomised control trial. *Resuscitation.* 2008;79:424–431. doi: 10.1016/j.resuscitation.2008.07.017
9. Jacobs IG, Finn JC, Oxer HF, Jelinek GA. CPR before defibrillation in out-of-hospital cardiac arrest: a randomized trial. *Emerg Med Australas.* 2005;17:39–45. doi: 10.1111/j.1742-6723.2005.00694.x
10. Ma MH, Chiang WC, Ko PC, Yang CW, Wang HC, Chen SY, Chang WT, Huang CH, Chou HC, Lai MS, Chien KL, Lee BC, Hwang CH, Wang YC, Hsiung GH, Hsiao YW, Chang AM, Chen WJ, Chen SC. A randomized trial of compression first or analyze first strategies in patients with out-of-hospital cardiac arrest: results from an Asian community. *Resuscitation.* 2012;83:806–812. doi: 10.1016/j.resuscitation.2012.01.009
11. Stiell IG, Nichol G, Leroux BG, Rea TD, Ornato JP, Powell J, Christenson J, Callaway CW, Kudenchuk PJ, Aufderheide TP, Idris AH, Daya MR, Wang HE, Morrison LJ, Davis D, Andrusiek D, Stephens S, Cheskes S, Schmicker RH, Fowler R, Vaillancourt C, Hostler D, Zive D, Pirrallo RG, Vilke GM, Sopko G, Weisfeldt M; ROC Investigators. Early versus later rhythm analysis in patients with out-of-hospital cardiac arrest. *N Engl J Med.* 2011;365:787–797. doi: 10.1056/NEJMoa1010076
12. Wik L, Hansen TB, Fylling F, Steen T, Vaagenes P, Auestad BH, Steen PA. Delaying defibrillation to give basic cardiopulmonary resuscitation to patients with out-of-hospital ventricular fibrillation: a randomized trial. *JAMA.* 2003;289:1389–1395. doi: 10.1001/jama.289.11.1389
13. Bobrow BJ, Clark LL, Ewy GA, Chikani V, Sanders AB, Berg RA, Richman PB, Kern KB. Minimally interrupted cardiac resuscitation by emergency medical services for out-of-hospital cardiac arrest. *JAMA.* 2008;299:1158–1165. doi: 10.1001/jama.299.10.1158
14. Rea TD, Helbock M, Perry S, Garcia M, Cloyd D, Becker L, Eisenberg M. Increasing use of cardiopulmonary resuscitation during out-of-hospital ventricular fibrillation arrest: survival implications of guideline changes. *Circulation.* 2006;114:2760–2765. doi: 10.1161/CIRCULATIONAHA.106.654715
15. Sutton RM, Case E, Brown SP, Atkins DL, Nadkarni VM, Kaltman J, Callaway C, Idris A, Nichol G, Hutchison J, Drennan IR, Austin M, Daya M, Cheskes S, Nuttall J, Herren H, Christenson J, Andrusiek D, Vaillancourt C, Menegazzi JJ, Rea TD, Berg RA; ROC Investigators. A quantitative analysis of out-of-hospital pediatric and adolescent resuscitation quality–A report from the ROC epistry-cardiac arrest. *Resuscitation.* 2015;93:150–157. doi: 10.1016/j.resuscitation.2015.04.010
16. Atkins DL, Kerber RE. Pediatric defibrillation: current flow is improved by using "adult" electrode paddles. *Pediatrics.* 1994;94:90–93.
17. Samson RA, Atkins DL, Kerber RE. Optimal size of self-adhesive preapplied electrode pads in pediatric defibrillation. *Am J Cardiol.* 1995;75:544–545. doi: 10.1016/s0002-9149(99)80606-7
18. Atkins DL, Sirna S, Kieso R, Charbonnier F, Kerber RE. Pediatric defibrillation: importance of paddle size in determining transthoracic impedance. *Pediatrics.* 1988;82:914–918.
19. Ristagno G, Yu T, Quan W, Freeman G, Li Y. Comparison of defibrillation efficacy between two pads placements in a pediatric porcine model of cardiac arrest. *Resuscitation.* 2012;83:755–759. doi: 10.1016/j.resuscitation.2011.12.010
20. Bhalala US, Balakumar N, Zamora M, Appachi E. Hands-On Defibrillation Skills of Pediatric Acute Care Providers During a Simulated Ventricular Fibrillation Cardiac Arrest Scenario. *Front Pediatr.* 2018;6:107. doi: 10.3389/fped.2018.00107
21. Atkins DL, Everson-Stewart S, Sears GK, Daya M, Osmond MH, Warden CR, Berg RA; Resuscitation Outcomes Consortium Investigators. Epidemiology and outcomes from out-of-hospital cardiac arrest in children: the Resuscitation Outcomes Consortium Epistry-Cardiac Arrest. *Circulation.* 2009;119:1484–1491. doi: 10.1161/CIRCULATIONAHA.108.802678
22. Samson RA, Nadkarni VM, Meaney PA, Carey SM, Berg MD, Berg RA; American Heart Association National Registry of CPR Investigators. Outcomes of in-hospital ventricular fibrillation in children. *N Engl J Med.* 2006;354:2328–2339. doi: 10.1056/NEJMoa052917
23. Cecchin F, Jorgenson DB, Berul CI, Perry JC, Zimmerman AA, Duncan BW, Lupinetti FM, Snyder D, Lyster TD, Rosenthal GL, Cross B, Atkins DL. Is arrhythmia detection by automatic external defibrillator accurate for children?: sensitivity and specificity of an automatic external defibrillator algorithm in 696 pediatric arrhythmias. *Circulation.* 2001;103:2483–2488. doi: 10.1161/01.cir.103.20.2483
24. Atkinson E, Mikysa B, Conway JA, Parker M, Christian K, Deshpande J, Knilans TK, Smith J, Walker C, Stickney RE, Hampton DR, Hazinski MF. Specificity and sensitivity of automated external defibrillator rhythm analysis in infants and children. *Ann Emerg Med.* 2003;42:185–196. doi: 10.1067/mem.2003.287
25. Atkins DL, Scott WA, Blaufox AD, Law IH, Dick M II, Geheb F, Sobh J, Brewer JE. Sensitivity and specificity of an automated external defibrillator algorithm designed for pediatric patients. *Resuscitation.* 2008;76:168–174. doi: 10.1016/j.resuscitation.2007.06.032
26. Atkins DL, Jorgenson DB. Attenuated pediatric electrode pads for automated external defibrillator use in children. *Resuscitation.* 2005;66:31–37. doi: 10.1016/j.resuscitation.2004.12.025
27. Bar-Cohen Y, Walsh EP, Love BA, Cecchin F. First appropriate use of automated external defibrillator in an infant. *Resuscitation.* 2005;67:135–137. doi: 10.1016/j.resuscitation.2005.05.003
28. Divekar A, Soni R. Successful parental use of an automated external defibrillator for an infant with long-QT syndrome. *Pediatrics.* 2006;118:e526–e529. doi: 10.1542/peds.2006-0129
29. Hoyt WJ Jr, Fish FA, Kannankeril PJ. Automated external defibrillator use in a previously healthy 31-day-old infant with out-of-hospital cardiac arrest due to ventricular fibrillation. *J Cardiovasc Electrophysiol.* 2019;30:2599–2602. doi: 10.1111/jce.14125
30. Gurnett CA, Atkins DL. Successful use of a biphasic waveform automated external defibrillator in a high-risk child. *Am J Cardiol.* 2000;86:1051–1053. doi: 10.1016/s0002-9149(00)01151-6
31. Mitani Y, Ohta K, Yodoya N, Otsuki S, Ohashi H, Sawada H, Nagashima M, Sumitomo N, Komada Y. Public access defibrillation improved the outcome after out-of-hospital cardiac arrest in school-age children: a nationwide, population-based, Utstein registry study in Japan. *Europace.* 2013;15:1259–1266. doi: 10.1093/europace/eut053
32. Pundi KN, Bos JM, Cannon BC, Ackerman MJ. Automated external defibrillator rescues among children with diagnosed and treated long QT syndrome. *Heart Rhythm.* 2015;12:776–781. doi: 10.1016/j.hrthm.2015.01.002
33. Chan PS, Krumholz HM, Spertus JA, Jones PG, Cram P, Berg RA, Peberdy MA, Nadkarni V, Mancini ME, Nallamothu BK. Automated external defibrillators and survival after in-hospital cardiac arrest. *JAMA.* 2010;304:2129–2136. doi: 10.1001/jama.2010.1576
34. Cheskes S, Schmicker RH, Christenson J, Salcido DD, Rea T, Powell J, Edelson DP, Sell R, May S, Menegazzi JJ, Van Ottingham L, Olsufka M, Pennington S, Simonini J, Berg RA, Stiell I, Idris A, Bigham B, Morrison L; Resuscitation Outcomes Consortium (ROC) Investigators. Perishock pause: an independent predictor of survival from out-of-hospital shockable cardiac arrest. *Circulation.* 2011;124:58–66. doi: 10.1161/CIRCULATIONAHA.110.010736
35. König B, Benger J, Goldsworthy L. Automatic external defibrillation in a 6 year old. *Arch Dis Child.* 2005;90:310–311. doi: 10.1136/adc.2004.054981

ASSESSMENT OF RESUSCITATION QUALITY

Initiating and maintaining high-quality CPR is associated with improved rates of ROSC, survival, and favorable neurological outcome, yet measured CPR quality is often suboptimal.[1–3] Noninvasive and invasive monitoring techniques may be used to assess and guide the quality of CPR. Invasive arterial blood pressure monitoring during CPR provides insight to blood pressures generated with compressions and medications.[4] End-tidal CO_2 ($ETCO_2$) reflects both the cardiac output produced and ventilation efficacy and may provide feedback on the quality of CPR.[5] A sudden rise in $ETCO_2$ may be an early sign of ROSC.[6] CPR feedback devices (ie, coaching, audio, and audiovisual devices) may improve compression rate, depth, and recoil within a system of training and quality assurance for high-quality CPR. Point of care ultrasound, specifically echocardiography, during CPR has been considered for identification of reversible causes of arrest. Technologies that are under evaluation to assess resuscitation quality include noninvasive measures of cerebral oxygenation, such as using near infrared spectroscopy during CPR.

Recommendations for the Assessment of Resuscitation Quality

COR	LOE	Recommendations
2a	C-LD	1. For patients with continuous invasive arterial blood pressure monitoring in place at the time of cardiac arrest, it is reasonable for providers to use diastolic blood pressure to assess CPR quality.[4]
2b	C-LD	2. $ETCO_2$ monitoring may be considered to assess the quality of chest compressions, but specific values to guide therapy have not been established in children.[7,8]
2b	C-EO	3. It may be reasonable for the rescuer to use CPR feedback devices to optimize adequate chest compression rate and depth as part of a continuous resuscitation quality improvement system.[9,10]
2b	C-EO	4. When appropriately trained personnel are available, echocardiography may be considered to identify potentially treatable causes of the arrest, such as pericardial tamponade and inadequate ventricular filling, but the potential benefits should be weighed against the known deleterious consequences of interrupting chest compressions.[11–13]

Recommendation-Specific Supportive Text

1. A prospective observational study of pediatric patients with invasive arterial blood pressure monitoring during the first 10 minutes of CPR demonstrated higher rates of favorable neurological outcome if the diastolic blood pressure was at least 25 mm Hg in infants and at least 30 mm Hg in children.[4] Of note, the cut points for diastolic blood pressure tracings were analyzed using post hoc waveform analysis; therefore, prospective evaluation is needed.
2. A single-center, retrospective study of in-hospital CPR in infants found that $ETCO_2$ values between 17 and 18 mm Hg had a positive predictive value for ROSC of 0.885.[7] A prospective, multicenter observational study of IHCA did not find an association between mean $ETCO_2$ and outcomes.[8]
3. A simulation trial of pediatric healthcare providers demonstrated a significant improvement in chest compression depth and rate compliance when they received visual feedback (compared to no feedback), although overall compression quality remained poor.[9] One small observational study of 8 children with IHCA did not find an association between CPR with or without audiovisual feedback and survival to discharge, although feedback decreased excessive compression rates.[10]
4. Several case series evaluated the use of bedside echocardiography to identify reversible causes of cardiac arrest, including pulmonary embolism.[11,12] One prospective observational study of children (without cardiac arrest) admitted to an ICU reported good agreement of estimates of shortening fraction and inferior vena cava volume between emergency physicians using bedside limited echocardiography and cardiologists performing formal echocardiography.[13]

REFERENCES

1. Niles DE, Duval-Arnould J, Skellett S, Knight L, Su F, Raymond TT, Sweberg T, Sen AI, Atkins DL, Friess SH, de Caen AR, Kurosawa H, Sutton RM, Wolfe H, Berg RA, Silver A, Hunt EA, Nadkarni VM; pediatric Resuscitation Quality (pediRES-Q) Collaborative Investigators. Characterization of Pediatric In-Hospital Cardiopulmonary Resuscitation Quality Metrics Across an International Resuscitation Collaborative. *Pediatr Crit Care Med.* 2018;19:421–432. doi: 10.1097/PCC.0000000000001520
2. Sutton RM, Case E, Brown SP, Atkins DL, Nadkarni VM, Kaltman J, Callaway C, Idris A, Nichol G, Hutchison J, Drennan IR, Austin M, Daya M, Cheskes S, Nuttall J, Herren H, Christenson J, Andrusiek D, Vaillancourt C, Menegazzi JJ, Rea TD, Berg RA; ROC Investigators. A quantitative analysis of out-of-hospital pediatric and adolescent resuscitation quality–A report from the ROC epistry-cardiac arrest. *Resuscitation.* 2015;93:150–157. doi: 10.1016/j.resuscitation.2015.04.010
3. Wolfe H, Zebuhr C, Topjian AA, Nishisaki A, Niles DE, Meaney PA, Boyle L, Giordano RT, Davis D, Priestley M, Apkon M, Berg RA, Nadkarni VM, Sutton RM. Interdisciplinary ICU cardiac arrest debriefing improves survival outcomes*. *Crit Care Med.* 2014;42:1688–1695. doi: 10.1097/CCM.0000000000000327
4. Berg RA, Sutton RM, Reeder RW, Berger JT, Newth CJ, Carcillo JA, McQuillen PS, Meert KL, Yates AR, Harrison RE, Moler FW, Pollack MM, Carpenter TC, Wessel DL, Jenkins TL, Notterman DA, Holubkov R, Tamburro RF, Dean JM, Nadkarni VM; Eunice Kennedy Shriver National Institute of Child Health and Human Development Collaborative Pediatric Critical Care Research Network (CPCCRN) PICqCPR (Pediatric Intensive Care Quality of Cardio-Pulmonary Resuscitation) Investigators. Association Between Diastolic Blood Pressure During Pediatric In-Hospital Cardiopulmonary Resuscitation and Survival. *Circulation.* 2018;137:1784–1795. doi: 10.1161/CIRCULATIONAHA.117.032270
5. Hamrick JL, Hamrick JT, Lee JK, Lee BH, Koehler RC, Shaffner DH. Efficacy of chest compressions directed by end-tidal CO2 feedback in a pediatric resuscitation model of basic life support. *J Am Heart Assoc.* 2014;3:e000450. doi: 10.1161/JAHA.113.000450
6. Hartmann SM, Farris RW, Di Gennaro JL, Roberts JS. Systematic Review and Meta-Analysis of End-Tidal Carbon Dioxide Values Associated With Return of Spontaneous Circulation During Cardiopulmonary Resuscitation. *J Intensive Care Med.* 2015;30:426–435. doi: 10.1177/0885066614530839

7. Stine CN, Koch J, Brown LS, Chalak L, Kapadia V, Wyckoff MH. Quantitative end-tidal CO2 can predict increase in heart rate during infant cardiopulmonary resuscitation. *Heliyon.* 2019;5:e01871. doi: 10.1016/j.heliyon.2019.e01871
8. Berg RA, Reeder RW, Meert KL, Yates AR, Berger JT, Newth CJ, Carcillo JA, McQuillen PS, Harrison RE, Moler FW, Pollack MM, Carpenter TC, Notterman DA, Holubkov R, Dean JM, Nadkarni VM, Sutton RM; Eunice Kennedy Shriver National Institute of Child Health and Human Development Collaborative Pediatric Critical Care Research Network (CPCCRN) Pediatric Intensive Care Quality of Cardio-Pulmonary Resuscitation (PICqCPR) investigators. End-tidal carbon dioxide during pediatric in-hospital cardiopulmonary resuscitation. *Resuscitation.* 2018;133:173–179. doi: 10.1016/j.resuscitation.2018.08.013
9. Cheng A, Brown LL, Duff JP, Davidson J, Overly F, Tofil NM, Peterson DT, White ML, Bhanji F, Bank I, et al; on behalf of the International Network for Simulation-Based Pediatric Innovation, Research, & Education (INSPIRE) CPR Investigators. Improving cardiopulmonary resuscitation with a CPR feedback device and refresher simulations (CPR CARES Study): a randomized clinical trial. *JAMA Pediatr.* 2015;169:137–144. doi: 10.1001/jamapediatrics.2014.2616
10. Sutton RM, Niles D, French B, Maltese MR, Leffelman J, Eilevstjonn J, Wolfe H, Nishisaki A, Meaney PA, Berg RA, et al. First quantitative analysis of cardiopulmonary resuscitation quality during in-hospital cardiac arrests of young children. *Resuscitation.* 2014;85:70–74. doi: 10.1016/j.resuscitation.2013.08.014
11. Steffen K, Thompson WR, Pustavoitau A, Su E. Return of Viable Cardiac Function After Sonographic Cardiac Standstill in Pediatric Cardiac Arrest. *Pediatr Emerg Care.* 2017;33:58–59. doi: 10.1097/PEC.0000000000001002
12. Morgan RW, Stinson HR, Wolfe H, Lindell RB, Topjian AA, Nadkarni VM, Sutton RM, Berg RA, Kilbaugh TJ. Pediatric In-Hospital Cardiac Arrest Secondary to Acute Pulmonary Embolism. *Crit Care Med.* 2018;46:e229–e234. doi: 10.1097/CCM.0000000000002921
13. Pershad J, Myers S, Plouman C, Rosson C, Elam K, Wan J, Chin T. Bedside limited echocardiography by the emergency physician is accurate during evaluation of the critically ill patient. *Pediatrics.* 2004;114:e667–e671. doi: 10.1542/peds.2004-0881

EXTRACORPOREAL CARDIOPULMONARY RESUSCITATION

Extracorporeal cardiopulmonary resuscitation (ECPR) is defined as the rapid deployment of venoarterial extracorporeal membrane oxygenation (ECMO) for patients who do not achieve sustained ROSC. It is a resource-intense, complex, multidisciplinary therapy that traditionally has been limited to large pediatric medical centers with providers who have expertise in the management of children with cardiac disease. Judicious use of ECPR for specific patient populations and within dedicated and highly practiced environments has proved successful, especially for IHCA with reversible causes.[1] ECPR use rates have increased, with single-center reports in both adults and children suggesting that application of this therapy across broader patient populations may improve survival after cardiac arrest.[2–4]

There are no studies of ECPR demonstrating improved outcomes following pediatric OHCA.

Recommendation for the Use of Extracorporeal Cardiopulmonary Resuscitation

COR	LOE	Recommendation
2b	C-LD	1. ECPR may be considered for pediatric patients with cardiac diagnoses who have IHCA in settings with existing ECMO protocols, expertise, and equipment.[5,6]

Recommendation-Specific Supportive Text

1. One observational registry study of ECPR for pediatric IHCA after cardiac surgery demonstrated that ECPR was associated with higher rates of survival to hospital discharge than conventional CPR.[5] A propensity-matched analysis of ECPR compared with conventional CPR using the same registry found that ECPR was associated with favorable neurological outcome in patients with IHCA of any etiology.[6] There is insufficient evidence to suggest for or against the use of ECPR for pediatric patients experiencing OHCA or pediatric patients with noncardiac disease experiencing IHCA refractory to conventional CPR.

This recommendation was reviewed in the "2019 American Heart Association Focused Update on Pediatric Advanced Life Support: An Update to the American Heart Association Guidelines for Cardiopulmonary Resuscitation and Emergency Cardiovascular Care."[7]

REFERENCES

1. Brunetti MA, Gaynor JW, Retzloff LB, Lehrich JL, Banerjee M, Amula V, Bailly D, Klugman D, Koch J, Lasa J, Pasquali SK, Gaies M. Characteristics, Risk Factors, and Outcomes of Extracorporeal Membrane Oxygenation Use in Pediatric Cardiac ICUs: A Report From the Pediatric Cardiac Critical Care Consortium Registry. *Pediatr Crit Care Med.* 2018;19:544–552. doi: 10.1097/PCC.0000000000001571
2. Sakamoto T, Morimura N, Nagao K, Asai Y, Yokota H, Nara S, Hase M, Tahara Y, Atsumi T; SAVE-J Study Group. Extracorporeal cardiopulmonary resuscitation versus conventional cardiopulmonary resuscitation in adults with out-of-hospital cardiac arrest: a prospective observational study. *Resuscitation.* 2014;85:762–768. doi: 10.1016/j.resuscitation.2014.01.031
3. Stub D, Bernard S, Pellegrino V, Smith K, Walker T, Sheldrake J, Hockings L, Shaw J, Duffy SJ, Burrell A, Cameron P, Smit de V, Kaye DM. Refractory cardiac arrest treated with mechanical CPR, hypothermia, ECMO and early reperfusion (the CHEER trial). *Resuscitation.* 2015;86:88–94. doi: 10.1016/j.resuscitation.2014.09.010
4. Conrad SJ, Bridges BC, Kalra Y, Pietsch JB, Smith AH. Extracorporeal Cardiopulmonary Resuscitation Among Patients with Structurally Normal Hearts. *ASAIO J.* 2017;63:781–786. doi: 10.1097/MAT.0000000000000568
5. Ortmann L, Prodhan P, Gossett J, Schexnayder S, Berg R, Nadkarni V, Bhutta A; American Heart Association's Get With the Guidelines–Resuscitation Investigators. Outcomes after in-hospital cardiac arrest in children with cardiac disease: a report from Get With the Guidelines–Resuscitation. *Circulation.* 2011;124:2329–2337. doi: 10.1161/CIRCULATIONAHA.110.013466
6. Lasa JJ, Rogers RS, Localio R, Shults J, Raymond T, Gaies M, Thiagarajan R, Laussen PC, Kilbaugh T, Berg RA, Nadkarni V, Topjian A. Extracorporeal Cardiopulmonary Resuscitation (E-CPR) During Pediatric In-Hospital Cardiopulmonary Arrest Is Associated With Improved Survival to Discharge: A Report from the American Heart Association's Get With The Guidelines-Resuscitation (GWTG-R) Registry. *Circulation.* 2016;133:165–176. doi: 10.1161/CIRCULATIONAHA.115.016082
7. Duff JP, Topjian AA, Berg MD, Chan M, Haskell SE, Joyner BL Jr, Lasa JJ, Ley SJ, Raymond TT, Sutton RM, Hazinski MF, Atkins DL. 2019 American Heart Association Focused Update on Pediatric Advanced Life Support: An Update to the American Heart Association Guidelines for Cardiopulmonary Resuscitation and Emergency Cardiovascular Care. *Circulation.* 2019;140:e904–e914. doi: 10.1161/CIR.0000000000000731

POST–CARDIAC ARREST CARE TREATMENT AND MONITORING

Successful resuscitation from cardiac arrest results in a post–cardiac arrest syndrome that can evolve in the days after ROSC. The components of post–cardiac arrest syndrome are (1) brain injury, (2) myocardial dysfunction, (3) systemic ischemia and reperfusion response, and (4) persistent precipitating pathophysiology.[1,2] Post–cardiac arrest brain injury remains a leading cause of morbidity and mortality in adults and children because the brain has limited tolerance of ischemia, hyperemia, or edema. Pediatric post–cardiac arrest care focuses on anticipating, identifying, and treating this complex physiology to improve survival and neurological outcomes.

Targeted temperature management (TTM) refers to continuous maintenance of patient temperature within a narrowly prescribed range while continuously monitoring temperature. All forms of TTM avoid fever, and hypothermic TTM attempts to treat reperfusion syndrome by decreasing metabolic demand, reducing free radical production, and decreasing apoptosis.[2]

Identification and treatment of derangements—such as hypotension, fever, seizures, acute kidney injury, and abnormalities of oxygenation, ventilation, and electrolytes—are important because they may impact outcomes.

Post–Cardiac Arrest Targeted Temperature Management

Recommendations for Post–Cardiac Arrest Targeted Temperature Management

COR	LOE	Recommendations
1	A	1. Continuous measurement of core temperature during TTM is recommended.[3,4]
2a	B-R	2. For infants and children between 24 h and 18 yr of age who remain comatose after OHCA or IHCA, it is reasonable to use either TTM of 32°C–34°C followed by TTM of 36°C–37.5°C or only TTM of 36°C–37.5°C.[3,4]

Recommendation-Specific Supportive Text

1 and 2. Two pediatric randomized clinical trials of TTM (32°C–34°C for 48 hours followed by 3 days of TTM 36°C–37.5°C versus TTM 36°C–37.5°C for a total of 5 days) after IHCA or OHCA in children with coma following ROSC found no difference in 1-year survival with a favorable neurological outcome.[3,4] Hyperthermia was actively prevented with TTM. Continuous core temperature monitoring was used for the 5 days of TTM in both trials.

Recommendations 1 and 2 were reviewed in the "2019 American Heart Association Focused Update on Pediatric Advanced Life Support: An Update to the American Heart Association Guidelines for Cardiopulmonary Resuscitation and Emergency Cardiovascular Care."[5]

Post–Cardiac Arrest Blood Pressure Management

Recommendations for Post–Cardiac Arrest Blood Pressure Management

COR	LOE	Recommendations
1	C-LD	1. After ROSC, we recommend that parenteral fluids and/or vasoactive drugs be used to maintain a systolic blood pressure greater than the fifth percentile for age.[6–9]
1	C-EO	2. When appropriate resources are available, continuous arterial pressure monitoring is recommended to identify and treat hypotension.[6–9]

Recommendation-Specific Supportive Text

1 and 2. Two observational studies demonstrated that systolic hypotension (below 5th percentile for age and sex) at approximately 6 to 12 hours following cardiac arrest is associated with decreased survival to discharge.[6,7] Another observational study found that patients who had longer periods of hypotension within the first 72 hours of ICU post–cardiac arrest care had decreased survival to discharge.[8] In an observational study of patients with arterial monitoring during and immediately after cardiac arrest, diastolic hypertension (above 90th percentile) in the first 20 minutes after ROSC was associated with an increased likelihood of survival to discharge.[9] Because blood pressure is often labile in the post–cardiac arrest period, continuous arterial pressure monitoring is recommended.

Post–Cardiac Arrest Oxygenation and Ventilation Management

Recommendations for Post–Cardiac Arrest Oxygenation and Ventilation Management

COR	LOE	Recommendations
2b	C-LD	1. It may be reasonable for rescuers to target normoxemia after ROSC that is appropriate to the specific patient's underlying condition.[10–13]
2b	C-LD	2. It may be reasonable for rescuers to wean oxygen to target an oxyhemoglobin saturation between 94% and 99%.[10–12,14]
2b	C-LD	3. It may be reasonable for practitioners to target a partial pressure of carbon dioxide ($Paco_2$) after ROSC that is appropriate to the specific patient's underlying condition, and limit exposure to severe hypercapnia or hypocapnia.[10,11,14]

Recommendation-Specific Supportive Text

1 and 2. Because an arterial oxyhemoglobin saturation of 100% may correspond to a Pao_2 between 80 and approximately 500 mm Hg, it is reasonable to target an oxyhemoglobin saturation between 94% and 99%. Three small observational studies

Circulation. 2020;142(suppl 2):S469–S523. DOI: 10.1161/CIR.0000000000000901

of pediatric IHCA and OHCA did not show an association between hyperoxemia and outcome.[10,11,13] In a larger observational study of pediatric IHCA and OHCA patients, the presence of normoxemia compared with hyperoxemia after ROSC was associated with improved survival to pediatric ICU discharge.[12]

3. One observational study demonstrated that both hypercapnia and hypocapnia after ROSC were associated with increased mortality.[11] One small observational study demonstrated no association between hypercapnia ($Paco_2$ greater than 50 mm Hg) or hypocapnia ($Paco_2$ less than 30 mm Hg) and outcome.[10] Another observational study of pediatric IHCA, showed hypercapnia ($Paco_2$ 50 mm Hg or greater) was associated with decreased survival to hospital discharge.[14] Because hypercapnia and hypocapnia impact cerebral blood flow, normocapnia should be the focus after ROSC while accounting for patients who have chronic hypercapnia.

Post–Cardiac Arrest EEG Monitoring and Seizure Treatment

Recommendations for Post–Cardiac Arrest EEG Monitoring and Seizure Treatment

COR	LOE	Recommendations
1	C-LD	1. When resources are available, continuous electroencephalography (EEG) monitoring is recommended for the detection of seizures following cardiac arrest in patients with persistent encephalopathy.[15–18]
1	C-LD	2. It is recommended to treat clinical seizures following cardiac arrest.[19,20]
2a	C-EO	3. It is reasonable to treat nonconvulsive status epilepticus following cardiac arrest in consultation with experts.[19,20]

Recommendation-Specific Supportive Text

1. Nonconvulsive seizures and nonconvulsive status epilepticus are common after pediatric cardiac arrest.[15–18] The American Clinical Neurophysiology Society recommends continuous EEG monitoring for encephalopathic patients after pediatric cardiac arrest.[15] Nonconvulsive seizures and nonconvulsive status epilepticus cannot be detected without EEG monitoring.[15]

2 and 3. There is insufficient evidence to determine whether treatment of convulsive or nonconvulsive seizures improves neurological and/or functional outcomes after pediatric cardiac arrest. Both convulsive and nonconvulsive status epilepticus are associated with worse outcomes.[17] The Neurocritical Care Society recommends treating status epilepticus with the goal of stopping convulsive and electrographic seizure activity.[19]

Figure 8 shows the checklist for post–cardiac arrest care.

REFERENCES

1. Neumar RW, Nolan JP, Adrie C, Aibiki M, Berg RA, Böttiger BW, Callaway C, Clark RS, Geocadin RG, Jauch EC, Kern KB, Laurent I, Longstreth WT Jr, Merchant RM, Morley P, Morrison LJ, Nadkarni V, Peberdy MA, Rivers EP, Rodriguez-Nunez A, Sellke FW, Spaulding C, Sunde K, Vanden Hoek T. Post-cardiac arrest syndrome: epidemiology, pathophysiology, treatment, and prognostication. A consensus statement from the International Liaison Committee on Resuscitation (American Heart Association, Australian and New Zealand Council on Resuscitation, European Resuscitation Council, Heart and Stroke Foundation of Canada, InterAmerican Heart Foundation, Resuscitation Council of Asia, and the Resuscitation Council of Southern Africa); the American Heart Association Emergency Cardiovascular Care Committee; the Council on Cardiovascular Surgery and Anesthesia; the Council on Cardiopulmonary, Perioperative, and Critical Care; the Council on Clinical Cardiology; and the Stroke Council. *Circulation.* 2008;118:2452–2483. doi: 10.1161/CIRCULATIONAHA.108.190652
2. Topjian AA, de Caen A, Wainwright MS, Abella BS, Abend NS, Atkins DL, Bembea MM, Fink EL, Guerguerian AM, Haskell SE, Kilgannon JH, Lasa JJ, Hazinski MF. Pediatric post-cardiac arrest care: a scientific statement from the American Heart Association. *Circulation.* 2019;140:e194–e233. doi: 10.1161/CIR.0000000000000697
3. Moler FW, Silverstein FS, Holubkov R, Slomine BS, Christensen JR, Nadkarni VM, Meert KL, Browning B, Pemberton VL, Page K, et al; on behalf of the THAPCA Trial Investigators. Therapeutic hypothermia after in-hospital cardiac arrest in children. *N Engl J Med.* 2017;376:318–329. doi: 10.1056/NEJMoa1610493
4. Moler FW, Silverstein FS, Holubkov R, Slomine BS, Christensen JR, Nadkarni VM, Meert KL, Clark AE, Browning B, Pemberton VL, Page K, Shankaran S, Hutchison JS, Newth CJ, Bennett KS, Berger JT, Topjian A, Pineda JA, Koch JD, Schleien CL, Dalton HJ, Ofori-Amanfo G, Goodman DM, Fink EL, McQuillen P, Zimmerman JJ, Thomas NJ, van der Jagt EW, Porter MB, Meyer MT, Harrison R, Pham N, Schwarz AJ, Nowak JE, Alten J, Wheeler DS, Bhalala US, Lidsky K, Lloyd E, Mathur M, Shah S, Wu T, Theodorou AA, Sanders RC Jr, Dean JM; THAPCA Trial Investigators. Therapeutic hypothermia after out-of-hospital cardiac arrest in children. *N Engl J Med.* 2015;372:1898–1908. doi: 10.1056/NEJMoa1411480
5. Duff JP, Topjian AA, Berg MD, Chan M, Haskell SE, Joyner BL Jr, Lasa JJ, Ley SJ, Raymond TT, Sutton RM, Hazinski MF, Atkins DL. 2019 American Heart Association focused update on pediatric advanced life support: an update to the American Heart Association Guidelines for Cardiopulmonary Resuscitation and Emergency Cardiovascular Care. *Circulation.* 2019;140:e904–e914. doi: 10.1161/CIR.0000000000000731
6. Topjian AA, Telford R, Holubkov R, Nadkarni VM, Berg RA, Dean JM, Moler FW; on behalf of the Therapeutic Hypothermia after Pediatric Cardiac Arrest (THAPCA) Trial Investigators. The association of early post-resuscitation hypotension with discharge survival following targeted temperature management for pediatric in-hospital cardiac arrest. *Resuscitation.* 2019;141:24–34. doi: 10.1016/j.resuscitation.2019.05.032
7. Topjian AA, Telford R, Holubkov R, Nadkarni VM, Berg RA, Dean JM, Moler FW; Therapeutic Hypothermia After Pediatric Cardiac Arrest (THAPCA) Trial Investigators. Association of Early Postresuscitation Hypotension With Survival to Discharge After Targeted Temperature Management for Pediatric Out-of-Hospital Cardiac Arrest: Secondary Analysis of a Randomized Clinical Trial. *JAMA Pediatr.* 2018;172:143–153. doi: 10.1001/jamapediatrics.2017.4043
8. Laverriere EK, Polansky M, French B, Nadkarni VM, Berg RA, Topjian AA. Association of Duration of Hypotension With Survival After Pediatric Cardiac Arrest. *Pediatr Crit Care Med.* 2020;21:143–149. doi: 10.1097/PCC.0000000000002119
9. Topjian AA, Sutton RM, Reeder RW, Telford R, Meert KL, Yates AR, Morgan RW, Berger JT, Newth CJ, Carcillo JA, McQuillen PS, Harrison RE, Moler FW, Pollack MM, Carpenter TC, Notterman DA, Holubkov R, Dean JM, Nadkarni VM, Berg RA, Zuppa AF, Graham K, Twelves C, Diliberto MA, Landis WP, Tomanio E, Kwok J, Bell MJ, Abraham A, Sapru A, Alkhouli MF, Heidemann S, Pawluszka A, Hall MW, Steele L, Shanley TP, Weber M, Dalton HJ, Bell A, Mourani PM, Malone K, Locandro C, Coleman W, Peterson A, Thelen J, Doctor A; Eunice Kennedy Shriver National Institute of Child Health and Human Development Collaborative Pediatric Critical Care Research Network (CPCCRN) Investigators. The association of immediate post cardiac arrest diastolic hypertension and survival following pediatric cardiac arrest. *Resuscitation.* 2019;141:88–95. doi: 10.1016/j.resuscitation.2019.05.033
10. Bennett KS, Clark AE, Meert KL, Topjian AA, Schleien CL, Shaffner DH, Dean JM, Moler FW; Pediatric Emergency Care Medicine Applied Research

Components of Post–Cardiac Arrest Care	Check
Oxygenation and ventilation	
Measure oxygenation and target normoxemia 94%-99% (or child's normal/appropriate oxygen saturation).	☐
Measure and target Pa_{CO_2} appropriate to the patient's underlying condition and limit exposure to severe hypercapnia or hypocapnia.	☐
Hemodynamic monitoring	
Set specific hemodynamic goals during post–cardiac arrest care and review daily.	☐
Monitor with cardiac telemetry.	☐
Monitor arterial blood pressure.	☐
Monitor serum lactate, urine output, and central venous oxygen saturation to help guide therapies.	☐
Use parenteral fluid bolus with or without inotropes or vasopressors to maintain a systolic blood pressure greater than the fifth percentile for age and sex.	☐
Targeted temperature management (TTM)	
Measure and continuously monitor core temperature.	☐
Prevent and treat fever immediately after arrest and during rewarming.	☐
If patient is comatose apply TTM (32°C-34°C) followed by (36°C-37.5°C) or only TTM (36°C-37.5°C).	☐
Prevent shivering.	☐
Monitor blood pressure and treat hypotension during rewarming.	☐
Neuromonitoring	
If patient has encephalopathy and resources are available, monitor with continuous electroencephalogram.	☐
Treat seizures.	☐
Consider early brain imaging to diagnose treatable causes of cardiac arrest.	☐
Electrolytes and glucose	
Measure blood glucose and avoid hypoglycemia.	☐
Maintain electrolytes within normal ranges to avoid possible life-threatening arrhythmias.	☐
Sedation	
Treat with sedatives and anxiolytics.	☐
Prognosis	
Always consider multiple modalities (clinical and other) over any single predictive factor.	☐
Remember that assessments may be modified by TTM or induced hypothermia.	☐
Consider electroencephalogram in conjunction with other factors within the first 7 days after cardiac arrest.	☐
Consider neuroimaging such as magnetic resonance imaging during the first 7 days.	☐

Figure 8. Post–cardiac arrest care checklist.

Network. Early oxygenation and ventilation measurements after pediatric cardiac arrest: lack of association with outcome. *Crit Care Med.* 2013;41:1534–1542. doi: 10.1097/CCM.0b013e318287f54c
11. López-Herce J, del Castillo J, Matamoros M, Canadas S, Rodriguez-Calvo A, Cecchetti C, Rodríguez-Núnez A, Carrillo Á; Iberoamerican Pediatric Cardiac Arrest Study Network RIBEPCI. Post return of spontaneous circulation factors associated with mortality in pediatric in-hospital cardiac arrest: a prospective multicenter multinational observational study. *Crit Care.* 2014;18:607. doi: 10.1186/s13054-014-0607-9
12. Ferguson LP, Durward A, Tibby SM. Relationship between arterial partial oxygen pressure after resuscitation from cardiac arrest and mortality in children. *Circulation.* 2012;126:335–342. doi: 10.1161/CIRCULATIONAHA.111.085100
13. van Zellem L, de Jonge R, van Rosmalen J, Reiss I, Tibboel D, Buysse C. High cumulative oxygen levels are associated with improved survival of children treated with mild therapeutic hypothermia after cardiac arrest. *Resuscitation.* 2015;90:150–157. doi: 10.1016/j.resuscitation.2014.12.013
14. Del Castillo J, López-Herce J, Matamoros M, Cañadas S, Rodriguez-Calvo A, Cechetti C, Rodriguez-Núñez A, Alvarez AC; Iberoamerican Pediatric Cardiac Arrest Study Network RIBEPCI. Hyperoxia, hypocapnia and hypercapnia as outcome factors after cardiac arrest in children. *Resuscitation.* 2012;83:1456–1461. doi: 10.1016/j.resuscitation.2012.07.019
15. Herman ST, Abend NS, Bleck TP, Chapman KE, Drislane FW, Emerson RG, Gerard EE, Hahn CD, Husain AM, Kaplan PW, et al. Consensus statement on continuous EEG in critically ill adults and children, part I: indications. *J Clin Neurophysiol.* 2015;32:87–95. doi: 10.1097/wnp.0000000000000166
16. Abend NS, Topjian A, Ichord R, Herman ST, Helfaer M, Donnelly M, Nadkarni V, Dlugos DJ, Clancy RR. Electroencephalographic monitoring during hypothermia after pediatric cardiac arrest. *Neurology.* 2009;72:1931–1940. doi: 10.1212/WNL.0b013e3181a82687
17. Topjian AA, Gutierrez-Colina AM, Sanchez SM, Berg RA, Friess SH, Dlugos DJ, Abend NS. Electrographic status epilepticus is associated with mortality and worse short-term outcome in critically ill children. *Crit Care Med.* 2013;41:215–223. doi: 10.1097/CCM.0b013e3182668035
18. Ostendorf AP, Hartman ME, Friess SH. Early Electroencephalographic Findings Correlate With Neurologic Outcome in Children Following Cardiac Arrest. *Pediatr Crit Care Med.* 2016;17:667–676. doi: 10.1097/PCC.0000000000000791
19. Brophy GM, Bell R, Claassen J, Alldredge B, Bleck TP, Glauser T, Laroche SM, Riviello JJ Jr, Shutter L, Sperling MR, Treiman DM, Vespa PM; Neurocritical Care Society Status Epilepticus Guideline Writing Committee. Guidelines for the evaluation and management of status epilepticus. *Neurocrit Care.* 2012;17:3–23. doi: 10.1007/s12028-012-9695-z
20. Topjian AA, Sánchez SM, Shults J, Berg RA, Dlugos DJ, Abend NS. Early Electroencephalographic Background Features Predict Outcomes in Children Resuscitated From Cardiac Arrest. *Pediatr Crit Care Med.* 2016;17:547–557. doi: 10.1097/PCC.0000000000000740

PROGNOSTICATION FOLLOWING CARDIAC ARREST

Early and reliable prognostication of neurological outcome in pediatric survivors of cardiac arrest is essential to guide treatment, enable effective planning, and provide family support. Clinicians use patient and cardiac arrest characteristics, postarrest neurological examination, laboratory results, neurological imaging (eg, brain computed tomography and MRI), and EEG to guide prognostication. At this time, no single factor or validated decision rule has been identified to reliably predict either favorable or unfavorable outcome within 24 to 48 hours of ROSC. EEG, neuroimaging, and serum biomarkers when used alone predict outcome with only moderate accuracy, and more data are needed before applying these to individual patients.

Recommendations for Prognostication Following Cardiac Arrest

COR	LOE	Recommendations
2a	B-NR	1. EEG in the first week post cardiac arrest can be useful as 1 factor for prognostication, augmented by other information.[1–8]
2a	B-NR	2. It is reasonable for providers to consider multiple factors when predicting outcomes in infants and children who survive cardiac arrests.[1,7,9–21]
2a	B-NR	3. It is reasonable for providers to consider multiple factors when predicting outcomes in infants and children who survive cardiac arrests after nonfatal drowning (ie, survival to hospital admission).[22–39]

Recommendation-Specific Supportive Text

1. Eight retrospective observational studies demonstrate that EEG background patterns are associated with neurological outcomes at discharge.[1–8] The presence of sleep spindles,[3,4,8] normal background,[2] and reactivity[7,8] is associated with favorable outcomes. Burst suppression and flat or attenuated EEG patterns are associated with unfavorable neurological outcome.[1,2,5,8] However, these associations do not reach the high degrees of sensitivity and specificity needed to use EEG as a stand-alone modality for neuroprognostication.
2. Several studies demonstrate the association of clinical history, patient characteristics, physical examination, imaging, and biomarker data with neurological outcome following cardiac arrest.[1,7,9–19] To date, no single factor has demonstrated sufficient accuracy to prognosticate outcome. Elevated serum lactate, pH, or base deficit measured within the first 24 hours after cardiac arrest are associated with unfavorable outcome;[9,11,12,16–18,20,21] however, specific cutoff values are unknown.
3. Shorter submersion times are associated with better outcomes after pediatric nonfatal drowning.[22–25] There is no clear association between patient age,[23,26–31,38]water type,[30,32,33] water temperature,[23,25,34,35] emergency medical services response times[35,36] or witnessed status,[36–39] and neurological outcome following nonfatal drowning. No single factor accurately predicts prognosis after nonfatal drowning.

REFERENCES

1. Brooks GA, Park JT. Clinical and Electroencephalographic Correlates in Pediatric Cardiac Arrest: Experience at a Tertiary Care Center. *Neuropediatrics.* 2018;49:324–329. doi: 10.1055/s-0038-1657757
2. Topjian AA, Sánchez SM, Shults J, Berg RA, Dlugos DJ, Abend NS. Early Electroencephalographic Background Features Predict Outcomes in Children Resuscitated From Cardiac Arrest. *Pediatr Crit Care Med.* 2016;17:547–557. doi: 10.1097/PCC.0000000000000740
3. Ostendorf AP, Hartman ME, Friess SH. Early Electroencephalographic Findings Correlate With Neurologic Outcome in Children Following Cardiac Arrest. *Pediatr Crit Care Med.* 2016;17:667–676. doi: 10.1097/PCC.0000000000000791

4. Ducharme-Crevier L, Press CA, Kurz JE, Mills MG, Goldstein JL, Wainwright MS. Early Presence of Sleep Spindles on Electroencephalography Is Associated With Good Outcome After Pediatric Cardiac Arrest. *Pediatr Crit Care Med.* 2017;18:452–460. doi: 10.1097/PCC.0000000000001137
5. Bourgoin P, Barrault V, Joram N, Leclair Visonneau L, Toulgoat F, Anthoine E, Loron G, Chenouard A. The Prognostic Value of Early Amplitude-Integrated Electroencephalography Monitoring After Pediatric Cardiac Arrest. *Pediatr Crit Care Med.* 2020;21:248–255. doi: 10.1097/PCC.0000000000002171
6. Lee S, Zhao X, Davis KA, Topjian AA, Litt B, Abend NS. Quantitative EEG predicts outcomes in children after cardiac arrest. *Neurology.* 2019;92:e2329–e2338. doi: 10.1212/WNL.0000000000007504
7. Yang D, Ryoo E, Kim HJ. Combination of Early EEG, Brain CT, and Ammonia Level Is Useful to Predict Neurologic Outcome in Children Resuscitated From Cardiac Arrest. *Front Pediatr.* 2019;7:223. doi: 10.3389/fped.2019.00223
8. Fung FW, Topjian AA, Xiao R, Abend NS. Early EEG Features for Outcome Prediction After Cardiac Arrest in Children. *J Clin Neurophysiol.* 2019;36:349–357. doi: 10.1097/WNP.0000000000000591
9. Meert K, Telford R, Holubkov R, Slomine BS, Christensen JR, Berger J, Ofori-Amanfo G, Newth CJL, Dean JM, Moler FW. Paediatric in-hospital cardiac arrest: Factors associated with survival and neurobehavioural outcome one year later. *Resuscitation.* 2018;124:96–105. doi: 10.1016/j.resuscitation.2018.01.013
10. Ichord R, Silverstein FS, Slomine BS, Telford R, Christensen J, Holubkov R, Dean JM, Moler FW; THAPCA Trial Group. Neurologic outcomes in pediatric cardiac arrest survivors enrolled in the THAPCA trials. *Neurology.* 2018;91:e123–e131. doi: 10.1212/WNL.0000000000005773
11. Meert KL, Telford R, Holubkov R, Slomine BS, Christensen JR, Dean JM, Moler FW; Therapeutic Hypothermia after Pediatric Cardiac Arrest (THAPCA) Trial Investigators. Pediatric Out-of-Hospital Cardiac Arrest Characteristics and Their Association With Survival and Neurobehavioral Outcome. *Pediatr Crit Care Med.* 2016;17:e543–e550. doi: 10.1097/PCC.0000000000000969
12. Del Castillo J, López-Herce J, Matamoros M, Cañadas S, Rodríguez-Calvo A, Cecchetti C, Rodriguez-Núñez A, Álvarez AC; Iberoamerican Pediatric Cardiac Arrest Study Network RIBEPCI. Long-term evolution after in-hospital cardiac arrest in children: Prospective multicenter multinational study. *Resuscitation.* 2015;96:126–134. doi: 10.1016/j.resuscitation.2015.07.037
13. Topjian AA, Telford R, Holubkov R, Nadkarni VM, Berg RA, Dean JM, Moler FW; Therapeutic Hypothermia After Pediatric Cardiac Arrest (THAPCA) Trial Investigators. Association of Early Postresuscitation Hypotension With Survival to Discharge After Targeted Temperature Management for Pediatric Out-of-Hospital Cardiac Arrest: Secondary Analysis of a Randomized Clinical Trial. *JAMA Pediatr.* 2018;172:143–153. doi: 10.1001/jamapediatrics.2017.4043
14. Conlon TW, Falkensammer CB, Hammond RS, Nadkarni VM, Berg RA, Topjian AA. Association of left ventricular systolic function and vasopressor support with survival following pediatric out-of-hospital cardiac arrest. *Pediatr Crit Care Med.* 2015;16:146–154. doi: 10.1097/pcc.0000000000000305
15. Starling RM, Shekdar K, Licht D, Nadkarni VM, Berg RA, Topjian AA. Early Head CT Findings Are Associated With Outcomes After Pediatric Out-of-Hospital Cardiac Arrest. *Pediatr Crit Care Med.* 2015;16:542–548. doi: 10.1097/PCC.0000000000000404
16. Alsoufi B, Awan A, Manlhiot C, Guechef A, Al-Halees Z, Al-Ahmadi M, McCrindle BW, Kalloghlian A. Results of rapid-response extracorporeal cardiopulmonary resuscitation in children with refractory cardiac arrest following cardiac surgery. *Eur J Cardiothorac Surg.* 2014;45:268–275. doi: 10.1093/ejcts/ezt319
17. Polimenakos AC, Rizzo V, El-Zein CF, Ilbawi MN. Post-cardiotomy Rescue Extracorporeal Cardiopulmonary Resuscitation in Neonates with Single Ventricle After Intractable Cardiac Arrest: Attrition After Hospital Discharge and Predictors of Outcome. *Pediatr Cardiol.* 2017;38:314–323. doi: 10.1007/s00246-016-1515-3
18. Scholefield BR, Gao F, Duncan HP, Tasker RC, Parslow RC, Draper ES, McShane P, Davies P, Morris KP. Observational study of children admitted to United Kingdom and Republic of Ireland Paediatric Intensive Care Units after out-of-hospital cardiac arrest. *Resuscitation.* 2015;97:122–128. doi: 10.1016/j.resuscitation.2015.07.011
19. Kramer P, Miera O, Berger F, Schmitt K. Prognostic value of serum biomarkers of cerebral injury in classifying neurological outcome after paediatric resuscitation. *Resuscitation.* 2018;122:113–120. doi: 10.1016/j.resuscitation.2017.09.012
20. López-Herce J, del Castillo J, Matamoros M, Canadas S, Rodriguez-Calvo A, Cecchetti C, Rodríguez-Núnez A, Carrillo Á; Iberoamerican Pediatric Cardiac Arrest Study Network RIBEPCI. Post return of spontaneous circulation factors associated with mortality in pediatric in-hospital cardiac arrest: a prospective multicenter multinational observational study. *Crit Care.* 2014;18:607. doi: 10.1186/s13054-014-0607-9
21. Topjian AA, Clark AE, Casper TC, Berger JT, Schleien CL, Dean JM, Moler FW; Pediatric Emergency Care Applied Research Network. Early lactate elevations following resuscitation from pediatric cardiac arrest are associated with increased mortality*. *Pediatr Crit Care Med.* 2013;14:e380–e387. doi: 10.1097/PCC.0b013e3182976402
22. Kyriacou DN, Arcinue EL, Peek C, Kraus JF. Effect of immediate resuscitation on children with submersion injury. *Pediatrics.* 1994;94(2 Pt 1):137–142.
23. Suominen P, Baillie C, Korpela R, Rautanen S, Ranta S, Olkkola KT. Impact of age, submersion time and water temperature on outcome in near-drowning. *Resuscitation.* 2002;52:247–254. doi: 10.1016/s0300-9572(01)00478-6
24. Panzino F, Quintillá JM, Luaces C, Pou J. [Unintentional drowning by immersion. Epidemiological profile of victims attended in 21 Spanish emergency departments]. *An Pediatr (Barc).* 2013;78:178–184. doi: 10.1016/j.anpedi.2012.06.014
25. Quan L, Mack CD, Schiff MA. Association of water temperature and submersion duration and drowning outcome. *Resuscitation.* 2014;85:790–794. doi: 10.1016/j.resuscitation.2014.02.024
26. Frates RC Jr. Analysis of predictive factors in the assessment of warm-water near-drowning in children. *Am J Dis Child.* 1981;135:1006–1008. doi: 10.1001/archpedi.1981.02130350010004
27. Nagel FO, Kibel SM, Beatty DW. Childhood near-drowning–factors associated with poor outcome. *S Afr Med J.* 1990;78:422–425.
28. Quan L, Wentz KR, Gore EJ, Copass MK. Outcome and predictors of outcome in pediatric submersion victims receiving prehospital care in King County, Washington. *Pediatrics.* 1990;86:586–593.
29. Niu YW, Cherng WS, Lin MT, Tsao LY. An analysis of prognostic factors for submersion accidents in children. *Zhonghua Min Guo Xiao Er Ke Yi Xue Hui Za Zhi.* 1992;33:81–88.
30. Mizuta R, Fujita H, Osamura T, Kidowaki T, Kiyosawa N. Childhood drownings and near-drownings in Japan. *Acta Paediatr Jpn.* 1993;35:186–192. doi: 10.1111/j.1442-200x.1993.tb03036.x
31. Al-Mofadda SM, Nassar A, Al-Turki A, Al-Sallounm AA. Pediatric near drowning: the experience of King Khalid University Hospital. *Ann Saudi Med.* 2001;21:300–303. doi: 10.5144/0256-4947.2001.300
32. Forler J, Carsin A, Arlaud K, Bosdure E, Viard L, Paut O, Camboulives J, Dubus JC. [Respiratory complications of accidental drownings in children]. *Arch Pediatr.* 2010;17:14–18. doi: 10.1016/j.arcped.2009.09.021
33. Al-Qurashi FO, Yousef AA, Aljoudi A, Alzahrani SM, Al-Jawder NY, Al-Ahmar AK, Al-Majed MS, Abouollo HM. A Review of Nonfatal Drowning in the Pediatric-Age Group: A 10-Year Experience at a University Hospital in Saudi Arabia. *Pediatr Emerg Care.* 2019;35:782–786. doi: 10.1097/PEC.0000000000001232
34. Kieboom JK, Verkade HJ, Burgerhof JG, Bierens JJ, Rheenen PF, Kneyber MC, Albers MJ. Outcome after resuscitation beyond 30 minutes in drowned children with cardiac arrest and hypothermia: Dutch nationwide retrospective cohort study. *BMJ.* 2015;350:h418. doi: 10.1136/bmj.h418
35. Claesson A, Lindqvist J, Ortenwall P, Herlitz J. Characteristics of lifesaving from drowning as reported by the Swedish Fire and Rescue Services 1996–2010. *Resuscitation.* 2012;83:1072–1077. doi: 10.1016/j.resuscitation.2012.05.025
36. Claesson A, Svensson L, Silfverstolpe J, Herlitz J. Characteristics and outcome among patients suffering out-of-hospital cardiac arrest due to drowning. *Resuscitation.* 2008;76:381–387. doi: 10.1016/j.resuscitation.2007.09.003
37. Dyson K, Morgans A, Bray J, Matthews B, Smith K. Drowning related out-of-hospital cardiac arrests: characteristics and outcomes. *Resuscitation.* 2013;84:1114–1118. doi: 10.1016/j.resuscitation.2013.01.020
38. Nitta M, Kitamura T, Iwami T, Nadkarni VM, Berg RA, Topjian AA, Okamoto Y, Nishiyama C, Nishiuchi T, Hayashi Y, Nishimoto Y, Takasu A. Out-of-hospital cardiac arrest due to drowning among children and adults from the Utstein Osaka Project. *Resuscitation.* 2013;84:1568–1573. doi: 10.1016/j.resuscitation.2013.06.017
39. Claesson A, Lindqvist J, Herlitz J. Cardiac arrest due to drowning–changes over time and factors of importance for survival. *Resuscitation.* 2014;85:644–648. doi: 10.1016/j.resuscitation.2014.02.006

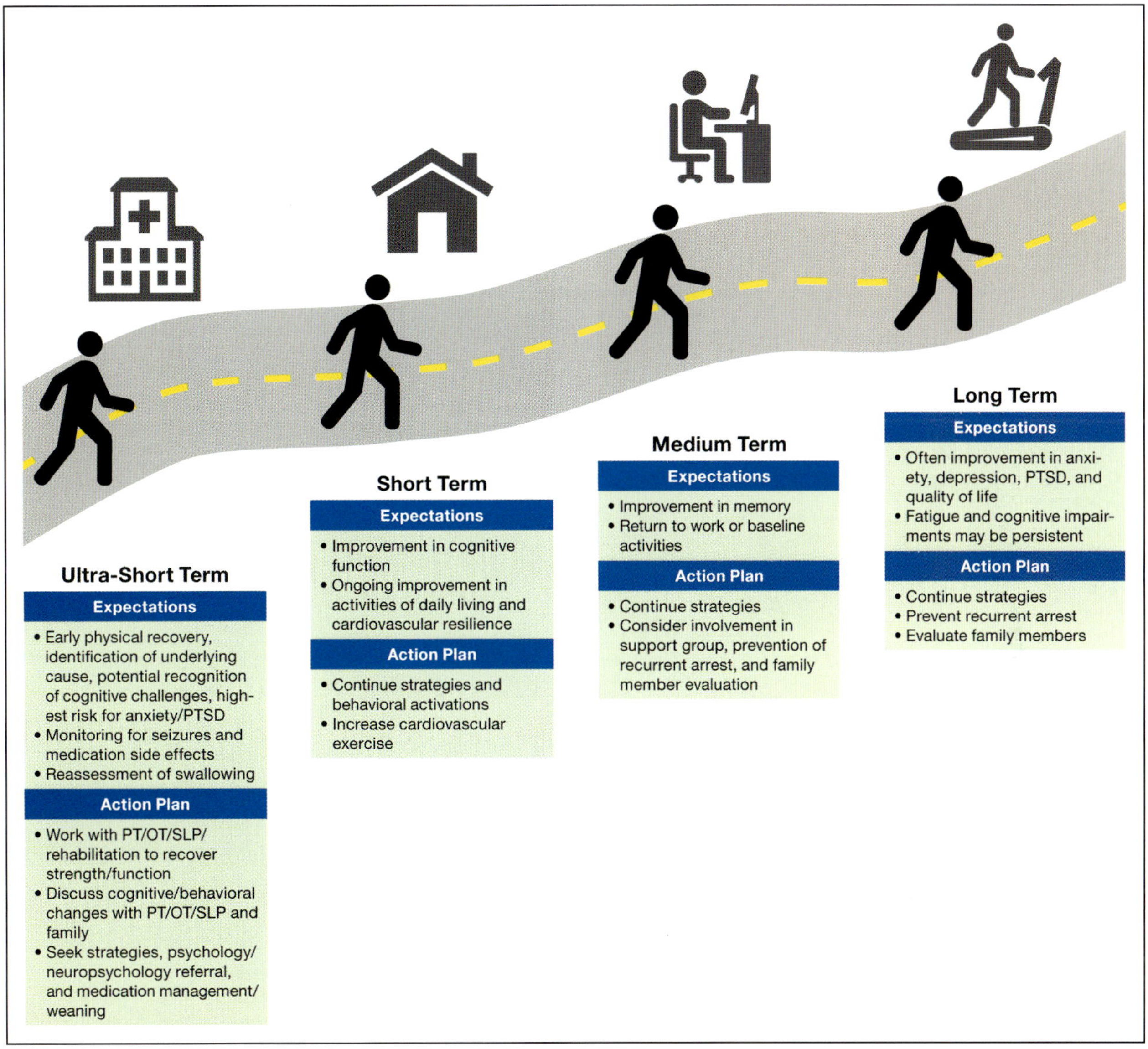

Figure 9. **Road map to recovery.**[3]

POST–CARDIAC ARREST RECOVERY

Survivors are at significant risk for both short-term and long-term physical, neurological, cognitive, emotional, and social morbidity.[3] Many children who survive a cardiac arrest with a grossly "favorable outcome" have more subtle and sustained neuropsychological impairment.[4] The full impact of brain injury on children's development may not be fully appreciated until months to years after the cardiac arrest. Furthermore, because children are raised by caregivers, the impact of morbidity following cardiac arrest affects not only the child but also the family.

Recovery has been introduced as the sixth link in the Chain of Survival to acknowledge that survivors of cardiac arrest may require ongoing integrated medical, rehabilitative, caregiver, and community support in the months to years after their cardiac arrest (see Figure 9).[3] Recent scientific statements from the AHA and ILCOR highlight the importance of studying long-term neurological and health-related quality-of-life outcomes.[5,6]

Recommendations for Post–Cardiac Arrest Recovery		
COR	**LOE**	**Recommendations**
1	C-LD	1. It is recommended that pediatric cardiac arrest survivors be evaluated for rehabilitation services.[4,7–11]
2a	C-LD	2. It is reasonable to refer pediatric cardiac arrest survivors for ongoing neurological evaluation for at least the first year after cardiac arrest.[3,5,10–15]

Recommendation-Specific Supportive Text

1. Two randomized controlled trials of TTM for comatose children after IHCA or OHCA with a primary outcome of neurobehavioral outcome at 1 year[7,8] showed that new morbidity is common.[9–11] Many children who survived to 1 year with a

favorable neurobehavioral outcome on Vineland Adaptive Behavior Scales-II (VABS-II) had global cognitive impairment or selective neuropsychological deficits.[4]

2. Two randomized controlled trials of TTM for pediatric cardiac arrest demonstrated that neurological function improves for some survivors during the first year after cardiac arrest.[10,11] Several case series of longer-term outcomes (more than 1 year after cardiac arrest) demonstrate ongoing cognitive, physical, and neuropsychological impairments.[12–14] Recent statements from the AHA highlight the importance of follow-up after discharge, because patient recovery continues during the first year after cardiac arrest.[3,5,6,15] It is unclear what impact ongoing childhood development has on recovery following pediatric cardiac arrest.

REFERENCES

1. Deleted in proof.
2. Deleted in proof.
3. Sawyer KN, Camp-Rogers TR, Kotini-Shah P, Del Rios M, Gossip MR, Moitra VK, Haywood KL, Dougherty CM, Lubitz SA, Rabinstein AA, Rittenberger JC, Callaway CW, Abella BS, Geocadin RG, Kurz MC; American Heart Association Emergency Cardiovascular Care Committee; Council on Cardiovascular and Stroke Nursing; Council on Genomic and Precision Medicine; Council on Quality of Care and Outcomes Research; and Stroke Council. Sudden Cardiac Arrest Survivorship: A Scientific Statement From the American Heart Association. *Circulation.* 2020;141:e654–e685. doi: 10.1161/CIR.0000000000000747
4. Slomine BS, Silverstein FS, Christensen JR, Page K, Holubkov R, Dean JM, Moler FW. Neuropsychological Outcomes of Children 1 Year After Pediatric Cardiac Arrest: Secondary Analysis of 2 Randomized Clinical Trials. *JAMA Neurol.* 2018;75:1502–1510. doi: 10.1001/jamaneurol.2018.2628
5. Geocadin RG, Callaway CW, Fink EL, Golan E, Greer DM, Ko NU, Lang E, Licht DJ, Marino BS, McNair ND, Peberdy MA, Perman SM, Sims DB, Soar J, Sandroni C; American Heart Association Emergency Cardiovascular Care Committee. Standards for Studies of Neurological Prognostication in Comatose Survivors of Cardiac Arrest: A Scientific Statement From the American Heart Association. *Circulation.* 2019;140:e517–e542. doi: 10.1161/CIR.0000000000000702
6. Topjian AA, Scholefield BR, Pinto NP, Fink EL, Buysse CMP, Haywood K, Maconochie I, Nadkarni VM, de Caen A, Escalante-Kanashiro R, Ng K-C, Nuthall G, Reis AG, Van de Voorde P, Suskauer SJ, Schexnayder SM, Hazinski MF, Slomine BS. P-COSCA (Pediatric Core Outcome Set for Cardiac Arrest) in children: an advisory statement from the International Liaison Committee on Resuscitation. *Circulation.* 2020;142:e000–e000. doi: 10.1161/CIR.0000000000000911
7. Moler FW, Silverstein FS, Holubkov R, Slomine BS, Christensen JR, Nadkarni VM, Meert KL, Clark AE, Browning B, Pemberton VL, Page K, Shankaran S, Hutchison JS, Newth CJ, Bennett KS, Berger JT, Topjian A, Pineda JA, Koch JD, Schleien CL, Dalton HJ, Ofori-Amanfo G, Goodman DM, Fink EL, McQuillen P, Zimmerman JJ, Thomas NJ, van der Jagt EW, Porter MB, Meyer MT, Harrison R, Pham N, Schwarz AJ, Nowak JE, Alten J, Wheeler DS, Bhalala US, Lidsky K, Lloyd E, Mathur M, Shah S, Wu T, Theodorou AA, Sanders RC Jr, Dean JM; THAPCA Trial Investigators. Therapeutic hypothermia after out-of-hospital cardiac arrest in children. *N Engl J Med.* 2015;372:1898–1908. doi: 10.1056/NEJMoa1411480
8. Moler FW, Silverstein FS, Holubkov R, Slomine BS, Christensen JR, Nadkarni VM, Meert KL, Browning B, Pemberton VL, Page K, et al; on behalf of the THAPCA Trial Investigators. Therapeutic hypothermia after in-hospital cardiac arrest in children. *N Engl J Med.* 2017;376:318–329. doi: 10.1056/NEJMoa1610493
9. Slomine BS, Silverstein FS, Page K, Holubkov R, Christensen JR, Dean JM, Moler FW; Therapeutic Hypothermia after Pediatric Cardiac Arrest (THAPCA) Trial Investigators. Relationships between three and twelve month outcomes in children enrolled in the therapeutic hypothermia after pediatric cardiac arrest trials. *Resuscitation.* 2019;139:329–336. doi: 10.1016/j.resuscitation.2019.03.020
10. Slomine BS, Silverstein FS, Christensen JR, Holubkov R, Telford R, Dean JM, Moler FW; Therapeutic Hypothermia after Paediatric Cardiac Arrest (THAPCA) Trial Investigators. Neurobehavioural outcomes in children after In-Hospital cardiac arrest. *Resuscitation.* 2018;124:80–89. doi: 10.1016/j.resuscitation.2018.01.002
11. Slomine BS, Silverstein FS, Christensen JR, Holubkov R, Page K, Dean JM, Moler FW; on behalf of the THAPCA Trial Group. Neurobehavioral outcomes in children after out-of-hospital cardiac arrest. *Pediatrics.* 2016;137:e20153412. doi: 10.1542/peds.2015-3412
12. van Zellem L, Buysse C, Madderom M, Legerstee JS, Aarsen F, Tibboel D, Utens EM. Long-term neuropsychological outcomes in children and adolescents after cardiac arrest. *Intensive Care Med.* 2015;41:1057–1066. doi: 10.1007/s00134-015-3789-y
13. van Zellem L, Utens EM, Legerstee JS, Cransberg K, Hulst JM, Tibboel D, Buysse C. Cardiac Arrest in Children: Long-Term Health Status and Health-Related Quality of Life. *Pediatr Crit Care Med.* 2015;16:693–702. doi: 10.1097/PCC.0000000000000452
14. van Zellem L, Utens EM, Madderom M, Legerstee JS, Aarsen F, Tibboel D, Buysse C. Cardiac arrest in infants, children, and adolescents: long-term emotional and behavioral functioning. *Eur J Pediatr.* 2016;175:977–986. doi: 10.1007/s00431-016-2728-4
15. Topjian AA, de Caen A, Wainwright MS, Abella BS, Abend NS, Atkins DL, Bembea MM, Fink EL, Guerguerian AM, Haskell SE, Kilgannon JH, Lasa JJ, Hazinski MF. Pediatric Post-Cardiac Arrest Care: A Scientific Statement From the American Heart Association. *Circulation.* 2019;140:e194–e233. doi: 10.1161/CIR.0000000000000697

FAMILY PRESENCE DURING RESUSCITATION

Over the past 20 years, the practice of maintaining family presence during resuscitation has increased. Most parents surveyed indicate that they would desire to be present during their child's resuscitation. Older data suggest a lower incidence of anxiety and depression and more constructive grief behaviors among parents who were present when their child died.[1]

Recommendations for Family Presence During Resuscitation

COR	LOE	Recommendations
1	B-NR	1. Whenever possible, provide family members with the option of being present during the resuscitation of their infant or child.[2–10]
1	B-NR	2. When family members are present during resuscitation, it is beneficial for a designated team member to provide comfort, answer questions, and support the family.[11,12]
1	C-LD	3. If the presence of family members is considered detrimental to the resuscitation, family members should be asked in a respectful manner to leave.[13,14]

Recommendation-Specific Supportive Text

1. Qualitative studies generally show that there can be benefits for families if they are permitted to be present during the resuscitation of their children. Parents stated that they believed their presence brought their child comfort and that it helped them to adjust to the loss of their child.[2] Other surveys of parents reported that they desired to be present to understand what was happening, to know that all that could be done was being done, and to

keep physical contact with their child.[3,4] However, not all parents who were present for their child's resuscitation would choose to do so again.[5] Some concerns have been raised about family presence during resuscitation, such as trauma for the family, interference with procedures, impact on technical performance, and concern for teaching and clinical decision-making, but these have not been supported by the available evidence.[6–8] Experienced providers are more likely than trainees to support family presence.[9,10]

2. The presence of a facilitator to support the family is helpful.[11,12] It is important that the family have a dedicated team member during the resuscitation to help process the traumatic event, but this is not always feasible. Lack of an available facilitator should not prevent family presence at the resuscitation.
3. Most surveys indicate family presence is not disruptive during resuscitation, although some providers feel increased stress.[13] Providers with significant experience with family presence acknowledge occasional negative experiences.[14]

REFERENCES

1. Robinson SM, Mackenzie-Ross S, Campbell Hewson GL, Egleston CV, Prevost AT. Psychological effect of witnessed resuscitation on bereaved relatives. *Lancet.* 1998;352:614–617. doi: 10.1016/s0140-6736(97)12179-1
2. Tinsley C, Hill JB, Shah J, Zimmerman G, Wilson M, Freier K, Abd-Allah S. Experience of families during cardiopulmonary resuscitation in a pediatric intensive care unit. *Pediatrics.* 2008;122:e799–e804. doi: 10.1542/peds.2007-3650
3. Maxton FJ. Parental presence during resuscitation in the PICU: the parents' experience. Sharing and surviving the resuscitation: a phenomenological study. *J Clin Nurs.* 2008;17:3168–3176. doi: 10.1111/j.1365-2702.2008.02525.x
4. Stewart SA. Parents' Experience During a Child's Resuscitation: Getting Through It. *J Pediatr Nurs.* 2019;47:58–67. doi: 10.1016/j.pedn.2019.04.019
5. Curley MA, Meyer EC, Scoppettuolo LA, McGann EA, Trainor BP, Rachwal CM, Hickey PA. Parent presence during invasive procedures and resuscitation: evaluating a clinical practice change. *Am J Respir Crit Care Med.* 2012;186:1133–1139. doi: 10.1164/rccm.201205-0915OC
6. McClenathan BM, Torrington KG, Uyehara CF. Family member presence during cardiopulmonary resuscitation: a survey of US and international critical care professionals. *Chest.* 2002;122:2204–2211. doi: 10.1378/chest.122.6.2204
7. Vavarouta A, Xanthos T, Papadimitriou L, Kouskouni E, Iacovidou N. Family presence during resuscitation and invasive procedures: physicians' and nurses' attitudes working in pediatric departments in Greece. *Resuscitation.* 2011;82:713–716. doi: 10.1016/j.resuscitation.2011.02.011
8. Pasek TA, Licata J. Parent Advocacy Group for Events of Resuscitation. *Crit Care Nurse.* 2016;36:58–64. doi: 10.4037/ccn2016759
9. Fein JA, Ganesh J, Alpern ER. Medical staff attitudes toward family presence during pediatric procedures. *Pediatr Emerg Care.* 2004;20:224–227. doi: 10.1097/01.pec.0000121241.99242.3b
10. Bradford KK, Kost S, Selbst SM, Renwick AE, Pratt A. Family member presence for procedures: the resident's perspective. *Ambul Pediatr.* 2005;5:294–297. doi: 10.1367/A04-024R1.1
11. Jarvis AS. Parental presence during resuscitation: attitudes of staff on a paediatric intensive care unit. *Intensive Crit Care Nurs.* 1998;14:3–7. doi: 10.1016/s0964-3397(98)80029-3
12. Zavotsky KE, McCoy J, Bell G, Haussman K, Joiner J, Marcoux KK, Magarelli K, Mahoney K, Maldonado L, Mastro KA, Milloria A, Tamburri LM, Tortajada D. Resuscitation team perceptions of family presence during CPR. *Adv Emerg Nurs J.* 2014;36:325–334. doi: 10.1097/TME.0000000000000027
13. Kuzin JK, Yborra JG, Taylor MD, Chang AC, Altman CA, Whitney GM, Mott AR. Family-member presence during interventions in the intensive care unit: perceptions of pediatric cardiac intensive care providers. *Pediatrics.* 2007;120:e895–e901. doi: 10.1542/peds.2006-2943
14. Fulbrook P, Latour JM, Albarran JW. Paediatric critical care nurses' attitudes and experiences of parental presence during cardiopulmonary resuscitation: a European survey. *Int J Nurs Stud.* 2007;44:1238–1249. doi: 10.1016/j.ijnurstu.2006.05.006

EVALUATION OF SUDDEN UNEXPLAINED CARDIAC ARREST

Hypertrophic cardiomyopathy, coronary artery anomalies, and arrhythmias are common causes of sudden unexplained cardiac arrest in infants and children. Up to one third of young patients who do not survive sudden unexplained cardiac arrest have no abnormalities found on gross and microscopic autopsy.[1–4] Postmortem genetic evaluation ("molecular autopsy") is increasingly used to inform etiology of sudden unexplained cardiac arrest.[5] In addition to providing an explanation for the arrest, genetic diagnosis can identify inheritable cardiac disease, such as channelopathy and cardiomyopathy, enabling screening and preventive measures for relatives.

Recommendations for the Evaluation of Sudden Unexplained Cardiac Arrest

COR	LOE	Recommendations
1	C-EO	1. All infants, children, and adolescents with sudden unexpected cardiac arrest should, when resources allow, have an unrestricted, complete autopsy, preferably performed by a pathologist with training and experience in cardiovascular pathology. Consider appropriate preservation of biological material for genetic analysis to determine the presence of inherited cardiac disease.[6–21]
1	C-EO	2. Refer families of patients who do not have a cause of death found on autopsy to a healthcare provider or center with expertise in inherited cardiac disease and cardiac genetic counseling.[6–12,17,18,20–25]
1	C-EO	3. For infants, children and adolescents who survive sudden unexplained cardiac arrest, obtain a complete past medical and family history (including a history of syncopal episodes, seizures, unexplained accidents or drowning, or sudden unexpected death before 50 yr of age), review previous electrocardiograms, and refer to a cardiologist.[16,17,19–21]

Recommendation-Specific Supportive Text

1. In 7 cohort studies, mutations causing channelopathies were identified in 2% to 10% of infants with sudden infant death syndrome.[6–12] Among children and adolescents with sudden unexplained cardiac arrest and a normal autopsy, 9 cohort studies report identification of genetic mutations associated with channelopathy or cardiomyopathy.[13–21]

2. In 7 cohort studies[17,18,20,22–25] and 1 population-based study[21] of screening using clinical and laboratory (electrocardiographic, molecular genetic screening) investigations, 14% to 53% of first- and second-degree relatives of patients with sudden unexplained cardiac arrest had inherited, arrhythmogenic disorders. In 7 cohort studies, mutations causing channelopathies were identified in 2% to 10% of infants with sudden infant death syndrome.[6–12]
3. Several cohort studies report the utility of obtaining a complete past medical and family history after sudden unexplained cardiac arrest as well as review of prior electrocardiograms. A small case series suggested that specific genetic screening of family members was directed by the clinical history.[20] Three small cohort studies and 1 population-based study reported relevant clinical symptoms or medical comorbidities, such as seizure, syncope, palpitations, chest pain, left arm pain, and shortness of breath, among patients who had a sudden unexplained cardiac arrest and their family members.[16,17,19,21]

REFERENCES

1. Doolan A, Langlois N, Semsarian C. Causes of sudden cardiac death in young Australians. *Med J Aust.* 2004;180:110–112.
2. Eckart RE, Scoville SL, Campbell CL, Shry EA, Stajduhar KC, Potter RN, Pearse LA, Virmani R. Sudden death in young adults: a 25-year review of autopsies in military recruits. *Ann Intern Med.* 2004;141:829–834. doi: 10.7326/0003-4819-141-11-200412070-00005
3. Ong ME, Stiell I, Osmond MH, Nesbitt L, Gerein R, Campbell S, McLellan B; OPALS Study Group. Etiology of pediatric out-of-hospital cardiac arrest by coroner's diagnosis. *Resuscitation.* 2006;68:335–342. doi: 10.1016/j.resuscitation.2005.05.026
4. Puranik R, Chow CK, Duflou JA, Kilborn MJ, McGuire MA. Sudden death in the young. *Heart Rhythm.* 2005;2:1277–1282. doi: 10.1016/j.hrthm.2005.09.008
5. Torkamani A, Muse ED, Spencer EG, Rueda M, Wagner GN, Lucas JR, Topol EJ. Molecular Autopsy for Sudden Unexpected Death. *JAMA.* 2016; 316:1492–1494. doi: 10.1001/jama.2016.11445
6. Ackerman MJ, Siu BL, Sturner WQ, Tester DJ, Valdivia CR, Makielski JC, Towbin JA. Postmortem molecular analysis of SCN5A defects in sudden infant death syndrome. *JAMA.* 2001;286:2264–2269. doi: 10.1001/jama.286.18.2264
7. Arnestad M, Crotti L, Rognum TO, Insolia R, Pedrazzini M, Ferrandi C, Vege A, Wang DW, Rhodes TE, George AL Jr, Schwartz PJ. Prevalence of long-QT syndrome gene variants in sudden infant death syndrome. *Circulation.* 2007;115:361–367. doi: 10.1161/CIRCULATIONAHA.106.658021
8. Cronk LB, Ye B, Kaku T, Tester DJ, Vatta M, Makielski JC, Ackerman MJ. Novel mechanism for sudden infant death syndrome: persistent late sodium current secondary to mutations in caveolin-3. *Heart Rhythm.* 2007;4:161–166. doi: 10.1016/j.hrthm.2006.11.030
9. Millat G, Kugener B, Chevalier P, Chahine M, Huang H, Malicier D, Rodriguez-Lafrasse C, Rousson R. Contribution of long-QT syndrome genetic variants in sudden infant death syndrome. *Pediatr Cardiol.* 2009;30:502–509. doi: 10.1007/s00246-009-9417-2
10. Otagiri T, Kijima K, Osawa M, Ishii K, Makita N, Matoba R, Umetsu K, Hayasaka K. Cardiac ion channel gene mutations in sudden infant death syndrome. *Pediatr Res.* 2008;64:482–487. doi: 10.1203/PDR.0b013e3181841eca
11. Plant LD, Bowers PN, Liu Q, Morgan T, Zhang T, State MW, Chen W, Kittles RA, Goldstein SA. A common cardiac sodium channel variant associated with sudden infant death in African Americans, SCN5A S1103Y. *J Clin Invest.* 2006;116:430–435. doi: 10.1172/JCI25618
12. Tester DJ, Dura M, Carturan E, Reiken S, Wronska A, Marks AR, Ackerman MJ. A mechanism for sudden infant death syndrome (SIDS): stress-induced leak via ryanodine receptors. *Heart Rhythm.* 2007;4:733–739. doi: 10.1016/j.hrthm.2007.02.026
13. Albert CM, Nam EG, Rimm EB, Jin HW, Hajjar RJ, Hunter DJ, MacRae CA, Ellinor PT. Cardiac sodium channel gene variants and sudden cardiac death in women. *Circulation.* 2008;117:16–23. doi: 10.1161/CIRCULATIONAHA.107.736330
14. Chugh SS, Senashova O, Watts A, Tran PT, Zhou Z, Gong Q, Titus JL, Hayflick SJ. Postmortem molecular screening in unexplained sudden death. *J Am Coll Cardiol.* 2004;43:1625–1629. doi: 10.1016/j.jacc.2003.11.052
15. Tester DJ, Spoon DB, Valdivia HH, Makielski JC, Ackerman MJ. Targeted mutational analysis of the RyR2-encoded cardiac ryanodine receptor in sudden unexplained death: a molecular autopsy of 49 medical examiner/coroner's cases. *Mayo Clin Proc.* 2004;79:1380–1384. doi: 10.4065/79.11.1380
16. Scheiper S, Ramos-Luis E, Blanco-Verea A, Niess C, Beckmann BM, Schmidt U, Kettner M, Geisen C, Verhoff MA, Brion M, Kauferstein S. Sudden unexpected death in the young - Value of massive parallel sequencing in postmortem genetic analyses. *Forensic Sci Int.* 2018;293:70–76. doi: 10.1016/j.forsciint.2018.09.034
17. Hellenthal N, Gaertner-Rommel A, Klauke B, Paluszkiewicz L, Stuhr M, Kerner T, Farr M, Püschel K, Milting H. Molecular autopsy of sudden unexplained deaths reveals genetic predispositions for cardiac diseases among young forensic cases. *Europace.* 2017;19:1881–1890. doi: 10.1093/europace/euw247
18. Jiménez-Jáimez J, Alcalde Martínez V, Jiménez Fernández M, Bermúdez Jiménez F, Rodríguez Vázquez Del Rey MDM, Perin F, Oyonarte Ramírez JM, López Fernández S, de la Torre I, García Orta R, González Molina M, Cabrerizo EM, Álvarez Abril B, Álvarez M, Macías Ruiz R, Correa C, Tercedor L. Clinical and Genetic Diagnosis of Nonischemic Sudden Cardiac Death. *Rev Esp Cardiol (Engl Ed).* 2017;70:808–816. doi: 10.1016/j.rec.2017.04.024
19. Lahrouchi N, Raju H, Lodder EM, Papatheodorou E, Ware JS, Papadakis M, Tadros R, Cole D, Skinner JR, Crawford J, Love DR, Pua CJ, Soh BY, Bhalshankar JD, Govind R, Tfelt-Hansen J, Winkel BG, van der Werf C, Wijeyeratne YD, Mellor G, Till J, Cohen MC, Tome-Esteban M, Sharma S, Wilde AAM, Cook SA, Bezzina CR, Sheppard MN, Behr ER. Utility of Post-Mortem Genetic Testing in Cases of Sudden Arrhythmic Death Syndrome. *J Am Coll Cardiol.* 2017;69:2134–2145. doi: 10.1016/j.jacc.2017.02.046
20. Anastasakis A, Papatheodorou E, Ritsatos K, Protonotarios N, Rentoumi V, Gatzoulis K, Antoniades L, Agapitos E, Koutsaftis P, Spiliopoulou C, Tousoulis D. Sudden unexplained death in the young: epidemiology, aetiology and value of the clinically guided genetic screening. *Europace.* 2018;20:472–480. doi: 10.1093/europace/euw362
21. Hendrix A, Borleffs CJ, Vink A, Doevendans PA, Wilde AA, van Langen IM, van der Smagt JJ, Bots ML, Mosterd A. Cardiogenetic screening of first-degree relatives after sudden cardiac death in the young: a population-based approach. *Europace.* 2011;13:716–722. doi: 10.1093/europace/euq460
22. Behr E, Wood DA, Wright M, Syrris P, Sheppard MN, Casey A, Davies MJ, McKenna W; Sudden Arrhythmic Death Syndrome Steering Group. Cardiological assessment of first-degree relatives in sudden arrhythmic death syndrome. *Lancet.* 2003;362:1457–1459. doi: 10.1016/s0140-6736(03)14692-2
23. Behr ER, Dalageorgou C, Christiansen M, Syrris P, Hughes S, Tome Esteban MT, Rowland E, Jeffery S, McKenna WJ. Sudden arrhythmic death syndrome: familial evaluation identifies inheritable heart disease in the majority of families. *Eur Heart J.* 2008;29:1670–1680. doi: 10.1093/eurheartj/ehn219
24. Hofman N, Tan HL, Clur SA, Alders M, van Langen IM, Wilde AA. Contribution of inherited heart disease to sudden cardiac death in childhood. *Pediatrics.* 2007;120:e967–e973. doi: 10.1542/peds.2006-3751
25. Tan HL, Hofman N, van Langen IM, van der Wal AC, Wilde AA. Sudden unexplained death: heritability and diagnostic yield of cardiological and genetic examination in surviving relatives. *Circulation.* 2005;112:207–213. doi: 10.1161/CIRCULATIONAHA.104.522581

RESUSCITATING THE PATIENT IN SHOCK

Shock is the failure of oxygen delivery to meet tissue metabolic demands and can be life threatening. The most common type of pediatric shock is hypovolemic, including shock due to hemorrhage. Distributive, cardiogenic, and obstructive shock occur less frequently. Often, multiple types of shock can occur simultaneously; thus, providers should be vigilant. Cardiogenic shock in its early stages can be difficult to diagnose, so a high index of suspicion is warranted.

Shock progresses over a continuum of severity, from a compensated to a decompensated (hypotensive) state. Compensatory mechanisms include tachycardia and increased systemic vascular resistance (vasoconstriction) in an effort to maintain cardiac output and end-organ perfusion. As compensatory mechanisms fail, hypotension and signs of inadequate end-organ perfusion develop, such as depressed mental status, decreased urine output, lactic acidosis, and weak central pulses.

Early administration of intravenous fluids to treat septic shock has been widely accepted based on limited evidence. Mortality from pediatric sepsis has declined in recent years, concurrent with implementation of guidelines emphasizing the role of early antibiotic and fluid administration.[1] Controversies in the management of septic shock include volume of fluid administration and how to assess the patient's response, the timing and choice of vasopressor agents, the use of corticosteroids, and modifications to treatment algorithms for patients in sepsis-related cardiac arrest. Previous AHA guidelines[2] have considered large studies of patients with malaria, sickle cell anemia, and dengue shock syndrome; however, these patients require special consideration that make generalization of results from these studies problematic.

Resuscitation guidance for children with hemorrhagic shock is evolving, as crystalloid-then-blood paradigms are being challenged by resuscitation protocols using blood products early in resuscitation. However, the ideal resuscitation strategy for a given type of injury is often unknown.

Fluid Resuscitation in Shock

Recommendations for Fluid Resuscitation in Shock

COR	LOE	Recommendations
1	C-LD	1. Providers should reassess the patient after every fluid bolus to assess for fluid responsiveness and for signs of volume overload.[3–5]
2a	B-R	2. Either isotonic crystalloids or colloids can be effective as the initial fluid choice for resuscitation.[6]
2a	B-NR	3. Either balanced or unbalanced solutions can be effective as the fluid choice for resuscitation.[7–9]
2a	C-LD	4. In patients with septic shock, it is reasonable to administer fluid in 10-mL/kg or 20-mL/kg aliquots with frequent reassessment.[4]

Recommendation-Specific Supportive Text

1. Although fluids remain the mainstay initial therapy for infants and children in shock, especially in hypovolemic and septic shock, fluid overload can lead to increased morbidity.[3] In 2 randomized trials of patients with septic shock, those who received higher fluid volumes[4] or faster fluid resuscitation[5] were more likely to develop clinically significant fluid overload characterized by increased rates of mechanical ventilation and worsening oxygenation.
2. In a systematic review, 12 relevant studies were identified, though 11 assessed colloid or crystalloid fluid resuscitation in patients with malaria, dengue shock syndrome, or "febrile illness" in sub-Saharan Africa.[6] There was no clear benefit to crystalloid or colloid solutions as first-line fluid therapy in any of the identified studies.
3. One pragmatic, randomized controlled trial compared the use of balanced (lactated Ringer's solution) to unbalanced (0.9% saline) crystalloid solutions as the initial resuscitation fluid and showed no difference in relevant clinical outcomes.[7] A matched retrospective cohort study of pediatric patients with septic shock showed no difference in outcomes,[8] though a propensity-matched database study showed an association with increased 72-hour mortality and vasoactive infusion days with unbalanced crystalloid fluid resuscitation.[9]
4. In a small, randomized controlled study, there were no significant differences in outcomes with the use of 20 mL/kg as the initial fluid bolus volume (compared with 10 mL/kg); however, the study was limited by a small sample size.[4]

Resuscitating a Patient in Septic Shock

Recommendations for Resuscitating a Patient in Septic Shock

COR	LOE	Recommendations
2a	C-LD	1. In infants and children with fluid-refractory septic shock, it is reasonable to use either epinephrine or norepinephrine as an initial vasoactive infusion.[1,10–14]
2a	C-EO	2. For infants and children with cardiac arrest and sepsis, it is reasonable to apply the standard pediatric advanced life support algorithm compared with any unique approach for sepsis-associated cardiac arrest.[15]
2b	B-NR	3. For infants and children with septic shock unresponsive to fluids and requiring vasoactive support, it may be reasonable to consider stress-dose corticosteroids.[12,16–19]
2b	C-LD	4. In infants and children with fluid-refractory septic shock, if epinephrine or norepinephrine are unavailable, dopamine may be considered.[10–12]

Recommendation-Specific Supportive Text

1. Two randomized controlled trials comparing escalating doses of dopamine or epinephrine demonstrated improvement in timing of resolution of shock[10] and 28-day mortality[11] with the use of epinephrine

over dopamine. Both studies were conducted in resource-limited settings, and the doses of inotropes used may not have been directly comparable, limiting conclusions from the studies. Medications that increase systemic vascular resistance, such as norepinephrine, may also be a reasonable initial vasopressor therapy in septic shock patients.[1,12–14] Recent international sepsis guidelines recommend the choice of the medications to be guided by patient physiology and clinician preferences.[1]

2. No studies support deviations from standard life-support algorithms to improve outcomes in patients with sepsis-associated cardiac arrest. Sepsis-associated cardiac arrest is associated with worse outcomes than other causes of cardiac arrest.[15]
3. A meta-analysis[20] showed no change in survival with corticosteroid use in pediatric septic shock, though a more recent randomized controlled trial suggested a shorter time to reversal of shock with steroid use.[17] Two observational studies[18,19] suggested there may be specific subpopulations, based on genomics, that would either benefit or experience harm from steroid administration, though these subpopulations are difficult to identify clinically. Patients at risk for adrenal insufficiency (eg, those on chronic steroids, patients with purpura fulminans) are more likely to benefit from steroid therapy.[12]
4. In situations when epinephrine or norepinephrine are not available, dopamine is a reasonable alternative initial vasoactive infusion in patients with fluid-refractory septic shock.[10,11] Patients with vasodilatory shock may require a higher dose of dopamine.[12]

Resuscitating the Patient in Cardiogenic Shock

Recommendations for Resuscitating the Patient in Cardiogenic Shock		
COR	**LOE**	**Recommendations**
1	C-EO	1. For infants and children with cardiogenic shock, early expert consultation is recommended.
2b	C-EO	2. For infants and children with cardiogenic shock, it may be reasonable to use epinephrine, dopamine, dobutamine, or milrinone as an inotropic infusion.

Recommendation-Specific Supportive Text

1 and 2. Cardiogenic shock in infants and children is uncommon and associated with high mortality rates. No studies were identified comparing outcomes between vasoactive medications. For patients with hypotension, medications such as epinephrine may be more appropriate as an initial inotropic therapy. Because of the rarity and complexity of these presentations, expert consultation is recommended when managing infants and children in cardiogenic shock.

Resuscitating the Patient in Traumatic Hemorrhagic Shock

Recommendation for Resuscitating the Patient in Traumatic Hemorrhagic Shock		
COR	**LOE**	**Recommendation**
2a	C-EO	1. Among infants and children with hypotensive hemorrhagic shock following trauma, it is reasonable to administer blood products, when available, instead of crystalloid for ongoing volume resuscitation.[21–27]

Recommendation-Specific Supportive Text

1. There are no prospective pediatric data comparing the administration of early blood products versus early crystalloid for traumatic hemorrhagic shock. A scoping review identified 6 recent retrospective studies that compared patient outcomes with the total volume of crystalloid resuscitation received in the first 24 to 48 hours among children with hemorrhagic shock[21–25,28] Four studies reported no differences in survival to 24 hours, survival at 30 days with good neurological outcome, or survival to discharge.[21,24,25,28] Large-volume resuscitation was associated with increased hospital/ICU length of stay in 5 of the 6 studies.[22–25,28] One study reported lower survival to hospital discharge among children who received more than 60 mL/kg crystalloid compared to lower volume groups.[22] Despite limited pediatric data, recent guidelines for adults from the Eastern Association for the Surgery of Trauma,[26] the American College of Surgeons, and the National Institute for Health and Care Excellence[27] suggest the early use of balanced ratios of packed red blood cells, fresh frozen plasma, and platelets for trauma-related hemorrhagic shock.[29]

REFERENCES

1. Weiss SL, Peters MJ, Alhazzani W, Agus MSD, Flori HR, Inwald DP, Nadel S, Schlapbach LJ, Tasker RC, Argent AC, Brierley J, Carcillo J, Carrol ED, Carroll CL, Cheifetz IM, Choong K, Cies JJ, Cruz AT, De Luca D, Deep A, Faust SN, De Oliveira CF, Hall MW, Ishimine P, Javouhey E, Joosten KFM, Joshi P, Karam O, Kneyber MCJ, Lemson J, MacLaren G, Mehta NM, Møller MH, Newth CJL, Nguyen TC, Nishisaki A, Nunnally ME, Parker MM, Paul RM, Randolph AG, Ranjit S, Romer LH, Scott HF, Tume LN, Verger JT, Williams EA, Wolf J, Wong HR, Zimmerman JJ, Kissoon N, Tissieres P. Surviving Sepsis Campaign International Guidelines for the Management of Septic Shock and Sepsis-Associated Organ Dysfunction in Children. *Pediatr Crit Care Med.* 2020;21:e52–e106. doi: 10.1097/PCC.0000000000002198
2. de Caen AR, Berg MD, Chameides L, Gooden CK, Hickey RW, Scott HF, Sutton RM, Tijssen JA, Topjian A, van der Jagt EW, et al. Part 12: pediatric advanced life support: 2015 American Heart Association Guidelines Update for Cardiopulmonary Resuscitation and Emergency Cardiovascular Care. *Circulation.* 2015;132(suppl 2):S526–S542. doi: 10.1161/CIR.0000000000000266
3. van Paridon BM, Sheppard C, Garcia Guerra G, Joffe AR; on behalf of the Alberta Sepsis Network. Timing of antibiotics, volume, and vasoactive infusions in children with sepsis admitted to intensive care. *Crit Care.* 2015;19:293. doi: 10.1186/s13054-015-1010-x
4. Inwald DP, Canter R, Woolfall K, Mouncey P, Zenasni Z, O'Hara C, Carter A, Jones N, Lyttle MD, Nadel S, et al; on behalf of PERUKI (Paediatric Emergency Research in the UK and Ireland) and PICS SG (Paediatric

Intensive Care Society Study Group). Restricted fluid bolus volume in early septic shock: results of the Fluids in Shock pilot trial. *Arch Dis Child.* 2019;104:426–431. doi: 10.1136/archdischild-2018–314924

5. Sankar J, Ismail J, Sankar MJ, C P S, Meena RS. Fluid Bolus Over 15-20 Versus 5-10 Minutes Each in the First Hour of Resuscitation in Children With Septic Shock: A Randomized Controlled Trial. *Pediatr Crit Care Med.* 2017;18:e435–e445. doi: 10.1097/PCC.0000000000001269
6. Medeiros DN, Ferranti JF, Delgado AF, de Carvalho WB. Colloids for the Initial Management of Severe Sepsis and Septic Shock in Pediatric Patients: A Systematic Review. *Pediatr Emerg Care.* 2015;31:e11–e16. doi: 10.1097/PEC.0000000000000601
7. Balamuth F, Kittick M, McBride P, Woodford AL, Vestal N, Casper TC, Metheney M, Smith K, Atkin NJ, Baren JM, Dean JM, Kuppermann N, Weiss SL. Pragmatic Pediatric Trial of Balanced Versus Normal Saline Fluid in Sepsis: The PRoMPT BOLUS Randomized Controlled Trial Pilot Feasibility Study. *Acad Emerg Med.* 2019;26:1346–1356. doi: 10.1111/acem.13815
8. Weiss SL, Keele L, Balamuth F, Vendetti N, Ross R, Fitzgerald JC, Gerber JS. Crystalloid Fluid Choice and Clinical Outcomes in Pediatric Sepsis: A Matched Retrospective Cohort Study. *J Pediatr.* 2017;182:304–310.e10. doi: 10.1016/j.jpeds.2016.11.075
9. Emrath ET, Fortenberry JD, Travers C, McCracken CE, Hebbar KB. Resuscitation With Balanced Fluids Is Associated With Improved Survival in Pediatric Severe Sepsis. *Crit Care Med.* 2017;45:1177–1183. doi: 10.1097/CCM.0000000000002365
10. Ventura AM, Shieh HH, Bousso A, Góes PF, de Cássia F O Fernandes I, de Souza DC, Paulo RL, Chagas F, Gilio AE. Double-Blind Prospective Randomized Controlled Trial of Dopamine Versus Epinephrine as First-Line Vasoactive Drugs in Pediatric Septic Shock. *Crit Care Med.* 2015;43:2292–2302. doi: 10.1097/CCM.0000000000001260
11. Ramaswamy KN, Singhi S, Jayashree M, Bansal A, Nallasamy K. Double-Blind Randomized Clinical Trial Comparing Dopamine and Epinephrine in Pediatric Fluid-Refractory Hypotensive Septic Shock. *Pediatr Crit Care Med.* 2016;17:e502–e512. doi: 10.1097/PCC.0000000000000954
12. Davis AL, Carcillo JA, Aneja RK, Deymann AJ, Lin JC, Nguyen TC, Okhuysen-Cawley RS, Relvas MS, Rozenfeld RA, Skippen PW, Stojadinovic BJ, Williams EA, Yeh TS, Balamuth F, Brierley J, de Caen AR, Cheifetz IM, Choong K, Conway E Jr, Cornell T, Doctor A, Dugas MA, Feldman JD, Fitzgerald JC, Flori HR, Fortenberry JD, Graciano AL, Greenwald BM, Hall MW, Han YY, Hernan LJ, Irazuzta JE, Iselin E, van der Jagt EW, Jeffries HE, Kache S, Katyal C, Kissoon N, Kon AA, Kutko MC, MacLaren G, Maul T, Mehta R, Odetola F, Parbuoni K, Paul R, Peters MJ, Ranjit S, Reuter-Rice KE, Schnitzler EJ, Scott HF, Torres A Jr, Weingarten-Arams J, Weiss SL, Zimmerman JJ, Zuckerberg AL. American College of Critical Care Medicine Clinical Practice Parameters for Hemodynamic Support of Pediatric and Neonatal Septic Shock. *Crit Care Med.* 2017;45:1061–1093. doi: 10.1097/CCM.0000000000002425
13. Lampin ME, Rousseaux J, Botte A, Sadik A, Cremer R, Leclerc F. Noradrenaline use for septic shock in children: doses, routes of administration and complications. *Acta Paediatr.* 2012;101:e426–e430. doi: 10.1111/j.1651-2227.2012.02725.x
14. Deep A, Goonasekera CD, Wang Y, Brierley J. Evolution of haemodynamics and outcome of fluid-refractory septic shock in children. *Intensive Care Med.* 2013;39:1602–1609. doi: 10.1007/s00134-013-3003-z
15. Del Castillo J, López-Herce J, Cañadas S, Matamoros M, Rodríguez-Núnez A, Rodríguez-Calvo A, Carrillo A; Iberoamerican Pediatric Cardiac Arrest Study Network RIBEPCI. Cardiac arrest and resuscitation in the pediatric intensive care unit: a prospective multicenter multinational study. *Resuscitation.* 2014;85:1380–1386. doi: 10.1016/j.resuscitation.2014.06.024
16. Menon K, Ward RE, Lawson ML, Gaboury I, Hutchison JS, Hébert PC; Canadian Critical Care Trials Group. A prospective multicenter study of adrenal function in critically ill children. *Am J Respir Crit Care Med.* 2010;182:246–251. doi: 10.1164/rccm.200911-1738OC
17. El-Nawawy A, Khater D, Omar H, Wali Y. Evaluation of Early Corticosteroid Therapy in Management of Pediatric Septic Shock in Pediatric Intensive Care Patients: A Randomized Clinical Study. *Pediatr Infect Dis J.* 2017;36:155–159. doi: 10.1097/INF.0000000000001380
18. Wong HR, Atkinson SJ, Cvijanovich NZ, Anas N, Allen GL, Thomas NJ, Bigham MT, Weiss SL, Fitzgerald JC, Checchia PA, et al. Combining prognostic and predictive enrichment strategies to identify children with septic shock responsive to corticosteroids. *Crit Care Med.* 2016;44:e1000–e1003. doi: 10.1097/CCM.0000000000001833
19. Wong HR, Cvijanovich NZ, Anas N, Allen GL, Thomas NJ, Bigham MT, Weiss SL, Fitzgerald JC, Checchia PA, Meyer K, et al. Endotype transitions during the acute phase of pediatric septic shock reflect changing risk and treatment response. *Crit Care Med.* 2018;46:e242–e249. doi: 10.1097/CCM.0000000000002932
20. Menon K, McNally D, Choong K, Sampson M. A systematic review and meta-analysis on the effect of steroids in pediatric shock. *Pediatr Crit Care Med.* 2013;14:474–480. doi: 10.1097/PCC.0b013e31828a8125
21. Hussmann B, Lefering R, Kauther MD, Ruchholtz S, Moldzio P, Lendemans S; and the TraumaRegister DGU. Influence of prehospital volume replacement on outcome in polytraumatized children. *Crit Care.* 2012;16:R201. doi: 10.1186/cc11809
22. Acker SN, Ross JT, Partrick DA, DeWitt P, Bensard DD. Injured children are resistant to the adverse effects of early high volume crystalloid resuscitation. *J Pediatr Surg.* 2014;49:1852–1855. doi: 10.1016/j.jpedsurg.2014.09.034
23. Edwards MJ, Lustik MB, Clark ME, Creamer KM, Tuggle D. The effects of balanced blood component resuscitation and crystalloid administration in pediatric trauma patients requiring transfusion in Afghanistan and Iraq 2002 to 2012. *J Trauma Acute Care Surg.* 2015;78:330–335. doi: 10.1097/TA.0000000000000469
24. Coons BE, Tam S, Rubsam J, Stylianos S, Duron V. High volume crystalloid resuscitation adversely affects pediatric trauma patients. *J Pediatr Surg.* 2018;53:2202–2208. doi: 10.1016/j.jpedsurg.2018.07.009
25. Elkbuli A, Zajd S, Ehrhardt JD Jr, McKenney M, Boneva D. Aggressive crystalloid resuscitation outcomes in low-severity pediatric trauma. *J Surg Res.* 2020;247:350–355. doi: 10.1016/j.jss.2019.10.009
26. Cannon JW, Khan MA, Raja AS, Cohen MJ, Como JJ, Cotton BA, Dubose JJ, Fox EE, Inaba K, Rodriguez CJ, Holcomb JB, Duchesne JC. Damage control resuscitation in patients with severe traumatic hemorrhage: A practice management guideline from the Eastern Association for the Surgery of Trauma. *J Trauma Acute Care Surg.* 2017;82:605–617. doi: 10.1097/TA.0000000000001333
27. Kanani AN, Hartshorn S. NICE clinical guideline NG39: Major trauma: assessment and initial management. *Arch Dis Child Educ Pract Ed.* 2017;102:20–23. doi: 10.1136/archdischild-2016-310869
28. Zhu H, Chen B, Guo C. Aggressive crystalloid adversely affects outcomes in a pediatric trauma population. *Eur J Trauma Emerg Surg.* 2019:Epub ahead of print. doi: 10.1007/s00068-019-01134-0
29. Henry S. *ATLS Advanced Trauma Life Support.* 10th Edition Student Course Manual. Chicago, IL: American College of Surgeons; 2018.

TREATMENT OF RESPIRATORY FAILURE

Respiratory failure occurs when a patient's breathing becomes inadequate and results in ineffective oxygenation and ventilation. This can occur due to disordered control of breathing, upper airway obstruction, lower airway obstruction, respiratory muscle failure, or parenchymal lung disease. Providing assisted ventilation when breathing is absent or inadequate, relieving foreign body airway obstruction (FBAO), and administering naloxone in opioid overdose can be lifesaving.

Suffocation (eg, FBAO) and poisoning are leading causes of death in infants and children. Balloons, foods (eg, hot dogs, nuts, grapes), and small household objects are the most common causes of FBAO in children,[1–3] whereas liquids are common among infants.[4] It is important to differentiate between mild FBAO (the patient is coughing and making sounds) and severe FBAO (the patient cannot make sounds). Patients with mild FBAO can attempt to clear the obstruction by coughing, but intervention is required in severe obstruction.

In the United States in 2017, opioid overdose caused 79 deaths in children less than 15 years old and 4094 deaths in people age 15 to 24 years.[5] Naloxone reverses the respiratory depression of narcotic overdose,[6] and, in 2014, the US Food and Drug Administration approved the use of a naloxone autoinjector by lay rescuers and healthcare providers. Naloxone intranasal delivery devices are also available.

Treatment of Inadequate Breathing With a Pulse

Recommendations for Treatment of Inadequate Breathing With a Pulse		
COR	**LOE**	**Recommendations**
1	C-EO	1. For infants and children with a pulse but absent or inadequate respiratory effort, provide rescue breathing.[7]
2a	C-EO	2. For infants and children with a pulse but absent or inadequate respiratory effort, it is reasonable to give 1 breath every 2 to 3 s (20–30 breaths/min).[7]

Recommendation-Specific Supportive Text

1 and 2. There are no pediatric-specific clinical studies evaluating the effect of different ventilation rates on outcomes in inadequate breathing with a pulse. One multicenter observational study found that high ventilation rates (at least 30/min in children younger than 1 year of age, at least 25/min in children older than 1 year) during CPR with an advanced airway for cardiac arrest were associated with improved ROSC and survival.[7] For the ease of training, the suggested respiratory rate for the patient with inadequate breathing and a pulse has been increased from 1 breath every 3 to 5 seconds to 1 breath every 2 to 3 seconds to be consistent with the new CPR guideline recommendation for ventilation in patients with an advanced airway.

Foreign Body Airway Obstruction

Recommendations for Foreign Body Airway Obstruction		
COR	**LOE**	**Recommendations**
1	C-LD	1. If the child has mild FBAO, allow the victim to clear the airway by coughing while observing for signs of severe FBAO.[4,8,9]
1	C-LD	2. For a child with severe FBAO, perform abdominal thrusts until the object is expelled or the victim becomes unresponsive.[4,8,9]
1	C-LD	3. For an infant with severe FBAO, deliver repeated cycles of 5 back blows (slaps) followed by 5 chest compressions until the object is expelled or the victim becomes unresponsive.[4,9–12]
1	C-LD	4. If the infant or child with severe FBAO becomes unresponsive, start CPR beginning with chest compressions (do not perform pulse check). After 2 min of CPR, activate the emergency response system if no one has done so.[11]
1	C-LD	5. For the infant or child with FBAO receiving CPR, remove any visible foreign body when opening the airway to provide breaths.[13–15]
3: Harm	C-LD	6. Do not perform blind finger sweeps.[13–15]

Recommendation-Specific Supportive Text

1 and 2. There are no high-quality data to support recommendations regarding FBAO in children. Many FBAOs are relieved by allowing the patient to cough or, if severe, are treated by bystanders using abdominal thrusts.[4,8,9]

3. Observational data primarily from case series support the use of back blows[4,9,10] or chest compressions[10,11] for infants. Abdominal thrusts are not recommended for infants given the potential to cause abdominal organ injury.[12]
4. Once the victim is unconscious, observational data support immediate provision of chest compressions whether or not the patient has a pulse.[11]

5 and 6. Observational data suggest that the risk of blind finger sweeps outweighs any potential benefit in the management of FBAO.[13–15]

Opioid-Related Respiratory and Cardiac Arrest

Recommendations for Opioid-Related Respiratory and Cardiac Arrest		
COR	**LOE**	**Recommendations**
1	C-LD	1. For patients in respiratory arrest, rescue breathing or bag-mask ventilation should be maintained until spontaneous breathing returns, and standard pediatric basic or advanced life support measures should continue if return of spontaneous breathing does not occur.[17,18]
1	C-EO	2. For patients known or suspected to be in cardiac arrest, in the absence of a proven benefit from the use of naloxone, standard resuscitative measures should take priority over naloxone administration, with a focus on high-quality CPR (compressions plus ventilation).[19,20]
1	C-EO	3. Lay and trained responders should not delay activating emergency response systems while awaiting the patient's response to naloxone or other interventions.[21,22]
2a	B-NR	4. For a patient with suspected opioid overdose who has a definite pulse but no normal breathing or only gasping (ie, a respiratory arrest), in addition to providing standard pediatric basic life support or advanced life support, it is reasonable for responders to administer intramuscular or intranasal naloxone.[23–36]

Recommendation-Specific Supportive Text

1. Initial management should focus on support of the patient's airway and breathing. This begins with opening the airway followed by delivery of rescue breaths, ideally with the use of a bag-mask or barrier device.[17,18] Provision of life support should continue if return of spontaneous breathing does not occur.
2. Because there are no studies demonstrating improvement in patient outcomes from administration of naloxone during cardiac arrest, provision of

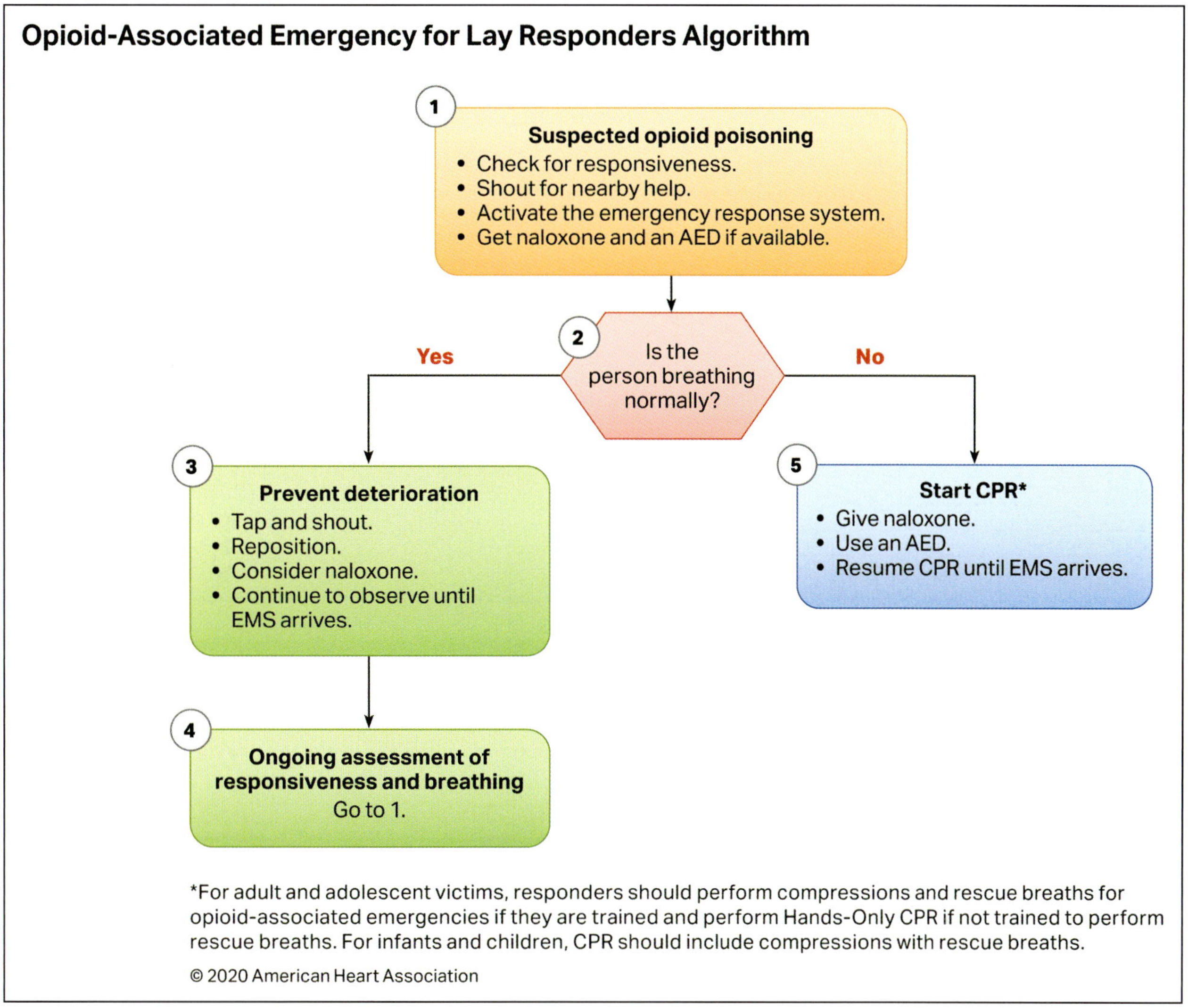
Opioid-Associated Emergency for Lay Responders Algorithm
1
Suspected opioid poisoning
• Check for responsiveness.
• Shout for nearby help.
• Activate the emergency response system.
• Get naloxone and an AED if available.
2
Is the person breathing normally?
Yes
No
3
Prevent deterioration
• Tap and shout.
• Reposition.
• Consider naloxone.
• Continue to observe until EMS arrives.
4
Ongoing assessment of responsiveness and breathing
Go to 1.
5
Start CPR*
• Give naloxone.
• Use an AED.
• Resume CPR until EMS arrives.
*For adult and adolescent victims, responders should perform compressions and rescue breaths for opioid-associated emergencies if they are trained and perform Hands-Only CPR if not trained to perform rescue breaths. For infants and children, CPR should include compressions with rescue breaths.
© 2020 American Heart Association

Figure 10. Opioid-Associated Emergency for Lay Responders Algorithm.
AED indicates automated external defibrillator; CPR, cardiopulmonary resuscitation; and EMS, emergency medical services.

CPR should be the focus of initial care.[20] Naloxone can be administered along with standard advanced cardiovascular life support care if it does not delay components of high-quality CPR.

3. Early activation of the emergency response system is critical for patients with suspected opioid overdose. Rescuers cannot be certain that the person's clinical condition is due to opioid-induced respiratory depression alone. This is particularly true in first aid and BLS, where determination of the presence of a pulse is unreliable.[21,22] Naloxone is ineffective in other medical conditions, including overdose involving nonopioids and cardiac arrest from any cause. Patients who respond to naloxone administration may develop recurrent central nervous system and/or respiratory depression and require longer periods of observation before safe discharge.[37–40]
4. Twelve studies examined the use of naloxone in respiratory arrest, of which 5 compared intramuscular, intravenous, and/or intranasal routes of naloxone administration (2 RCT[23,24] and 3 non-RCT[25–27]) and 9 assessed the safety of naloxone use or were observational studies of naloxone use.[28–36] These studies report that naloxone is safe and effective in treatment of opioid-induced respiratory depression and that complications are rare and dose related.

These recommendations were taken from Part 3: Adult Basic and Advanced Life Support[41] and further supported by a 2020 ILCOR evidence update.[42] There were no pediatric data supporting these recommendations; however, due to the urgency of the opioid crisis, the adult recommendations should be applied to children.

Figures 10 and 11 are algorithms for opioid-associated emergencies for lay responders and healthcare providers.

REFERENCES

1. Morley RE, Ludemann JP, Moxham JP, Kozak FK, Riding KH. Foreign body aspiration in infants and toddlers: recent trends in British Columbia. *J Otolaryngol.* 2004;33:37–41. doi: 10.2310/7070.2004.00310

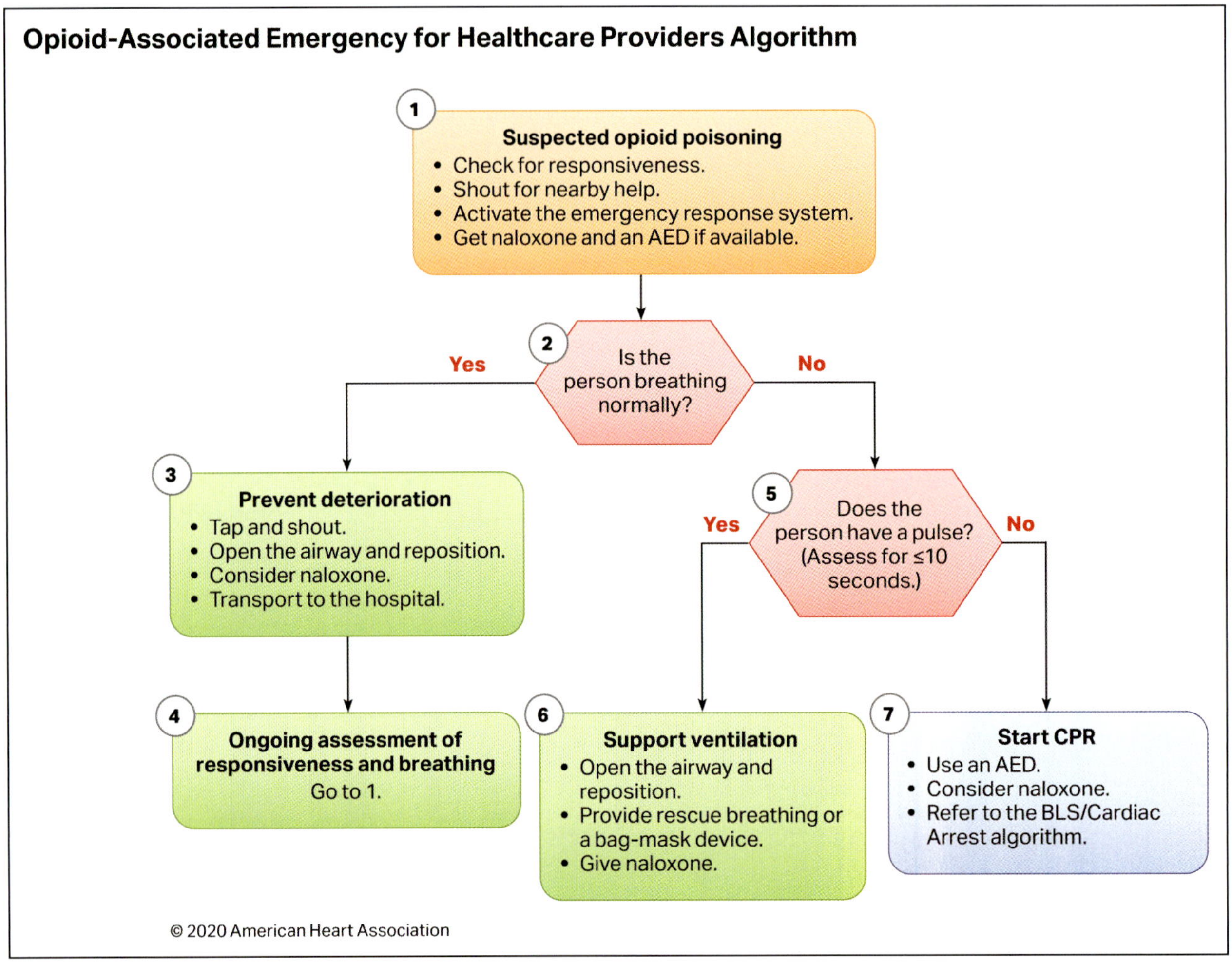
Opioid-Associated Emergency for Healthcare Providers Algorithm
1
Suspected opioid poisoning
• Check for responsiveness.
• Shout for nearby help.
• Activate the emergency response system.
• Get naloxone and an AED if available.
2
Is the person breathing normally?
Yes
No
3
Prevent deterioration
• Tap and shout.
• Open the airway and reposition.
• Consider naloxone.
• Transport to the hospital.
5
Does the person have a pulse? (Assess for ≤10 seconds.)
Yes
No
4
Ongoing assessment of responsiveness and breathing
Go to 1.
6
Support ventilation
• Open the airway and reposition.
• Provide rescue breathing or a bag-mask device.
• Give naloxone.
7
Start CPR
• Use an AED.
• Consider naloxone.
• Refer to the BLS/Cardiac Arrest algorithm.
© 2020 American Heart Association

Figure 11. Opioid-Associated Emergency for Healthcare Providers Algorithm.
AED indicates automated external defibrillator; BLS, basic life support; and CPR, cardiopulmonary resuscitation.

2. Harris CS, Baker SP, Smith GA, Harris RM. Childhood asphyxiation by food. A national analysis and overview. *JAMA.* 1984;251:2231–2235.
3. Rimell FL, Thome A Jr, Stool S, Reilly JS, Rider G, Stool D, Wilson CL. Characteristics of objects that cause choking in children. *JAMA.* 1995;274:1763–1766.
4. Vilke GM, Smith AM, Ray LU, Steen PJ, Murrin PA, Chan TC. Airway obstruction in children aged less than 5 years: the prehospital experience. *Prehosp Emerg Care.* 2004;8:196–199. doi: 10.1016/j.prehos.2003.12.014
5. Scholl L, Seth P, Kariisa M, Wilson N, Baldwin G. Drug and opioid-involved overdose deaths—United States, 2013–2017. *MMWR Morb Mortal Wkly Rep.* 2018;67:1419–1427. doi: 10.15585/mmwr.mm675152e1
6. Fischer CG, Cook DR. The respiratory and narcotic antagonistic effects of naloxone in infants. *Anesth Analg.* 1974;53:849–852. doi: 10.1213/00000539-197453060-00007
7. Sutton RM, Reeder RW, Landis WP, Meert KL, Yates AR, Morgan RW, Berger JT, Newth CJ, Carcillo JA, McQuillen PS, Harrison RE, Moler FW, Pollack MM, Carpenter TC, Notterman DA, Holubkov R, Dean JM, Nadkarni VM, Berg RA; Eunice Kennedy Shriver National Institute of Child Health and Human Development Collaborative Pediatric Critical Care Research Network (CPCCRN). Ventilation Rates and Pediatric In-Hospital Cardiac Arrest Survival Outcomes. *Crit Care Med.* 2019;47:1627–1636. doi: 10.1097/CCM.0000000000003898
8. Heimlich HJ. A life-saving maneuver to prevent food-choking. *JAMA.* 1975;234:398–401.
9. Sternbach G, Kiskaddon RT. Henry Heimlich: a life-saving maneuver for food choking. *J Emerg Med.* 1985;3:143–148. doi: 10.1016/0736-4679(85)90047-2
10. Redding JS. The choking controversy: critique of evidence on the Heimlich maneuver. *Crit Care Med.* 1979;7:475–479.
11. Kinoshita K, Azuhata T, Kawano D, Kawahara Y. Relationships between pre-hospital characteristics and outcome in victims of foreign body airway obstruction during meals. *Resuscitation.* 2015;88:63–67. doi: 10.1016/j.resuscitation.2014.12.018
12. Lee SL, Kim SS, Shekherdimian S, Ledbetter DJ. Complications as a result of the Heimlich maneuver. *J Trauma.* 2009;66:E34–E35. doi: 10.1097/01.ta.0000219291.27245.90
13. Abder-Rahman HA. Infants choking following blind finger sweep. *J Pediatr (Rio J).* 2009;85:273–275. doi: 10.2223/JPED.1892
14. Hartrey R, Bingham RM. Pharyngeal trauma as a result of blind finger sweeps in the choking child. *J Accid Emerg Med.* 1995;12:52–54. doi: 10.1136/emj.12.1.52
15. Kabbani M, Goodwin SR. Traumatic epiglottis following blind finger sweep to remove a pharyngeal foreign body. *Clin Pediatr (Phila).* 1995;34:495–497. doi: 10.1177/000992289503400908
16. Deleted in proof.
17. Guildner CW. Resuscitation—opening the airway: a comparative study of techniques for opening an airway obstructed by the tongue. *JACEP.* 1976;5:588–590. doi: 10.1016/s0361-1124(76)80217-1
18. Wenzel V, Keller C, Idris AH, Dörges V, Lindner KH, Brimacombe JR. Effects of smaller tidal volumes during basic life support ventilation in patients with respiratory arrest: good ventilation, less risk? *Resuscitation.* 1999;43:25–29. doi: 10.1016/s0300-9572(99)00118-5
19. Saybolt MD, Alter SM, Dos Santos F, Calello DP, Rynn KO, Nelson DA, Merlin MA. Naloxone in cardiac arrest with suspected opioid overdoses. *Resuscitation.* 2010;81:42–46. doi: 10.1016/j.resuscitation.2009.09.016
20. Dezfulian C, Orkin AM, Maron BA, Elmer J, Girota S, Gladwin MT, Merchant RM, Panchal AR, Perman SM, Starks M, et al; on behalf of the American Heart Association Council on Cardiopulmonary, Critical Care,

Perioperative and Resuscitation; Council on Arteriosclerosis, Thrombosis and Vascular Biology; Council on Cardiovascular and Stroke Nursing; and Council on Clinical Cardiology. Opioid-associated out-of-hospital cardiac arrest: distinctive clinical features and implications for healthcare and public responses: a scientific statement from the American Heart Association. *Circulation*. In press.

21. Bahr J, Klingler H, Panzer W, Rode H, Kettler D. Skills of lay people in checking the carotid pulse. *Resuscitation*. 1997;35:23–26. doi: 10.1016/s0300-9572(96)01092-1
22. Eberle B, Dick WF, Schneider T, Wisser G, Doetsch S, Tzanova I. Checking the carotid pulse check: diagnostic accuracy of first responders in patients with and without a pulse. *Resuscitation*. 1996;33:107–116. doi: 10.1016/s0300-9572(96)01016-7
23. Kelly AM, Kerr D, Dietze P, Patrick I, Walker T, Koutsogiannis Z. Randomised trial of intranasal versus intramuscular naloxone in prehospital treatment for suspected opioid overdose. *Med J Aust*. 2005;182:24–27.
24. Kerr D, Kelly AM, Dietze P, Jolley D, Barger B. Randomized controlled trial comparing the effectiveness and safety of intranasal and intramuscular naloxone for the treatment of suspected heroin overdose. *Addiction*. 2009;104:2067–2074. doi: 10.1111/j.1360-0443.2009.02724.x
25. Wanger K, Brough L, Macmillan I, Goulding J, MacPhail I, Christenson JM. Intravenous vs subcutaneous naloxone for out-of-hospital management of presumed opioid overdose. *Acad Emerg Med*. 1998;5:293–299. doi: 10.1111/j.1553-2712.1998.tb02707.x
26. Barton ED, Colwell CB, Wolfe T, Fosnocht D, Gravitz C, Bryan T, Dunn W, Benson J, Bailey J. Efficacy of intranasal naloxone as a needleless alternative for treatment of opioid overdose in the prehospital setting. *J Emerg Med*. 2005;29:265–271. doi: 10.1016/j.jemermed.2005.03.007
27. Robertson TM, Hendey GW, Stroh G, Shalit M. Intranasal naloxone is a viable alternative to intravenous naloxone for prehospital narcotic overdose. *Prehosp Emerg Care*. 2009;13:512–515. doi: 10.1080/10903120903144866
28. Cetrullo C, Di Nino GF, Melloni C, Pieri C, Zanoni A. [Naloxone antagonism toward opiate analgesic drugs. Clinical experimental study]. *Minerva Anestesiol*. 1983;49:199–204.
29. Osterwalder JJ. Naloxone–for intoxications with intravenous heroin and heroin mixtures–harmless or hazardous? A prospective clinical study. *J Toxicol Clin Toxicol*. 1996;34:409–416. doi: 10.3109/15563659609013811
30. Sporer KA, Firestone J, Isaacs SM. Out-of-hospital treatment of opioid overdoses in an urban setting. *Acad Emerg Med*. 1996;3:660–667. doi: 10.1111/j.1553-2712.1996.tb03487.x
31. Stokland O, Hansen TB, Nilsen JE. [Prehospital treatment of heroin intoxication in Oslo in 1996]. *Tidsskr Nor Laegeforen*. 1998;118:3144–3146.
32. Buajordet I, Naess AC, Jacobsen D, Brørs O. Adverse events after naloxone treatment of episodes of suspected acute opioid overdose. *Eur J Emerg Med*. 2004;11:19–23. doi: 10.1097/00063110-200402000-00004
33. Cantwell K, Dietze P, Flander L. The relationship between naloxone dose and key patient variables in the treatment of non-fatal heroin overdose in the prehospital setting. *Resuscitation*. 2005;65:315–319. doi: 10.1016/j.resuscitation.2004.12.012
34. Boyd JJ, Kuisma MJ, Alaspää AO, Vuori E, Repo JV, Randell TT. Recurrent opioid toxicity after pre-hospital care of presumed heroin overdose patients. *Acta Anaesthesiol Scand*. 2006;50:1266–1270. doi: 10.1111/j.1399-6576.2006.01172.x
35. Nielsen K, Nielsen SL, Siersma V, Rasmussen LS. Treatment of opioid overdose in a physician-based prehospital EMS: frequency and long-term prognosis. *Resuscitation*. 2011;82:1410–1413. doi: 10.1016/j.resuscitation.2011.05.027
36. Wampler DA, Molina DK, McManus J, Laws P, Manifold CA. No deaths associated with patient refusal of transport after naloxone-reversed opioid overdose. *Prehosp Emerg Care*. 2011;15:320–324. doi: 10.3109/10903127.2011.569854
37. Clarke SF, Dargan PI, Jones AL. Naloxone in opioid poisoning: walking the tightrope. *Emerg Med J*. 2005;22:612–616. doi: 10.1136/emj.2003.009613
38. Etherington J, Christenson J, Innes G, Grafstein E, Pennington S, Spinelli JJ, Gao M, Lahiffe B, Wanger K, Fernandes C. Is early discharge safe after naloxone reversal of presumed opioid overdose? *CJEM*. 2000;2:156–162. doi: 10.1017/s1481803500004863
39. Zuckerman M, Weisberg SN, Boyer EW. Pitfalls of intranasal naloxone. *Prehosp Emerg Care*. 2014;18:550–554. doi: 10.3109/10903127.2014.896961
40. Heaton JD, Bhandari B, Faryar KA, Huecker MR. Retrospective Review of Need for Delayed Naloxone or Oxygen in Emergency Department Patients Receiving Naloxone for Heroin Reversal. *J Emerg Med*. 2019;56:642–651. doi: 10.1016/j.jemermed.2019.02.015
41. Panchal AR, Bartos JA, Cabañas JG, Donnino MW, Drennan IR, Hirsch KG, Kudenchuk PJ, Kurz MC, Lavonas EJ, Morley PT, et al; on behalf of the Adult Basic and Advanced Life Support Writing Group. Part 3: adult basic and advanced life support: 2020 American Heart Association Guidelines for Cardiopulmonary Resuscitation and Emergency Cardiovascular Care. *Circulation*. 2020;142(suppl 2):S366–S468 doi: 10.1161/CIR.0000000000000916
42. Olasveengen TM, Mancini ME, Perkins GD, Avis S, Brooks S, Castrén M, Chung SP, Considine J, Couper K, Escalante R, et al; on behalf of the Adult Basic Life Support Collaborators. Adult basic life support: 2020 International Consensus on Cardiopulmonary Resuscitation and Emergency Cardiovascular Care Science With Treatment Recommendations. *Circulation*. 2020;142(suppl 1):S41–S91. doi: 10.1161/CIR.0000000000000892

INTUBATION

It is important to select appropriate equipment and medications for pediatric intubation. Uncuffed ETTs were historically preferred for young children because the normal pediatric airway narrows below the vocal cords, creating an anatomic seal around the distal tube. In the acute setting and with poor pulmonary compliance, uncuffed ETTs may need to be changed to cuffed ETTs. Cuffed tubes improve capnography accuracy, reduce the need for ETT changes (resulting in high-risk reintubations or delayed compressions), and improve pressure and tidal volume delivery. However, high pressure in the cuff can cause airway mucosal damage. Although several studies have identified that cuffed tube use may actually decrease airway trauma by decreasing tube changes, attention must be made to selecting the correct tube size and cuff inflation pressure.[1] ETT cuff pressures are dynamic during transport at altitude[2] and with increasing airway edema.

Intubation is a high-risk procedure. Depending on the patient's hemodynamics, respiratory mechanics, and airway status, the patient can be at increased risk for cardiac arrest during intubation. Therefore, it is important to provide adequate resuscitation before intubation.

Cricoid pressure during bag-mask ventilation and intubation has historically been used to minimize the risk of gastric contents refluxing into the airway, but there are concerns that tracheal compression may impede effective bag-mask ventilation and intubation success.

Confirmation of ETT placement in patients with a perfusing rhythm is not reliably achieved by auscultation of breath sounds, mist in the tube, or chest rise. Either colorimetric detector or capnography ($ETCO_2$) can be used to assess initial ETT placement. In patients with decreased pulmonary blood flow from low cardiac output or cardiac arrest, $ETCO_2$ may not be as reliable.

Use of Cuffed Endotracheal Tubes for Intubation

Recommendations for the Use of Cuffed Endotracheal Tubes for Intubation		
COR	LOE	Recommendations
1	C-EO	1. When a cuffed ETT is used, attention should be paid to ETT size, position, and cuff inflation pressure (usually <20–25 cm H_2O).[3]
2a	C-LD	2. It is reasonable to choose cuffed ETTs over uncuffed ETTs for intubating infants and children.[4–15]

Recommendation-Specific Supportive Text

1. A retrospective study including 2953 children noted that, with 25 cm H_2O of pressure to the airway and a slight leak around the ETT, there were no cases of clinically significant subglottic stenosis, and the incidence of stridor requiring reintubation was less than 1%.[3]
2. Three systematic reviews, 2 randomized controlled trials, and 2 retrospective reviews support the safety of cuffed ETTs and the decreased need for ETT changes.[4–10] These studies were almost entirely performed in the perioperative patient population, and intubation was performed by highly skilled airway providers. Thus, ETT duration may have been shorter than in critically ill patients. The use of cuffed ETTs is associated with lower reintubation rates, more successful ventilation, and improved accuracy of capnography without increased risk of complications.[7,9–13] Cuffed ETTs may decrease the risk of aspiration.[14,15]

The Use of Cricoid Pressure During Intubation

Recommendations for the Use of Cricoid Pressure During Intubation		
COR	LOE	Recommendations
2b	C-LD	1. Cricoid pressure during bag-mask ventilation may be considered to reduce gastric insufflation.[16,17]
3: No Benefit	C-LD	2. Routine use of cricoid pressure is not recommended during endotracheal intubation of pediatric patients.[16,17]
3: Harm	C-LD	3. If cricoid pressure is used, discontinue if it interferes with ventilation or the speed or ease of intubation.[16,17]

Recommendation-Specific Supportive Text

1, 2, and 3. A retrospective, propensity score–matched study from a large pediatric ICU intubation registry showed that cricoid pressure during induction and bag-mask ventilation before tracheal intubation was not associated with lower rates of regurgitation.[17] A study from the same pediatric ICU database reported external laryngeal manipulation was associated with lower initial tracheal intubation success.[16]

Atropine Use for Intubation

Recommendations for Atropine Use for Intubation		
COR	LOE	Recommendations
2b	C-LD	1. It may be reasonable for practitioners to use atropine as a premedication to prevent bradycardia during emergency intubations when there is higher risk of bradycardia (eg, when giving succinylcholine).[18,19]
2b	C-LD	2. When atropine is used as a premedication for emergency intubation, a dose of 0.02 mg/kg of atropine, with no minimum dose, may be considered.[20]

Recommendation-Specific Supportive Text

1. The 2019 French Society of Anesthesia and Intensive Care Medicine guidelines state that atropine "should probably" be used as a preintubation drug in children 28 days to 8 years with septic shock, with hypovolemia, or with succinylcholine administration.[18,19]
2. One nonrandomized, single-center intervention study did not identify an association between atropine dosing less than 0.1 mg and bradycardia or arrhythmias.[20]

Monitoring Exhaled CO_2 in Patients With Advanced Airways

Recommendations for Monitoring Exhaled CO_2 in Patients With Advanced Airways		
COR	LOE	Recommendations
1	C-LD	1. In all settings, for infants and children with a perfusing rhythm, use exhaled CO_2 detection (colorimetric detector or capnography) for confirmation of ETT placement.[21–27]
2a	C-LD	2. In infants and children with a perfusing rhythm, it is beneficial to monitor exhaled CO_2 (colorimetric detector or capnography) during out-of-hospital and intra/interhospital transport.[21,22,28–30]

Recommendation-Specific Supportive Text

1. Although there are no randomized controlled trials linking use of $ETCO_2$ detection with clinical outcomes, the Fourth National Audit Project of the Royal College of Anesthetists and Difficult Airway Society concluded that the failure to use or inability to properly interpret capnography contributed to adverse events, including ICU-related deaths (mixed adult and pediatric data).[21,22] One small randomized study showed that capnography was faster than clinical assessment in premature newborns intubated in the delivery room.[23] There was no difference in patient outcomes between qualitative (colorimetric) and quantitative (capnography or numeric display) $ETCO_2$ detectors.[24–27]
2. Adult literature suggests monitoring and correct interpretation of capnography in intubated patients may prevent adverse events.[21,22,28] This

has been demonstrated in simulated pediatric scenarios, in which capnography increased provider recognition of possible ETT dislodgement.[29,30]

REFERENCES

1. Tobias JD. Pediatric airway anatomy may not be what we thought: implications for clinical practice and the use of cuffed endotracheal tubes. *Paediatr Anaesth.* 2015;25:9–19. doi: 10.1111/pan.12528
2. Orsborn J, Graham J, Moss M, Melguizo M, Nick T, Stroud M. Pediatric Endotracheal Tube Cuff Pressures During Aeromedical Transport. *Pediatr Emerg Care.* 2016;32:20–22. doi: 10.1097/PEC.0000000000000365
3. Black AE, Hatch DJ, Nauth-Misir N. Complications of nasotracheal intubation in neonates, infants and children: a review of 4 years' experience in a children's hospital. *Br J Anaesth.* 1990;65:461–467. doi: 10.1093/bja/65.4.461
4. Chen L, Zhang J, Pan G, Li X, Shi T, He W. Cuffed versus uncuffed endotracheal tubes in pediatrics: a meta-analysis. *Open Med (Wars).* 2018;13:366–373. doi: 10.1515/med-2018-0055
5. Shi F, Xiao Y, Xiong W, Zhou Q, Huang X. Cuffed versus uncuffed endotracheal tubes in children: a meta-analysis. *J Anesth.* 2016;30:3–11. doi: 10.1007/s00540-015-2062-4
6. De Orange FA, Andrade RG, Lemos A, Borges PS, Figueiroa JN, Kovatsis PG. Cuffed versus uncuffed endotracheal tubes for general anaesthesia in children aged eight years and under. *Cochrane Database Syst Rev.* 2017;11:CD011954. doi: 10.1002/14651858.CD011954.pub2
7. Chambers NA, Ramgolam A, Sommerfield D, Zhang G, Ledowski T, Thurm M, Lethbridge M, Hegarty M, von Ungern-Sternberg BS. Cuffed vs. uncuffed tracheal tubes in children: a randomised controlled trial comparing leak, tidal volume and complications. *Anaesthesia.* 2018;73:160–168. doi: 10.1111/anae.14113
8. de Wit M, Peelen LM, van Wolfswinkel L, de Graaff JC. The incidence of postoperative respiratory complications: A retrospective analysis of cuffed vs uncuffed tracheal tubes in children 0-7 years of age. *Paediatr Anaesth.* 2018;28:210–217. doi: 10.1111/pan.13340
9. Schweiger C, Marostica PJ, Smith MM, Manica D, Carvalho PR, Kuhl G. Incidence of post-intubation subglottic stenosis in children: prospective study. *J Laryngol Otol.* 2013;127:399–403. doi: 10.1017/S002221511300025X
10. Dorsey DP, Bowman SM, Klein MB, Archer D, Sharar SR. Perioperative use of cuffed endotracheal tubes is advantageous in young pediatric burn patients. *Burns.* 2010;36:856–860. doi: 10.1016/j.burns.2009.11.011
11. Khine HH, Corddry DH, Kettrick RG, Martin TM, McCloskey JJ, Rose JB, Theroux MC, Zagnoev M. Comparison of cuffed and uncuffed endotracheal tubes in young children during general anesthesia. *Anesthesiology.* 1997;86:627–31; discussion 27A. doi: 10.1097/00000542-199703000-00015
12. Weiss M, Dullenkopf A, Fischer JE, Keller C, Gerber AC; European Paediatric Endotracheal Intubation Study Group. Prospective randomized controlled multi-centre trial of cuffed or uncuffed endotracheal tubes in small children. *Br J Anaesth.* 2009;103:867–873. doi: 10.1093/bja/aep290
13. James I. Cuffed tubes in children. *Paediatr Anaesth.* 2001;11:259–263. doi: 10.1046/j.1460-9592.2001.00675.x
14. Gopalareddy V, He Z, Soundar S, Bolling L, Shah M, Penfil S, McCloskey JJ, Mehta DI. Assessment of the prevalence of microaspiration by gastric pepsin in the airway of ventilated children. *Acta Paediatr.* 2008;97:55–60. doi: 10.1111/j.1651-2227.2007.00578.x
15. Browning DH, Graves SA. Incidence of aspiration with endotracheal tubes in children. *J Pediatr.* 1983;102:582–584. doi: 10.1016/s0022-3476(83)80191-7
16. Kojima T, Laverriere EK, Owen EB, Harwayne-Gidansky I, Shenoi AN, Napolitano N, Rehder KJ, Adu-Darko MA, Nett ST, Spear D, et al; and the National Emergency Airway Registry for Children (NEAR4KIDS) Collaborators and Pediatric Acute Lung Injury and Sepsis Investigators (PALISI). Clinical impact of external laryngeal manipulation during laryngoscopy on tracheal intubation success in critically ill children. *Pediatr Crit Care Med.* 2018;19:106–114. doi: 10.1097/PCC.0000000000001373
17. Kojima T, Harwayne-Gidansky I, Shenoi AN, Owen EB, Napolitano N, Rehder KJ, Adu-Darko MA, Nett ST, Spear D, Meyer K, Giuliano JS Jr, Tarquinio KM, Sanders RC Jr, Lee JH, Simon DW, Vanderford PA, Lee AY, Brown CA III, Skippen PW, Breuer RK, Toedt-Pingel I, Parsons SJ, Gradidge EA, Glater LB, Culver K, Nadkarni VM, Nishisaki A; National Emergency Airway Registry for Children (NEAR4KIDS) and Pediatric Acute Lung Injury and Sepsis Investigators (PALISI). Cricoid Pressure During Induction for Tracheal Intubation in Critically Ill Children: A Report From National Emergency Airway Registry for Children. *Pediatr Crit Care Med.* 2018;19:528–537. doi: 10.1097/PCC.0000000000001531
18. Quintard H, l'Her E, Pottecher J, Adnet F, Constantin JM, De Jong A, Diemunsch P, Fesseau R, Freynet A, Girault C, Guitton C, Hamonic Y, Maury E, Mekontso-Dessap A, Michel F, Nolent P, Perbet S, Prat G, Roquilly A, Tazarourte K, Terzi N, Thille AW, Alves M, Gayat E, Donetti L. Experts' guidelines of intubation and extubation of the ICU patient of French Society of Anaesthesia and Intensive Care Medicine (SFAR) and French-speaking Intensive Care Society (SRLF): In collaboration with the pediatric Association of French-speaking Anaesthetists and Intensivists (ADARPEF), French-speaking Group of Intensive Care and Paediatric emergencies (GFRUP) and Intensive Care physiotherapy society (SKR). *Ann Intensive Care.* 2019;9:13. doi: 10.1186/s13613-019-0483-1
19. Jones P, Ovenden N, Dauger S, Peters MJ. Estimating 'lost heart beats' rather than reductions in heart rate during the intubation of critically-ill children. *PLoS One.* 2014;9:e86766. doi: 10.1371/journal.pone.0086766
20. Eisa L, Passi Y, Lerman J, Raczka M, Heard C. Do small doses of atropine (<0.1 mg) cause bradycardia in young children? *Arch Dis Child.* 2015;100:684–688. doi: 10.1136/archdischild-2014-307868
21. Cook TM, Woodall N, Harper J, Benger J; on behalf of the Fourth National Audit Project. Major complications of airway management in the UK: results of the Fourth National Audit Project of the Royal College of Anaesthetists and the Difficult Airway Society, part 2: intensive care and emergency departments. *Br J Anaesth.* 2011;106:632–642. doi: 10.1093/bja/aer059
22. Cook TM. Strategies for the prevention of airway complications - a narrative review. *Anaesthesia.* 2018;73:93–111. doi: 10.1111/anae.14123
23. Hosono S, Inami I, Fujita H, Minato M, Takahashi S, Mugishima H. A role of end-tidal CO(2) monitoring for assessment of tracheal intubations in very low birth weight infants during neonatal resuscitation at birth. *J Perinat Med.* 2009;37:79–84. doi: 10.1515/JPM.2009.017
24. Hawkes GA, Finn D, Kenosi M, Livingstone V, O'Toole JM, Boylan GB, O'Halloran KD, Ryan AC, Dempsey EM. A Randomized Controlled Trial of End-Tidal Carbon Dioxide Detection of Preterm Infants in the Delivery Room. *J Pediatr.* 2017;182:74–78.e2. doi: 10.1016/j.jpeds.2016.11.006
25. Hunt KA, Yamada Y, Murthy V, Srihari Bhat P, Campbell M, Fox GF, Milner AD, Greenough A. Detection of exhaled carbon dioxide following intubation during resuscitation at delivery. *Arch Dis Child Fetal Neonatal Ed.* 2019;104:F187–F191. doi: 10.1136/archdischild-2017-313982
26. Langhan ML, Emerson BL, Nett S, Pinto M, Harwayne-Gidansky I, Rehder KJ, Krawiec C, Meyer K, Giuliano JS Jr, Owen EB, Tarquinio KM, Sanders RC Jr, Shepherd M, Bysani GK, Shenoi AN, Napolitano N, Gangadharan S, Parsons SJ, Simon DW, Nadkarni VM, Nishisaki A; for Pediatric Acute Lung Injury and Sepsis Investigators (PALISI) and National Emergency Airway Registry for Children (NEAR4KIDS) Investigators. End-Tidal Carbon Dioxide Use for Tracheal Intubation: Analysis From the National Emergency Airway Registry for Children (NEAR4KIDS) Registry. *Pediatr Crit Care Med.* 2018;19:98–105. doi: 10.1097/PCC.0000000000001372
27. Hawkes GA, Kenosi M, Ryan CA, Dempsey EM. Quantitative or qualitative carbon dioxide monitoring for manual ventilation: a mannequin study. *Acta Paediatr.* 2015;104:e148–e151. doi: 10.1111/apa.12868
28. Fanara B, Manzon C, Barbot O, Desmettre T, Capellier G. Recommendations for the intra-hospital transport of critically ill patients. *Crit Care.* 2010;14:R87. doi: 10.1186/cc9018
29. Langhan ML, Ching K, Northrup V, Alletag M, Kadia P, Santucci K, Chen L. A randomized controlled trial of capnography in the correction of simulated endotracheal tube dislodgement. *Acad Emerg Med.* 2011;18:590–596. doi: 10.1111/j.1553-2712.2011.01090.x
30. Langhan ML, Auerbach M, Smith AN, Chen L. Improving detection by pediatric residents of endotracheal tube dislodgement with capnography: a randomized controlled trial. *J Pediatr.* 2012;160:1009–14.e1. doi: 10.1016/j.jpeds.2011.12.012

MANAGEMENT OF BRADYCARDIA

Bradycardia associated with hemodynamic compromise, even with a palpable pulse, may be a harbinger for cardiac arrest. As such, bradycardia with a heart rate of less than 60 beats per minute requires emergent evaluation for cardiopulmonary compromise. If cardiopulmonary compromise is present, the initial management in the pediatric patient requires simultaneous assessment of the etiology and treatment by supporting airway, ventilation, and oxygenation. If bradycardia with cardiopulmonary compromise is present despite effective oxygenation and ventilation, CPR should be initiated immediately. Outcomes are better for children who receive CPR for bradycardia before progressing to pulseless arrest.[1] Correctable factors that contribute to bradycardia (ie, hypoxia, hypotension, hypoglycemia, hypothermia, acidosis, or toxic ingestions) should be identified and treated immediately.

Recommendations for the Management of Bradycardia		
COR	LOE	Recommendations
1	C-LD	1. If bradycardia is due to increased vagal tone or primary atrioventricular conduction block (ie, not secondary to factors such as hypoxia), give atropine.[2,4,6,7]
1	C-LD	2. If the heart rate is <60 beats/min with cardiopulmonary compromise despite effective ventilation with oxygen, start CPR.[1,10]
1	C-EO	3. If bradycardia persists after correction of other factors (eg, hypoxia) or responds only transiently, give epinephrine IV/IO. If IV/IO access is not available, give endotracheally if present.[1,11]
2b	C-LD	4. Emergency transcutaneous pacing may be considered if bradycardia is due to complete heart block or sinus node dysfunction unresponsive to ventilation, oxygenation, chest compressions, and medications, especially in children with congenital or acquired heart disease.[12–16]

Recommendation-Specific Supportive Text

1. Two adult studies[2,4] and 2 pediatric studies[6,7] demonstrate that atropine is effective to treat bradycardia due to vagal stimulation, atrioventricular block, and intoxication. There is no evidence that atropine should be used for bradycardia due to other causes.
2. Two retrospective analyses from the same database showed children who received CPR for bradycardia and poor perfusion had better outcomes than children who suffered pulseless cardiac arrest and received CPR.[1,10] The longer the time between the initiation of CPR for bradycardia and the loss of a pulse, the lower the chance of survival.
3. There are limited pediatric data regarding the treatment of bradycardia. A recent retrospective, propensity-matched study of pediatric patients with bradycardia with a pulse found that patients who received epinephrine had worse outcomes than patients who did not receive epinephrine.[11] However, due to limitations of the study, further research on the impact of epinephrine on patients with bradycardia and a pulse is required.
4. There are limited data about transcutaneous pacing for refractory bradycardia in children.[12–16] In patients with complete heart block or sinus node dysfunction, especially when caused by congenital or acquired heart disease, emergency transcutaneous pacing may be considered. Pacing is not useful for asystole or bradycardia due to postarrest hypoxic or ischemic myocardial insult or respiratory failure.

Figure 12 shows the algorithm for pediatric bradycardia with a pulse.

REFERENCES

1. Khera R, Tang Y, Girotra S, Nadkarni VM, Link MS, Raymond TT, Guerguerian AM, Berg RA, Chan PS; on behalf of the American Heart Association's Get With the Guidelines-Resuscitation Investigators. Pulselessness after initiation of cardiopulmonary resuscitation for bradycardia in hospitalized children. *Circulation.* 2019;140:370–378. doi: 10.1161/CIRCULATIONAHA.118.039048
2. Smith I, Monk TG, White PF. Comparison of transesophageal atrial pacing with anticholinergic drugs for the treatment of intraoperative bradycardia. *Anesth Analg.* 1994;78:245–252. doi: 10.1213/00000539-199402000-00009
3. Deleted in proof.
4. Brady WJ, Swart G, DeBehnke DJ, Ma OJ, Aufderheide TP. The efficacy of atropine in the treatment of hemodynamically unstable bradycardia and atrioventricular block: prehospital and emergency department considerations. *Resuscitation.* 1999;41:47–55. doi: 10.1016/s0300-9572(99)00032-5
5. Deleted in proof.
6. Zimmerman G, Steward DJ. Bradycardia delays the onset of action of intravenous atropine in infants. *Anesthesiology.* 1986;65:320–322.
7. Fullerton DA, St Cyr JA, Clarke DR, Campbell DN, Toews WH, See WM. Bezold-Jarisch reflex in postoperative pediatric cardiac surgical patients. *Ann Thorac Surg.* 1991;52:534–536. doi: 10.1016/0003-4975(91)90919-h
8. Deleted in proof.
9. Deleted in proof.
10. Donoghue A, Berg RA, Hazinski MF, Praestgaard AH, Roberts K, Nadkarni VM; American Heart Association National Registry of CPR Investigators. Cardiopulmonary resuscitation for bradycardia with poor perfusion versus pulseless cardiac arrest. *Pediatrics.* 2009;124:1541–1548. doi: 10.1542/peds.2009-0727
11. Holmberg MJ, Ross CE, Yankama T, Roberts JS, Andersen LW; on behalf of the American Heart Association's Get With The Guidelines-Resuscitation Investigators. Epinephrine in children receiving cardiopulmonary resuscitation for bradycardia with poor perfusion. *Resuscitation.* 2020:180–190. doi: 10.1016/j.resuscitation.2019.12.032
12. Pirasath S, Arulnithy K. Yellow oleander poisoning in eastern province: an analysis of admission and outcome. *Indian J Med Sci.* 2013;67:178–183. doi: 10.4103/0019-5359.125879
13. Singh HR, Batra AS, Balaji S. Pacing in children. *Ann Pediatr Cardiol.* 2013;6:46–51. doi: 10.4103/0974-2069.107234
14. Kugler JD, Danford DA. Pacemakers in children: an update. *Am Heart J.* 1989;117:665–679. doi: 10.1016/0002-8703(89)90743-6
15. Bolourchi M, Silver ES, Liberman L. Advanced heart block in children with Lyme disease. *Pediatr Cardiol.* 2019;40:513–517. doi: 10.1007/s00246-018-2003-8
16. Nazif TM, Vazquez J, Honig LS, Dizon JM. Anti-N-methyl-D-aspartate receptor encephalitis: an emerging cause of centrally mediated sinus node dysfunction. *Europace.* 2012;14:1188–1194. doi: 10.1093/europace/eus014

TACHYARRHYTHMIAS

Regular, narrow-complex tachyarrhythmias (QRS duration 0.09 seconds or less) are most commonly caused by re-entrant circuits, although other mechanisms (eg, ectopic atrial tachycardia, atrial fibrillation) sometimes occur. Regular, wide-complex tachyarrhythmias (greater than 0.09 seconds) can have multiple mechanisms, including supraventricular tachycardia (SVT) with aberrant conduction or ventricular tachycardia.

The hemodynamic impact of SVT in the pediatric patient can be variable, with cardiovascular compromise

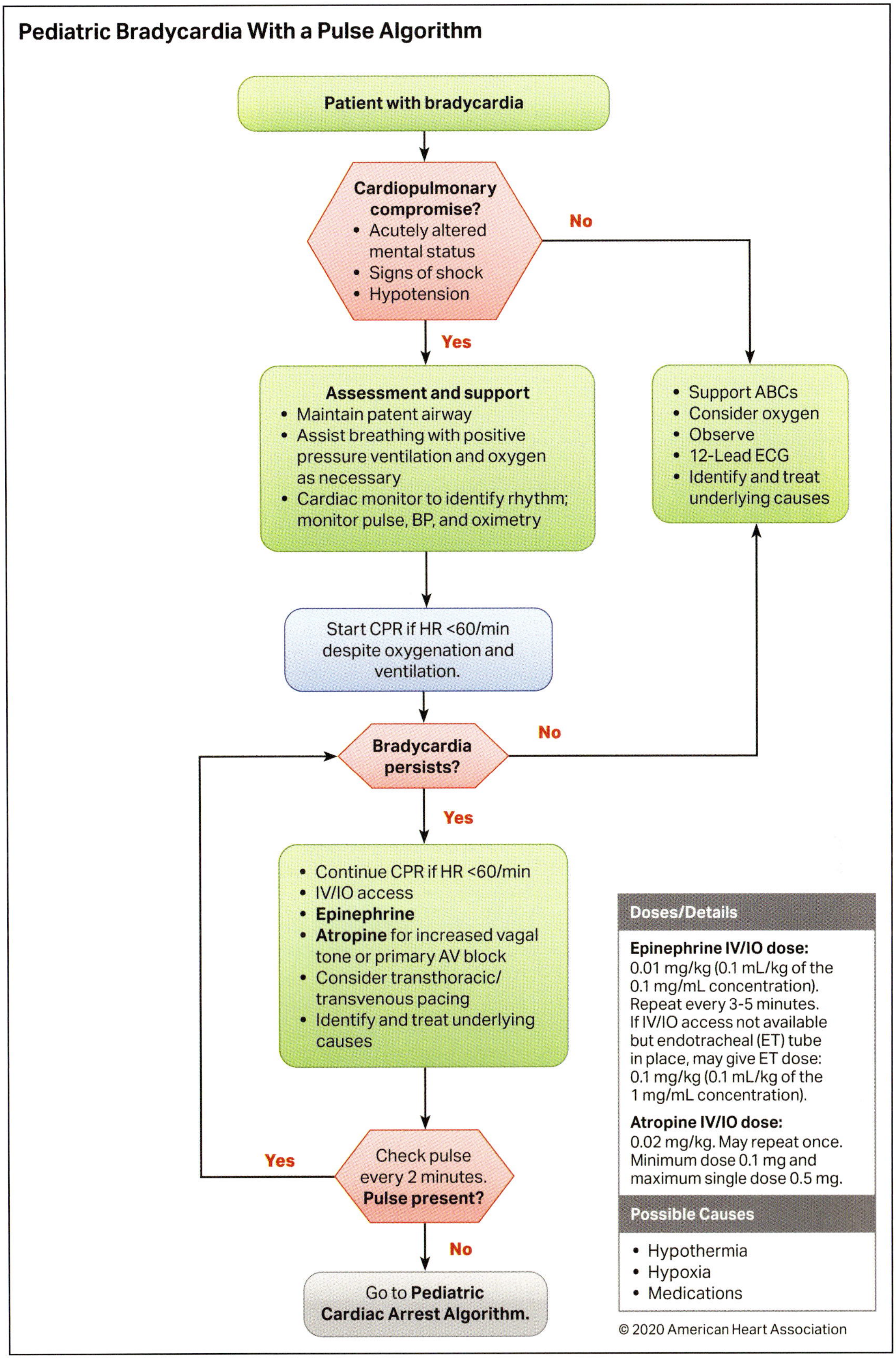

Figure 12. Pediatric Bradycardia With a Pulse Algorithm.
ABC indicates airway, breathing, and circulation; AV, atrioventricular; BP, blood pressure; CPR, cardiopulmonary resuscitation; ECG, electrocardiogram; HR, heart rate; IO, intraosseous; and IV, intravenous.

(ie, altered mental status, signs of shock, hypotension) occurring in the minority of patients. In hemodynamically stable patients, re-entrant SVT can often be terminated with vagal maneuvers.[1,2] Adenosine remains the preferred medication to treat SVT in infants and children with a palpable pulse who do not respond to vagal maneuvers. For patients with hemodynamically stable wide-complex tachycardia and those in whom SVT recurs after initial successful treatment, expert consultation is important to diagnose etiology and customize treatment.

In hemodynamically unstable patients with SVT or wide-complex tachycardia, synchronized cardioversion should be considered.

Treatment of Supraventricular Tachycardia With A Pulse

Recommendations for Treatment of Supraventricular Tachycardia With A Pulse

COR	LOE	Recommendations
1	C-LD	1. If IV/IO access is readily available, adenosine is recommended for the treatment of SVT.[3–9]
1	C-EO	2. For hemodynamically stable patients whose SVT is unresponsive to vagal maneuvers and/or IV adenosine, expert consultation is recommended.[5–15,17]
2a	C-LD	3. It is reasonable to attempt vagal stimulation first, unless the patient is hemodynamically unstable or it will delay chemical or electric synchronized cardioversion.[1,2,4]
2a	C-LD	4. If the patient with SVT is hemodynamically unstable with evidence of cardiovascular compromise (ie. altered mental status, signs of shock, hypotension) it is reasonable to perform electric synchronized cardioversion starting with a dose of 0.5 to 1 J/kg. If unsuccessful, increase the dose to 2 J/kg.[5,8,15]
2b	C-LD	5. For a patient with unstable SVT unresponsive to vagal maneuvers, IV adenosine, electric synchronized cardioversion and for whom expert consultation is not available, it may be reasonable to consider either procainamide or amiodarone.[12,15]

Recommendation-Specific Supportive Text

1. Intravenous adenosine remains generally effective for terminating re-entrant SVT within the first 2 doses.[3–6] Of 5 retrospective observational studies on the management of tachyarrhythmias (4 single center, 1 multicenter), none directly compared adenosine to other drugs.[6–9,17]
2. For patients with hemodynamically stable SVT that is refractory to vagal maneuvers or adenosine, consideration of alternative second-line agents should be guided by expert consultation, given potential proarrhythmic and life-threatening hemodynamic collapse with the administration of multiple antiarrhythmic agents. Multiple medications have been used as second-line agents for the management of adenosine-refractory SVT, including intravenous verapamil, β-blockers, amiodarone, procainamide, and sotalol.[5–15,17] Few comparative studies exist.
3. Vagal maneuvers are noninvasive, have few adverse effects, and effectively terminate SVT in many cases; exact success rates for each type of maneuver (ie, ice water to face, postural modification) are unknown.[4] Although improved success rates have been reported with a postural modification to the standard Valsalva maneuver in adults,[1] published pediatric experience with this technique is very limited. Upside-down positioning may be an additional form of a vagal maneuver that is effective in children.[2]
4. Direct current synchronized cardioversion remains the treatment of choice for patients with hemodynamically unstable SVT (ie, with cardiovascular compromise characterized by altered mental status, signs of shock, or hypotension) and those with SVT unresponsive to standard measures. However, these cases are uncommon, and there are few data reporting outcomes from cardioversion of SVT.[5,8,15] Consider administering sedation prior to synchronized cardioversion if resources are available and definitive therapy is not delayed.
5. Procainamide and amiodarone are moderately effective treatments for adenosine-resistant SVT.[12] There may be a small efficacy advantage favoring procainamide; adverse effects are frequent with both therapies. Intravenous sotalol was approved by the US Food and Drug Administration for the treatment of SVT in 2009. Only 3 reports describe its use in acute or subacute supraventricular tachyarrhythmias, with a 60% to 100% termination rate of SVT and atrial tachyarrhythmias.[9,13,14] In the aforementioned studies, IV sotalol was administered under the guidance of pediatric electrophysiologists in the critical care or pediatric cardiology unit. Due to its potential proarrhythmic properties, it is unknown whether IV sotalol can be safely given in other settings. There is currently insufficient evidence in support for or against the use of IV sotalol for refractory SVT.

Treatment of Wide-Complex Tachycardia With a Pulse

Recommendations for Treatment of Wide-Complex Tachycardia With a Pulse

COR	LOE	Recommendations
1	C-LD	1. If the patient with a wide-complex tachycardia is hemodynamically stable, expert consultation is recommended prior to administration of antiarrhythmic agents.[18]
2a	C-EO	2. If the patient with a wide-complex tachycardia is hemodynamically unstable with evidence of cardiovascular compromise (ie, altered mental status, signs of shock, hypotension), it is reasonable to perform electric synchronized cardioversion starting with a dose of 0.5–1 J/kg. If unsuccessful, increase the dose to 2 J/kg.

Circulation. 2020;142(suppl 2):S469–S523. DOI: 10.1161/CIR.0000000000000901

Recommendation-Specific Supportive Text

1. The occurrence of wide-complex tachycardia (QRS duration more than 0.09 s) with a pulse is rare in children and may originate from either the ventricle (ventricular tachycardia) or atria (SVT with aberrant conduction).[18] Both pediatric and adult studies have identified potential populations at risk of proarrhythmic complications from antiarrhythmic therapies, including patients with underlying cardiomyopathies, long-QT syndrome, Brugada syndrome, and Wolff-Parkinson-White syndrome.[19–23]
2. Electric direct current synchronized cardioversion should be provided urgently for the treatment of children with wide-complex tachycardia of either atrial or ventricular origin who are hemodynamically unstable with a pulse. Cardiovascular compromise is a key factor in determining the use of electric therapy instead of primary pharmacological management. There is insufficient evidence describing the incidence of wide-complex tachycardias with a pulse and hemodynamic stability, and there is no support for or against the use of specific antiarrhythmic drugs in the management of children with wide-complex tachycardia with a pulse.

Figure 13 shows the algorithm for pediatric tachycardia with a pulse.

REFERENCES

1. Appelboam A, Reuben A, Mann C, Gagg J, Ewings P, Barton A, Lobban T, Dayer M, Vickery J, Benger J; REVERT trial collaborators. Postural modification to the standard Valsalva manoeuvre for emergency treatment of supraventricular tachycardias (REVERT): a randomised controlled trial. *Lancet.* 2015;386:1747–1753. doi: 10.1016/S0140-6736(15)61485-4
2. Bronzetti G, Brighenti M, Mariucci E, Fabi M, Lanari M, Bonvicini M, Gargiulo G, Pession A. Upside-down position for the out of hospital management of children with supraventricular tachycardia. *Int J Cardiol.* 2018;252:106–109. doi: 10.1016/j.ijcard.2017.10.120
3. Losek JD, Endom E, Dietrich A, Stewart G, Zempsky W, Smith K. Adenosine and pediatric supraventricular tachycardia in the emergency department: multicenter study and review. *Ann Emerg Med.* 1999;33:185–191. doi: 10.1016/s0196-0644(99)70392-6
4. Campbell M, Buitrago SR. BET 2: Ice water immersion, other vagal manoeuvres or adenosine for SVT in children. *Emerg Med J.* 2017;34:58–60. doi: 10.1136/emermed-2016–206487.2
5. Clausen H, Theophilos T, Jackno K, Babl FE. Paediatric arrhythmias in the emergency department. *Emerg Med J.* 2012;29:732–737. doi: 10.1136/emermed-2011-200242
6. Díaz-Parra S, Sánchez-Yañez P, Zabala-Argüelles I, Picazo-Angelin B, Conejo-Muñoz L, Cuenca-Peiró V, Durán-Hidalgo I, García-Soler P. Use of adenosine in the treatment of supraventricular tachycardia in a pediatric emergency department. *Pediatr Emerg Care.* 2014;30:388–393. doi: 10.1097/PEC.0000000000000144
7. Chu PY, Hill KD, Clark RH, Smith PB, Hornik CP. Treatment of supraventricular tachycardia in infants: Analysis of a large multicenter database. *Early Hum Dev.* 2015;91:345–350. doi: 10.1016/j.earlhumdev.2015.04.001
8. Lewis J, Arora G, Tudorascu DL, Hickey RW, Saladino RA, Manole MD. Acute management of refractory and unstable pediatric supraventricular tachycardia. *J Pediatr.* 2017;181;177.e2–182.e2. doi: 10.1016/j.jpeds.2016.10.051
9. Borquez AA, Aljohani OA, Williams MR, Perry JC. Intravenous sotalol in the young. *J Am Coll Cardiol EP.* 2020;6:425–432. doi: 10.1016/j.jacep.2019.11.019
10. Lim SH, Anantharaman V, Teo WS, Chan YH. Slow infusion of calcium channel blockers compared with intravenous adenosine in the emergency treatment of supraventricular tachycardia. *Resuscitation.* 2009;80:523–528. doi: 10.1016/j.resuscitation.2009.01.017
11. Lapage MJ, Bradley DJ, Dick M II. Verapamil in infants: an exaggerated fear? *Pediatr Cardiol.* 2013;34:1532–1534. doi: 10.1007/s00246-013-0739-8
12. Chang PM, Silka MJ, Moromisato DY, Bar-Cohen Y. Amiodarone versus procainamide for the acute treatment of recurrent supraventricular tachycardia in pediatric patients. *Circ Arrhythm Electrophysiol.* 2010;3:134–140. doi: 10.1161/CIRCEP.109.901629
13. Li X, Zhang Y, Liu H, Jiang H, Ge H, Zhang Y. Efficacy of intravenous sotalol for treatment of incessant tachyarrhythmias in children. *Am J Cardiol.* 2017;119:1366–1370. doi: 10.1016/j.amjcard.2017.01.034
14. Valdés SO, Landstrom AP, Schneider AE, Miyake CY, de la Uz CM, Kim JJ. Intravenous sotalol for the management of postoperative junctional ectopic tachycardia. *HeartRhythm Case Rep.* 2018;4:375–377. doi: 10.1016/j.hrcr.2018.05.007
15. Sacchetti A, Moyer V, Baricella R, Cameron J, Moakes ME. Primary cardiac arrhythmias in children. *Pediatr Emerg Care.* 1999;15:95–98. doi: 10.1097/00006565-199904000-00004
16. Deleted in proof.
17. Chandler SF, Chu E, Whitehill RD, Bevilacqua LM, Bezzerides VJ, DeWitt ES, Alexander ME, Abrams DJ, Triedman JK, Walsh EP, et al. Adverse event rate during inpatient sotalol initiation for the management of supraventricular and ventricular tachycardia in the pediatric and young adult population. *Heart Rhythm.* 2020;17:984-990. doi: 10.1016/j.hrthm.2020.01.022
18. Brady WJ, Mattu A, Tabas J, Ferguson JD. The differential diagnosis of wide QRS complex tachycardia. *Am J Emerg Med.* 2017;35:1525–1529. doi: 10.1016/j.ajem.2017.07.056
19. Ramusovic S, Läer S, Meibohm B, Lagler FB, Paul T. Pharmacokinetics of intravenous amiodarone in children. *Arch Dis Child.* 2013;98:989–993. doi: 10.1136/archdischild-2013-304483
20. Sarganas G, Garbe E, Klimpel A, Hering RC, Bronder E, Haverkamp W. Epidemiology of symptomatic drug-induced long QT syndrome and Torsade de Pointes in Germany. *Europace.* 2014;16:101–108. doi: 10.1093/europace/eut214
21. Chen S, Motonaga KS, Hollander SA, Almond CS, Rosenthal DN, Kaufman BD, May LJ, Avasarala K, Dao DT, Dubin AM, Ceresnak SR. Electrocardiographic repolarization abnormalities and increased risk of life-threatening arrhythmias in children with dilated cardiomyopathy. *Heart Rhythm.* 2016;13:1289–1296. doi: 10.1016/j.hrthm.2016.02.014
22. Coughtrie AL, Behr ER, Layton D, Marshall V, Camm AJ, Shakir SAW. Drugs and life-threatening ventricular arrhythmia risk: results from the DARE study cohort. *BMJ Open.* 2017;7:e016627. doi: 10.1136/bmjopen-2017-016627
23. Ortiz M, Martín A, Arribas F, Coll-Vinent B, Del Arco C, Peinado R, Almendral J; PROCAMIO Study Investigators. Randomized comparison of intravenous procainamide vs. intravenous amiodarone for the acute treatment of tolerated wide QRS tachycardia: the PROCAMIO study. *Eur Heart J.* 2017;38:1329–1335. doi: 10.1093/eurheartj/ehw230

TREATMENT OF MYOCARDITIS AND CARDIOMYOPATHY

Fulminant myocarditis can result in decreased cardiac output with end-organ compromise; conduction system disease, including complete heart block; and persistent supraventricular or ventricular arrhythmias, which can ultimately result in cardiac arrest.[1] Because patients can present with nonspecific symptoms such as abdominal pain, diarrhea, vomiting, or fatigue, myocarditis can be confused with other, more common disease presentations. Outcomes can be optimized by early diagnosis and prompt intervention, including ICU monitoring and therapy. Sudden onset of heart block and multifocal ventricular ectopy in the patient with fulminant myocarditis should be considered a prearrest state. Treatment with external or intracardiac pacing or antiarrhythmic drugs may not be successful, and early transfer to a center capable of providing extracorporeal life support (ECLS) or mechanical

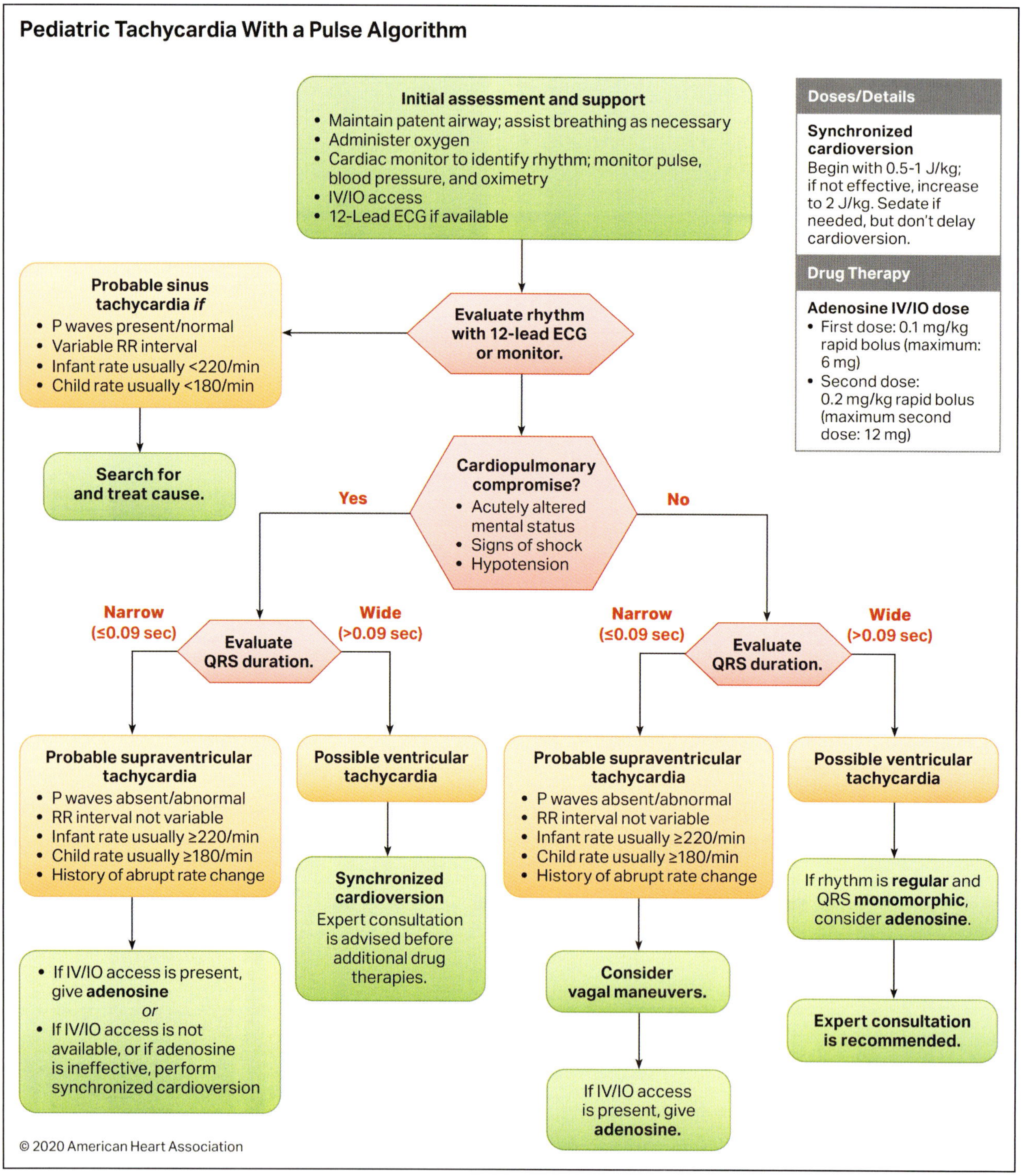

Figure 13. Pediatric Tachycardia With a Pulse Algorithm.
CPR indicates cardiopulmonary resuscitation; ECG, electrocardiogram; IO, intraosseous; and IV, intravenous.

circulatory support (MCS), such as temporary or implanted ventricular assist devices, is recommended.[2,3]

Noninfectious causes of cardiomyopathy in children include dilated cardiomyopathy, hypertrophic cardiomyopathy, restrictive cardiomyopathy, and miscellaneous (rare) forms of cardiomyopathy that include arrhythmogenic right ventricular dysplasia and mitochondrial and left ventricular noncompaction cardiomyopathies. Cardiomyopathy patients who present in acute decompensated heart failure refractory to mechanical ventilation and vasoactive administration have undergone preemptive MCS in the form of ECMO, short-term percutaneous ventricular assist device, or long-term implantable ventricular assist device prior to or during cardiac arrest.[4,5]

For patients who have worsening clinical status or incessant ventricular arrhythmias, ECLS can be lifesaving when initiated prior to cardiac arrest. ECLS also offers an opportunity to wean inotropic support, assist myocardial recovery, and serve as a bridge to cardiac transplantation if needed. The use of ECLS and MCS have improved outcomes from acute myocarditis, with a high possibility of partial or complete recovery of myocardial function.[2,6]

Recommendations for Treatment of Myocarditis and Cardiomyopathy

COR	LOE	Recommendations
1	C-LD	1. Given the high risk of cardiac arrest in children with acute myocarditis who demonstrate arrhythmias, heart block, ST-segment changes, and/or low cardiac output, early consideration of transfer to ICU monitoring and therapy is recommended.[1,7,8]
2a	B-NR	2. For children with myocarditis or cardiomyopathy and refractory low cardiac output, prearrest use of ECLS or MCS can be beneficial to provide end-organ support and prevent cardiac arrest.[9,10]
2a	B-NR	3. Given the challenges to successful resuscitation of children with myocarditis and cardiomyopathy, once cardiac arrest occurs, early consideration of ECPR can be beneficial.[9]

Recommendation-Specific Supportive Text

1. Three retrospective studies have evaluated predictors of worse outcome in fulminant myocarditis, noting increased incidence of cardiac arrest and the need for ECLS in this high-risk population.[1,7,8] In 1 study, nearly half of fulminant myocarditis patients required CPR, and nearly one third received MCS.[7] Even modest decreases in left ventricular ejection fraction are associated with the need for invasive circulatory support.[8]
2. The prognosis for patients with fulminant myocarditis who receive ECLS or MCS can be good. In 1 study, 13 (46%) of 28 children requiring MCS survived without transplant.[9] One study noted that outcomes for ECPR patients cannulated with a diagnosis of myocarditis are superior to other arrest and illness categories leading to ECPR (ie, patients without congenital heart disease), noting myocarditis as a precannulation factor associated with improved survival.[10] In the pre–cardiac arrest cardiomyopathy patient, newer forms of temporary circulatory support devices provide alternate and potentially improved support for decompensated heart failure requiring bridge to transplantation. These devices may provide a survival benefit over ECMO.[4,5]
3. In 1 study, 95% of children with myocarditis who were placed on ECLS (n=15) or MCS (n=1) after cardiac arrest were alive 6 months later.[9]

REFERENCES

1. Miyake CY, Teele SA, Chen L, Motonaga KS, Dubin AM, Balasubramanian S, Balise RR, Rosenthal DN, Alexander ME, Walsh EP, Mah DY. In-hospital arrhythmia development and outcomes in pediatric patients with acute myocarditis. *Am J Cardiol.* 2014;113:535–540. doi: 10.1016/j.amjcard.2013.10.021
2. Wilmot I, Morales DL, Price JF, Rossano JW, Kim JJ, Decker JA, McGarry MC, Denfield SW, Dreyer WJ, Towbin JA, Jefferies JL. Effectiveness of mechanical circulatory support in children with acute fulminant and persistent myocarditis. *J Card Fail.* 2011;17:487–494. doi: 10.1016/j.cardfail.2011.02.008
3. Teele SA, Allan CK, Laussen PC, Newburger JW, Gauvreau K, Thiagarajan RR. Management and outcomes in pediatric patients presenting with acute fulminant myocarditis. *J Pediatr.* 2011;158:638–643.e1. doi: 10.1016/j.jpeds.2010.10.015
4. Lorts A, Eghtesady P, Mehegan M, Adachi I, Villa C, Davies R, Gossett JG, Kanter K, Alejos J, Koehl D, Cantor RS, Morales DLS. Outcomes of children supported with devices labeled as "temporary" or short term: A report from the Pediatric Interagency Registry for Mechanical Circulatory Support. *J Heart Lung Transplant.* 2018;37:54–60. doi: 10.1016/j.healun.2017.10.023
5. Yarlagadda VV, Maeda K, Zhang Y, Chen S, Dykes JC, Gowen MA, Shuttleworth P, Murray JM, Shin AY, Reinhartz O, Rosenthal DN, McElhinney DB, Almond CS. Temporary Circulatory Support in U.S. Children Awaiting Heart Transplantation. *J Am Coll Cardiol.* 2017;70:2250–2260. doi: 10.1016/j.jacc.2017.08.072
6. Rajagopal SK, Almond CS, Laussen PC, Rycus PT, Wypij D, Thiagarajan RR. Extracorporeal membrane oxygenation for the support of infants, children, and young adults with acute myocarditis: a review of the Extracorporeal Life Support Organization registry. *Crit Care Med.* 2010;38:382–387. doi: 10.1097/CCM.0b013e3181bc8293
7. Casadonte JR, Mazwi ML, Gambetta KE, Palac HL, McBride ME, Eltayeb OM, Monge MC, Backer CL, Costello JM. Risk Factors for Cardiac Arrest or Mechanical Circulatory Support in Children with Fulminant Myocarditis. *Pediatr Cardiol.* 2017;38:128–134. doi: 10.1007/s00246-016-1493-5
8. Wu HP, Lin MJ, Yang WC, Wu KH, Chen CY. Predictors of Extracorporeal Membrane Oxygenation Support for Children with Acute Myocarditis. *Biomed Res Int.* 2017;2017:2510695. doi: 10.1155/2017/2510695
9. Schubert S, Opgen-Rhein B, Boehne M, Weigelt A, Wagner R, Müller G, Rentzsch A, Zu Knyphausen E, Fischer M, Papakostas K, Wiegand G, Ruf B, Hannes T, Reineker K, Kiski D, Khalil M, Steinmetz M, Fischer G, Pickardt T, Klingel K, Messroghli DR, Degener F; MYKKE consortium. Severe heart failure and the need for mechanical circulatory support and heart transplantation in pediatric patients with myocarditis: Results from the prospective multicenter registry "MYKKE". *Pediatr Transplant.* 2019;23:e13548. doi: 10.1111/petr.13548
10. Conrad SJ, Bridges BC, Kalra Y, Pietsch JB, Smith AH. Extracorporeal Cardiopulmonary Resuscitation Among Patients with Structurally Normal Hearts. *ASAIO J.* 2017;63:781–786. doi: 10.1097/MAT.0000000000000568

RESUSCITATION OF THE PATIENT WITH A SINGLE VENTRICLE

The complexity and variability in pediatric congenital heart disease pose unique challenges during resuscitation. Children with single-ventricle heart disease typically undergo a series of staged palliative operations. The objectives of the first palliative procedure, typically performed during the neonatal period, are (1) to create unobstructed systemic blood flow, (2) to create an effective atrial communication to allow for atrial level mixing, and (3) to regulate pulmonary blood flow to prevent overcirculation and decrease the volume load on the systemic ventricle (Figure 14). During the second stage of palliation, a superior cavopulmonary anastomosis, or bidirectional Glenn/hemi-Fontan operation, is performed to create an anastomosis, which aids in the redistribution of systemic venous return directly to the pulmonary circulation (Figure 15). The Fontan is the final palliation, in which inferior vena caval blood flow is baffled directly to the pulmonary circulation, thereby making the single (systemic) ventricle preload dependent on passive flow across the pulmonary vascular bed (Figure 16).

Neonates and infants with single-ventricle physiology have an increased risk of cardiac arrest as a result of (1) increased myocardial work as a consequence of volume overload, (2) imbalances in relative systemic (Qs) and pulmonary (Qp) blood flow, and (3) potential shunt occlusion.[1,2] Depending on the stage of repair, resuscitation may require control of pulmonary vascular resistance, oxygenation, systemic vascular resistance, or ECLS.

Preoperative and Postoperative Stage I Palliation (Norwood/Blalock-Taussig Shunt or Sano Shunt)

Recommendations for the Treatment of Preoperative and Postoperative Stage I Palliation (Norwood/Blalock-Taussig Shunt or Sano Shunt)

COR	LOE	Recommendations
2a	B-NR	1. Direct (superior vena cava catheter) and/or indirect (near infrared spectroscopy) oxygen saturation monitoring can be beneficial to trend and direct management in the critically ill neonate after stage I Norwood palliation or shunt placement.[3]
2a	C-LD	2. In the patient with an appropriately restrictive shunt, manipulation of pulmonary vascular resistance may have little effect, whereas lowering systemic vascular resistance with the use of systemic vasodilators (α-adrenergic antagonists and/or phosphodiesterase type III inhibitors), with or without the use of oxygen, can be useful to increase systemic oxygen delivery (DO_2).[4,5]
2a	C-LD	3. For neonates prior to stage I repair with pulmonary overcirculation and symptomatic low systemic cardiac output and delivery of oxygen (DO_2), it is reasonable to target a $Pa{CO_2}$ of 50–60 mm Hg. This can be achieved during mechanical ventilation by reducing minute ventilation or by administering analgesia/sedation with or without neuromuscular blockade.[6,7]
2a	C-LD	4. ECLS after Stage I Norwood palliation can be useful to treat low systemic DO_2.[8,9]
2a	C-EO	5. In the situation of known or suspected shunt obstruction, it is reasonable to administer oxygen, vasoactive agents to increase shunt perfusion pressure, and heparin (50–100 U/kg bolus) while preparing for catheter-based or surgical intervention.[2]

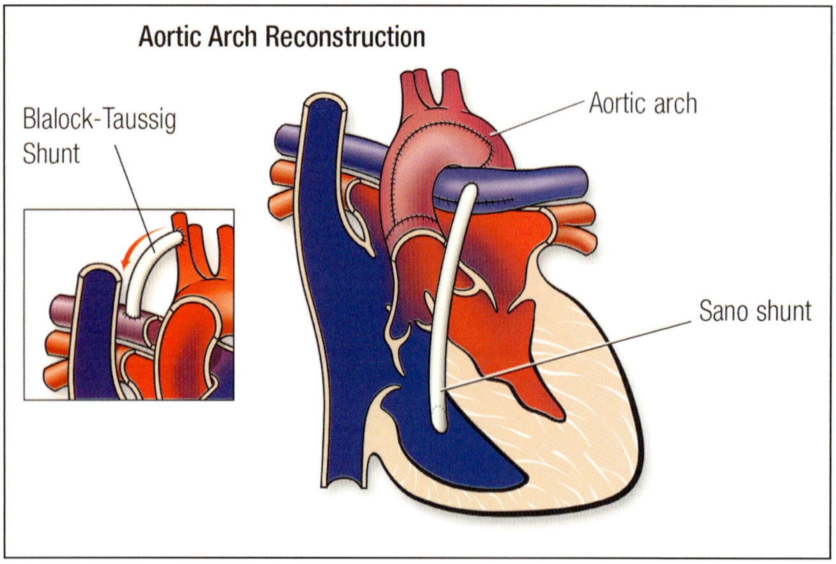

Figure 14. Stage I palliation for single ventricle with a Norwood repair and either a Blalock-Taussig Shunt from the right subclavian artery to the right pulmonary artery or a Sano shunt from the right ventricle to pulmonary artery.

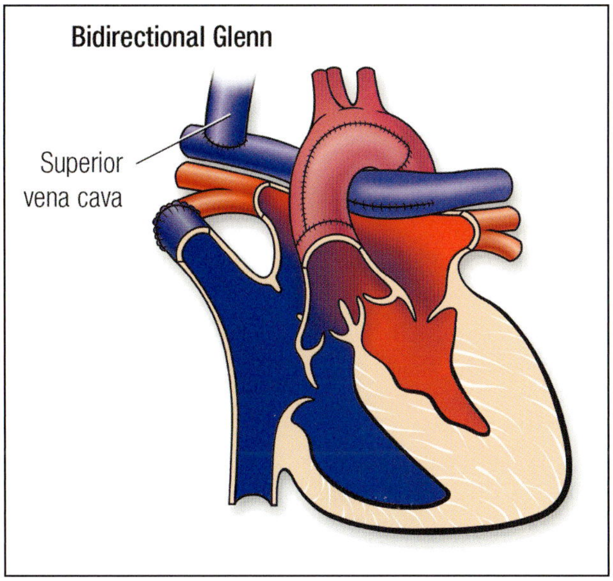

Figure 15. Stage II palliation for single ventricle with a bidirectional Glenn shunt connecting the superior vena cava to the right pulmonary artery.

Recommendation-Specific Supportive Text

1. In the early postoperative period, noninvasively measured regional cerebral and somatic saturations, via near infrared spectroscopy, can predict outcomes of early mortality and ECLS use following stage I Norwood palliation. There are retrospective data that postoperative near infrared spectroscopy measures may be targets for goal-directed interventions.[3]
2. Afterload reduction using vasodilators (sodium nitroprusside or phentolamine), with or without a phosphodiesterase type III inhibitor (eg, milrinone), reduces systemic vascular resistance, serum lactate, arterial venous oxygen difference, and the need for ECPR in the postoperative period for shunt-dependent single-ventricle patients.[4,5]
3. In the period before single-ventricle palliation, cautious use of controlled hypoventilation can reduce Qp:Qs by increasing pulmonary vascular resistance, narrowing the arterial-venous oxygen difference, and increasing cerebral oxygen delivery. Simple hypoventilation can also increase the pulmonary vascular resistance but can be associated with unwanted atelectasis or respiratory acidosis.[6,7]
4. For cardiac arrest before or after Stage I palliation repair, the use of ECPR is associated with improved survival. In 2 observational studies, 32% to 54% of neonates requiring ECPR survived, and, in 1 study, the odds of survival improved in cardiac arrest patients managed with ECPR.[8,9]
5. Treatment of acute shunt obstruction can include administration of oxygen, vasoactive agents (eg, phenylephrine, norepinephrine, epinephrine) to maximize shunt perfusion pressure, anticoagulation with heparin (50–100 U/kg bolus), shunt intervention by catheterization or surgery, and ECLS.[2]

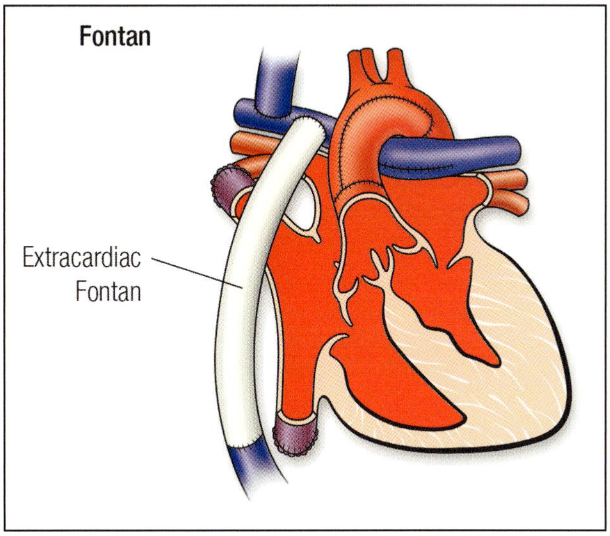

Figure 16. Stage III Fontan single ventricle palliation with an extracardiac conduit connecting the inferior vena cava to the right pulmonary artery.

Postoperative Stage II (Bidirectional Glenn/Hemi-Fontan) and III (Fontan) Palliation

Recommendations for the Treatment of Postoperative Stage II (Bidirectional Glenn/Hemi-Fontan) and III (Fontan) Palliation

COR	LOE	Recommendations
2a	B-NR	1. For patients in a prearrest state with superior cavopulmonary anastomosis physiology and severe hypoxemia due to inadequate Qp, ventilatory strategies that target a mild respiratory acidosis and a minimum mean airway pressure without atelectasis can be useful to increase cerebral and systemic arterial oxygenation.[10]
2b	B-NR	2. ECLS in patients with superior cavopulmonary anastomosis or Fontan circulation may be considered to treat low DO_2 from reversible causes or as a bridge to a ventricular assist device or surgical revision.[11]

Recommendation-Specific Supportive Text

1. In patients immediately following bidirectional Glenn placement, a ventilation strategy with higher Pa_{CO_2} improved oxygenation.[10]
2. In 1 retrospective analysis of the Extracorporeal Life Support Organization database, among infants in whom a bidirectional Glenn had been placed and in whom ECLS was required, survival was similar in patients who had cardiac arrest before ECLS (16/39, 41%) and those who did not (26/64, 41%).[11]

These topics were reviewed previously in "Cardiopulmonary Resuscitation in Infants and Children With Cardiac Disease: A Scientific Statement From the American Heart Association."[12]

REFERENCES

1. Feinstein JA, Benson DW, Dubin AM, Cohen MS, Maxey DM, Mahle WT, Pahl E, Villafañe J, Bhatt AB, Peng LF, et al. Hypoplastic left heart syndrome: current considerations and expectations. *J Am Coll Cardiol.* 2012;59(suppl 1):S1–S42. doi: 10.1016/j.jacc.2011.09.022
2. Marino BS, Tibby SM, Hoffman GM. Resuscitation of the patient with the functionally univentricular heart. *Curr Pediatr Rev.* 2013;9:148–157. doi: 10.2174/1573396311309020008
3. Hoffman GM, Ghanayem NS, Scott JP, Tweddell JS, Mitchell ME, Mussatto KA. Postoperative Cerebral and Somatic Near-Infrared Spectroscopy Saturations and Outcome in Hypoplastic Left Heart Syndrome. *Ann Thorac Surg.* 2017;103:1527–1535. doi: 10.1016/j.athoracsur.2016.09.100
4. Mills KI, Kaza AK, Walsh BK, Bond HC, Ford M, Wypij D, Thiagarajan RR, Almodovar MC, Quinonez LG, Baird CW, et al. Phosphodiesterase inhibitor-based vasodilation improves oxygen delivery and clinical outcomes following stage 1 palliation. *J Am Heart Assoc.* 2016;5 doi: 10.1161/JAHA.116.003554
5. Hansen JH, Schlangen J, Voges I, Jung O, Wegmann A, Scheewe J, Kramer HH. Impact of afterload reduction strategies on regional tissue oxygenation after the Norwood procedure for hypoplastic left heart syndrome. *Eur J Cardiothorac Surg.* 2014;45:e13–e19. doi: 10.1093/ejcts/ezt538
6. Ramamoorthy C, Tabbutt S, Kurth CD, Steven JM, Montenegro LM, Durning S, Wernovsky G, Gaynor JW, Spray TL, Nicolson SC. Effects of inspired hypoxic and hypercapnic gas mixtures on cerebral oxygen saturation in neonates with univentricular heart defects. *Anesthesiology.* 2002;96:283–288. doi: 10.1097/00000542-200202000-00010
7. Tabbutt S, Ramamoorthy C, Montenegro LM, Durning SM, Kurth CD, Steven JM, Godinez RI, Spray TL, Wernovsky G, Nicolson SC. Impact of inspired gas mixtures on preoperative infants with hypoplastic left heart syndrome during controlled ventilation. *Circulation.* 2001;104(suppl 1):I159–I164. doi: 10.1161/hc37t1.094818
8. Alsoufi B, Awan A, Manlhiot C, Guechef A, Al-Halees Z, Al-Ahmadi M, McCrindle BW, Kalloghlian A. Results of rapid-response extracorporeal cardiopulmonary resuscitation in children with refractory cardiac arrest following cardiac surgery. *Eur J Cardiothorac Surg.* 2014;45:268–275. doi: 10.1093/ejcts/ezt319
9. Alsoufi B, Awan A, Manlhiot C, Al-Halees Z, Al-Ahmadi M, McCrindle BW, Alwadai A. Does single ventricle physiology affect survival of children requiring extracorporeal membrane oxygenation support following cardiac surgery? *World J Pediatr Congenit Heart Surg.* 2014;5:7–15. doi: 10.1177/2150135113507292
10. Zhu L, Xu Z, Gong X, Zheng J, Sun Y, Liu L, Han L, Zhang H, Xu Z, Liu J, et al. Mechanical ventilation after bidirectional superior cavopulmonary anastomosis for single-ventricle physiology: a comparison of pressure support ventilation and neurally adjusted ventilatory assist. *Pediatr Cardiol.* 2016;37:1064–1071. doi: 10.1007/s00246-016-1392-9
11. Jolley M, Thiagarajan RR, Barrett CS, Salvin JW, Cooper DS, Rycus PT, Teele SA. Extracorporeal membrane oxygenation in patients undergoing superior cavopulmonary anastomosis. *J Thorac Cardiovasc Surg.* 2014;148:1512–1518. doi: 10.1016/j.jtcvs.2014.04.028
12. Marino BS, Tabbutt S, MacLaren G, Hazinski MF, Adatia I, Atkins DL, Checchia PA, DeCaen A, Fink EL, Hoffman GM, Jefferies JL, Kleinman M, Krawczeski CD, Licht DJ, Macrae D, Ravishankar C, Samson RA, Thiagarajan RR, Toms R, Tweddell J, Laussen PC; American Heart Association Congenital Cardiac Defects Committee of the Council on Cardiovascular Disease in the Young; Council on Clinical Cardiology; Council on Cardiovascular and Stroke Nursing; Council on Cardiovascular Surgery and Anesthesia; and Emergency Cardiovascular Care Committee. Cardiopulmonary Resuscitation in Infants and Children With Cardiac Disease: A Scientific Statement From the American Heart Association. *Circulation.* 2018;137:e691–e782. doi: 10.1161/CIR.0000000000000524

RECOMMENDATION FOR TREATMENT OF THE CHILD WITH PULMONARY HYPERTENSION

Pulmonary hypertension is a rare disease in infants and children that is associated with significant morbidity and mortality. In the majority of pediatric patients, pulmonary hypertension is idiopathic or associated with chronic lung disease; congenital heart disease; and, rarely, other conditions, such as connective tissue or thromboembolic disease.[1] Pulmonary hypertension occurs in 2% to 20% of patients following congenital heart disease surgery, with substantial morbidity and mortality.[2] Pulmonary hypertension occurs in 2% to 5% of pediatric patients after cardiac surgery,[3] and 0.7% to 5% of all cardiovascular surgical patients experience postoperative pulmonary hypertensive crises.[4] Pulmonary hypertensive crises are acute rapid increases in pulmonary artery pressure accompanied by right-sided (or single-ventricle) heart failure. During pulmonary hypertensive crises, the right ventricle fails, and the increased afterload on the right ventricle produces increased myocardial oxygen demand at the same time that the coronary perfusion pressure and coronary blood flow decrease. The elevated left ventricle and right ventricle pressures lead to a fall in pulmonary blood flow and left-sided heart filling, with a resultant fall in cardiac output. Inotropic agents can be administered to improve right ventricle function, and vasopressors can be administered to treat systemic hypotension and improve coronary artery perfusion pressure. Once cardiac arrest has occurred, outcomes can be improved in the presence of an anatomic right-to-left shunt that permits left ventricle preload to be maintained without pulmonary blood flow.[2] These crises are life threatening and may lead to systemic hypotension, myocardial ischemia, cardiac arrest, and death. Because acidosis and hypoxemia are both potent pulmonary vasoconstrictors, careful monitoring and management of these conditions are critical in the management of pulmonary hypertension. Treatment should also include the provision of adequate analgesics, sedatives, and muscle relaxants. Pulmonary vasodilators, including inhaled nitric oxide, inhaled prostacyclin, inhaled and intravenous prostacyclin analogs, and intravenous and oral phosphodiesterase type V inhibitors (eg, sildenafil) are used to prevent and treat pulmonary hypertensive crises.[5–8]

Recommendations for Treatment of the Child With Pulmonary Hypertension

COR	LOE	Recommendations
1	B-R	1. Inhaled nitric oxide or prostacyclin should be used as the initial therapy to treat pulmonary hypertensive crises or acute right-sided heart failure secondary to increased pulmonary vascular resistance.[7,9–12]
1	B-NR	2. Provide careful respiratory management and monitoring to avoid hypoxia and acidosis in the postoperative care of the child with pulmonary hypertension.[13–15]
1	C-EO	3. For pediatric patients who are at high risk for pulmonary hypertensive crises, provide adequate analgesics, sedatives, and neuromuscular blocking agents.[2,11,16,17]
2a	C-LD	4. For the initial treatment of pulmonary hypertensive crises, oxygen administration and induction of alkalosis through hyperventilation or alkali administration can be useful while pulmonary-specific vasodilators are administered.[13–15]
2b	C-LD	5. For children who develop refractory pulmonary hypertension, including signs of low cardiac output or profound respiratory failure despite optimal medical therapy, ECLS may be considered.[11,18–23]

Recommendation-Specific Supportive Text

1. Treatment with inhaled nitric oxide reduces the frequency of pulmonary hypertensive crises and shortens time to extubation.[9] In patients with atrioventricular septal defect repair and severe postoperative pulmonary hypertension, inhaled nitric oxide administration is associated with reduced mortality.[7,10] Inhaled prostacyclin transiently produces pulmonary vasodilation and improves oxygenation, but the alkalinity of the drug can irritate airways, and precise dosing can be complicated by drug loss in the nebulization circuit.[11,12]
2. Two physiological reviews and 1 randomized clinical trial have demonstrated that hypercarbia, hypoxemia, acidosis, atelectasis, and ventilation-perfusion mismatch can all lead to increases in pulmonary vascular resistance and, hence, elevation of pulmonary artery pressures in the immediate postoperative period.[13–15]
3. Two observational studies looking at select high-risk postoperative cardiac patients found an attenuation in the stress response in those patients receiving fentanyl in the postoperative period.[2,11,16,17]
4. Two physiological reviews and 1 randomized clinical trial have demonstrated that hypercarbia, hypoxemia, acidosis, atelectasis, and ventilation-perfusion mismatch can all lead to increases in pulmonary vascular resistance and, hence, elevation of pulmonary artery pressures in the immediate postoperative period.[13–15]
5. ECLS has been used in children with pulmonary vascular disease after cardiopulmonary collapse or low cardiac output.[18,19] Although outcomes remain poor in certain populations,[20] advances in technology of extracorporeal devices may allow for bridging to MCS or to transplantation.[21] Although patients with pulmonary hypertension who require ECLS have a high mortality rate, provision of ECLS can be lifesaving.[11,22,23]

These topics were reviewed previously in "Cardiopulmonary Resuscitation in Infants and Children With Cardiac Disease: A Scientific Statement From the American Heart Association"[2] and "Pediatric Pulmonary Hypertension: Guidelines From the American Heart Association and American Thoracic Society."[11]

REFERENCES

1. Ivy DD, Abman SH, Barst RJ, Berger RM, Bonnet D, Fleming TR, Haworth SG, Raj JU, Rosenzweig EB, Schulze Neick I, et al. Pediatric pulmonary hypertension. *J Am Coll Cardiol.* 2013;62(suppl):D117–D126. doi: 10.1016/j.jacc.2013.10.028
2. Marino BS, Tabbutt S, MacLaren G, Hazinski MF, Adatia I, Atkins DL, Checchia PA, DeCaen A, Fink EL, Hoffman GM, Jefferies JL, Kleinman M, Krawczeski CD, Licht DJ, Macrae D, Ravishankar C, Samson RA, Thiagarajan RR, Toms R, Tweddell J, Laussen PC; American Heart Association Congenital Cardiac Defects Committee of the Council on Cardiovascular Disease in the Young; Council on Clinical Cardiology; Council on Cardiovascular and Stroke Nursing; Council on Cardiovascular Surgery and Anesthesia; and Emergency Cardiovascular Care Committee. Cardiopulmonary Resuscitation in Infants and Children With Cardiac Disease: A Scientific Statement From the American Heart Association. *Circulation.* 2018;137:e691–e782. doi: 10.1161/CIR.0000000000000524
3. Bando K, Turrentine MW, Sharp TG, Sekine Y, Aufiero TX, Sun K, Sekine E, Brown JW. Pulmonary hypertension after operations for congenital heart disease: analysis of risk factors and management. *J Thorac Cardiovasc Surg.* 1996;112:1600–7; discussion 1607. doi: 10.1016/S0022-5223(96)70019-3
4. Lindberg L, Olsson AK, Jögi P, Jonmarker C. How common is severe pulmonary hypertension after pediatric cardiac surgery? *J Thorac Cardiovasc Surg.* 2002;123:1155–1163. doi: 10.1067/mtc.2002.121497
5. Avila-Alvarez A, Del Cerro Marin MJ, Bautista-Hernandez V. Pulmonary Vasodilators in the Management of Low Cardiac Output Syndrome After Pediatric Cardiac Surgery. *Curr Vasc Pharmacol.* 2016;14:37–47. doi: 10.2174/1570161113666151014124912
6. Sabri MR, Bigdelian H, Hosseinzadeh M, Ahmadi A, Ghaderian M, Shoja M. Comparison of the therapeutic effects and side effects of tadalafil and sildenafil after surgery in young infants with pulmonary arterial hypertension due to systemic-to-pulmonary shunts. *Cardiol Young.* 2017;27:1686–1693. doi: 10.1017/S1047951117000981
7. Bizzarro M, Gross I, Barbosa FT. Inhaled nitric oxide for the postoperative management of pulmonary hypertension in infants and children with congenital heart disease. *Cochrane Database Syst Rev.* 2014:CD005055. doi: 10.1002/14651858.CD005055.pub3
8. Unegbu C, Noje C, Coulson JD, Segal JB, Romer L. Pulmonary hypertension therapy and a systematic review of efficacy and safety of PDE-5 inhibitors. *Pediatrics.* 2017;139:e20161450. doi: 10.1542/peds.2016-1450
9. Miller OI, Tang SF, Keech A, Pigott NB, Beller E, Celermajer DS. Inhaled nitric oxide and prevention of pulmonary hypertension after congenital heart surgery: a randomised double-blind study. *Lancet.* 2000;356:1464–1469. doi: 10.1016/S0140-6736(00)02869-5
10. Journois D, Baufreton C, Mauriat P, Pouard P, Vouhé P, Safran D. Effects of inhaled nitric oxide administration on early postoperative mortality in patients operated for correction of atrioventricular canal defects. *Chest.* 2005;128:3537–3544. doi: 10.1378/chest.128.5.3537
11. Abman SH, Hansmann G, Archer SL, Ivy DD, Adatia I, Chung WK, Hanna BD, Rosenzweig EB, Raj JU, Cornfield D, Stenmark KR, Steinhorn R, Thébaud B, Fineman JR, Kuehne T, Feinstein JA, Friedberg MK, Earing M, Barst RJ, Keller RL, Kinsella JP, Mullen M, Deterding R, Kulik T, Mallory G, Humpl T, Wessel DL; American Heart Association Council on Cardiopulmonary, Critical Care, Perioperative and Resuscitation; Council on Clinical

Cardiology; Council on Cardiovascular Disease in the Young; Council on Cardiovascular Radiology and Intervention; Council on Cardiovascular Surgery and Anesthesia; and the American Thoracic Society. Pediatric Pulmonary Hypertension: Guidelines From the American Heart Association and American Thoracic Society. *Circulation.* 2015;132:2037–2099. doi: 10.1161/CIR.0000000000000329
12. Kelly LK, Porta NF, Goodman DM, Carroll CL, Steinhorn RH. Inhaled prostacyclin for term infants with persistent pulmonary hypertension refractory to inhaled nitric oxide. *J Pediatr.* 2002;141:830–832. doi: 10.1067/mpd.2002.129849
13. Morris K, Beghetti M, Petros A, Adatia I, Bohn D. Comparison of hyperventilation and inhaled nitric oxide for pulmonary hypertension after repair of congenital heart disease. *Crit Care Med.* 2000;28:2974–2978. doi: 10.1097/00003246-200008000-00048
14. Nair J, Lakshminrusimha S. Update on PPHN: mechanisms and treatment. *Semin Perinatol.* 2014;38:78–91. doi: 10.1053/j.semperi.2013.11.004
15. Moudgil R, Michelakis ED, Archer SL. Hypoxic pulmonary vasoconstriction. *J Appl Physiol (1985).* 2005;98:390–403. doi: 10.1152/japplphysiol.00733.2004
16. Hopkins RA, Bull C, Haworth SG, de Leval MR, Stark J. Pulmonary hypertensive crises following surgery for congenital heart defects in young children. *Eur J Cardiothorac Surg.* 1991;5:628–634. doi: 10.1016/1010-7940(91)90118-4
17. Anand KJ, Hansen DD, Hickey PR. Hormonal-metabolic stress responses in neonates undergoing cardiac surgery. *Anesthesiology.* 1990;73:661–670. doi: 10.1097/00000542-199010000-00012
18. Kolovos NS, Bratton SL, Moler FW, Bove EL, Ohye RG, Bartlett RH, Kulik TJ. Outcome of pediatric patients treated with extracorporeal life support after cardiac surgery. *Ann Thorac Surg.* 2003;76:1435–41; discussion 1441. doi: 10.1016/s0003-4975(03)00898-1
19. Dhillon R, Pearson GA, Firmin RK, Chan KC, Leanage R. Extracorporeal membrane oxygenation and the treatment of critical pulmonary hypertension in congenital heart disease. *Eur J Cardiothorac Surg.* 1995;9:553–556. doi: 10.1016/s1010-7940(05)80004-1
20. Puri V, Epstein D, Raithel SC, Gandhi SK, Sweet SC, Faro A, Huddleston CB. Extracorporeal membrane oxygenation in pediatric lung transplantation. *J Thorac Cardiovasc Surg.* 2010;140:427–432. doi: 10.1016/j.jtcvs.2010.04.012
21. Ricci M, Gaughan CB, Rossi M, Andreopoulos FM, Novello C, Salerno TA, Rosenkranz ER, Panos AL. Initial experience with the TandemHeart circulatory support system in children. *ASAIO J.* 2008;54:542–545. doi: 10.1097/MAT.0b013e31818312f1
22. Morrell NW, Aldred MA, Chung WK, Elliott CG, Nichols WC, Soubrier F, Trembath RC, Loyd JE. Genetics and genomics of pulmonary arterial hypertension. *Eur Respir J.* 2019;53:Epub ahead of print. doi: 10.1183/13993003.01899-2018
23. Frank DB, Crystal MA, Morales DL, Gerald K, Hanna BD, Mallory GB Jr, Rossano JW. Trends in pediatric pulmonary hypertension-related hospitalizations in the United States from 2000–2009. *Pulm Circ.* 2015;5:339–348. doi: 10.1086/681226

MANAGEMENT OF TRAUMATIC CARDIAC ARREST

Unintentional injuries are the most common cause of death among children and adolescents.[1] Although many organizations have established trauma care guidelines,[2–4] the management of traumatic cardiac arrest is often inconsistent. Cardiac arrest due to major blunt or penetrating injury in children has a very high mortality rate.[5–8] Thoracic injury should be suspected in all thoracoabdominal trauma because tension pneumothorax, hemothorax, pulmonary contusion, or pericardial tamponade may impair hemodynamics, oxygenation, and ventilation.

Recommendations for the Management of Traumatic Cardiac Arrest

COR	LOE	Recommendations
1	C-EO	1. In pediatric traumatic cardiac arrest, evaluate for and treat potential reversible causes, such as hemorrhage, tension pneumothorax, and pericardial tamponade.[9,10]
2b	C-LD	2. In pediatric cardiac arrest secondary to penetrating injury with a short transport time, it may be reasonable to perform resuscitative thoracotomy.[11–18]

Recommendation-Specific Supportive Text

1. Early correction of reversible causes by reducing delays in the delivery of trauma-specific interventions may increase survival following penetrating traumatic cardiac arrest.[9,10] Guidelines for cardiac arrest due to trauma recommend hemorrhage control, restoration of circulating blood volume, opening the airway, and relieving tension pneumothorax. These measures should be performed simultaneously with conventional resuscitation.
2. Recent systematic reviews,[11–14] multicenter retrospective studies,[15,16] and single-center retrospective studies[17] recommend emergent thoracotomy for pediatric patients who present pulseless after penetrating thoracic injury. There is no evidence to support emergent thoracotomy for infants and children with blunt injury who are without signs of life.[12,18]

REFERENCES

1. Heron M. Deaths: leading causes for 2010. *Natl Vital Stat Rep.* 2013;62:1–96.
2. Western Trauma Association. Western Trauma Association algorithms. 2011. https://www.westerntrauma.org/algorithms/algorithms.html. Accessed March 6, 2020.
3. Eastern Association for the Surgery of Trauma. EAST practice management guidelines. https://www.east.org/education/practice-management-guidelines. Accessed February 3, 2020.
4. Pediatric Trauma Society. Pediatric trauma society clinical practice guidelines. https://pediatrictraumasociety.org/resources/clinical-resources.cgi. Accessed February 3, 2020.
5. Calkins CM, Bensard DD, Partrick DA, Karrer FM. A critical analysis of outcome for children sustaining cardiac arrest after blunt trauma. *J Pediatr Surg.* 2002;37:180–184. doi: 10.1053/jpsu.2002.30251
6. Crewdson K, Lockey D, Davies G. Outcome from paediatric cardiac arrest associated with trauma. *Resuscitation.* 2007;75:29–34. doi: 10.1016/j.resuscitation.2007.02.018
7. Perron AD, Sing RF, Branas CC, Huynh T. Predicting survival in pediatric trauma patients receiving cardiopulmonary resuscitation in the prehospital setting. *Prehosp Emerg Care.* 2001;5:6–9. doi: 10.1080/10903120190940245
8. Lopez-Herce Cid J, Dominguez Sampedro P, Rodriguez Nunez A, Garcia Sanz C, Carrillo Alvarez A, Calvo Macias C, Bellon Cano JM. [Cardiorespiratory arrest in children with trauma]. *An Pediatr (Barc).* 2006;65:439–447. doi: 10.1157/13094250
9. Shibahashi K, Sugiyama K, Hamabe Y. Pediatric Out-of-Hospital Traumatic Cardiopulmonary Arrest After Traffic Accidents and Termination of Resuscitation. *Ann Emerg Med.* 2020;75:57–65. doi: 10.1016/j.annemergmed.2019.05.036
10. Alqudah Z, Nehme Z, Williams B, Oteir A, Bernard S, Smith K. A descriptive analysis of the epidemiology and management of paediatric traumatic out-of-hospital cardiac arrest. *Resuscitation.* 2019;140:127–134. doi: 10.1016/j.resuscitation.2019.05.020

11. Nevins EJ, Bird NTE, Malik HZ, Mercer SJ, Shahzad K, Lunevicius R, Taylor JV, Misra N. A systematic review of 3251 emergency department thoracotomies: is it time for a national database? *Eur J Trauma Emerg Surg*. 2019;45:231–243. doi: 10.1007/s00068-018-0982-z
12. Moskowitz EE, Burlew CC, Kulungowski AM, Bensard DD. Survival after emergency department thoracotomy in the pediatric trauma population: a review of published data. *Pediatr Surg Int*. 2018;34:857–860. doi: 10.1007/s00383-018-4290-9
13. Seamon MJ, Haut ER, Van Arendonk K, Barbosa RR, Chiu WC, Dente CJ, Fox N, Jawa RS, Khwaja K, Lee JK, Magnotti LJ, Mayglothling JA, McDonald AA, Rowell S, To KB, Falck-Ytter Y, Rhee P. An evidence-based approach to patient selection for emergency department thoracotomy: A practice management guideline from the Eastern Association for the Surgery of Trauma. *J Trauma Acute Care Surg*. 2015;79:159–173. doi: 10.1097/TA.0000000000000648
14. Moore HB, Moore EE, Bensard DD. Pediatric emergency department thoracotomy: A 40-year review. *J Pediatr Surg*. 2016;51:315–318. doi: 10.1016/j.jpedsurg.2015.10.040
15. Flynn-O'Brien KT, Stewart BT, Fallat ME, Maier RV, Arbabi S, Rivara FP, McIntyre LK. Mortality after emergency department thoracotomy for pediatric blunt trauma: analysis of the National Trauma Data Bank 2007–2012. *J Pediatr Surg*. 2016;51:163–167. doi: 10.1016/j.jpedsurg.2015.10.034
16. Nicolson NG, Schwulst S, Esposito TA, Crandall ML. Resuscitative thoracotomy for pediatric trauma in Illinois, 1999 to 2009. *Am J Surg*. 2015;210:720–723. doi: 10.1016/j.amjsurg.2015.05.007
17. Easter JS, Vinton DT, Haukoos JS. Emergent pediatric thoracotomy following traumatic arrest. *Resuscitation*. 2012;83:1521–1524. doi: 10.1016/j.resuscitation.2012.05.024
18. Duron V, Burke RV, Bliss D, Ford HR, Upperman JS. Survival of pediatric blunt trauma patients presenting with no signs of life in the field. *J Trauma Acute Care Surg*. 2014;77:422–426. doi: 10.1097/TA.0000000000000394

CRITICAL KNOWLEDGE GAPS AND ONGOING RESEARCH

During the literature review process, we identified several critical knowledge gaps related to pediatric basic and advanced life support. These topics are either current areas of ongoing research or lack significant pediatric evidence to support evidence-based recommendations. In addition, we identified topics for which systematic or scoping reviews are in process by the ILCOR Basic Life Support or Pediatric Life Support Task Forces and elected not to make premature recommendations until these reviews are available.

As is so often the case in pediatric medicine, many recommendations are extrapolated from adult data. This is particularly true for the BLS components of pediatric resuscitation. The causes of pediatric cardiac arrest are very different from cardiac arrest in adults, and pediatric studies are critically needed. Furthermore, infants, children, and adolescents are distinct patient populations. Dedicated pediatric resuscitation research is a priority given the more than 20 000 infants, children, and adolescents who suffer cardiac arrest in the United States each year.

Critical knowledge gaps are summarized in Table 2.

Table 2. Critical Knowledge Gaps Due to Insufficient Pediatric Data

What is the optimal method of medication delivery during CPR: IO or IV?
What is the optimal method to determine body weight for medication administration?
In what time frame should the first dose of epinephrine be administered during pulseless cardiac arrest?
With what frequency should subsequent doses of epinephrine be administered?
With what frequency should epinephrine be administered in infants and children during CPR who are awaiting ECMO cannulation?
Are alternative compression techniques (cough CPR, fist pacing, interposed abdominal compression CPR) more effective alternatives to CPR?
With what frequency should the rhythm be checked during CPR?
What is the optimal method of airway management during OHCA—bag-mask ventilation, supraglottic airway, or endotracheal tube?
What is the optimal FIO_2 to administer during CPR?
What is the optimal ventilation rate during CPR in patients with or without an advanced airway? Is it age dependent?
What is the optimal chest compression rate during CPR? Is it age dependent?
What are the optimal blood pressure targets during CPR? Are they age dependent?
Can echocardiography improve CPR quality or outcomes from cardiac arrest?
Are there specific situations in which advanced airway placement is beneficial or harmful in OHCA?
What is the appropriate timing of advanced airway placement in IHCA?
What is the role of ECPR for patients with OHCA and IHCA due to noncardiac causes?
What is the optimal timing and dosing of defibrillation for VF/pVT?
What clinical tools can be used to help in the decision to terminate pediatric IHCA and OHCA resuscitation?
What is the optimal blood pressure target during the post–cardiac arrest period?
Should seizure prophylaxis be administered post cardiac arrest?
Does the treatment of postarrest convulsive and nonconvulsive seizure improve outcomes?
What are the reliable methods for postarrest prognostication?
What rehabilitation therapies and follow-up should be provided to improve outcomes post arrest?
What are the most effective and safe medications for adenosine-refractory SVT?
What is the appropriate age and setting to transition from (1) neonatal resuscitation protocols to pediatric resuscitation protocols and (2) from pediatric resuscitation protocols to adult resuscitation protocols?

CPR indicates cardiopulmonary resuscitation; ECMO, extracorporeal membrane oxygenation; ECPR, extracorporeal cardiopulmonary resuscitation; FIO_2, fraction of inspired oxygen; IHCA, in-hospital cardiac arrest; IO, intraosseous; IV, intravenous; OHCA, out-of-hospital cardiac arrest; pVT, pulseless ventricular tachycardia; SVT, supraventricular tachycardia; and VF, ventricular fibrillation.

ARTICLE INFORMATION

The American Heart Association requests that this document be cited as follows: Topjian AA, Raymond TT, Atkins D, Chan M, Duff JP, Joyner BL Jr, Lasa JJ, Lavonas EJ, Levy A, Mahgoub M, Meckler GD, Roberts KE, Sutton RM, Schexnayder SM; on behalf of the Pediatric Basic and Advanced Life Support Collaborators. Part 4: pediatric basic and advanced life support: 2020 American Heart Association Guidelines for Cardiopulmonary Resuscitation and Emergency Cardiovascular Care. *Circulation*. 2020;142(suppl 2):S469–S523. doi: 10.1161/CIR.0000000000000901

Acknowledgments

The authors thank the following individuals (the Pediatric Basic and Advanced Life Support Collaborators) for their contributions: Ronald A. Bronicki, MD; Allan R. de Caen, MD; Anne Marie Guerguerian, MD, PhD; Kelly D. Kadlec, MD, MEd; Monica E. Kleinman, MD; Lynda J. Knight, MSN, RN; Taylor N. McCormick, MD, MSc; Ryan W. Morgan, MD, MTR; Joan S. Roberts, MD; Barnaby R. Scholefield, MBBS, PhD; Sarah Tabbutt, MD, PhD; Ravi Thiagarajan, MBBS, MPH; Janice Tijssen, MD, MSc; Brian Walsh, PhD, RRT, RRT-NPS; and Arno Zaritsky, MD.

Disclosures

Appendix 1. Writing Group Disclosures

Writing Group Member	Employment	Research Grant	Other Research Support	Speakers' Bureau/ Honoraria	Expert Witness	Ownership Interest	Consultant/ Advisory Board	Other
Alexis A. Topjian	The Children's Hospital of Philadelphia, University of Pennsylvania School of Medicine Anesthesia and Critical Care	NIH*	None	None	Plaintiff*	None	None	None
Dianne Atkins	University of Iowa Pediatrics	None	None	None	None	None	None	None
Melissa Chan	University of British Columbia Pediatrics BC Children's Hospital	None	None	None	None	None	None	None
Jonathan P. Duff	University of Alberta and Stollery Children's Hospital Pediatrics	None	None	None	None	None	None	None
Benny L. Joyner Jr	University of North Carolina Pediatrics	None	None	None	None	None	None	None
Javier J. Lasa	Texas Children's Hospital, Baylor College of Medicine Pediatrics/Critical Care Medicine and Cardiology	None	None	None	None	None	None	None
Eric J. Lavonas	Denver Health Emergency Medicine	BTG Pharmaceuticals (Denver Health (Dr Lavonas' employer) has research, call center, consulting, and teaching agreements with BTG Pharmaceuticals. BTG manufactures the digoxin antidote, DigiFab. Dr Lavonas does not receive bonus or incentive compensation, and these agreements involve an unrelated product. When these guidelines were developed, Dr Lavonas recused from discussions related to digoxin poisoning.)†	None	None	None	None	None	American Heart Association (Senior Science Editor)†
Arielle Levy	University of Montreal Pediatric	None	None	None	None	None	None	None
Melissa Mahgoub	American Heart Association	None	None	None	None	None	None	None
Garth D. Meckler	University of British Columbia Pediatrics and Emergency Medicine Ambulatory Care Building, BC Children's	None	None	None	None	None	None	None
Tia T. Raymond	Medical City Children's Hospital Pediatric Cardiac Intensive Care Unit	None	None	None	None	None	None	None
Kathryn E. Roberts	Joe DiMaggio Children's Hospital	None	None	None	None	None	None	None

(Continued)

Appendix 1. Continued

Writing Group Member	Employment	Research Grant	Other Research Support	Speakers' Bureau/ Honoraria	Expert Witness	Ownership Interest	Consultant/ Advisory Board	Other
Stephen M. Schexnayder	Univ. of Arkansas/ Arkansas Children's Hospital Pediatric Critical Care	None	None	None	None	None	None	None
Robert M. Sutton	The Children's Hospital of Philadelphia, University of Pennsylvania School of Medicine Anesthesia and Critical Care Medicine	NIH†	None	None	Roberts & Durkee, Plantiff, 2019†	None	None	None

This table represents the relationships of writing group members that may be perceived as actual or reasonably perceived conflicts of interest as reported on the Disclosure Questionnaire, which all members of the writing group are required to complete and submit. A relationship is considered to be "significant" if (a) the person receives $10 000 or more during any 12-month period, or 5% or more of the person's gross income; or (b) the person owns 5% or more of the voting stock or share of the entity, or owns $10 000 or more of the fair market value of the entity. A relationship is considered to be "modest" if it is less than "significant" under the preceding definition.

*Modest.

†Significant.

Appendix 2. Reviewer Disclosures

Reviewer	Employment	Research Grant	Other Research Support	Speakers' Bureau/ Honoraria	Expert Witness	Ownership Interest	Consultant/ Advisory Board	Other
Nandini Calamur	Saint Louis University	None	None	None	None	None	None	None
Leon Chameides	Connecticut Children's Medical Center	None	None	None	None	None	None	None
Todd P. Chang	Children's Hospital Los Angeles & Keck School Of Medicine	None	None	None	None	None	None	Oculus from FaceBook†
Ericka L. Fink	Primary Work Children's Hospital of Pittsburgh	NIH†	None	None	None	None	None	None
Monica E. Kleinman	Children's Hospital Boston	None	None	None	None	None	International Liaison Committee on Resuscitation*	None
Michael-Alice Moga	The Hospital for Sick Children, Labatt Family Heart Center and University of Toronto (Canada)	CIHR*; CIHR/ NSERC†	None	None	None	None	None	None
Tara Neubrand	Children's Hospital Colorado, University of Colorado	None	None	None	None	None	None	None
Ola Didrik Saugstad	University of Oslo (Norway)	None	None	None	None	None	None	None

This table represents the relationships of reviewers that may be perceived as actual or reasonably perceived conflicts of interest as reported on the Disclosure Questionnaire, which all reviewers are required to complete and submit. A relationship is considered to be "significant" if (a) the person receives $10 000 or more during any 12-month period, or 5% or more of the person's gross income; or (b) the person owns 5% or more of the voting stock or share of the entity, or owns $10 000 or more of the fair market value of the entity. A relationship is considered to be "modest" if it is less than "significant" under the preceding definition.

*Modest.

†Significant.

Circulation

Part 5: Neonatal Resuscitation

2020 American Heart Association Guidelines for Cardiopulmonary Resuscitation and Emergency Cardiovascular Care

Khalid Aziz, MBBS, MA, MEd(IT), Chair
Henry C. Lee, MD, Vice Chair
Marilyn B. Escobedo, MD
Amber V. Hoover, RN, MSN
Beena D. Kamath-Rayne, MD, MPH
Vishal S. Kapadia, MD, MSCS
David J. Magid, MD, MPH
Susan Niermeyer, MD, MPH
Georg M. Schmölzer, MD, PhD
Edgardo Szyld, MD, MSc
Gary M. Weiner, MD
Myra H. Wyckoff, MD
Nicole K. Yamada, MD, MS
Jeanette Zaichkin, RN, MN, NNP-BC

TOP 10 TAKE-HOME MESSAGES FOR NEONATAL LIFE SUPPORT

1. Newborn resuscitation requires anticipation and preparation by providers who train individually and as teams.
2. Most newly born infants do not require immediate cord clamping or resuscitation and can be evaluated and monitored during skin-to-skin contact with their mothers after birth.
3. Inflation and ventilation of the lungs are the priority in newly born infants who need support after birth.
4. A rise in heart rate is the most important indicator of effective ventilation and response to resuscitative interventions.
5. Pulse oximetry is used to guide oxygen therapy and meet oxygen saturation goals.
6. Chest compressions are provided if there is a poor heart rate response to ventilation after appropriate ventilation corrective steps, which preferably include endotracheal intubation.
7. The heart rate response to chest compressions and medications should be monitored electrocardiographically.
8. If the response to chest compressions is poor, it may be reasonable to provide epinephrine, preferably via the intravenous route.
9. Failure to respond to epinephrine in a newborn with history or examination consistent with blood loss may require volume expansion.
10. If all these steps of resuscitation are effectively completed and there is no heart rate response by 20 minutes, redirection of care should be discussed with the team and family.

PREAMBLE

It is estimated that approximately 10% of newly born infants need help to begin breathing at birth,[1–3] and approximately 1% need intensive resuscitative measures to restore cardiorespiratory function.[4,5] The neonatal mortality rate in the United States and Canada has fallen from almost 20 per 1000 live births[6,7] in the 1960s to the current rate of approximately 4 per 1000 live births. The inability of newly born infants to establish and sustain adequate or spontaneous respiration contributes significantly to these early deaths and to the burden of adverse neurodevelopmental outcome among survivors. Effective and timely resuscitation at birth could therefore improve neonatal outcomes further.

Successful neonatal resuscitation efforts depend on critical actions that must occur in rapid succession to maximize the chances of survival. The International Liaison Committee on Resuscitation (ILCOR) Formula for Survival emphasizes 3 essential components for good resuscitation outcomes: guidelines based on sound resuscitation science,

Key Words: AHA Scientific Statements ■ cardiopulmonary resuscitation ■ neonatal resuscitation ■ neonate

https://www.ahajournals.org/journal/circ

effective education of resuscitation providers, and implementation of effective and timely resuscitation.[8] The 2020 neonatal guidelines contain recommendations, based on the best available resuscitation science, for the most impactful steps to perform in the birthing room and in the neonatal period. In addition, specific recommendations about the training of resuscitation providers and systems of care are provided in their respective guideline Parts.[9,10]

INTRODUCTION

Scope of Guideline

This guideline is designed for North American healthcare providers who are looking for an up-to-date summary for clinical care, as well as for those who are seeking more in-depth information on resuscitation science and gaps in current knowledge. The science of neonatal resuscitation applies to newly born infants transitioning from the fluid-filled environment of the womb to the air-filled environment of the birthing room and to newborns in the days after birth. In circumstances of altered or impaired transition, effective neonatal resuscitation reduces the risk of mortality and morbidity. Even healthy babies who breathe well after birth benefit from facilitation of normal transition, including appropriate cord management and thermal protection with skin-to-skin care.

The 2015 Neonatal Resuscitation Algorithm and the major concepts based on sections of the algorithm continue to be relevant in 2020 (Figure). The following sections are worth special attention.

- Positive-pressure ventilation (PPV) remains the main intervention in neonatal resuscitation. While the science and practices surrounding monitoring and other aspects of neonatal resuscitation continue to evolve, the development of skills and practice surrounding PPV should be emphasized.
- Supplemental oxygen should be used judiciously, guided by pulse oximetry.
- Prevention of hypothermia continues to be an important focus for neonatal resuscitation. The importance of skin-to-skin care in healthy babies is reinforced as a means of promoting parental bonding, breast feeding, and normothermia.
- Team training remains an important aspect of neonatal resuscitation, including anticipation, preparation, briefing, and debriefing. Rapid and effective response and performance are critical to good newborn outcomes.
- Delayed umbilical cord clamping was recommended for both term and preterm neonates in 2015. This guideline affirms the previous recommendations.
- The *2015 American Heart Association* (AHA) *Guidelines Update for Cardiopulmonary Resuscitation* (CPR) *and Emergency Cardiovascular Care* (ECC) recommended against routine endotracheal suctioning for both vigorous and nonvigorous infants born with meconium-stained amniotic fluid (MSAF). This guideline reinforces initial steps and PPV as priorities.

It is important to recognize that there are several significant gaps in knowledge relating to neonatal resuscitation. Many current recommendations are based on weak evidence with a lack of well-designed human studies. This is partly due to the challenges of performing large randomized controlled trials (RCTs) in the delivery room. The current guideline, therefore, concludes with a summary of current gaps in neonatal research and some potential strategies to address these gaps.

COVID-19 Guidance

Together with other professional societies, the AHA has provided interim guidance for basic and advanced life support in adults, children, and neonates with suspected or confirmed coronavirus disease 2019 (COVID-19) infection. Because evidence and guidance are evolving with the COVID-19 situation, this interim guidance is maintained separately from the ECC guidelines. Readers are directed to the AHA website for the most recent guidance.[12]

Evidence Evaluation and Guidelines Development

The following sections briefly describe the process of evidence review and guideline development. See "Part 2: Evidence Evaluation and Guidelines Development" for more details on this process.[11]

Organization of the Writing Committee

The Neonatal Life Support Writing Group includes neonatal physicians and nurses with backgrounds in clinical medicine, education, research, and public health. Volunteers with recognized expertise in resuscitation are nominated by the writing group chair and selected by the AHA ECC Committee. The AHA has rigorous conflict of interest policies and procedures to minimize the risk of bias or improper influence during development of the guidelines.[13] Before appointment, writing group members and peer reviewers disclosed all commercial relationships and other potential (including intellectual) conflicts. Disclosure information for writing group members is listed in Appendix 1.

Methodology and Evidence Review

These 2020 AHA neonatal resuscitation guidelines are based on the extensive evidence evaluation performed in conjunction with the ILCOR and affiliated ILCOR member councils. Three different types of evidence reviews (systematic reviews, scoping reviews, and evidence updates) were used in the 2020 process. Each of these resulted in a description of the literature that facilitated guideline development.[14–17]

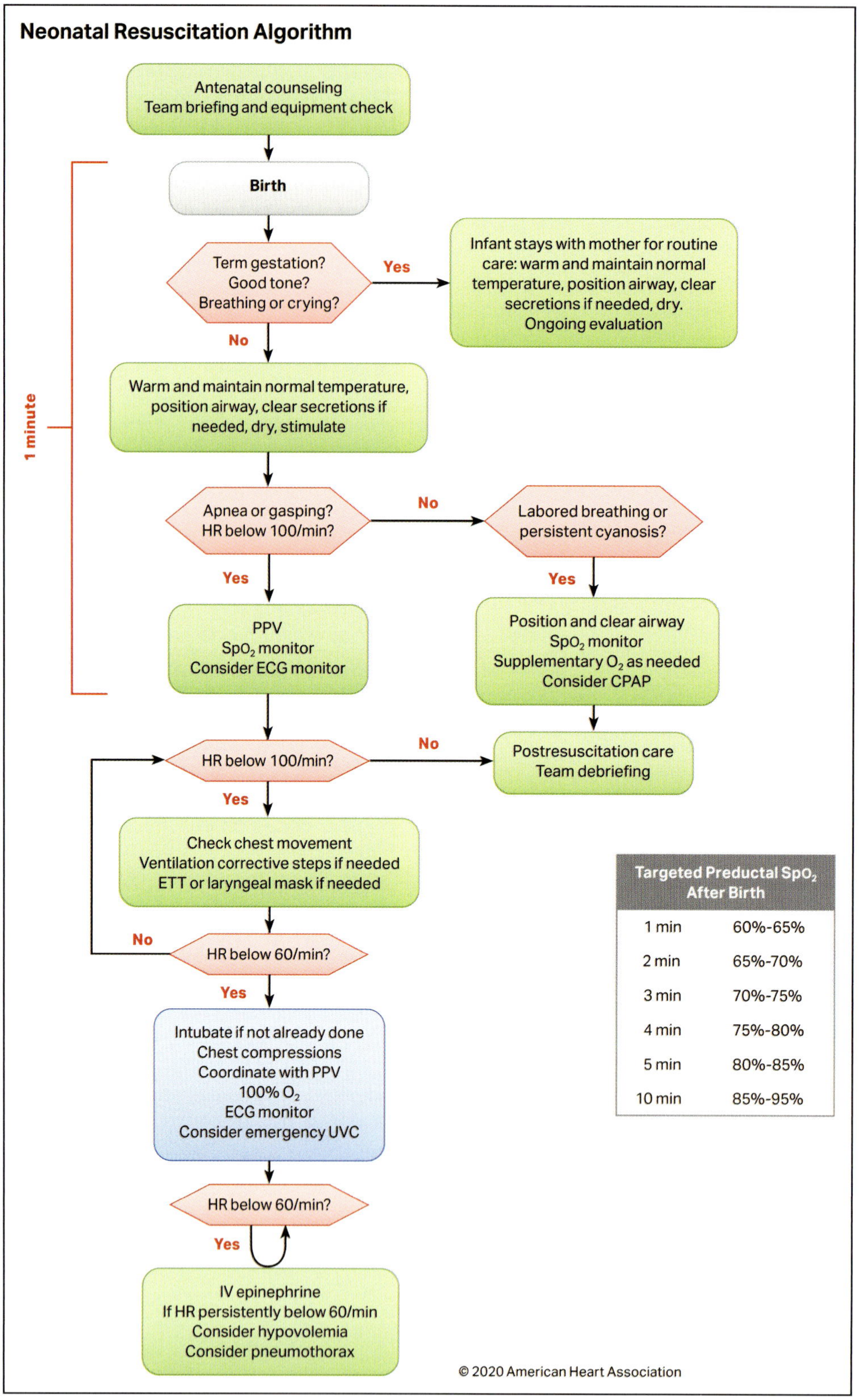
Neonatal Resuscitation Algorithm
Antenatal counseling
Team briefing and equipment check
Birth
1 minute
Term gestation?
Good tone?
Breathing or crying?
Yes
Infant stays with mother for routine care: warm and maintain normal temperature, position airway, clear secretions if needed, dry.
Ongoing evaluation
No
Warm and maintain normal temperature, position airway, clear secretions if needed, dry, stimulate
Apnea or gasping?
HR below 100/min?
No
Labored breathing or persistent cyanosis?
Yes
PPV
SpO_2 monitor
Consider ECG monitor
Yes
Position and clear airway
SpO_2 monitor
Supplementary O_2 as needed
Consider CPAP
HR below 100/min?
No
Postresuscitation care
Team debriefing
Yes
Check chest movement
Ventilation corrective steps if needed
ETT or laryngeal mask if needed
No
HR below 60/min?
Yes
Intubate if not already done
Chest compressions
Coordinate with PPV
100% O_2
ECG monitor
Consider emergency UVC
HR below 60/min?
Yes
IV epinephrine
If HR persistently below 60/min
Consider hypovolemia
Consider pneumothorax
Targeted Preductal SpO_2 After Birth
1 min 60%-65%
2 min 65%-70%
3 min 70%-75%
4 min 75%-80%
5 min 80%-85%
10 min 85%-95%
© 2020 American Heart Association

Figure. Neonatal Resuscitation Algorithm.
CPAP indicates continuous positive airway pressure; ECG, electrocardiographic; ETT, endotracheal tube; HR, heart rate; IV, intravenous; O_2, oxygen; SpO_2, oxygen saturation; and UVC, umbilical venous catheter.

Class of Recommendation and Level of Evidence

Each AHA writing group reviewed all relevant and current AHA guidelines for CPR and ECC[18–20] and all relevant *2020 ILCOR International Consensus on CPR and ECC Science With Treatment Recommendations* evidence and recommendations[21] to determine if current guidelines should be reaffirmed, revised, or retired, or if new

Table. Applying Class of Recommendation and Level of Evidence to Clinical Strategies, Interventions, Treatments, or Diagnostic Testing in Patient Care (Updated May 2019)*

CLASS (STRENGTH) OF RECOMMENDATION	
CLASS 1 (STRONG)	**Benefit >>> Risk**
Suggested phrases for writing recommendations: • Is recommended • Is indicated/useful/effective/beneficial • Should be performed/administered/other • Comparative-Effectiveness Phrases†: – Treatment/strategy A is recommended/indicated in preference to treatment B – Treatment A should be chosen over treatment B	
CLASS 2a (MODERATE)	**Benefit >> Risk**
Suggested phrases for writing recommendations: • Is reasonable • Can be useful/effective/beneficial • Comparative-Effectiveness Phrases†: – Treatment/strategy A is probably recommended/indicated in preference to treatment B – It is reasonable to choose treatment A over treatment B	
CLASS 2b (WEAK)	**Benefit ≥ Risk**
Suggested phrases for writing recommendations: • May/might be reasonable • May/might be considered • Usefulness/effectiveness is unknown/unclear/uncertain or not well-established	
CLASS 3: No Benefit (MODERATE) **(Generally, LOE A or B use only)**	**Benefit = Risk**
Suggested phrases for writing recommendations: • Is not recommended • Is not indicated/useful/effective/beneficial • Should not be performed/administered/other	
Class 3: Harm (STRONG)	**Risk > Benefit**
Suggested phrases for writing recommendations: • Potentially harmful • Causes harm • Associated with excess morbidity/mortality • Should not be performed/administered/other	

LEVEL (QUALITY) OF EVIDENCE‡	
LEVEL A	
• High-quality evidence‡ from more than 1 RCT • Meta-analyses of high-quality RCTs • One or more RCTs corroborated by high-quality registry studies	
LEVEL B-R	**(Randomized)**
• Moderate-quality evidence‡ from 1 or more RCTs • Meta-analyses of moderate-quality RCTs	
LEVEL B-NR	**(Nonrandomized)**
• Moderate-quality evidence‡ from 1 or more well-designed, well-executed nonrandomized studies, observational studies, or registry studies • Meta-analyses of such studies	
LEVEL C-LD	**(Limited Data)**
• Randomized or nonrandomized observational or registry studies with limitations of design or execution • Meta-analyses of such studies • Physiological or mechanistic studies in human subjects	
LEVEL C-EO	**(Expert Opinion)**
• Consensus of expert opinion based on clinical experience	

COR and LOE are determined independently (any COR may be paired with any LOE).

A recommendation with LOE C does not imply that the recommendation is weak. Many important clinical questions addressed in guidelines do not lend themselves to clinical trials. Although RCTs are unavailable, there may be a very clear clinical consensus that a particular test or therapy is useful or effective.

* The outcome or result of the intervention should be specified (an improved clinical outcome or increased diagnostic accuracy or incremental prognostic information).

† For comparative-effectiveness recommendations (COR 1 and 2a; LOE A and B only), studies that support the use of comparator verbs should involve direct comparisons of the treatments or strategies being evaluated.

‡ The method of assessing quality is evolving, including the application of standardized, widely-used, and preferably validated evidence grading tools; and for systematic reviews, the incorporation of an Evidence Review Committee.

COR indicates Class of Recommendation; EO, expert opinion; LD, limited data; LOE, Level of Evidence; NR, nonrandomized; R, randomized; and RCT, randomized controlled trial.

recommendations were needed. The writing groups then drafted, reviewed, and approved recommendations, assigning to each a Level of Evidence (LOE; ie, quality) and Class of Recommendation (COR; ie, strength) (Table).[11]

Guideline Structure

The 2020 guidelines are organized into "knowledge chunks," grouped into discrete modules of information on specific topics or management issues.[22] Each modular knowledge chunk includes a table of recommendations using standard AHA nomenclature of COR and LOE. A brief introduction or short synopsis is provided to put the recommendations into context with important background information and overarching management or treatment concepts. Recommendation-specific text clarifies the rationale and key study data supporting the recommendations. When appropriate, flow diagrams or additional tables are included. Hyperlinked references are provided to facilitate quick access and review.

Document Review and Approval

Each *2020 AHA Guidelines for CPR and ECC* document was submitted for blinded peer review to 5 subject matter experts nominated by the AHA. Before appointment, all peer reviewers were required to disclose relationships with industry and any other potential conflicts of interest, and all disclosures were reviewed by AHA staff. Peer reviewer feedback was provided for guidelines in draft format and again in final format. All guidelines were reviewed and approved for publication by the AHA

Science Advisory and Coordinating Committee and AHA Executive Committee. Disclosure information for peer reviewers is listed in Appendix 2.

REFERENCES

1. Little MP, Järvelin MR, Neasham DE, Lissauer T, Steer PJ. Factors associated with fall in neonatal intubation rates in the United Kingdom–prospective study. *BJOG*. 2007;114:156–164. doi: 10.1111/j.1471-0528.2006.01188.x
2. Niles DE, Cines C, Insley E, Foglia EE, Elci OU, Skåre C, Olasveengen T, Ades A, Posencheg M, Nadkarni VM, Kramer-Johansen J. Incidence and characteristics of positive pressure ventilation delivered to newborns in a US tertiary academic hospital. *Resuscitation*. 2017;115:102–109. doi: 10.1016/j.resuscitation.2017.03.035
3. Aziz K, Chadwick M, Baker M, Andrews W. Ante- and intra-partum factors that predict increased need for neonatal resuscitation. *Resuscitation*. 2008;79:444–452. doi: 10.1016/j.resuscitation.2008.08.004
4. Perlman JM, Risser R. Cardiopulmonary resuscitation in the delivery room. Associated clinical events. *Arch Pediatr Adolesc Med*. 1995;149:20–25. doi: 10.1001/archpedi.1995.02170130022005
5. Barber CA, Wyckoff MH. Use and efficacy of endotracheal versus intravenous epinephrine during neonatal cardiopulmonary resuscitation in the delivery room. *Pediatrics*. 2006;118:1028–1034. doi: 10.1542/peds.2006-0416
6. MacDorman MF, Rosenberg HM. Trends in infant mortality by cause of death and other characteristics, 1960–88. *Vital Health Stat 20*. 1993:1–57.
7. Kochanek KD, Murphy SL, Xu JQ, Arias E; Division of Vital Statistics. *National Vital Statistics Reports: Deaths: Final Data for 2017* Hyattsville, MD: National Center for Health Statistics; 2019(68). https://www.cdc.gov/nchs/data/nvsr/nvsr68/nvsr68_09-508.pdf. Accessed February 28, 2020.
8. Søreide E, Morrison L, Hillman K, Monsieurs K, Sunde K, Zideman D, Eisenberg M, Sterz F, Nadkarni VM, Soar J, Nolan JP; Utstein Formula for Survival Collaborators. The formula for survival in resuscitation. *Resuscitation*. 2013;84:1487–1493. doi: 10.1016/j.resuscitation.2013.07.020
9. Cheng A, Magid DJ, Auerbach M, Bhanji F, Bigham BL, Blewer AL, Dainty KN, Diederich E, Lin Y, Leary M, et al. Part 6: resuscitation education science: 2020 American Heart Association Guidelines for Cardiopulmonary Resuscitation and Emergency Cardiovascular Care. *Circulation*. 2020;142(suppl 2):S551–S579. doi: 10.1161/CIR.0000000000000903
10. Berg KM, Cheng A, Panchal AR, Topjian AA, Aziz K, Bhanji F, Bigham BL, Hirsch KG, Hoover AV, Kurz MC, et al; on behalf of the Adult Basic and Advanced Life Support, Pediatric Basic and Advanced Life Support, Neonatal Life Support, and Resuscitation Education Science Writing Groups. Part 7: systems of care: 2020 American Heart Association Guidelines for Cardiopulmonary Resuscitation and Emergency Cardiovascular Care. *Circulation*. 2020;142(suppl 2):S580–S604. doi: 10.1161/CIR.0000000000000899
11. Magid DJ, Aziz K, Cheng A, Hazinski MF, Hoover AV, Mahgoub M, Panchal AR, Sasson C, Topjian AA, Rodriguez AJ, et al. Part 2: evidence evaluation and guidelines development: 2020 American Heart Association Guidelines for Cardiopulmonary Resuscitation and Emergency Cardiovascular Care. *Circulation*. 2020;142(suppl 2):S358–S365. doi: 10.1161/CIR.0000000000000898
12. American Heart Association. CPR & ECC. https://cpr.heart.org/. Accessed June 19, 2020.
13. American Heart Association. Conflict of interest policy. https://www.heart.org/en/about-us/statements-and-policies/conflict-of-interest-policy. Accessed December 31, 2019.
14. International Liaison Committee on Resuscitation. Continuous evidence evaluation guidance and templates. https://www.ilcor.org/documents/continuous-evidence-evaluation-guidance-and-templates. Accessed December 31, 2019.
15. Institute of Medicine (US) Committee of Standards for Systematic Reviews of Comparative Effectiveness Research. *Finding What Works in Health Care: Standards for Systematic Reviews*. Eden J, Levit L, Berg A, Morton S, eds. Washington, DC: The National Academies Press; 2011.
16. PRISMA. Preferred Reporting Items for Systematic Reviews and Meta-Analyses (PRISMA) website. http://www.prisma-statement.org/. Accessed December 31, 2019.
17. Tricco AC, Lillie E, Zarin W, O'Brien KK, Colquhoun H, Levac D, Moher D, Peters MDJ, Horsley T, Weeks L, Hempel S, Akl EA, Chang C, McGowan J, Stewart L, Hartling L, Aldcroft A, Wilson MG, Garritty C, Lewin S, Godfrey CM, Macdonald MT, Langlois EV, Soares-Weiser K, Moriarty J, Clifford T, Tunçalp Ö, Straus SE. PRISMA Extension for Scoping Reviews (PRISMA-ScR): Checklist and Explanation. *Ann Intern Med*. 2018;169:467–473. doi: 10.7326/M18-0850
18. Kattwinkel J, Perlman JM, Aziz K, Colby C, Fairchild K, Gallagher J, Hazinski MF, Halamek LP, Kumar P, Little G, et al. Part 15: neonatal resuscitation: 2010 American Heart Association Guidelines for Cardiopulmonary Resuscitation and Emergency Cardiovascular Care. *Circulation*. 2010;122(suppl 3):S909–S919. doi: 10.1161/CIRCULATIONAHA.110.971119
19. Wyckoff MH, Aziz K, Escobedo MB, Kapadia VS, Kattwinkel J, Perlman JM, Simon WM, Weiner GM, Zaichkin JG. Part 13: neonatal resuscitation: 2015 American Heart Association Guidelines Update for Cardiopulmonary Resuscitation and Emergency Cardiovascular Care. *Circulation*. 2015;132(suppl 2):S543–S560. doi: 10.1161/CIR.0000000000000267
20. Escobedo MB, Aziz K, Kapadia VS, Lee HC, Niermeyer S, Schmölzer GM, Szyld E, Weiner GM, Wyckoff MH, Yamada NK, Zaichkin JG. 2019 American Heart Association Focused Update on Neonatal Resuscitation: An Update to the American Heart Association Guidelines for Cardiopulmonary Resuscitation and Emergency Cardiovascular Care. *Circulation*. 2019;140:e922–e930. doi: 10.1161/CIR.0000000000000729
21. Wyckoff MH, Wyllie J, Aziz K, de Almeida MF, Fabres J, Fawke J, Guinsburg R, Hosono S, Isayama T, Kapadia VS, et al; on behalf of the Neonatal Life Support Collaborators. Neonatal life support: 2020 International Consensus on Cardiopulmonary Resuscitation and Emergency Cardiovascular Care Science With Treatment Recommendations. *Circulation*. 2020;142(suppl 1):S185–S221. doi: 10.1161/CIR.0000000000000895
22. Levine GN, O'Gara PT, Beckman JA, Al-Khatib SM, Birtcher KK, Cigarroa JE, de Las Fuentes L, Deswal A, Fleisher LA, Gentile F, Goldberger ZD, Hlatky MA, Joglar JA, Piano MR, Wijeysundera DN. Recent Innovations, Modifications, and Evolution of ACC/AHA Clinical Practice Guidelines: An Update for Our Constituencies: A Report of the American College of Cardiology/American Heart Association Task Force on Clinical Practice Guidelines. *Circulation*. 2019;139:e879–e886. doi: 10.1161/CIR.0000000000000651

MAJOR CONCEPTS

These guidelines apply primarily to the "newly born" baby who is transitioning from the fluid-filled womb to the air-filled room. The "newly born" period extends from birth to the end of resuscitation and stabilization in the delivery area. However, the concepts in these guidelines may be applied to newborns during the neonatal period (birth to 28 days).

The primary goal of neonatal care at birth is to facilitate transition. The most important priority for newborn survival is the establishment of adequate lung inflation and ventilation after birth. Consequently, all newly born babies should be attended to by at least 1 person skilled and equipped to provide PPV. Other important goals include establishment and maintenance of cardiovascular and temperature stability as well as the promotion of mother-infant bonding and breast feeding, recognizing that healthy babies transition naturally.

The Neonatal Resuscitation Algorithm remains unchanged from 2015 and is the organizing framework for major concepts that reflect the needs of the baby, the family, and the surrounding team of perinatal caregivers.

Anticipation and Preparation

Every healthy newly born baby should have a trained and equipped person assigned to facilitate transition. Identification of risk factors for resuscitation may indicate the need for additional personnel and equipment. Effective team behaviors, such as anticipation, communication, briefing, equipment checks, and assignment of roles, result in improved team performance and neonatal outcome.

Cord Management

After an uncomplicated term or late preterm birth, it is reasonable to delay cord clamping until after the baby is placed on the mother, dried, and assessed for breathing, tone, and activity. In other situations, clamping and cutting of the cord may also be deferred while respiratory, cardiovascular, and thermal transition is evaluated and initial steps are undertaken. In preterm birth, there are also potential advantages from delaying cord clamping.

Initial Actions

When possible, healthy term babies should be managed skin-to-skin with their mothers. After birth, the baby should be dried and placed directly skin-to-skin with attention to warm coverings and maintenance of normal temperature. There should be ongoing evaluation of the baby for normal respiratory transition. Radiant warmers and other warming adjuncts are suggested for babies who require resuscitation at birth, especially very preterm and very low-birth-weight babies.

Stimulation may be provided to facilitate respiratory effort. Suctioning may be considered for suspected airway obstruction.

Assessment of Heart Rate

Heart rate is assessed initially by auscultation and/or palpation. Oximetry and electrocardiography are important adjuncts in babies requiring resuscitation.

Positive-Pressure Ventilation

PPV remains the primary method for providing support for newborns who are apneic, bradycardic, or demonstrate inadequate respiratory effort. Most babies will respond to this intervention. An improvement in heart rate and establishment of breathing or crying are all signs of effective PPV.

Oxygen Therapy

PPV may be initiated with air (21% oxygen) in term and late preterm babies, and up to 30% oxygen in preterm babies. Oximetry is used to target the natural range of oxygen saturation levels that occur in term babies.

Chest Compressions

If the heart rate remains less than 60/min despite 30 seconds of adequate PPV, chest compressions should be provided. The suggested ratio is 3 chest compressions synchronized to 1 inflation (with 30 inflations per minute and 90 compressions per minute) using the 2 thumb–encircling hands technique for chest compressions.

Vascular Access

When vascular access is required in the newly born, the umbilical venous route is preferred. When intravenous access is not feasible, the intraosseous route may be considered.

Medications

If the heart rate remains less than 60/min despite 60 seconds of chest compressions and adequate PPV, epinephrine should be administered, ideally via the intravenous route.

Volume Expansion

When blood loss is known or suspected based on history and examination, and there is no response to epinephrine, volume expansion is indicated.

Withholding and Discontinuing Resuscitation

It may be possible to identify conditions in which withholding or discontinuation of resuscitative efforts may be reasonably considered by families and care providers. Appropriate and timely support should be provided to all involved.

Human Factors and Systems

Teams and individuals who provide neonatal resuscitation are faced with many challenges with respect to the knowledge, skills, and behaviors needed to perform effectively. Neonatal resuscitation teams may therefore benefit from ongoing booster training, briefing, and debriefing.

Abbreviations

AHA	American Heart Association
COR	Class of Recommendation
CPAP	continuous positive airway pressure
ECC	emergency cardiovascular care
ECG	electrocardiogram/electrocardiographic
H_2O	water
HIE	hypoxic-ischemic encephalopathy
ILCOR	International Liaison Committee on Resuscitation
LOE	Level of Evidence
MSAF	meconium-stained amniotic fluid
PEEP	positive end-expiratory pressure
PPV	positive pressure ventilation
RCT	randomized controlled trial
ROSC	return of spontaneous circulation

ANTICIPATION OF RESUSCITATION NEED

Recommendations for Anticipating Resuscitation Need

COR	LOE	Recommendations
1	B-NR	1. Every birth should be attended by at least 1 person who can perform the initial steps of newborn resuscitation and initiate PPV, and whose only responsibility is the care of the newborn.[1–4]
1	B-NR	2. Before every birth, a standardized risk factors assessment tool should be used to assess perinatal risk and assemble a qualified team on the basis of that risk.[5–7]
1	C-LD	3. Before every birth, a standardized equipment checklist should be used to ensure the presence and function of supplies and equipment necessary for a complete resuscitation.[8,9]
1	C-LD	4. When anticipating a high-risk birth, a preresuscitation team briefing should be completed to identify potential interventions and assign roles and responsibilities.[8,10–12]

Synopsis

Approximately 10% of newborns require assistance to breathe after birth.[1–3,5,13] Newborn resuscitation requires training, preparation, and teamwork. When the need for resuscitation is not anticipated, delays in assisting a newborn who is not breathing may increase the risk of death.[1,5,13] Therefore, every birth should be attended by at least 1 person whose primary responsibility is the newborn and who is trained to begin PPV without delay.[2–4]

A risk assessment tool that evaluates risk factors present during pregnancy and labor can identify newborns likely to require advanced resuscitation; in these cases, a team with more advanced skills should be mobilized and present at delivery.[5,7] In the absence of risk stratification, up to half of babies requiring PPV may not be identified before delivery.[6,13]

A standardized equipment checklist is a comprehensive list of critical supplies and equipment needed in a given clinical setting. In the birth setting, a standardized checklist should be used before every birth to ensure that supplies and equipment for a complete resuscitation are present and functional.[8,9,14,15]

A predelivery team briefing should be completed to identify the leader, assign roles and responsibilities, and plan potential interventions. Team briefings promote effective teamwork and communication, and support patient safety.[8,10–12]

Recommendation-Specific Supportive Text

1. A large observational study found that delaying PPV increases risk of death and prolonged hospitalization.[1] A systematic review and meta-analysis showed neonatal resuscitation training reduced stillbirths and improved 7-day neonatal survival in low-resource countries.[3] A retrospective cohort study demonstrated improved Apgar scores among high-risk newborns after neonatal resuscitation training.[16]
2. A multicenter, case-control study identified 10 perinatal risk factors that predict the need for advanced neonatal resuscitation.[7] An audit study done before the use of risk stratification showed that resuscitation was anticipated in less than half of births requiring PPV.[6] A prospective cohort study showed that risk stratification based on perinatal risk factors increased the likelihood of skilled team attendance at high-risk births.[5]
3. A multicenter quality improvement study demonstrated high staff compliance with the use of a neonatal resuscitation bundle that included briefing and an equipment checklist.[8] A management bundle for preterm infants that included team briefing and equipment checks resulted in clear role assignments, consistent equipment checks, and improved thermoregulation and oxygen saturation.[9]
4. A single-center RCT found that role confusion during simulated neonatal resuscitation was avoided and teamwork skills improved by conducting a team briefing.[11] A statewide collaborative quality initiative demonstrated that team briefing improved team communication and clinical outcomes.[10] A single-center study demonstrated that team briefing and an equipment checklist improved team communication but showed no improvement in equipment preparation.[12]

REFERENCES

1. Ersdal HL, Mduma E, Svensen E, Perlman JM. Early initiation of basic resuscitation interventions including face mask ventilation may reduce birth asphyxia related mortality in low-income countries: a prospective descriptive observational study. *Resuscitation.* 2012;83:869–873. doi: 10.1016/j.resuscitation.2011.12.011
2. Dempsey E, Pammi M, Ryan AC, Barrington KJ. Standardised formal resuscitation training programmes for reducing mortality and morbidity in newborn infants. *Cochrane Database Syst Rev.* 2015:CD009106. doi: 10.1002/14651858.CD009106.pub2
3. Patel A, Khatib MN, Kurhe K, Bhargava S, Bang A. Impact of neonatal resuscitation trainings on neonatal and perinatal mortality: a systematic review and meta-analysis. *BMJ Paediatr Open.* 2017;1:e000183. doi: 10.1136/bmjpo-2017-000183
4. Wyckoff MH, Aziz K, Escobedo MB, Kapadia VS, Kattwinkel J, Perlman JM, Simon WM, Weiner GM, Zaichkin JG. Part 13: neonatal resuscitation: 2015 American Heart Association Guidelines Update for Cardiopulmonary Resuscitation and Emergency Cardiovascular Care. *Circulation.* 2015;132(suppl 2):S543–S560. doi: 10.1161/CIR.0000000000000267
5. Aziz K, Chadwick M, Baker M, Andrews W. Ante- and intra-partum factors that predict increased need for neonatal resuscitation. *Resuscitation.* 2008;79:444–452. doi: 10.1016/j.resuscitation.2008.08.004
6. Mitchell A, Niday P, Boulton J, Chance G, Dulberg C. A prospective clinical audit of neonatal resuscitation practices in Canada. *Adv Neonatal Care.* 2002;2:316–326. doi: 10.1053/adnc.2002.36831
7. Berazategui JP, Aguilar A, Escobedo M, Dannaway D, Guinsburg R, de Almeida MF, Saker F, Fernández A, Albornoz G, Valera M, Amado D, Puig G, Althabe F, Szyld E; ANR study group. Risk factors

for advanced resuscitation in term and near-term infants: a case-control study. *Arch Dis Child Fetal Neonatal Ed.* 2017;102:F44–F50. doi: 10.1136/archdischild-2015-309525
8. Bennett SC, Finer N, Halamek LP, Mickas N, Bennett MV, Nisbet CC, Sharek PJ. Implementing Delivery Room Checklists and Communication Standards in a Multi-Neonatal ICU Quality Improvement Collaborative. *Jt Comm J Qual Patient Saf.* 2016;42:369–376. doi: 10.1016/s1553-7250(16)42052-0
9. Balakrishnan M, Falk-Smith N, Detman LA, Miladinovic B, Sappenfield WM, Curran JS, Ashmeade TL. Promoting teamwork may improve infant care processes during delivery room management: Florida perinatal quality collaborative's approach. *J Perinatol.* 2017;37:886–892. doi: 10.1038/jp.2017.27
10. Talati AJ, Scott TA, Barker B, Grubb PH; Tennessee Initiative for Perinatal Quality Care Golden Hour Project Team. Improving neonatal resuscitation in Tennessee: a large-scale, quality improvement project. *J Perinatol.* 2019;39:1676–1683. doi: 10.1038/s41372-019-0461-3
11. Litke-Wager C, Delaney H, Mu T, Sawyer T. Impact of task-oriented role assignment on neonatal resuscitation performance: a simulation-based randomized controlled trial. *Am J Perinatol.* 2020; doi: 10.1055/s-0039-3402751
12. Katheria A, Rich W, Finer N. Development of a strategic process using checklists to facilitate team preparation and improve communication during neonatal resuscitation. *Resuscitation.* 2013;84:1552–1557. doi: 10.1016/j.resuscitation.2013.06.012
13. Niles DE, Cines C, Insley E, Foglia EE, Elci OU, Skåre C, Olasveengen T, Ades A, Posencheg M, Nadkarni VM, Kramer-Johansen J. Incidence and characteristics of positive pressure ventilation delivered to newborns in a US tertiary academic hospital. *Resuscitation.* 2017;115:102–109. doi: 10.1016/j.resuscitation.2017.03.035
14. Brown T, Tu J, Profit J, Gupta A, Lee HC. Optimal Criteria Survey for Preresuscitation Delivery Room Checklists. *Am J Perinatol.* 2016;33:203–207. doi: 10.1055/s-0035-1564064
15. The Joint Commission. Sentinel Event Alert: Preventing infant death and injury during delivery. 2004. https://www.jointcommission.org/resources/patient-safety-topics/sentinel-event/sentinel-event-alert-newsletters/sentinel-event-alert-issue-30-preventing-infant-death-and-injury-during-delivery/. Accessed February 28, 2020.
16. Patel D, Piotrowski ZH, Nelson MR, Sabich R. Effect of a statewide neonatal resuscitation training program on Apgar scores among high-risk neonates in Illinois. *Pediatrics.* 2001;107:648–655. doi: 10.1542/peds.107.4.648

UMBILICAL CORD MANAGEMENT

Recommendations for Umbilical Cord Management

COR	LOE	Recommendations
2a	B-R	1. For preterm infants who do not require resuscitation at birth, it is reasonable to delay cord clamping for longer than 30 s.[1–8]
2b	C-LD	2. For term infants who do not require resuscitation at birth, it may be reasonable to delay cord clamping for longer than 30 s.[9–21]
2b	C-EO	3. For term and preterm infants who require resuscitation at birth, there is insufficient evidence to recommend early cord clamping versus delayed cord clamping.[22]
3: No Benefit	B-R	4. For infants born at less than 28 wk of gestation, cord milking is not recommended.[23]

Synopsis

During an uncomplicated term or late preterm birth, it may be reasonable to defer cord clamping until after the infant is placed on the mother and assessed for breathing and activity. Early cord clamping (within 30 seconds) may interfere with healthy transition because it leaves fetal blood in the placenta rather than filling the newborn's circulating volume. Delayed cord clamping is associated with higher hematocrit after birth and better iron levels in infancy.[9–21] While developmental outcomes have not been adequately assessed, iron deficiency is associated with impaired motor and cognitive development.[24–26] It is reasonable to delay cord clamping (longer than 30 seconds) in preterm babies because it reduces need for blood pressure support and transfusion and may improve survival.[1–8]

There are insufficient studies in babies requiring PPV before cord clamping to make a recommendation.[22] Early cord clamping should be considered for cases when placental transfusion is unlikely to occur, such as maternal hemorrhage or hemodynamic instability, placental abruption, or placenta previa.[27] There is no evidence of maternal harm from delayed cord clamping compared with early cord clamping.[10–12,28–34] Cord milking is being studied as an alternative to delayed cord clamping but should be avoided in babies less than 28 weeks' gestational age, because it is associated with brain injury.[23]

Recommendation-Specific Supportive Text

1. Compared with preterm infants receiving early cord clamping, those receiving delayed cord clamping were less likely to receive medications for hypotension in a meta-analysis of 6 RCTs[1–6] and receive transfusions in a meta-analysis of 5 RCTs.[7] Among preterm infants not requiring resuscitation, delayed cord clamping may be associated with higher survival than early cord clamping is.[8] Ten RCTs found no difference in postpartum hemorrhage rates with delayed cord clamping versus early cord clamping.[10–12,28–34]
2. Compared with term infants receiving early cord clamping, term infants receiving delayed cord clamping had increased hemoglobin concentration within the first 24 hours and increased ferritin concentration in the first 3 to 6 months in meta-analyses of 12 and 6 RCTs,[9–21] respectively. Compared with term and late preterm infants receiving early cord clamping, those receiving delayed cord clamping showed no significant difference in mortality, admission to the neonatal intensive care unit, or hyperbilirubinemia leading to phototherapy in meta-analyses of 4,[10,13,29,35] 10,[10,12,17,19,21,28,31,34,36,37] and 15 RCTs, respectively.[9,12,14,18–21,28–30,32–34,38,39] Compared with term infants receiving early cord clamping, those receiving delayed cord clamping had increased polycythemia in meta-analyses of 13[10,11,13,14,17,18,21,29,30,33,39–41] and 8 RCTs,[9,10,13,19,20,28,30,34] respectively.

3. For infants requiring PPV at birth, there is currently insufficient evidence to recommend delayed cord clamping versus early cord clamping.
4. A large multicenter RCT found higher rates of intraventricular hemorrhage with cord milking in preterm babies born at less than 28 weeks' gestational age.[23]

REFERENCES

1. Dong XY, Sun XF, Li MM, Yu ZB, Han SP. [Influence of delayed cord clamping on preterm infants with a gestational age of <32 weeks]. *Zhongguo Dang Dai Er Ke Za Zhi.* 2016;18:635–638.
2. Gokmen Z, Ozkiraz S, Tarcan A, Kozanoglu I, Ozcimen EE, Ozbek N. Effects of delayed umbilical cord clamping on peripheral blood hematopoietic stem cells in premature neonates. *J Perinat Med.* 2011;39:323–329. doi: 10.1515/jpm.2011.021
3. McDonnell M, Henderson-Smart DJ. Delayed umbilical cord clamping in preterm infants: a feasibility study. *J Paediatr Child Health.* 1997;33:308–310. doi: 10.1111/j.1440-1754.1997.tb01606.x
4. Oh W, Fanaroff A, Carlo WA, Donovan EF, McDonald SA, Poole WK; on behalf of the Eunice Kennedy Shriver National Institute of Child Health and Human Development Neonatal Research Network. Effects of delayed cord clamping in very-low-birth-weight infants. *J Perinatol.* 2011;31(suppl 1):S68–71. doi: 10.1038/jp.2010.186
5. Rabe H, Wacker A, Hülskamp G, Hörnig-Franz I, Schulze-Everding A, Harms E, Cirkel U, Louwen F, Witteler R, Schneider HP. A randomised controlled trial of delayed cord clamping in very low birth weight preterm infants. *Eur J Pediatr.* 2000;159:775–777. doi: 10.1007/pl00008345
6. Ruangkit C, Bumrungphuet S, Panburana P, Khositseth A, Nuntnarumit P. A Randomized Controlled Trial of Immediate versus Delayed Umbilical Cord Clamping in Multiple-Birth Infants Born Preterm. *Neonatology.* 2019;115:156–163. doi: 10.1159/000494132
7. Rabe H, Diaz-Rossello JL, Duley L, Dowswell T. Effect of timing of umbilical cord clamping and other strategies to influence placental transfusion at preterm birth on maternal and infant outcomes. *Cochrane Database Syst Rev.* 2012:CD003248. doi: 10.1002/14651858.CD003248.pub3
8. Fogarty M, Osborn DA, Askie L, Seidler AL, Hunter K, Lui K, Simes J, Tarnow-Mordi W. Delayed vs early umbilical cord clamping for preterm infants: a systematic review and meta-analysis. *Am J Obstet Gynecol.* 2018;218:1–18. doi: 10.1016/j.ajog.2017.10.231
9. Al-Tawil MM, Abdel-Aal MR, Kaddah MA. A randomized controlled trial on delayed cord clamping and iron status at 3–5 months in term neonates held at the level of maternal pelvis. *J Neonatal Perinat Med.* 2012;5:319–326. doi: 10.3233/NPM-1263112
10. Ceriani Cernadas JM, Carroli G, Pellegrini L, Otaño L, Ferreira M, Ricci C, Casas O, Giordano D, Lardizábal J. The effect of timing of cord clamping on neonatal venous hematocrit values and clinical outcome at term: a randomized, controlled trial. *Pediatrics.* 2006;117:e779–e786. doi: 10.1542/peds.2005-1156
11. Chaparro CM, Neufeld LM, Tena Alavez G, Eguia-Líz Cedillo R, Dewey KG. Effect of timing of umbilical cord clamping on iron status in Mexican infants: a randomised controlled trial. *Lancet.* 2006;367:1997–2004. doi: 10.1016/S0140-6736(06)68889-2
12. Chen X, Li X, Chang Y, Li W, Cui H. Effect and safety of timing of cord clamping on neonatal hematocrit values and clinical outcomes in term infants: A randomized controlled trial. *J Perinatol.* 2018;38:251–257. doi: 10.1038/s41372-017-0001-y
13. Chopra A, Thakur A, Garg P, Kler N, Gujral K. Early versus delayed cord clamping in small for gestational age infants and iron stores at 3 months of age - a randomized controlled trial. *BMC Pediatr.* 2018;18:234. doi: 10.1186/s12887-018-1214-8
14. Emhamed MO, van Rheenen P, Brabin BJ. The early effects of delayed cord clamping in term infants born to Libyan mothers. *Trop Doct.* 2004;34:218–222. doi: 10.1177/004947550403400410
15. Jahazi A, Kordi M, Mirbehbahani NB, Mazloom SR. The effect of early and late umbilical cord clamping on neonatal hematocrit. *J Perinatol.* 2008;28:523–525. doi: 10.1038/jp.2008.55
16. Philip AG. Further observations on placental transfusion. *Obstet Gynecol.* 1973;42:334–343.
17. Salari Z, Rezapour M, Khalili N. Late umbilical cord clamping, neonatal hematocrit and Apgar scores: a randomized controlled trial. *J Neonatal Perinatal Med.* 2014;7:287–291. doi: 10.3233/NPM-1463913
18. Ultee CA, van der Deure J, Swart J, Lasham C, van Baar AL. Delayed cord clamping in preterm infants delivered at 34 36 weeks' gestation: a randomised controlled trial. *Arch Dis Child Fetal Neonatal Ed.* 2008;93:F20–F23. doi: 10.1136/adc.2006.100354
19. Vural I, Ozdemir H, Teker G, Yoldemir T, Bilgen H, Ozek E. Delayed cord clamping in term large-for-gestational age infants: A prospective randomised study. *J Paediatr Child Health.* 2019;55:555–560. doi: 10.1111/jpc.14242
20. Yadav AK, Upadhyay A, Gothwal S, Dubey K, Mandal U, Yadav CP. Comparison of three types of intervention to enhance placental redistribution in term newborns: randomized control trial. *J Perinatol.* 2015;35:720–724. doi: 10.1038/jp.2015.65
21. Mercer JS, Erickson-Owens DA, Collins J, Barcelos MO, Parker AB, Padbury JF. Effects of delayed cord clamping on residual placental blood volume, hemoglobin and bilirubin levels in term infants: a randomized controlled trial. *J Perinatol.* 2017;37:260–264. doi: 10.1038/jp.2016.222
22. Wyckoff MH, Aziz K, Escobedo MB, Kapadia VS, Kattwinkel J, Perlman JM, Simon WM, Weiner GM, Zaichkin JG. Part 13: Neonatal Resuscitation: 2015 American Heart Association Guidelines Update for Cardiopulmonary Resuscitation and Emergency Cardiovascular Care (Reprint). *Pediatrics.* 2015;136 Suppl 2:S196–S218. doi: 10.1542/peds.2015-3373G
23. Katheria A, Reister F, Essers J, Mendler M, Hummler H, Subramaniam A, Carlo W, Tita A, Truong G, Davis-Nelson S, Schmölzer G, Chari R, Kaempf J, Tomlinson M, Yanowitz T, Beck S, Simhan H, Dempsey E, O'Donoghue K, Bhat S, Hoffman M, Faksh A, Arnell K, Rich W, Finer N, Vaucher Y, Khanna P, Meyers M, Varner M, Allman P, Szychowski J, Cutter G. Association of Umbilical Cord Milking vs Delayed Umbilical Cord Clamping With Death or Severe Intraventricular Hemorrhage Among Preterm Infants. *JAMA.* 2019;322:1877–1886. doi: 10.1001/jama.2019.16004
24. Gunnarsson BS, Thorsdottir I, Palsson G, Gretarsson SJ. Iron status at 1 and 6 years versus developmental scores at 6 years in a well-nourished affluent population. *Acta Paediatr.* 2007;96:391–395. doi: 10.1111/j.1651-2227.2007.00086.x
25. Grantham-McGregor S, Ani C. A review of studies on the effect of iron deficiency on cognitive development in children. *J Nutr.* 2001;131(2S-2):649S–666S; discussion 666S. doi: 10.1093/jn/131.2.649S
26. Lozoff B, Beard J, Connor J, Barbara F, Georgieff M, Schallert T. Long-lasting neural and behavioral effects of iron deficiency in infancy. *Nutr Rev.* 2006;64(5 Pt 2):S34–43; discussion S72. doi: 10.1301/nr.2006.may.s34-s43
27. Committee on Obstetric Practice. Committee opinion no. 684: delayed umbilical cord clamping after birth. *Obstet Gynecol.* 2017;129:e5–e10. doi: 10.1097/aog.0000000000001860
28. Andersson O, Hellström-Westas L, Andersson D, Domellöf M. Effect of delayed versus early umbilical cord clamping on neonatal outcomes and iron status at 4 months: a randomised controlled trial. *BMJ.* 2011;343:d7157. doi: 10.1136/bmj.d7157
29. Backes CH, Huang H, Cua CL, Garg V, Smith CV, Yin H, Galantowicz M, Bauer JA, Hoffman TM. Early versus delayed umbilical cord clamping in infants with congenital heart disease: a pilot, randomized, controlled trial. *J Perinatol.* 2015;35:826–831. doi: 10.1038/jp.2015.89
30. Krishnan U, Rosenzweig EB. Pulmonary hypertension in chronic lung disease of infancy. *Curr Opin Pediatr.* 2015;27:177–183. doi: 10.1097/MOP.0000000000000205
31. Mohammad K, Tailakh S, Fram K, Creedy D. Effects of early umbilical cord clamping versus delayed clamping on maternal and neonatal outcomes: a Jordanian study. *J Matern Fetal Neonatal Med.* 2019:1–7. doi: 10.1080/14767058.2019.1602603
32. Oxford Midwives Research Group. A study of the relationship between the delivery to cord clamping interval and the time of cord separation. *Midwifery.* 1991;7:167–176. doi: 10.1016/s0266-6138(05)80195-0
33. van Rheenen P, de Moor L, Eschbach S, de Grooth H, Brabin B. Delayed cord clamping and haemoglobin levels in infancy: a randomised controlled trial in term babies. *Trop Med Int Health.* 2007;12:603–616. doi: 10.1111/j.1365-3156.2007.01835.x
34. Withanathantrige M, Goonewardene I. Effects of early versus delayed umbilical cord clamping during antepartum lower segment caesarean section on placental delivery and postoperative haemorrhage: a randomised controlled trial. *Ceylon Med J.* 2017;62:5–11. doi: 10.4038/cmj.v62i1.8425
35. Datta BV, Kumar A, Yadav R. A Randomized Controlled Trial to Evaluate the Role of Brief Delay in Cord Clamping in Preterm Neonates (34-36 weeks) on Short-term Neurobehavioural Outcome. *J Trop Pediatr.* 2017;63:418–424. doi: 10.1093/tropej/fmx004
36. De Paco C, Florido J, Garrido MC, Prados S, Navarrete L. Umbilical cord blood acid-base and gas analysis after early versus delayed cord clamping

in neonates at term. *Arch Gynecol Obstet.* 2011;283:1011–1014. doi: 10.1007/s00404-010-1516-z
37. De Paco C, Herrera J, Garcia C, Corbalán S, Arteaga A, Pertegal M, Checa R, Prieto MT, Nieto A, Delgado JL. Effects of delayed cord clamping on the third stage of labour, maternal haematological parameters and acid-base status in fetuses at term. *Eur J Obstet Gynecol Reprod Biol.* 2016;207:153–156. doi: 10.1016/j.ejogrb.2016.10.031
38. Cavallin F, Galeazzo B, Loretelli V, Madella S, Pizzolato M, Visentin S, Trevisanuto D. Delayed Cord Clamping versus Early Cord Clamping in Elective Cesarean Section: A Randomized Controlled Trial. *Neonatology.* 2019;116:252–259. doi: 10.1159/000500325
39. Salae R, Tanprasertkul C, Somprasit C, Bhamarapravatana K, Suwannarurk K. Efficacy of Delayed versus Immediate Cord Clamping in Late Preterm Newborns following Normal Labor: A Randomized Control Trial. *J Med Assoc Thai.* 2016;99 Suppl 4:S159–S165.
40. Grajeda R, Pérez-Escamilla R, Dewey KG. Delayed clamping of the umbilical cord improves hematologic status of Guatemalan infants at 2 mo of age. *Am J Clin Nutr.* 1997;65:425–431. doi: 10.1093/ajcn/65.2.425
41. Saigal S, O'Neill A, Surainder Y, Chua LB, Usher R. Placental transfusion and hyperbilirubinemia in the premature. *Pediatrics.* 1972;49:406–419.

INITIAL ACTIONS

Temperature at Birth

Recommendations for Temperature Management

COR	LOE	Recommendations
1	B-NR	1. Admission temperature should be routinely recorded.[1,2]
1	C-EO	2. The temperature of newly born babies should be maintained between 36.5°C and 37.5°C after birth through admission and stabilization.[2]
1	B-NR	3. Hypothermia (temperature less than 36°C) should be prevented due to an increased risk of adverse outcomes.[3–5]
2a	B-NR	4. Prevention of hyperthermia (temperature greater than 38°C) is reasonable due to an increased risk of adverse outcomes.[4,6]

Synopsis

Temperature should be measured and recorded after birth and monitored as a measure of quality.[1] The temperature of newly born babies should be maintained between 36.5°C and 37.5°C.[2] Hypothermia (less than 36°C) should be prevented as it is associated with increased neonatal mortality and morbidity, especially in very preterm (less than 33 weeks) and very low-birth-weight babies (less than 1500 g), who are at increased risk for hypothermia.[3–5,7] It is also reasonable to prevent hyperthermia as it may be associated with harm.[4,6]

Recommendation-Specific Supportive Text

1. Hypothermia after birth is common worldwide, with a higher incidence in babies of lower gestational age and birth weight.[3–5]
2. There are long-standing worldwide recommendations for routine temperature management for the newborn.[2]
3. In observational studies in both preterm (less than 37 weeks) and low-birth-weight babies (less than 2500 g), the presence and degree of hypothermia after birth is strongly associated with increased neonatal mortality and morbidity.[3–5]
4. Two observational studies found an association between hyperthermia and increased morbidity and mortality in very preterm (moderate quality) and very low-birth-weight neonates (very low quality).[4,6]

Temperature Management for Newly Born Infants

Additional Recommendations for Interventions to Maintain or Normalize Temperature

COR	LOE	Recommendations
2a	B-R	1. Placing healthy newborn infants who do not require resuscitation skin-to-skin after birth can be effective in improving breastfeeding, temperature control and blood glucose stability.[8]
2a	C-LD	2. It is reasonable to perform all resuscitation procedures, including endotracheal intubation, chest compressions, and insertion of intravenous lines with temperature-controlling interventions in place.[9]
2a	B-R	3. The use of radiant warmers, plastic bags and wraps (with a cap), increased room temperature, and warmed humidified inspired gases can be effective in preventing hypothermia in preterm babies in the delivery room.[10,11]
2b	B-R	4. Exothermic mattresses may be effective in preventing hypothermia in preterm babies.[11]
2b	B-NR	5. Various combinations of warming strategies (or "bundles") may be reasonable to prevent hypothermia in very preterm babies.[12]
2b	C-LD	6. In resource-limited settings, it may be reasonable to place newly born babies in a clean food-grade plastic bag up to the level of the neck and swaddle them in order to prevent hypothermia.[13]

Synopsis

Healthy babies should be skin-to-skin after birth.[8] For preterm and low-birth-weight babies or babies requiring resuscitation, warming adjuncts (increased ambient temperature [greater than 23°C], skin-to-skin care, radiant warmers, plastic wraps or bags, hats, blankets, exothermic mattresses, and warmed humidified inspired gases)[10,11,14] individually or in combination may reduce the risk of hypothermia. Exothermic mattresses have been reported to cause local heat injury and hyperthermia.[15]

When babies are born in out-of-hospital, resource-limited, or remote settings, it may be reasonable to prevent hypothermia by using a clean food-grade plastic bag[13] as an alternative to skin-to-skin contact.[8]

Recommendation-Specific Supportive Text

1. A systematic review (low to moderate certainty) of 6 RCTs showed that early skin-to-skin contact promotes normothermia in healthy neonates.[8] Two meta-analyses reviewed RCTs and observational studies of extended skin-to-skin care after initial resuscitation and/or stabilization, some in resource-limited settings, showing reduced mortality, improved breastfeeding, shortened length of stay, and improved weight gain in preterm and low-birth-weight babies (moderate quality evidence).[16,17]
2. Most RCTs in well-resourced settings would routinely manage at-risk babies under a radiant warmer.[11]
3. RCTs and observational studies of warming adjuncts, alone and in combination, demonstrate reduced rates of hypothermia in very preterm and very low-birth-weight babies.[10,11] However, meta-analysis of RCTs of interventions that reduce hypothermia in very preterm or very low-birth-weight babies (low certainty) show no impact on neonatal morbidity or mortality.[11] Two RCTs and expert opinion support ambient temperatures of 23°C and above.[2,14,18]
4. One moderate quality RCT found higher rates of hyperthermia with exothermic mattresses.[15]
5. Numerous nonrandomized quality improvement (very low to low certainty) studies support the use of warming adjunct "bundles."[12]
6. One RCT in resource-limited settings found that plastic coverings reduced the incidence of hypothermia, but they were not directly compared with uninterrupted skin-to-skin care.[13]

Clearing the Airway and Tactile Stimulation in Newly Born Infants

Recommendation for Tactile Stimulation and Clearing the Airway in Newly Born Infants

COR	LOE	Recommendation
3: No Benefit	C-LD	1. Routine oral, nasal, oropharyngeal, or endotracheal suctioning of newly born babies is not recommended.[7,19]

Synopsis

The immediate care of newly born babies involves an initial assessment of gestation, breathing, and tone. Babies who are breathing well and/or crying are cared for skin-to-skin with their mothers and should not need interventions such as routine tactile stimulation or suctioning, even if the amniotic fluid is meconium stained.[7,19] Avoiding unnecessary suctioning helps prevent the risk of induced bradycardia as a result of suctioning of the airway.

Recommendation-Specific Supportive Text

1. A meta-analysis of 8 RCTs[19] (low certainty of evidence) suggest no benefit from routine suctioning after birth.[7] Subsequently, 2 additional studies supported this conclusion.[7]

Recommendations for Tactile Stimulation and Clearing the Airway in Newly Born Infants With Ineffective Respiratory Effort

COR	LOE	Recommendations
2a	B-NR	1. In babies who appear to have ineffective respiratory effort after birth, tactile stimulation is reasonable.[20,21]
2b	C-EO	2. Suctioning may be considered if PPV is required and the airway appears obstructed.[20]

Synopsis

If there is ineffective breathing effort or apnea after birth, tactile stimulation may stimulate breathing. Tactile stimulation should be limited to drying an infant and rubbing the back and soles of the feet.[21,22] There may be some benefit from repeated tactile stimulation in preterm babies during or after providing PPV, but this requires further study.[23] If, at initial assessment, there is visible fluid obstructing the airway or a concern about obstructed breathing, the mouth and nose may be suctioned. Suction should also be considered if there is evidence of airway obstruction during PPV.

Recommendation-Specific Supportive Text

1. Limited observational studies suggest that tactile stimulation may improve respiratory effort. One RCT (low certainty of evidence) suggests improved oxygenation after resuscitation in preterm babies who received repeated tactile stimulation.[23]
2. Suctioning for suspected airway obstruction during PPV is based on expert opinion.[7]

Recommendations for Clearing the Airway in Newly Born Infants Delivered Through MSAF

COR	LOE	Recommendations
2a	C-EO	1. For nonvigorous newborns delivered through MSAF who have evidence of airway obstruction during PPV, intubation and tracheal suction can be beneficial.
3: No Benefit	C-LD	2. For nonvigorous newborns (presenting with apnea or ineffective breathing effort) delivered through MSAF, routine laryngoscopy with or without tracheal suctioning is not recommended.[7]

Synopsis

Direct laryngoscopy and endotracheal suctioning are not routinely required for babies born through MSAF but can be beneficial in babies who have evidence of airway obstruction while receiving PPV.[7]

Recommendation-Specific Supportive Text

1. Endotracheal suctioning for apparent airway obstruction with MSAF is based on expert opinion.
2. A meta-analysis of 3 RCTs (low certainty of evidence) and a further single RCT suggest that nonvigorous newborns delivered through MSAF have the same outcomes (survival, need for respiratory support, or neurodevelopment) whether they are suctioned before or after the initiation of PPV.[7]

REFERENCES

1. Perlman JM, Wyllie J, Kattwinkel J, Wyckoff MH, Aziz K, Guinsburg R, Kim HS, Liley HG, Mildenhall L, Simon WM, et al; on behalf of the Neonatal Resuscitation Chapter Collaborators. Part 7: neonatal resuscitation: 2015 International Consensus on Cardiopulmonary Resuscitation and Emergency Cardiovascular Care Science With Treatment Recommendations. *Circulation.* 2015;132(suppl 1):S204–S241. doi: 10.1161/CIR.0000000000000276
2. Department of Reproductive Health and Research (RHR) WHO. *Thermal Protection of the Newborn: A Practical Guide (WHO/RHT/MSM/97.2)* Geneva, Switzerland: World Health Organisation; 1997. https://apps.who.int/iris/bitstream/handle/10665/63986/WHO_RHT_MSM_97.2.pdf;jsessionid=9CF1FA8ABF2E8CE1955D96C1315D9799?sequence=1. Accessed March 1, 2020.
3. Laptook AR, Bell EF, Shankaran S, Boghossian NS, Wyckoff MH, Kandefer S, Walsh M, Saha S, Higgins R; Generic and Moderate Preterm Subcommittees of the NICHD Neonatal Research Network. Admission Temperature and Associated Mortality and Morbidity among Moderately and Extremely Preterm Infants. *J Pediatr.* 2018;192:53–59.e2. doi: 10.1016/j.jpeds.2017.09.021
4. Lyu Y, Shah PS, Ye XY, Warre R, Piedboeuf B, Deshpandey A, Dunn M, Lee SK; Canadian Neonatal Network. Association between admission temperature and mortality and major morbidity in preterm infants born at fewer than 33 weeks' gestation. *JAMA Pediatr.* 2015;169:e150277. doi: 10.1001/jamapediatrics.2015.0277
5. Lunze K, Bloom DE, Jamison DT, Hamer DH. The global burden of neonatal hypothermia: systematic review of a major challenge for newborn survival. *BMC Med.* 2013;11:24. doi: 10.1186/1741-7015-11-24
6. Amadi HO, Olateju EK, Alabi P, Kawuwa MB, Ibadin MO, Osibogun AO. Neonatal hyperthermia and thermal stress in low- and middle-income countries: a hidden cause of death in extremely low-birthweight neonates. *Paediatr Int Child Health.* 2015;35:273–281. doi: 10.1179/2046905515Y.0000000030
7. Wyckoff MH, Wyllie J, Aziz K, de Almeida MF, Fabres J, Fawke J, Guinsburg R, Hosono S, Isayama T, Kapadia VS, et al; on behalf of the Neonatal Life Support Collaborators. Neonatal life support: 2020 International Consensus on Cardiopulmonary Resuscitation and Emergency Cardiovascular Care Science With Treatment Recommendations. *Circulation.* 2020;142(suppl 1):S185–S221. doi: 10.1161/CIR.0000000000000895
8. Moore ER, Bergman N, Anderson GC, Medley N. Early skin-to-skin contact for mothers and their healthy newborn infants. *Cochrane Database Syst Rev.* 2016;11:CD003519. doi: 10.1002/14651858.CD003519.pub4
9. Kattwinkel J, Perlman JM, Aziz K, Colby C, Fairchild K, Gallagher J, Hazinski MF, Halamek LP, Kumar P, Little G, et al. Part 15: neonatal resuscitation: 2010 American Heart Association Guidelines for Cardiopulmonary Resuscitation and Emergency Cardiovascular Care. *Circulation.* 2010;122(suppl 3):S909–S919. doi: 10.1161/CIRCULATIONAHA.110.971119
10. Meyer MP, Owen LS, Te Pas AB. Use of Heated Humidified Gases for Early Stabilization of Preterm Infants: A Meta-Analysis. *Front Pediatr.* 2018;6:319. doi: 10.3389/fped.2018.00319
11. McCall EM, Alderdice F, Halliday HL, Vohra S, Johnston L. Interventions to prevent hypothermia at birth in preterm and/or low birth weight infants. *Cochrane Database Syst Rev.* 2018;2:CD004210. doi: 10.1002/14651858.CD004210.pub5
12. Donnellan D, Moore Z, Patton D, O'Connor T, Nugent L. The effect of thermoregulation quality improvement initiatives on the admission temperature of premature/very low birth-weight infants in neonatal intensive care units: a systematic review. *J Spec Pediatr Nurs.* 2020:e12286. doi: 10.1111/jspn.12286
13. Belsches TC, Tilly AE, Miller TR, Kambeyanda RH, Leadford A, Manasyan A, Chomba E, Ramani M, Ambalavanan N, Carlo WA. Randomized trial of plastic bags to prevent term neonatal hypothermia in a resource-poor setting. *Pediatrics.* 2013;132:e656–e661. doi: 10.1542/peds.2013-0172
14. Duryea EL, Nelson DB, Wyckoff MH, Grant EN, Tao W, Sadana N, Chalak LF, McIntire DD, Leveno KJ. The impact of ambient operating room temperature on neonatal and maternal hypothermia and associated morbidities: a randomized controlled trial. *Am J Obstet Gynecol.* 2016;214:505.e1–505.e7. doi: 10.1016/j.ajog.2016.01.190
15. McCarthy LK, Molloy EJ, Twomey AR, Murphy JF, O'Donnell CP. A randomized trial of exothermic mattresses for preterm newborns in polyethylene bags. *Pediatrics.* 2013;132:e135–e141. doi: 10.1542/peds.2013-0279
16. Boundy EO, Dastjerdi R, Spiegelman D, Fawzi WW, Missmer SA, Lieberman E, Kajeepeta S, Wall S, Chan GJ. Kangaroo mother care and neonatal outcomes: a meta-analysis. *Pediatrics.* 2016;137 doi: 10.1542/peds.2015–2238
17. Conde-Agudelo A, Díaz-Rossello JL. Kangaroo mother care to reduce morbidity and mortality in low birthweight infants. *Cochrane Database Syst Rev.* 2016:CD002771. doi: 10.1002/14651858.CD002771.pub4
18. Jia YS, Lin ZL, Lv H, Li YM, Green R, Lin J. Effect of delivery room temperature on the admission temperature of premature infants: a randomized controlled trial. *J Perinatol.* 2013;33:264–267. doi: 10.1038/jp.2012.100
19. Foster JP, Dawson JA, Davis PG, Dahlen HG. Routine oro/nasopharyngeal suction versus no suction at birth. *Cochrane Database Syst Rev.* 2017;4:CD010332. doi: 10.1002/14651858.CD010332.pub2
20. Ersdal HL, Mduma E, Svensen E, Perlman JM. Early initiation of basic resuscitation interventions including face mask ventilation may reduce birth asphyxia related mortality in low-income countries: a prospective descriptive observational study. *Resuscitation.* 2012;83:869–873. doi: 10.1016/j.resuscitation.2011.12.011
21. Lee AC, Cousens S, Wall SN, Niermeyer S, Darmstadt GL, Carlo WA, Keenan WJ, Bhutta ZA, Gill C, Lawn JE. Neonatal resuscitation and immediate newborn assessment and stimulation for the prevention of neonatal deaths: a systematic review, meta-analysis and Delphi estimation of mortality effect. *BMC Public Health.* 2011;11(suppl 3):S12. doi: 10.1186/1471-2458-11-S3-S12
22. World Health Organization. *Guidelines on Basic Newborn Resuscitation.* Geneva, Switzerland: World Health Organization; 2012. https://apps.who.int/iris/bitstream/handle/10665/75157/9789241503693_eng.pdf;jsessionid=EA13BF490E4D349E12B4DAF16BA64A8D?sequence=1. Accessed March 1, 2020.
23. Dekker J, Hooper SB, Martherus T, Cramer SJE, van Geloven N, Te Pas AB. Repetitive versus standard tactile stimulation of preterm infants at birth - A randomized controlled trial. *Resuscitation.* 2018;127:37–43. doi: 10.1016/j.resuscitation.2018.03.030

ASSESSMENT OF HEART RATE DURING NEONATAL RESUSCITATION

After birth, the newborn's heart rate is used to assess the effectiveness of spontaneous respiratory effort, the need for interventions, and the response to interventions. In addition, accurate, fast, and continuous heart rate assessment is necessary for newborns in whom chest compressions are initiated. Therefore, identifying a rapid and reliable method to measure the newborn's heart rate is critically important during neonatal resuscitation.

Recommendation for Assessment of Heart Rate

COR	LOE	Recommendation
2b	C-LD	1. During resuscitation of term and preterm newborns, the use of electrocardiography (ECG) for the rapid and accurate measurement of the newborn's heart rate may be reasonable.[1–8]

Synopsis

Auscultation of the precordium remains the preferred physical examination method for the initial assessment of the heart rate.[9] Pulse oximetry and ECG remain important adjuncts to provide continuous heart rate assessment in babies needing resuscitation.

ECG provides the most rapid and accurate measurement of the newborn's heart rate at birth and during resuscitation. Clinical assessment of heart rate by auscultation or palpation may be unreliable and inaccurate.[1–4] Compared to ECG, pulse oximetry is both slower in detecting the heart rate and tends to be inaccurate during the first few minutes after birth.[5,6,10–12] Underestimation of heart rate can lead to potentially unnecessary interventions. On the other hand, overestimation of heart rate when a newborn is bradycardic may delay necessary interventions. There are limited data comparing the different approaches to heart rate assessment during neonatal resuscitation on other neonatal outcomes. Use of ECG for heart rate detection does not replace the need for pulse oximetry to evaluate oxygen saturation or the need for supplemental oxygen.

Recommendation-Specific Supportive Text

1. In one RCT and one observational study, there were no reports of technical difficulties with ECG monitoring during neonatal resuscitation, supporting its feasibility as a tool for monitoring heart rate during neonatal resuscitation.[6,7]
2. One observational study compared neonatal outcomes before (historical cohort) and after implementation of ECG monitoring in the delivery room.[8] Compared with the newborns in the historical cohort, newborns with the ECG monitoring had lower rates of endotracheal intubation and higher 5-minute Apgar scores. However, newborns with ECG monitoring also had higher odds of receiving chest compressions in the delivery room.
3. Very low-quality evidence from 8 nonrandomized studies[2,5,6,10,12–15] enrolling 615 newborns and 2 small RCTs[7,16] suggests that at birth, ECG is faster and more accurate for newborn heart assessment compared with pulse oximetry.
4. Very low-quality evidence from 2 nonrandomized studies and 1 randomized trial show that auscultation is not as accurate as ECG for heart rate assessment during newborn stabilization immediately after birth.[2–4]

Recommendation for Assessment of Heart Rate

COR	LOE	Recommendation
1	C-EO	1. During chest compressions, an ECG should be used for the rapid and accurate assessment of heart rate.[1–7,10,12–16]

Synopsis

When chest compressions are initiated, an ECG should be used to confirm heart rate. When ECG heart rate is greater than 60/min, a palpable pulse and/or audible heart rate rules out pulseless electric activity.[17–21]

Recommendation-Specific Supportive Text

1. Given the evidence for ECG during initial steps of PPV, expert opinion is that ECG should be used when providing chest compressions.

REFERENCES

1. Chitkara R, Rajani AK, Oehlert JW, Lee HC, Epi MS, Halamek LP. The accuracy of human senses in the detection of neonatal heart rate during standardized simulated resuscitation: implications for delivery of care, training and technology design. *Resuscitation.* 2013;84:369–372. doi: 10.1016/j.resuscitation.2012.07.035
2. Kamlin CO, O'Donnell CP, Everest NJ, Davis PG, Morley CJ. Accuracy of clinical assessment of infant heart rate in the delivery room. *Resuscitation.* 2006;71:319–321. doi: 10.1016/j.resuscitation.2006.04.015
3. Owen CJ, Wyllie JP. Determination of heart rate in the baby at birth. *Resuscitation.* 2004;60:213–217. doi: 10.1016/j.resuscitation.2003.10.002
4. Voogdt KG, Morrison AC, Wood FE, van Elburg RM, Wyllie JP. A randomised, simulated study assessing auscultation of heart rate at birth. *Resuscitation.* 2010;81:1000–1003. doi: 10.1016/j.resuscitation.2010.03.021
5. Kamlin CO, Dawson JA, O'Donnell CP, Morley CJ, Donath SM, Sekhon J, Davis PG. Accuracy of pulse oximetry measurement of heart rate of newborn infants in the delivery room. *J Pediatr.* 2008;152:756–760. doi: 10.1016/j.jpeds.2008.01.002
6. Katheria A, Rich W, Finer N. Electrocardiogram provides a continuous heart rate faster than oximetry during neonatal resuscitation. *Pediatrics.* 2012;130:e1177–e1181. doi: 10.1542/peds.2012-0784
7. Katheria A, Arnell K, Brown M, Hassen K, Maldonado M, Rich W, Finer N. A pilot randomized controlled trial of EKG for neonatal resuscitation. *PLoS One.* 2017;12:e0187730. doi: 10.1371/journal.pone.0187730
8. Shah BA, Wlodaver AG, Escobedo MB, Ahmed ST, Blunt MH, Anderson MP, Szyld EG. Impact of electronic cardiac (ECG) monitoring on delivery room resuscitation and neonatal outcomes. *Resuscitation.* 2019;143:10–16. doi: 10.1016/j.resuscitation.2019.07.031
9. Wyckoff MH, Aziz K, Escobedo MB, Kapadia VS, Kattwinkel J, Perlman JM, Simon WM, Weiner GM, Zaichkin JG. Part 13: neonatal resuscitation: 2015 American Heart Association Guidelines Update for Cardiopulmonary Resuscitation and Emergency Cardiovascular Care. *Circulation.* 2015;132(suppl 2):S543–S560. doi: 10.1161/CIR.0000000000000267
10. Mizumoto H, Tomotaki S, Shibata H, Ueda K, Akashi R, Uchio H, Hata D. Electrocardiogram shows reliable heart rates much earlier than pulse oximetry during neonatal resuscitation. *Pediatr Int.* 2012;54:205–207. doi: 10.1111/j.1442-200X.2011.03506.x
11. Narayen IC, Smit M, van Zwet EW, Dawson JA, Blom NA, te Pas AB. Low signal quality pulse oximetry measurements in newborn infants are reliable for oxygen saturation but underestimate heart rate. *Acta Paediatr.* 2015;104:e158–e163. doi: 10.1111/apa.12932
12. van Vonderen JJ, Hooper SB, Kroese JK, Roest AA, Narayen IC, van Zwet EW, te Pas AB. Pulse oximetry measures a lower heart rate at birth compared with electrocardiography. *J Pediatr.* 2015;166:49–53. doi: 10.1016/j.jpeds.2014.09.015
13. Dawson JA, Saraswat A, Simionato L, Thio M, Kamlin CO, Owen LS, Schmölzer GM, Davis PG. Comparison of heart rate and oxygen saturation measurements from Masimo and Nellcor pulse oximeters in newly born term infants. *Acta Paediatr.* 2013;102:955–960. doi: 10.1111/apa.12329
14. Gulati R, Zayek M, Eyal F. Presetting ECG electrodes for earlier heart rate detection in the delivery room. *Resuscitation.* 2018;128:83–87. doi: 10.1016/j.resuscitation.2018.03.038
15. Iglesias B, Rodrí Guez MAJ, Aleo E, Criado E, Martí Nez-Orgado J, Arruza L. 3-lead electrocardiogram is more reliable than pulse oximetry to detect bradycardia during stabilisation at birth of very preterm infants. *Arch Dis Child Fetal Neonatal Ed.* 2018;103:F233–F237. doi: 10.1136/archdischild-2016-311492
16. Murphy MC, De Angelis L, McCarthy LK, O'Donnell CPF. Randomised study comparing heart rate measurement in newly born infants using a monitor incorporating electrocardiogram and pulse oximeter versus pulse oximeter alone. *Arch Dis Child Fetal Neonatal Ed.* 2019;104:F547–F550. doi: 10.1136/archdischild-2017-314366
17. Luong D, Cheung PY, Barrington KJ, Davis PG, Unrau J, Dakshinamurti S, Schmölzer GM. Cardiac arrest with pulseless electrical activity rhythm in newborn infants: a case series. *Arch Dis Child Fetal Neonatal Ed.* 2019;104:F572–F574. doi: 10.1136/archdischild-2018-316087

18. Luong DH, Cheung PY, O'Reilly M, Lee TF, Schmolzer GM. Electrocardiography vs. Auscultation to Assess Heart Rate During Cardiac Arrest With Pulseless Electrical Activity in Newborn Infants. *Front Pediatr.* 2018;6:366. doi: 10.3389/fped.2018.00366
19. Patel S, Cheung PY, Solevåg AL, Barrington KJ, Kamlin COF, Davis PG, Schmölzer GM. Pulseless electrical activity: a misdiagnosed entity during asphyxia in newborn infants? *Arch Dis Child Fetal Neonatal Ed.* 2019;104:F215–F217. doi: 10.1136/archdischild-2018-314907
20. Sillers L, Handley SC, James JR, Foglia EE. Pulseless Electrical Activity Complicating Neonatal Resuscitation. *Neonatology.* 2019;115:95–98. doi: 10.1159/000493357
21. Solevåg AL, Luong D, Lee TF, O'Reilly M, Cheung PY, Schmölzer GM. Nonperfusing cardiac rhythms in asphyxiated newborn piglets. *PLoS One.* 2019;14:e0214506. doi: 10.1371/journal.pone.0214506

VENTILATORY SUPPORT AFTER BIRTH: PPV AND CONTINUOUS POSITIVE AIRWAY PRESSURE

Initial Breaths (When and How to Provide PPV)

The vast majority of newborns breathe spontaneously within 30 to 60 seconds after birth, sometimes after drying and tactile stimulation.[1] Newborns who do not breathe within the first 60 seconds after birth or are persistently bradycardic (heart rate less than 100/min) despite appropriate initial actions (including tactile stimulation) may receive PPV at a rate of 40 to 60/min.[2,3] The order of resuscitative procedures in newborns differs from pediatric and adult resuscitation algorithms. On the basis of animal research, the progression from primary apnea to secondary apnea in newborns results in the cessation of respiratory activity before the onset of cardiac failure.[4] This cycle of events differs from that of asphyxiated adults, who experience concurrent respiratory and cardiac failure. For this reason, neonatal resuscitation should begin with PPV rather than with chest compressions.[2,3] Delays in initiating ventilatory support in newly born infants increase the risk of death.[1]

Recommendations About Pressure for Providing PPV

COR	LOE	Recommendations
1	B-NR	1. In newly born infants who are gasping or apneic within 60 s after birth or who are persistently bradycardic (heart rate less than 100/min) despite appropriate initial actions (including tactile stimulation), PPV should be provided without delay.[1]
2a	C-LD	2. In newly born infants who require PPV, it is reasonable to use peak inflation pressure to inflate the lung and achieve a rise in heart rate. This can usually be achieved with a peak inflation pressure of 20 to 25 cm water (H_2O). Occasionally, higher peak inflation pressures are required.[5–14]
2b	C-LD	3. In newly born infants receiving PPV, it may be reasonable to provide positive end-expiratory pressure (PEEP).[15–23]
3: Harm	C-LD	4. Excessive peak inflation pressures are potentially harmful and should be avoided.[24,25]

Synopsis

The adequacy of ventilation is measured by a rise in heart rate and, less reliably, chest expansion. Peak inflation pressures of up to 30 cm H_2O in term newborns and 20 to 25 cm H_2O in preterm newborns are usually sufficient to inflate the lungs.[5–7,9,11–14] In some cases, however, higher inflation pressures are required.[5,7–10] Peak inflation pressures or tidal volumes greater than what is required to increase heart rate and achieve chest expansion should be avoided.[24,26–28]

The lungs of sick or preterm infants tend to collapse because of immaturity and surfactant deficiency.[15] PEEP provides low-pressure inflation of the lungs during expiration. PEEP has been shown to maintain lung volume during PPV in animal studies, thus improving lung function and oxygenation.[16] PEEP may be beneficial during neonatal resuscitation, but the evidence from human studies is limited. Optimal PEEP has not been determined, because all human studies used a PEEP level of 5 cm H_2O.[18–22]

Recommendation-Specific Supportive Text

1. A large observational study showed that most nonvigorous newly born infants respond to stimulation and PPV. The same study demonstrated that the risk of death or prolonged admission increases 16% for every 30-second delay in initiating PPV.[1]
2. Animal studies in newborn mammals show that heart rate decreases during asphyxia. Ventilation of the lungs results in a rapid increase in heart rate.[3,4] Several case series found that most term newborns can be resuscitated using peak inflation pressures of 30 cm H_2O, delivered without PEEP.[5–8] Occasionally, higher peak pressures are required.[5,7–10]
3. Case series in preterm infants have found that most preterm infants can be resuscitated using PPV inflation pressures in the range of 20 to 25 cm H_2O,[11–14] but higher pressures may be required.[10,11]
4. An observational study including 1962 infants between 23 and 33 weeks' gestational age reported lower rates of mortality and chronic lung disease when giving PPV with PEEP versus no PEEP.[19]
5. Two randomized trials and 1 quasi-randomized trial (very low quality) including 312 infants compared PPV with a T-piece (with PEEP) versus a self-inflating bag (no PEEP) and reported similar rates of death and chronic lung disease.[20–22] One trial (very low quality) compared PPV using a T-piece and PEEP of 5 cm H_2O versus 0 cm H_2O and reported similar rates of death and chronic lung disease.[23]
6. Studies of newly born animals showed that PEEP facilitates lung aeration and accumulation of functional residual capacity, prevents distal airway collapse, increases lung surface area and

compliance, decreases expiratory resistance, conserves surfactant, and reduces hyaline membrane formation, alveolar collapse, and the expression of proinflammatory mediators.[16,18]

7. One observational study in newly born infants associated high tidal volumes during resuscitation with brain injury.[25]
8. Several animal studies found that ventilation with high volumes caused lung injury, impaired gas exchange, and reduced lung compliance in immature animals.[24,26–28]

Recommendations for Rate and Inspiratory Time During PPV

COR	LOE	Recommendations
2a	C-EO	1. It is reasonable to provide PPV at a rate of 40 to 60 inflations per minute.
2a	C-LD	2. In term and preterm newly born infants, it is reasonable to initiate PPV with an inspiratory time of 1 s or less.[2]
3: Harm	B-R	3. In preterm newly born infants, the routine use of sustained inflations to initiate resuscitation is potentially harmful and should not be performed.[29]

Synopsis

It is reasonable to initiate PPV at a rate of 40 to 60/min to newly born infants who have ineffective breathing, are apneic, or are persistently bradycardic (heart rate less than 100/min) despite appropriate initial actions (including tactile stimulation).[1]

To match the natural breathing pattern of both term and preterm newborns, the inspiratory time while delivering PPV should be 1 second or less. While there has been research to study the potential effectiveness of providing longer, sustained inflations, there may be potential harm in providing sustained inflations greater than 10 seconds for preterm newborns. The potential benefit or harm of sustained inflations between 1 and 10 seconds is uncertain.[2,29]

Recommendation-Specific Supportive Text

1. Providing PPV at a rate of 40 to 60 inflations per minute is based on expert opinion.
2. The ILCOR task force review, when comparing PPV with sustained inflation breaths, defined PPV to have an inspiratory time of 1 second or less, based on expert opinion. One observational study describes the initial pattern of breathing in term and preterm newly born infants to have an inspiratory time of around 0.3 seconds.[2]
3. Two systematic reviews[29,30] in preterm newborns (low to moderate certainty) found no significant benefit from sustained lung inflation over PPV; one review found a higher risk of death in the first 48 hours. One large RCT[31] was stopped early when an increased rate of early mortality was identified in babies less than 28 weeks' gestational age who received sustained inflations; no significant difference was found in the primary outcome of death or bronchopulmonary dysplasia.

Continuous Positive Airway Pressure Administration

Recommendation for Providing CPAP

COR	LOE	Recommendation
2a	A	1. For spontaneously breathing preterm infants who require respiratory support immediately after delivery, it is reasonable to use CPAP rather than intubation.[32]

Synopsis

Newly born infants who breathe spontaneously need to establish a functional residual capacity after birth.[8] Some newly born infants experience respiratory distress, which manifests as labored breathing or persistent cyanosis. CPAP, a form of respiratory support, helps newly born infants keep their lungs open. CPAP is helpful for preterm infants with breathing difficulty after birth or after resuscitation[33] and may reduce the risk of bronchopulmonary dysplasia in very preterm infants when compared with endotracheal ventilation.[34–36] CPAP is also a less invasive form of respiratory support than intubation and PPV are.

Recommendation-Specific Supportive Text

1. Four RCTs and 1 meta-analysis[32,34–37] (high quality) showed reduction in the combined outcome of death and bronchopulmonary dysplasia when starting treatment with CPAP compared with intubation and ventilation in very preterm infants (less than 30 weeks of gestation) with respiratory distress (the number needed to prevent was 25). The meta-analysis reported no differences in the individual outcomes of mortality, bronchopulmonary dysplasia, pneumothorax, interventricular hemorrhage, necrotizing enterocolitis, or retinopathy of prematurity.[32]

REFERENCES

1. Ersdal HL, Mduma E, Svensen E, Perlman JM. Early initiation of basic resuscitation interventions including face mask ventilation may reduce birth asphyxia related mortality in low-income countries: a prospective descriptive observational study. *Resuscitation.* 2012;83:869–873. doi: 10.1016/j.resuscitation.2011.12.011
2. te Pas AB, Wong C, Kamlin CO, Dawson JA, Morley CJ, Davis PG. Breathing patterns in preterm and term infants immediately after birth. *Pediatr Res.* 2009;65:352–356. doi: 10.1203/PDR.0b013e318193f117
3. Milner AD. Resuscitation of the newborn. *Arch Dis Child.* 1991;66(1 Spec No):66–69. doi: 10.1136/adc.66.1_spec_no.66
4. Dawes GS, Jacobson HN, Mott JC, Shelley HJ, Stafford A. The treatment of asphyxiated, mature foetal lambs and rhesus monkeys with intravenous glucose and sodium carbonate. *J Physiol.* 1963;169:167–184. doi: 10.1113/jphysiol.1963.sp007248
5. Hull D. Lung expansion and ventilation during resuscitation of asphyxiated newborn infants. *J Pediatr.* 1969;75:47–58. doi: 10.1016/s0022-3476(69)80100-9
6. Hoskyns EW, Milner AD, Hopkin IE. A simple method of face mask resuscitation at birth. *Arch Dis Child.* 1987;62:376–378. doi: 10.1136/adc.62.4.376

7. Field D, Milner AD, Hopkin IE. Efficiency of manual resuscitators at birth. *Arch Dis Child.* 1986;61:300–302. doi: 10.1136/adc.61.3.300
8. Boon AW, Milner AD, Hopkin IE. Lung expansion, tidal exchange, and formation of the functional residual capacity during resuscitation of asphyxiated neonates. *J Pediatr.* 1979;95:1031–1036. doi: 10.1016/s0022-3476(79)80304-2
9. Vyas H, Milner AD, Hopkin IE, Boon AW. Physiologic responses to prolonged and slow-rise inflation in the resuscitation of the asphyxiated newborn infant. *J Pediatr.* 1981;99:635–639. doi: 10.1016/s0022-3476(81)80279-x
10. Upton CJ, Milner AD. Endotracheal resuscitation of neonates using a rebreathing bag. *Arch Dis Child.* 1991;66(1 Spec No):39–42. doi: 10.1136/adc.66.1_spec_no.39
11. Hoskyns EW, Milner AD, Boon AW, Vyas H, Hopkin IE. Endotracheal resuscitation of preterm infants at birth. *Arch Dis Child.* 1987;62:663–666. doi: 10.1136/adc.62.7.663
12. Hird MF, Greenough A, Gamsu HR. Inflating pressures for effective resuscitation of preterm infants. *Early Hum Dev.* 1991;26:69–72. doi: 10.1016/0378-3782(91)90045-5
13. Lindner W, Vossbeck S, Hummler H, Pohlandt F. Delivery room management of extremely low birth weight infants: spontaneous breathing or intubation? *Pediatrics.* 1999;103(5 Pt 1):961–967. doi: 10.1542/peds.103.5.961
14. Menakaya J, Andersen C, Chirla D, Wolfe R, Watkins A. A randomised comparison of resuscitation with an anaesthetic rebreathing circuit or an infant ventilator in very preterm infants. *Arch Dis Child Fetal Neonatal Ed.* 2004;89:F494–F496. doi: 10.1136/adc.2003.033340
15. te Pas AB, Davis PG, Hooper SB, Morley CJ. From liquid to air: breathing after birth. *J Pediatr.* 2008;152:607–611. doi: 10.1016/j.jpeds.2007.10.041
16. Siew ML, Te Pas AB, Wallace MJ, Kitchen MJ, Lewis RA, Fouras A, Morley CJ, Davis PG, Yagi N, Uesugi K, et al. Positive end-expiratory pressure enhances development of a functional residual capacity in preterm rabbits ventilated from birth. *J Appl Physiol (1985).* 2009;106:1487–1493. doi: 10.1152/japplphysiol.91591.2008
17. Wyckoff MH, Aziz K, Escobedo MB, Kapadia VS, Kattwinkel J, Perlman JM, Simon WM, Weiner GM, Zaichkin JG. Part 13: neonatal resuscitation: 2015 American Heart Association Guidelines Update for Cardiopulmonary Resuscitation and Emergency Cardiovascular Care. *Circulation.* 2015;132(suppl 2):S543–S560. doi: 10.1161/CIR.0000000000000267
18. Probyn ME, Hooper SB, Dargaville PA, McCallion N, Crossley K, Harding R, Morley CJ. Positive end expiratory pressure during resuscitation of premature lambs rapidly improves blood gases without adversely affecting arterial pressure. *Pediatr Res.* 2004;56:198–204. doi: 10.1203/01.PDR.0000132752.94155.13
19. Guinsburg R, de Almeida MFB, de Castro JS, Gonçalves-Ferri WA, Marques PF, Caldas JPS, Krebs VLJ, Souza Rugolo LMS, de Almeida JHCL, Luz JH, Procianoy RS, Duarte JLMB, Penido MG, Ferreira DMLM, Alves Filho N, Diniz EMA, Santos JP, Acquesta AL, Santos CND, Gonzalez MRC, da Silva RPVC, Meneses J, Lopes JMA, Martinez FE. T-piece versus self-inflating bag ventilation in preterm neonates at birth. *Arch Dis Child Fetal Neonatal Ed.* 2018;103:F49–F55. doi: 10.1136/archdischild-2016-312360
20. Dawson JA, Schmölzer GM, Kamlin CO, Te Pas AB, O'Donnell CP, Donath SM, Davis PG, Morley CJ. Oxygenation with T-piece versus self-inflating bag for ventilation of extremely preterm infants at birth: a randomized controlled trial. *J Pediatr.* 2011;158:912–918.e1-2 doi: 10.1016/j.jpeds.2010.12.003
21. Szyld E, Aguilar A, Musante GA, Vain N, Prudent L, Fabres J, Carlo WA; Delivery Room Ventilation Devices Trial Group. Comparison of devices for newborn ventilation in the delivery room. *J Pediatr.* 2014;165:234–239.e3. doi: 10.1016/j.jpeds.2014.02.035
22. Thakur A, Saluja S, Modi M, Kler N, Garg P, Soni A, Kaur A, Chetri S. T-piece or self inflating bag for positive pressure ventilation during delivery room resuscitation: an RCT. *Resuscitation.* 2015;90:21–24. doi: 10.1016/j.resuscitation.2015.01.021
23. Finer NN, Carlo WA, Duara S, Fanaroff AA, Donovan EF, Wright LL, Kandefer S, Poole WK; National Institute of Child Health and Human Development Neonatal Research Network. Delivery room continuous positive airway pressure/positive end-expiratory pressure in extremely low birth weight infants: a feasibility trial. *Pediatrics.* 2004;114:651–657. doi: 10.1542/peds.2004-0394
24. Hillman NH, Moss TJ, Kallapur SG, Bachurski C, Pillow JJ, Polglase GR, Nitsos I, Kramer BW, Jobe AH. Brief, large tidal volume ventilation initiates lung injury and a systemic response in fetal sheep. *Am J Respir Crit Care Med.* 2007;176:575–581. doi: 10.1164/rccm.200701-051OC
25. Mian Q, Cheung PY, O'Reilly M, Barton SK, Polglase GR, Schmölzer GM. Impact of delivered tidal volume on the occurrence of intraventricular haemorrhage in preterm infants during positive pressure ventilation in the delivery room. *Arch Dis Child Fetal Neonatal Ed.* 2019;104:F57–F62. doi: 10.1136/archdischild-2017-313864
26. Björklund LJ, Ingimarsson J, Curstedt T, John J, Robertson B, Werner O, Vilstrup CT. Manual ventilation with a few large breaths at birth compromises the therapeutic effect of subsequent surfactant replacement in immature lambs. *Pediatr Res.* 1997;42:348–355. doi: 10.1203/00006450-199709000-00016
27. Björklund LJ, Ingimarsson J, Curstedt T, Larsson A, Robertson B, Werner O. Lung recruitment at birth does not improve lung function in immature lambs receiving surfactant. *Acta Anaesthesiol Scand.* 2001;45:986–993. doi: 10.1034/j.1399-6576.2001.450811.x
28. Wada K, Jobe AH, Ikegami M. Tidal volume effects on surfactant treatment responses with the initiation of ventilation in preterm lambs. *J Appl Physiol (1985).* 1997;83:1054–1061. doi: 10.1152/jappl.1997.83.4.1054
29. Wyckoff MH, Wyllie J, Aziz K, de Almeida MF, Fabres J, Fawke J, Guinsburg R, Hosono S, Isayama T, Kapadia VS, et al; on behalf of the Neonatal Life Support Collaborators. Neonatal life support: 2020 International Consensus on Cardiopulmonary Resuscitation and Emergency Cardiovascular Care Science With Treatment Recommendations. *Circulation.* 2020;142(suppl 1):S185–S221. doi: 10.1161/CIR.0000000000000895
30. Foglia EE, Te Pas AB, Kirpalani H, Davis PG, Owen LS, van Kaam AH, Onland W, Keszler M, Schmölzer GM, Hummler H, et al. Sustained inflation vs standard resuscitation for preterm infants: a systematic review and meta-analysis. *JAMA Pediatr.* 2020:e195897. doi: 10.1001/jamapediatrics.2019.5897
31. Kirpalani H, Ratcliffe SJ, Keszler M, Davis PG, Foglia EE, Te Pas A, Fernando M, Chaudhary A, Localio R, van Kaam AH, Onland W, Owen LS, Schmölzer GM, Katheria A, Hummler H, Lista G, Abbasi S, Klotz D, Simma B, Nadkarni V, Poulain FR, Donn SM, Kim HS, Park WS, Cadet C, Kong JY, Smith A, Guillen U, Liley HG, Hopper AO, Tamura M; on behalf of the SAIL Site Investigators. Effect of Sustained Inflations vs Intermittent Positive Pressure Ventilation on Bronchopulmonary Dysplasia or Death Among Extremely Preterm Infants: The SAIL Randomized Clinical Trial. *JAMA.* 2019;321:1165–1175. doi: 10.1001/jama.2019.1660
32. Schmölzer GM, Kumar M, Pichler G, Aziz K, O'Reilly M, Cheung PY. Non-invasive versus invasive respiratory support in preterm infants at birth: systematic review and meta-analysis. *BMJ.* 2013;347:f5980. doi: 10.1136/bmj.f5980
33. Hooper SB, Polglase GR, Roehr CC. Cardiopulmonary changes with aeration of the newborn lung. *Paediatr Respir Rev.* 2015;16:147–150. doi: 10.1016/j.prrv.2015.03.003
34. Dunn MS, Kaempf J, de Klerk A, de Klerk R, Reilly M, Howard D, Ferrelli K, O'Conor J, Soll RF; Vermont Oxford Network DRM Study Group. Randomized trial comparing 3 approaches to the initial respiratory management of preterm neonates. *Pediatrics.* 2011;128:e1069–e1076. doi: 10.1542/peds.2010-3848
35. Morley CJ, Davis PG, Doyle LW, Brion LP, Hascoet JM, Carlin JB; COIN Trial Investigators. Nasal CPAP or intubation at birth for very preterm infants. *N Engl J Med.* 2008;358:700–708. doi: 10.1056/NEJMoa072788
36. SUPPORT Study Group of the Eunice Kennedy Shriver NICHD Neonatal Research Network. Early CPAP versus surfactant in extremely preterm infants. *N Engl J Med.* 2010;362:1970–1979. doi: 10.1056/NEJMoa0911783
37. Sandri F, Plavka R, Ancora G, Simeoni U, Stranak Z, Martinelli S, Mosca F, Nona J, Thomson M, Verder H, Fabbri L, Halliday H; CURPAP Study Group. Prophylactic or early selective surfactant combined with nCPAP in very preterm infants. *Pediatrics.* 2010;125:e1402–e1409. doi: 10.1542/peds.2009-2131

OXYGEN ADMINISTRATION

Recommendations for Oxygen Administration During Neonatal Resuscitation

COR	LOE	Recommendations
2a	B-R	1. In term and late preterm newborns (35 wk or more of gestation) receiving respiratory support at birth, the initial use of 21% oxygen is reasonable.[1]
2b	C-LD	2. In preterm newborns (less than 35 wk of gestation) receiving respiratory support at birth, it may be reasonable to begin with 21% to 30% oxygen with subsequent oxygen titration based on pulse oximetry.[2,3]
3: Harm	B-R	3. In term and late preterm newborns (35 wk or more of gestation) receiving respiratory support at birth, 100% oxygen should not be used because it is associated with excess mortality.[1]

Synopsis

During an uncomplicated delivery, the newborn transitions from the low oxygen environment of the womb to room air (21% oxygen) and blood oxygen levels rise over several minutes. During resuscitation, supplemental oxygen may be provided to prevent harm from inadequate oxygen supply to tissues (hypoxemia).[4] However, overexposure to oxygen (hyperoxia) may be associated with harm.[5]

Term and late preterm newborns have lower short-term mortality when respiratory support during resuscitation is started with 21% oxygen (air) versus 100% oxygen.[1] No difference was found in neurodevelopmental outcome of survivors.[1] During resuscitation, pulse oximetry may be used to monitor oxygen saturation levels found in healthy term infants after vaginal birth at sea level.[3]

In more preterm newborns, there were no differences in mortality or other important outcomes when respiratory support was started with low (50% or less) versus high (greater than 50%) oxygen concentrations.[2] Given the potential for harm from hyperoxia, it may be reasonable to start with 21% to 30% oxygen. Pulse oximetry with oxygen targeting is recommended in this population.[3]

Recommendation-Specific Supportive Text

1. A meta-analysis of 5 randomized and quasi-randomized trials enrolling term and late preterm newborns showed no difference in rates of hypoxic-ischemic encephalopathy (HIE). Similarly, meta-analysis of 2 quasi-randomized trials showed no difference in moderate-to-severe neurodevelopmental impairment at 1 to 3 years of age[1] for newborns administered 21% versus 100% oxygen.[1]
2. Meta-analysis of 10 randomized trials enrolling preterm newborns, including subanalysis of 7 trials reporting outcomes for newborns 28 weeks' gestational age or less, showed no difference in short-term mortality when respiratory support was started with low compared with high oxygen.[2] In the included studies, low oxygen was generally 21% to 30% and high oxygen was always 60% to 100%. Furthermore, no differences were found in long-term mortality, neurodevelopmental outcome, retinopathy of prematurity, bronchopulmonary dysplasia, necrotizing enterocolitis, or major cerebral hemorrhage.[2] In a systematic review of 8 trials that used oxygen saturation targeting as a cointervention, all preterm babies in whom respiratory support was initiated with 21% oxygen (air) required supplemental oxygen to achieve the predetermined oxygen saturation target.[2] The recommendation to initiate respiratory support with a lower oxygen concentration reflects a preference to avoid exposing preterm newborns to additional oxygen (beyond what is necessary to achieve the predetermined oxygen saturation target) without evidence demonstrating a benefit for important outcomes.[3]
3. Meta-analysis of 7 randomized and quasi-randomized trials enrolling term and late preterm newborns showed decreased short-term mortality when using 21% oxygen compared with 100% oxygen for delivery room resuscitation.[1] No studies looked at starting with intermediate oxygen concentrations (ie, 22% to 99% oxygen).

REFERENCES

1. Welsford M, Nishiyama C, Shortt C, Isayama T, Dawson JA, Weiner G, Roehr CC, Wyckoff MH, Rabi Y; on behalf of the International Liaison Committee on Resuscitation Neonatal Life Support Task Force. Room air for initiating term newborn resuscitation: a systematic review with meta-analysis. *Pediatrics*. 2019;143. doi: 10.1542/peds.2018-1825
2. Welsford M, Nishiyama C, Shortt C, Weiner G, Roehr CC, Isayama T, Dawson JA, Wyckoff MH, Rabi Y; on behalf of the International Liaison Committee on Resuscitation Neonatal Life Support Task Force. Initial oxygen use for preterm newborn resuscitation: a systematic review with meta-analysis. *Pediatrics*. 2019;143 doi: 10.1542/peds.2018-1828
3. Escobedo MB, Aziz K, Kapadia VS, Lee HC, Niermeyer S, Schmölzer GM, Szyld E, Weiner GM, Wyckoff MH, Yamada NK, Zaichkin JG. 2019 American Heart Association Focused Update on Neonatal Resuscitation: An Update to the American Heart Association Guidelines for Cardiopulmonary Resuscitation and Emergency Cardiovascular Care. *Circulation*. 2019;140:e922–e930. doi: 10.1161/CIR.0000000000000729
4. Saugstad OD. Resuscitation of newborn infants: from oxygen to room air. *Lancet*. 2010;376:1970–1971. doi: 10.1016/S0140-6736(10)60543-0
5. Weinberger B, Laskin DL, Heck DE, Laskin JD. Oxygen toxicity in premature infants. *Toxicol Appl Pharmacol*. 2002;181:60–67. doi: 10.1006/taap.2002.9387

CHEST COMPRESSIONS

CPR Timing

Recommendations for Initiating CPR

COR	LOE	Recommendations
2a	C-EO	1. If heart rate after birth remains at less than 60/min despite adequate ventilation for at least 30 s, initiating chest compressions is reasonable.[1,2]
2b	C-EO	2. The benefit of 100% oxygen compared with 21% oxygen (air) or any other oxygen concentration for ventilation during chest compressions is uncertain. It may be reasonable to use higher concentrations of oxygen during chest compressions.[1,2]

Synopsis

Most newborns who are apneic or have ineffective breathing at birth will respond to initial steps of newborn resuscitation (positioning to open the airway, clearing secretions, drying, and tactile stimulation) or to effective PPV with a rise in heart rate and improved breathing. If the heart rate remains less than 60/min despite these interventions, chest compressions can supply oxygenated blood to the brain until the heart rate rises. Ventilation should be optimized before starting chest compressions, with endotracheal intubation if possible. Chest compressions should be started if the heart rate remains less than 60/min after at least 30 seconds of adequate PPV.[1]

Oxygen is essential for organ function; however, excess inspired oxygen during resuscitation may be harmful. Although current guidelines recommend using 100% oxygen while providing chest compressions, no studies have confirmed a benefit of using 100% oxygen compared to any other oxygen concentration, including air (21%). However, it may be reasonable to increase inspired oxygen to 100% if there was no response to PPV with lower concentrations. Once return of spontaneous circulation (ROSC) is achieved, the supplemental oxygen concentration may be decreased to target a physiological level based on pulse oximetry to reduce the risks associated with hyperoxia.[1,2]

Recommendation-Specific Supportive Text

1. The initiation of chest compressions in newborn babies with a heart rate less than 60/min is based on expert opinion because there are no clinical or physiological human studies addressing this question.
2. A meta-analysis (very low quality) of 8 animal studies (n=323 animals) that compared air with 100% oxygen during chest compressions showed equivocal results.[3] Two animal studies (very low quality) compared the tissue oxidative stress or damage between air (21%) and 100% oxygen and reported no difference in brain or lung inflammatory markers.[3] The use of 100% oxygen during chest compressions is therefore expert opinion.

Compression-to-Ventilation Ratio and Techniques (Newborn)

Recommendations for Providing Chest Compressions		
COR	LOE	Recommendations
2b	C-EO	1. When providing chest compressions in a newborn, it may be reasonable to repeatedly deliver 3 compressions followed by an inflation (3:1 ratio).[4–8]
2b	C-LD	2. When providing chest compressions to a newborn, it may be reasonable to choose the 2 thumb–encircling hands technique over the 2-finger technique, as the 2 thumb–encircling hands technique is associated with improved blood pressure and less provider fatigue.[9,10]

Synopsis

Chest compressions are a rare event in full-term newborns (approximately 0.1%) but are provided more frequently to preterm newborns.[11] When providing chest compressions to a newborn, it may be reasonable to deliver 3 compressions before or after each inflation: providing 30 inflations and 90 compressions per minute (3:1 ratio for 120 total events per minute).

Alternative compression-to-ventilation ratios to 3:1, as well as asynchronous PPV (administration of inflations to a patient that are not coordinated with chest compressions), are routinely utilized outside the newborn period, but the preferred method in the newly born is 3:1 in synchrony. Newer methods of chest compression, using a sustained inflation that maintains lung inflation while providing chest compressions, are under investigation and cannot be recommended at this time outside research protocols.[12,13]

When providing chest compressions to a newborn, the 2 thumb–encircling hands technique may have benefit over the 2-finger technique with respect to blood pressure generation and provider fatigue. When providing chest compressions with the 2 thumb–encircling hands technique, the hands encircle the chest while the thumbs depress the sternum.[1,2] The 2 thumb–encircling hands technique can be performed from the side of the infant or from above the head of the newborn.[1] Performing chest compressions with the 2 thumb–encircling hands technique from above the head facilitates placement of an umbilical venous catheter.

Recommendation-Specific Supportive Text

1. In animal studies (very low quality), the use of alternative compression-to-inflation ratios to 3:1 (eg, 2:1, 4:1, 5:1, 9:3, 15:2, and continuous chest compressions with asynchronous PPV) are associated with similar times to ROSC and mortality rates.[4–8]
2. In a small number of newborns (n=2) with indwelling catheters, the 2 thumb–encircling hands technique generated higher systolic and mean blood pressures compared with the 2-finger technique.[9]
3. One small manikin study (very low quality), compared the 2 thumb–encircling hands technique and 2-finger technique during 60 seconds of uninterrupted chest compressions. The 2 thumb–encircling hands technique achieved greater depth, less fatigue, and less variability with each compression compared with the 2-finger technique.[10]

REFERENCES

1. Wyckoff MH, Aziz K, Escobedo MB, Kapadia VS, Kattwinkel J, Perlman JM, Simon WM, Weiner GM, Zaichkin JG. Part 13: neonatal resuscitation: 2015 American Heart Association Guidelines Update for Cardiopulmonary Resuscitation and Emergency Cardiovascular Care. *Circulation.* 2015;132(suppl 2):S543–S560. doi: 10.1161/CIR.0000000000000267
2. Perlman JM, Wyllie J, Kattwinkel J, Wyckoff MH, Aziz K, Guinsburg R, Kim HS, Liley HG, Mildenhall L, Simon WM, et al; on behalf of the Neonatal Resuscitation Chapter Collaborators. Part 7: neonatal resuscitation: 2015 International Consensus on Cardiopulmonary Resuscitation and Emergency Cardiovascular Care Science With Treatment Recommendations. *Circulation.* 2015;132(suppl 1):S204–S241. doi: 10.1161/CIR.0000000000000276
3. Garcia-Hidalgo C, Cheung PY, Solevåg AL, Vento M, O'Reilly M, Saugstad O, Schmölzer GM. A Review of Oxygen Use During Chest Compressions in Newborns-A Meta-Analysis of Animal Data. *Front Pediatr.* 2018;6:400. doi: 10.3389/fped.2018.00400
4. Solevåg AL, Schmölzer GM, O'Reilly M, Lu M, Lee TF, Hornberger LK, Nakstad B, Cheung PY. Myocardial perfusion and oxidative stress after

21% vs. 100% oxygen ventilation and uninterrupted chest compressions in severely asphyxiated piglets. *Resuscitation.* 2016;106:7–13. doi: 10.1016/j.resuscitation.2016.06.014
5. Schmölzer GM, O'Reilly M, Labossiere J, Lee TF, Cowan S, Nicoll J, Bigam DL, Cheung PY. 3:1 compression to ventilation ratio versus continuous chest compression with asynchronous ventilation in a porcine model of neonatal resuscitation. *Resuscitation.* 2014;85:270–275. doi: 10.1016/j.resuscitation.2013.10.011
6. Solevåg AL, Dannevig I, Wyckoff M, Saugstad OD, Nakstad B. Extended series of cardiac compressions during CPR in a swine model of perinatal asphyxia. *Resuscitation.* 2010;81:1571–1576. doi: 10.1016/j.resuscitation.2010.06.007
7. Solevag AL, Dannevig I, Wyckoff M, Saugstad OD, Nakstad B. Return of spontaneous circulation with a compression:ventilation ratio of 15:2 versus 3:1 in newborn pigs with cardiac arrest due to asphyxia. *Arch Dis Child Fetal Neonatal Ed.* 2011;96:F417–F421. doi: 10.1136/adc.2010.200386
8. Pasquin MP, Cheung PY, Patel S, Lu M, Lee TF, Wagner M, O'Reilly M, Schmolzer GM. Comparison of Different Compression to Ventilation Ratios (2: 1, 3: 1, and 4: 1) during Cardiopulmonary Resuscitation in a Porcine Model of Neonatal Asphyxia. *Neonatology.* 2018;114:37–45. doi: 10.1159/000487988
9. David R. Closed chest cardiac massage in the newborn infant. *Pediatrics.* 1988;81:552–554.
10. Christman C, Hemway RJ, Wyckoff MH, Perlman JM. The two-thumb is superior to the two-finger method for administering chest compressions in a manikin model of neonatal resuscitation. *Arch Dis Child Fetal Neonatal Ed.* 2011;96:F99–F101. doi: 10.1136/adc.2009.180406
11. Handley SC, Sun Y, Wyckoff MH, Lee HC. Outcomes of extremely preterm infants after delivery room cardiopulmonary resuscitation in a population-based cohort. *J Perinatol.* 2015;35:379–383. doi: 10.1038/jp.2014.222
12. Schmölzer GM, M OR, Fray C, van Os S, Cheung PY. Chest compression during sustained inflation versus 3:1 chest compression:ventilation ratio during neonatal cardiopulmonary resuscitation: a randomised feasibility trial. *Arch Dis Child Fetal Neonatal Ed.* 2018;103:F455–F460. doi: 10.1136/archdischild-2017–313037
13. Schmölzer GM, O'Reilly M, Labossiere J, Lee TF, Cowan S, Qin S, Bigam DL, Cheung PY. Cardiopulmonary resuscitation with chest compressions during sustained inflations: a new technique of neonatal resuscitation that improves recovery and survival in a neonatal porcine model. *Circulation.* 2013;128:2495–2503. doi: 10.1161/circulationaha.113.002289

INTRAVASCULAR ACCESS

Recommendations for Vascular Access		
COR	LOE	Recommendations
1	C-EO	1. For babies requiring vascular access at the time of delivery, the umbilical vein is the recommended route.[1]
2b	C-EO	2. If intravenous access is not feasible, it may be reasonable to use the intraosseous route.[1]

Synopsis

Babies who have failed to respond to PPV and chest compressions require vascular access to infuse epinephrine and/or volume expanders. In the delivery room setting, the primary method of vascular access is umbilical venous catheterization. Outside the delivery room, or if intravenous access is not feasible, the intraosseous route may be a reasonable alternative, determined by the local availability of equipment, training, and experience.

Recommendation-Specific Supportive Text

1. Umbilical venous catheterization has been the accepted standard route in the delivery room for decades.[2] There are no human neonatal studies to support one route over others.[1]
2. There are 6 case reports indicating local complications of intraosseous needle placement.[3–8]
3. Practitioners outside of the delivery room setting, and when umbilical venous catheterization is not feasible, may secure vascular access with the intraosseous route.

REFERENCES

1. Wyckoff MH, Wyllie J, Aziz K, de Almeida MF, Fabres J, Fawke J, Guinsburg R, Hosono S, Isayama T, Kapadia VS, et al; on behalf of the Neonatal Life Support Collaborators. Neonatal life support: 2020 International Consensus on Cardiopulmonary Resuscitation and Emergency Cardiovascular Care Science With Treatment Recommendations. *Circulation.* 2020;142(suppl 1):S185–S221. doi: 10.1161/CIR.0000000000000895
2. Niermeyer S, Kattwinkel J, Van Reempts P, Nadkarni V, Phillips B, Zideman D, Azzopardi D, Berg R, Boyle D, Boyle R, Burchfield D, Carlo W, Chameides L, Denson S, Fallat M, Gerardi M, Gunn A, Hazinski MF, Keenan W, Knaebel S, Milner A, Perlman J, Saugstad OD, Schleien C, Solimano A, Speer M, Toce S, Wiswell T, Zaritsky A. International Guidelines for Neonatal Resuscitation: An excerpt from the Guidelines 2000 for Cardiopulmonary Resuscitation and Emergency Cardiovascular Care: International Consensus on Science. Contributors and Reviewers for the Neonatal Resuscitation Guidelines. *Pediatrics.* 2000;106:E29. doi: 10.1542/peds.106.3.e29
3. Vidal R, Kissoon N, Gayle M. Compartment syndrome following intraosseous infusion. *Pediatrics.* 1993;91:1201–1202.
4. Katz DS, Wojtowycz AR. Tibial fracture: a complication of intraosseous infusion. *Am J Emerg Med.* 1994;12:258–259. doi: 10.1016/0735-6757(94)90261-5
5. Ellemunter H, Simma B, Trawöger R, Maurer H. Intraosseous lines in preterm and full term neonates. *Arch Dis Child Fetal Neonatal Ed.* 1999;80:F74–F75. doi: 10.1136/fn.80.1.f74
6. Carreras-González E, Brió-Sanagustín S, Guimerá I, Crespo C. Complication of the intraosseous route in a newborn infant [in Spanish]. *Med Intensiva.* 2012;36:233–234. doi: 10.1016/j.medin.2011.05.004
7. Oesterlie GE, Petersen KK, Knudsen L, Henriksen TB. Crural amputation of a newborn as a consequence of intraosseous needle insertion and calcium infusion. *Pediatr Emerg Care.* 2014;30:413–414. doi: 10.1097/PEC.0000000000000150
8. Suominen PK, Nurmi E, Lauerma K. Intraosseous access in neonates and infants: risk of severe complications - a case report. *Acta Anaesthesiol Scand.* 2015;59:1389–1393. doi: 10.1111/aas.12602

MEDICATIONS (EPINEPHRINE) IN NEONATAL RESUSCITATION

Recommendations for Epinephrine Administration in Neonatal Resuscitation		
COR	LOE	Recommendations
2b	C-LD	1. If the heart rate has not increased to 60/min or more after optimizing ventilation and chest compressions, it may be reasonable to administer intravascular* epinephrine (0.01 to 0.03 mg/kg).[1–3]
2b	C-LD	2. While vascular access is being obtained, it may be reasonable to administer endotracheal epinephrine at a larger dose (0.05 to 0.1 mg/kg).[1–3]
2b	C-LD	3. If endotracheal epinephrine is given before vascular access is available and response is inadequate, it may be reasonable to give an intravascular* dose as soon as access is obtained, regardless of the interval.[1,2]
2b	C-LD	4. It may be reasonable to administer further doses of epinephrine every 3 to 5 min, preferably intravascularly,* if the heart rate remains less than 60/min.[2,3]

*In this situation, "intravascular" means intravenous or intraosseous. Intra-arterial epinephrine is not recommended.

Synopsis

Medications are rarely needed in resuscitation of the newly born infant because low heart rate usually results from a very low oxygen level in the fetus or inadequate lung inflation after birth. Establishing ventilation is the most important step to correct low heart rate. However, if heart rate remains less than 60/min after ventilating with 100% oxygen (preferably through an endotracheal tube) and chest compressions, administration of epinephrine is indicated.

Administration of epinephrine via a low-lying umbilical venous catheter provides the most rapid and reliable medication delivery. The intravenous dose of epinephrine is 0.01 to 0.03 mg/kg, followed by a normal saline flush.[4] If umbilical venous access has not yet been obtained, epinephrine may be given by the endotracheal route in a dose of 0.05 to 0.1 mg/kg. The dosage interval for epinephrine is every 3 to 5 minutes if the heart rate remains less than 60/min, although an intravenous dose may be given as soon as umbilical access is obtained if response to endotracheal epinephrine has been inadequate.

Recommendation-Specific Supportive Text

1. The very limited observational evidence in human infants does not demonstrate greater efficacy of endotracheal or intravenous epinephrine; however, most babies received at least 1 intravenous dose before ROSC.[1,2] In a perinatal model of cardiac arrest using term lambs undergoing transition with asphyxia-induced cardiopulmonary arrest, central venous epinephrine was associated with shorter time to ROSC and higher rates of ROSC than endotracheal epinephrine was.[3] Intravenous epinephrine followed by a normal saline flush improves medication delivery.[4]
2. One very limited observational study (human) showed 0.03 mg/kg to be an inadequate endotracheal dose.[1] In the perinatal model of cardiac arrest, peak plasma epinephrine concentrations in animals were higher and were achieved sooner after central or low-lying umbilical venous administration compared with the endotracheal route, despite a lower intravenous dose (0.03 mg/kg intravenous versus 0.1 mg/kg endotracheal route).[3]
3. In one very limited observational study, most infants who received an endotracheal dose achieved ROSC after a subsequent intravenous dose.[2] Although the more rapid response to intravenous epinephrine warrants its immediate administration once umbilical access is obtained, repetitive endotracheal doses or higher intravenous doses may result in potentially harmful plasma levels that lead to associated hypertension and tachycardia.[5–8]
4. In one very limited observational study, many infants received multiple doses of epinephrine before ROSC.[2] The perinatal model of cardiac arrest documented peak plasma epinephrine concentrations at 1 minute after intravenous administration, but not until 5 minutes after endotracheal administration.[3]

REFERENCES

1. Barber CA, Wyckoff MH. Use and efficacy of endotracheal versus intravenous epinephrine during neonatal cardiopulmonary resuscitation in the delivery room. *Pediatrics.* 2006;118:1028–1034. doi: 10.1542/peds.2006-0416
2. Halling C, Sparks JE, Christie L, Wyckoff MH. Efficacy of Intravenous and Endotracheal Epinephrine during Neonatal Cardiopulmonary Resuscitation in the Delivery Room. *J Pediatr.* 2017;185:232–236. doi: 10.1016/j.jpeds.2017.02.024
3. Vali P, Chandrasekharan P, Rawat M, Gugino S, Koenigsknecht C, Helman J, Jusko WJ, Mathew B, Berkelhamer S, Nair J, et al. Evaluation of timing and route of epinephrine in a neonatal model of asphyxial arrest. *J Am Heart Assoc.* 2017;6:e004402. doi: 10.1161/JAHA.116.004402
4. Vali P, Sankaran D, Rawat M, Berkelhamer S, Lakshminrusimha S. Epinephrine in neonatal resuscitation. *Children (Basel).* 2019;6:E51. doi: 10.3390/children6040051
5. Perondi MB, Reis AG, Paiva EF, Nadkarni VM, Berg RA. A comparison of high-dose and standard-dose epinephrine in children with cardiac arrest. *N Engl J Med.* 2004;350:1722–1730. doi: 10.1056/NEJMoa032440
6. Vandycke C, Martens P. High dose versus standard dose epinephrine in cardiac arrest - a meta-analysis. *Resuscitation.* 2000;45:161–166. doi: 10.1016/s0300-9572(00)00188-x
7. Berg RA, Otto CW, Kern KB, Hilwig RW, Sanders AB, Henry CP, Ewy GA. A randomized, blinded trial of high-dose epinephrine versus standard-dose epinephrine in a swine model of pediatric asphyxial cardiac arrest. *Crit Care Med.* 1996;24:1695–1700. doi: 10.1097/00003246-199610000-00016
8. Burchfield DJ, Preziosi MP, Lucas VW, Fan J. Effects of graded doses of epinephrine during asphxia-induced bradycardia in newborn lambs. *Resuscitation.* 1993;25:235–244. doi: 10.1016/0300-9572(93)90120-f

VOLUME REPLACEMENT

Recommendations for Volume Resuscitation		
COR	LOE	Recommendations
2b	C-EO	1. It may be reasonable to administer a volume expander to newly born infants with suspected hypovolemia, based on history and physical examination, who remain bradycardic (heart rate less than 60/min) despite ventilation, chest compressions, and epinephrine.[1–3]
2b	C-EO	2. It may be reasonable to provide volume expansion with normal saline (0.9% sodium chloride) or blood at 10 to 20 mL/kg.[4,5]

Synopsis

A newly born infant in shock from blood loss may respond poorly to the initial resuscitative efforts of ventilation, chest compressions, and/or epinephrine. History and physical examination findings suggestive of blood loss include a pale appearance, weak pulses, and persistent bradycardia (heart rate less than 60/min). Blood may be lost from the placenta into the mother's circulation, from the cord, or from the infant.

When blood loss is suspected in a newly born infant who responds poorly to resuscitation (ventilation, chest compressions, and/or epinephrine), it may be reasonable to administer a volume expander without delay. Normal saline (0.9% sodium chloride) is the crystalloid fluid of choice. Uncrossmatched type O, Rh-negative blood (or crossmatched, if immediately available) is preferred when blood loss is substantial.[4,5] An initial volume of 10 mL/kg over 5 to 10 minutes may be reasonable and may be repeated if there is inadequate response. The recommended route is intravenous, with the intraosseous route being an alternative.

Recommendation-Specific Supportive Text

1. There is no evidence from randomized trials to support the use of volume resuscitation at delivery. One large retrospective review found that 0.04% of newborns received volume resuscitation in the delivery room, confirming that it is a relatively uncommon event.[1] Those newborns who received volume resuscitation in the delivery room had lower blood pressure on admission to the neonatal intensive care unit compared with those who did not, indicating that factors other than blood loss may be important.[1]
2. There is insufficient clinical evidence to determine what type of volume expander (crystalloid or blood) is more beneficial during neonatal resuscitation. Extrapolation from studies in hypotensive newborns shortly after birth[6–8] and studies in animals (piglets) support the use of crystalloid over albumin expanders[5] and blood over crystalloid solutions.[4] One review discussed recommendations for the use of volume expanders.[2]

REFERENCES

1. Wyckoff MH, Perlman JM, Laptook AR. Use of volume expansion during delivery room resuscitation in near-term and term infants. *Pediatrics*. 2005;115:950–955. doi: 10.1542/peds.2004-0913
2. Finn D, Roehr CC, Ryan CA, Dempsey EM. Optimising intravenous volume resuscitation of the newborn in the delivery room: practical considerations and gaps in knowledge. *Neonatology*. 2017;112:163–171. doi: 10.1159/000475456
3. Conway-Orgel M. Management of hypotension in the very low-birth-weight infant during the golden hour. *Adv Neonatal Care*. 2010;10:241–5; quiz 246. doi: 10.1097/ANC.0b013e3181f0891c
4. Mendler MR, Schwarz S, Hechenrieder L, Kurth S, Weber B, Hofler S, Kalbitz M, Mayer B, Hummler HD. Successful resuscitation in a model of asphyxia and hemorrhage to test different volume resuscitation strategies. a study in newborn piglets after transition. *Front Pediatr*. 2018;6:192. doi: 10.3389/fped.2018.00192
5. Wyckoff M, Garcia D, Margraf L, Perlman J, Laptook A. Randomized trial of volume infusion during resuscitation of asphyxiated neonatal piglets. *Pediatr Res*. 2007;61:415–420. doi: 10.1203/pdr.0b013e3180332c45
6. Niermeyer S. Volume resuscitation: crystalloid versus colloid. *Clin Perinatol*. 2006;33:133–140. doi: 10.1016/j.clp.2005.12.002
7. Shalish W, Olivier F, Aly H, Sant'Anna G. Uses and misuses of albumin during resuscitation and in the neonatal intensive care unit. *Semin Fetal Neonatal Med*. 2017;22:328–335. doi: 10.1016/j.siny.2017.07.009
8. Keir AK, Karam O, Hodyl N, Stark MJ, Liley HG, Shah PS, Stanworth SJ; NeoBolus Study Group. International, multicentre, observational study of fluid bolus therapy in neonates. *J Paediatr Child Health*. 2019;55:632–639. doi: 10.1111/jpc.14260

POSTRESUSCITATION CARE

Recommendations for Postresuscitation Care

COR	LOE	Recommendations
1	A	1. Newly born infants born at 36 wk or more estimated gestational age with evolving moderate-to-severe HIE should be offered therapeutic hypothermia under clearly defined protocols.[1]
1	C-EO	2. Newly born infants who receive prolonged PPV or advanced resuscitation (intubation, chest compressions, or epinephrine) should be maintained in or transferred to an environment where close monitoring can be provided.[2–7]
1	C-LD	3. Glucose levels should be monitored as soon as practical after advanced resuscitation, with treatment as indicated.[8–14]
2b	C-LD	4. For newly born infants who are unintentionally hypothermic (temperature less than 36°C) after resuscitation, it may be reasonable to rewarm either rapidly (0.5°C/h) or slowly (less than 0.5°C/h).[15–19]

Synopsis

Newly born infants who receive prolonged PPV or advanced resuscitation (eg, intubation, chest compressions ± epinephrine) should be closely monitored after stabilization in a neonatal intensive care unit or a monitored triage area because these infants are at risk for further deterioration.

Infants 36 weeks' or greater estimated gestational age who receive advanced resuscitation should be examined for evidence of HIE to determine if they meet criteria for therapeutic hypothermia. Therapeutic hypothermia is provided under defined protocols similar to those used in published clinical trials and in facilities capable of multidisciplinary care and longitudinal follow-up. The impact of therapeutic hypothermia on infants less than 36 weeks' gestational age with HIE is unclear and is a subject of ongoing research trials.

Hypoglycemia is common in infants who have received advanced resuscitation and is associated with poorer outcomes.[8] These infants should be monitored for hypoglycemia and treated appropriately.

Infants with unintentional hypothermia (temperature less than 36°C) immediately after stabilization should be rewarmed to avoid complications associated with low body temperature (including increased mortality, brain injury, hypoglycemia, and respiratory distress). Evidence suggests that warming can be done rapidly (0.5°C/h) or slowly (less than 0.5°C/h) with no significant difference in outcomes.[15–19] Caution should be taken to avoid overheating.

Recommendation-Specific Supportive Text

1. In a meta-analysis of 8 RCTs involving 1344 term and late preterm infants with moderate-to-severe encephalopathy and evidence of intrapartum asphyxia, therapeutic hypothermia resulted in a significant reduction in the combined outcome of mortality or major neurodevelopmental disability to 18 months of age (odds ratio 0.75; 95% CI, 0.68–0.83).[1]
2. Newly born infants who required advanced resuscitation are at significant risk of developing moderate-to-severe HIE[2–4] and other morbidities.[5–7]
3. Newly born infants with abnormal glucose levels (both low and high) are at increased risk for brain injury and adverse outcomes after a hypoxic-ischemic insult.[8–14]
4. Two small RCTs[16,19] and 4 observational studies[15,17,18,20] of infants with hypothermia after delivery room stabilization found no difference between rapid or slow rewarming for outcomes of mortality,[15,17] convulsions/seizures,[19] intraventricular or pulmonary hemorrhage,[15,17,19,20] hypoglycemia,[16,17,19] or apnea.[16,17,19] One observational study found less respiratory distress in infants who were slowly rewarmed,[18] while a separate study found less respiratory distress syndrome in infants who were rapidly rewarmed.[17]

REFERENCES

1. Jacobs SE, Berg M, Hunt R, Tarnow-Mordi WO, Inder TE, Davis PG. Cooling for newborns with hypoxic ischaemic encephalopathy. *Cochrane Database Syst Rev.* 2013:CD003311. doi: 10.1002/14651858.CD003311.pub3
2. Laptook AR, Shankaran S, Ambalavanan N, Carlo WA, McDonald SA, Higgins RD, Das A; Hypothermia Subcommittee of the NICHD Neonatal Research Network. Outcome of term infants using apgar scores at 10 minutes following hypoxic-ischemic encephalopathy. *Pediatrics.* 2009;124:1619–1626. doi: 10.1542/peds.2009-0934
3. Ayrapetyan M, Talekar K, Schwabenbauer K, Carola D, Solarin K, McElwee D, Adeniyi-Jones S, Greenspan J, Aghai ZH. Apgar scores at 10 minutes and outcomes in term and late preterm neonates with hypoxic-ischemic encephalopathy in the cooling era. *Am J Perinatol.* 2019;36:545–554. doi: 10.1055/s-0038-1670637
4. Kasdorf E, Laptook A, Azzopardi D, Jacobs S, Perlman JM. Improving infant outcome with a 10 min Apgar of 0. *Arch Dis Child Fetal Neonatal Ed.* 2015;100:F102–F105. doi: 10.1136/archdischild-2014-306687
5. Barber CA, Wyckoff MH. Use and efficacy of endotracheal versus intravenous epinephrine during neonatal cardiopulmonary resuscitation in the delivery room. *Pediatrics.* 2006;118:1028–1034. doi: 10.1542/peds.2006-0416
6. Harrington DJ, Redman CW, Moulden M, Greenwood CE. The long-term outcome in surviving infants with Apgar zero at 10 minutes: a systematic review of the literature and hospital-based cohort. *Am J Obstet Gynecol.* 2007;196:463.e1–463.e5. doi: 10.1016/j.ajog.2006.10.877
7. Wyckoff MH, Salhab WA, Heyne RJ, Kendrick DE, Stoll BJ, Laptook AR; National Institute of Child Health and Human Development Neonatal Research Network. Outcome of extremely low birth weight infants who received delivery room cardiopulmonary resuscitation. *J Pediatr.* 2012;160:239–244.e2. doi: 10.1016/j.jpeds.2011.07.041
8. Salhab WA, Wyckoff MH, Laptook AR, Perlman JM. Initial hypoglycemia and neonatal brain injury in term infants with severe fetal acidemia. *Pediatrics.* 2004;114:361–366. doi: 10.1542/peds.114.2.361
9. Castrodale V, Rinehart S. The golden hour: improving the stabilization of the very low birth-weight infant. *Adv Neonatal Care.* 2014;14:9–14; quiz 15. doi: 10.1097/ANC.0b013e31828d0289
10. Nadeem M, Murray DM, Boylan GB, Dempsey EM, Ryan CA. Early blood glucose profile and neurodevelopmental outcome at two years in neonatal hypoxic-ischaemic encephalopathy. *BMC Pediatr.* 2011;11:10. doi: 10.1186/1471-2431-11-10
11. McKinlay CJ, Alsweiler JM, Ansell JM, Anstice NS, Chase JG, Gamble GD, Harris DL, Jacobs RJ, Jiang Y, Paudel N, Signal M, Thompson B, Wouldes TA, Yu TY, Harding JE; CHYLD Study Group. Neonatal Glycemia and Neurodevelopmental Outcomes at 2 Years. *N Engl J Med.* 2015;373:1507–1518. doi: 10.1056/NEJMoa1504909
12. Tan JKG, Minutillo C, McMichael J, Rao S. Impact of hypoglycaemia on neurodevelopmental outcomes in hypoxic ischaemic encephalopathy: a retrospective cohort study. *BMJ Paediatr Open.* 2017;1:e000175. doi: 10.1136/bmjpo-2017-000175
13. Shah BR, Sharifi F. Perinatal outcomes for untreated women with gestational diabetes by IADPSG criteria: a population-based study. *BJOG.* 2020;127:116–122. doi: 10.1111/1471-0528.15964
14. Pinchefsky EF, Hahn CD, Kamino D, Chau V, Brant R, Moore AM, Tam EWY. Hyperglycemia and Glucose Variability Are Associated with Worse Brain Function and Seizures in Neonatal Encephalopathy: A Prospective Cohort Study. *J Pediatr.* 2019;209:23–32. doi: 10.1016/j.jpeds.2019.02.027
15. Feldman A, De Benedictis B, Alpan G, La Gamma EF, Kase J. Morbidity and mortality associated with rewarming hypothermic very low birth weight infants. *J Neonatal Perinatal Med.* 2016;9:295–302. doi: 10.3233/NPM-16915143
16. Motil KJ, Blackburn MG, Pleasure JR. The effects of four different radiant warmer temperature set-points used for rewarming neonates. *J Pediatr.* 1974;85:546–550. doi: 10.1016/s0022-3476(74)80467-1
17. Rech Morassutti F, Cavallin F, Zaramella P, Bortolus R, Parotto M, Trevisanuto D. Association of Rewarming Rate on Neonatal Outcomes in Extremely Low Birth Weight Infants with Hypothermia. *J Pediatr.* 2015;167:557–61.e1. doi: 10.1016/j.jpeds.2015.06.008
18. Sofer S, Yagupsky P, Hershkowits J, Bearman JE. Improved outcome of hypothermic infants. *Pediatr Emerg Care.* 1986;2:211–214. doi: 10.1097/00006565-198612000-00001
19. Tafari N, Gentz J. Aspects of rewarming newborn infants with severe accidental hypothermia. *Acta Paediatr Scand.* 1974;63:595–600. doi: 10.1111/j.1651-2227.1974.tb04853.x
20. Racine J, Jarjoui E. Severe hypothermia in infants. *Helv Paediatr Acta.* 1982;37:317–322.

WITHHOLDING AND DISCONTINUING RESUSCITATION

Recommendations for Withholding and Discontinuing Resuscitation

COR	LOE	Recommendations
1	C-EO	1. Noninitiation of resuscitation and discontinuation of life-sustaining treatment during or after resuscitation should be considered ethically equivalent.[1,2]
1	C-LD	2. In newly born babies receiving resuscitation, if there is no heart rate and all the steps of resuscitation have been performed, cessation of resuscitation efforts should be discussed with the team and the family. A reasonable time frame for this change in goals of care is around 20 min after birth.[3]
2a	C-EO	3. If a birth is at the lower limit of viability or involves a condition likely to result in early death or severe morbidity, noninitiation or limitation of neonatal resuscitation is reasonable after expert consultation and parental involvement in decision-making.[1,2,4,5]

Synopsis

Expert neonatal and bioethical committees have agreed that, in certain clinical conditions, it is reasonable not to initiate or to discontinue life-sustaining efforts while continuing to provide supportive care for babies and families.[1,2,4]

If the heart rate remains undetectable and all steps of resuscitation have been completed, it may be reasonable to redirect goals of care. Case series show small numbers of intact survivors after 20 minutes of no detectable heart rate. The decision to continue or discontinue resuscitative efforts should be individualized and should be considered at about 20 minutes after birth. Variables to be considered may include whether the resuscitation was considered optimal, availability of advanced neonatal care (such as therapeutic hypothermia), specific circumstances before delivery, and wishes expressed by the family.[3,6]

Some babies are so sick or immature at birth that survival is unlikely, even if neonatal resuscitation and intensive care are provided. In addition, some conditions are so severe that the burdens of the illness and treatment greatly outweigh the likelihood of survival or a healthy outcome. If it is possible to identify such conditions at or before birth, it is reasonable not to initiate resuscitative efforts. These situations benefit from expert consultation, parental involvement in decision-making, and, if indicated, a palliative care plan.[1,2,4–6]

Recommendation-Specific Supportive Text

1. It is the expert opinion of national medical societies that conditions exist for which it is reasonable to not initiate resuscitation or to discontinue resuscitation once these conditions are identified.[1,2,4,5]
2. Randomized controlled studies and observational studies in settings where therapeutic hypothermia is available (with very low certainty of evidence) describe variable rates of survival without moderate-to-severe disability in babies who achieve ROSC after 10 minutes or more despite continued resuscitation. None of these studies evaluate outcomes of resuscitation that extends beyond 20 minutes of age, by which time the likelihood of intact survival was very low. The studies were too heterogeneous to be amenable to meta-analysis.[3]
3. Conditions in which noninitiation or discontinuation of resuscitation may be considered include extremely preterm birth and certain severe congenital anomalies. National guidelines recommend individualization of parent-informed decisions based on social, maternal, and fetal/neonatal factors.[1,2,4] A systematic review showed that international guidelines variably described periviability between 22 and 24 weeks' gestational age.[7]

REFERENCES

1. American Academy of Pediatrics Committee on Fetus and Newborn, Bell EF. Noninitiation or withdrawal of intensive care for high-risk newborns. *Pediatrics*. 2007;119:401–403. doi: 10.1542/peds.2006-3180
2. Cummings J; and the Committee on Fetus and Newborn. Antenatal Counseling Regarding Resuscitation and Intensive Care Before 25 Weeks of Gestation. *Pediatrics*. 2015;136:588–595. doi: 10.1542/peds.2015-2336
3. Wyckoff MH, Wyllie J, Aziz K, de Almeida MF, Fabres J, Fawke J, Guinsburg R, Hosono S, Isayama T, Kapadia VS, et al; on behalf of the Neonatal Life Support Collaborators. Neonatal life support: 2020 International Consensus on Cardiopulmonary Resuscitation and Emergency Cardiovascular Care Science With Treatment Recommendations. *Circulation*. 2020;142(suppl 1):S185–S221. doi: 10.1161/CIR.0000000000000895
4. American College of Obstetricians and Gynecologists; Society for Maternal-Fetal M. Obstetric Care Consensus No. 6: periviable birth. *Obstet Gynecol*. 2017;130:e187–e199. doi: 10.1097/AOG.0000000000002352
5. Lemyre B, Moore G. Counselling and management for anticipated extremely preterm birth. *Paediatr Child Health*. 2017;22:334–341. doi: 10.1093/pch/pxx058
6. Wyckoff MH, Aziz K, Escobedo MB, Kapadia VS, Kattwinkel J, Perlman JM, Simon WM, Weiner GM, Zaichkin JG. Part 13: neonatal resuscitation: 2015 American Heart Association Guidelines Update for Cardiopulmonary Resuscitation and Emergency Cardiovascular Care. *Circulation*. 2015;132(suppl 2):S543–S560. doi: 10.1161/CIR.0000000000000267
7. Guillén Ú, Weiss EM, Munson D, Maton P, Jefferies A, Norman M, Naulaers G, Mendes J, Justo da Silva L, Zoban P, Hansen TW, Hallman M, Delivoria-Papadopoulos M, Hosono S, Albersheim SG, Williams C, Boyle E, Lui K, Darlow B, Kirpalani H. Guidelines for the Management of Extremely Premature Deliveries: A Systematic Review. *Pediatrics*. 2015;136:343–350. doi: 10.1542/peds.2015-0542

HUMAN AND SYSTEM PERFORMANCE

Training Frequency

Recommendation for Training Frequency

COR	LOE	Recommendation
1	C-LD	1. For participants who have been trained in neonatal resuscitation, individual or team booster training should occur more frequently than every 2 yr at a frequency that supports retention of knowledge, skills, and behaviors.[1–5]

Synopsis

To perform neonatal resuscitation effectively, individual providers and teams need training in the required knowledge, skills, and behaviors. Historically, the repeat training has occurred every 2 years.[6–9] However, adult, pediatric, and neonatal studies suggest that without practice, CPR knowledge and skills decay within 3 to 12 months[10–12] after training. Short, frequent practice (booster training) has been shown to improve neonatal resuscitation outcomes.[5] Educational programs and perinatal facilities should develop strategies to ensure that individual and team training is frequent enough to sustain knowledge and skills.

Recommendation-Specific Supportive Text

1. In a randomized controlled simulation study, medical students who underwent booster training retained improved neonatal intubation skills over a 6-week period compared with medical students who did not receive booster training. There was no difference in neonatal intubation performance after weekly booster practice for 4 weeks compared with daily booster practice for 4 consecutive days.[1]

   In a randomized controlled simulation study, pediatric and family practice residents who underwent booster training 9 months after an initial

Neonatal Resuscitation Program course demonstrated better procedural skills and teamwork behaviors at a follow-up assessment at 16 months compared with residents who did not receive booster training.[2]

In a prospective cohort study, physicians and nurses trained in Helping Babies Breathe demonstrated a rapid loss of resuscitation skills by 1 month after training. Subjects who received monthly practice sessions were more likely to pass an objective structured clinical evaluation than those who practiced less frequently.[3]

In a prospective observational study, implementation of weekly, brief Helping Babies Breathe simulation training after a 1-day Helping Babies Breathe training course resulted in increased frequency of stimulation of newborns, decrease in bag-mask ventilation, and decreased neonatal mortality at 24 hours.[4]

REFERENCES

1. Ernst KD, Cline WL, Dannaway DC, Davis EM, Anderson MP, Atchley CB, Thompson BM. Weekly and consecutive day neonatal intubation training: comparable on a pediatrics clerkship. *Acad Med.* 2014;89:505–510. doi: 10.1097/ACM.0000000000000150
2. Bender J, Kennally K, Shields R, Overly F. Does simulation booster impact retention of resuscitation procedural skills and teamwork? *J Perinatol.* 2014;34:664–668. doi: 10.1038/jp.2014.72
3. Tabangin ME, Josyula S, Taylor KK, Vasquez JC, Kamath-Rayne BD. Resuscitation skills after Helping Babies Breathe training: a comparison of varying practice frequency and impact on retention of skills in different types of providers. *Int Health.* 2018;10:163–171. doi: 10.1093/inthealth/ihy017
4. Mduma E, Ersdal H, Svensen E, Kidanto H, Auestad B, Perlman J. Frequent brief on-site simulation training and reduction in 24-h neonatal mortality–an educational intervention study. *Resuscitation.* 2015;93:1–7. doi: 10.1016/j.resuscitation.2015.04.019
5. Reisman J, Arlington L, Jensen L, Louis H, Suarez-Rebling D, Nelson BD. Newborn resuscitation training in resource-limited settings: a systematic literature review. *Pediatrics.* 2016;138:e20154490. doi: 10.1542/peds.2015–4490
6. American Academy of Pediatrics and American Heart Association. *Textbook of Neonatal Resuscitation (NRP)* 7th ed. Elk Grove Village, IL: American Academy of Pediatrics; 2016.
7. American Heart Association. *Basic Life Support Provider Manual.* Dallas, TX: American Heart Association; 2016.
8. American Heart Association. *Pediatric Advanced Life Support Provider Manual.* Dallas, TX: American Heart Association; 2016.
9. American Heart Association. *Advanced Cardiovascular Life Support Provider Manual.* Dallas, TX: American Heart Association; 2016.
10. Soar J, Mancini ME, Bhanji F, Billi JE, Dennett J, Finn J, Ma MH, Perkins GD, Rodgers DL, Hazinski MF, et al; on behalf of the Education, Implementation, and Teams Chapter Collaborators. Part 12: education, implementation, and teams: 2010 International Consensus on Cardiopulmonary Resuscitation and Emergency Cardiovascular Care Science with Treatment Recommendations. *Resuscitation.* 2010;81(suppl 1):e288–e330. doi: 10.1016/j.resuscitation.2010.08.030
11. Bang A, Patel A, Bellad R, Gisore P, Goudar SS, Esamai F, Liechty EA, Meleth S, Goco N, Niermeyer S, Keenan W, Kamath-Rayne BD, Little GA, Clarke SB, Flanagan VA, Bucher S, Jain M, Mujawar N, Jain V, Rukunga J, Mahantshetti N, Dhaded S, Bhandankar M, McClure EM, Carlo WA, Wright LL, Hibberd PL. Helping Babies Breathe (HBB) training: What happens to knowledge and skills over time? *BMC Pregnancy Childbirth.* 2016;16:364. doi: 10.1186/s12884-016-1141-3
12. Arlington L, Kairuki AK, Isangula KG, Meda RA, Thomas E, Temu A, Mponzi V, Bishanga D, Msemo G, Azayo M, et al. Implementation of "Helping Babies Breathe": a 3-year experience in Tanzania. *Pediatrics.* 2017;139:e20162132. doi: 10.1542/peds.2016–2132

Briefing and Debriefing

Recommendation for Training Frequency		
COR	**LOE**	**Recommendation**
2b	C-LD	1. For neonatal resuscitation providers, it may be reasonable to brief before delivery and debrief after neonatal resuscitation.[1–3]

Synopsis

Briefing has been defined as "a discussion about an event that is yet to happen to prepare those who will be involved and thereby reduce the risk of failure or harm."[4] *Debriefing* has been defined as "a discussion of actions and thought processes after an event to promote reflective learning and improve clinical performance"[5] or "a facilitated discussion of a clinical event focused on learning and performance improvement."[6] Briefing and debriefing have been recommended for neonatal resuscitation training since 2010[7] and have been shown to improve a variety of educational and clinical outcomes in neonatal, pediatric, and adult simulation-based and clinical studies. The effect of briefing and debriefing on longer-term and critical outcomes remains uncertain.

Recommendation-Specific Supportive Text

Multiple clinical and simulation studies examining briefings or debriefings of resuscitation team performance have shown improved knowledge or skills.[8–12]

1. In a prospective interventional clinical study, video-based debriefing of neonatal resuscitations was associated with improved preparation and adherence to the initial steps of the Neonatal Resuscitation Algorithm, improved quality of PPV, and improved team function and communication.[1]

   In 2 pre–quality improvement/post–quality improvement initiatives, use of a team briefing, debriefing, and predelivery checklist was associated with an improvement in team communication in the delivery room and short-term clinical outcomes, such as decreased frequency of intubation in the delivery room and increased frequency of normothermia on admission to the neonatal intensive care unit. There was no significant effect on other in-hospital clinical outcomes such as bronchopulmonary dysplasia, necrotizing enterocolitis, retinopathy of prematurity, intraventricular hemorrhage, or length of stay.[2,3]

REFERENCES

1. Skåre C, Calisch TE, Saeter E, Rajka T, Boldingh AM, Nakstad B, Niles DE, Kramer-Johansen J, Olasveengen TM. Implementation and effectiveness of a video-based debriefing programme for neonatal resuscitation. *Acta Anaesthesiol Scand.* 2018;62:394–403. doi: 10.1111/aas.13050

2. Sauer CW, Boutin MA, Fatayerji AN, Proudfoot JA, Fatayerji NI, Golembeski DJ. Delivery Room Quality Improvement Project Improved Compliance with Best Practices for a Community NICU. *Sci Rep.* 2016;6:37397. doi: 10.1038/srep37397
3. Katheria A, Rich W, Finer N. Development of a strategic process using checklists to facilitate team preparation and improve communication during neonatal resuscitation. *Resuscitation.* 2013;84:1552–1557. doi: 10.1016/j.resuscitation.2013.06.012
4. Halamek LP, Cady RAH, Sterling MR. Using briefing, simulation and debriefing to improve human and system performance. *Semin Perinatol.* 2019;43:151178. doi: 10.1053/j.semperi.2019.08.007
5. Mullan PC, Kessler DO, Cheng A. Educational opportunities with postevent debriefing. *JAMA.* 2014;312:2333–2334. doi: 10.1001/jama.2014.15741
6. Sawyer T, Loren D, Halamek LP. Post-event debriefings during neonatal care: why are we not doing them, and how can we start? *J Perinatol.* 2016;36:415–419. doi: 10.1038/jp.2016.42
7. Kattwinkel J, Perlman JM, Aziz K, Colby C, Fairchild K, Gallagher J, Hazinski MF, Halamek LP, Kumar P, Little G, et al. Part 15: neonatal resuscitation: 2010 American Heart Association Guidelines for Cardiopulmonary Resuscitation and Emergency Cardiovascular Care. *Circulation.* 2010;122(suppl 3):S909–S919. doi: 10.1161/CIRCULATIONAHA.110.971119
8. Savoldelli GL, Naik VN, Park J, Joo HS, Chow R, Hamstra SJ. Value of debriefing during simulated crisis management: oral versus video-assisted oral feedback. *Anesthesiology.* 2006;105:279–285. doi: 10.1097/00000542-200608000-00010
9. Edelson DP, Litzinger B, Arora V, Walsh D, Kim S, Lauderdale DS, Vanden Hoek TL, Becker LB, Abella BS. Improving in-hospital cardiac arrest process and outcomes with performance debriefing. *Arch Intern Med.* 2008;168:1063–1069. doi: 10.1001/archinte.168.10.1063
10. Morgan PJ, Tarshis J, LeBlanc V, Cleave-Hogg D, DeSousa S, Haley MF, Herold-McIlroy J, Law JA. Efficacy of high-fidelity simulation debriefing on the performance of practicing anaesthetists in simulated scenarios. *Br J Anaesth.* 2009;103:531–537. doi: 10.1093/bja/aep222
11. Dine CJ, Gersh RE, Leary M, Riegel BJ, Bellini LM, Abella BS. Improving cardiopulmonary resuscitation quality and resuscitation training by combining audiovisual feedback and debriefing. *Crit Care Med.* 2008;36:2817–2822. doi: 10.1097/CCM.0b013e318186fe37
12. Wolfe H, Zebuhr C, Topjian AA, Nishisaki A, Niles DE, Meaney PA, Boyle L, Giordano RT, Davis D, Priestley M, Apkon M, Berg RA, Nadkarni VM, Sutton RM. Interdisciplinary ICU cardiac arrest debriefing improves survival outcomes*. *Crit Care Med.* 2014;42:1688–1695. doi: 10.1097/CCM.0000000000000327

KNOWLEDGE GAPS

Neonatal resuscitation science has advanced significantly over the past 3 decades, with contributions by many researchers in laboratories, in the delivery room, and in other clinical settings. While this research has led to substantial improvements in the Neonatal Resuscitation Algorithm, it has also highlighted that we still have more to learn to optimize resuscitation for both preterm and term infants. With growing enthusiasm for clinical studies in neonatology, elements of the Neonatal Resuscitation Algorithm continue to evolve as new evidence emerges.

The current guidelines have focused on clinical activities described in the resuscitation algorithm, rather than on the most appropriate devices for each step. Reviews in 2021 and later will address choice of devices and aids, including those required for ventilation (T-piece, self-inflating bag, flow-inflating bag), ventilation interface (face mask, laryngeal mask), suction (bulb syringe, meconium aspirator), monitoring (respiratory function monitors, heart rate monitoring, near infrared spectroscopy), feedback, and documentation.

Review of the knowledge chunks during this update identified numerous questions and practices for which evidence was weak, uncertain, or absent. The following knowledge gaps require further research:

Resuscitation Preparedness

- The frequency and format of booster training or refresher training that best supports retention of neonatal resuscitation knowledge, technical skills, and behavioral skills
- The effects of briefing and debriefing on team performance

During and Just After Delivery

- Optimal cord management strategies for various populations, including nonvigorous infants and those with congenital heart or lung disease
- Optimal management of nonvigorous infants with MSAF

Early Resuscitation

- The most effective device(s) and interface(s) for providing PPV
- Impact of routine use of the ECG during neonatal resuscitation on resuscitation
- Feasibility and effectiveness of new technologies for rapid heart rate measurement (such as electric, ultrasonic, or optical devices)
- Optimal oxygen management during and after resuscitation

Advanced Resuscitation

- Novel techniques for effective delivery of CPR, such as chest compressions accompanied by sustained inflation
- Optimal timing, dosing, dose interval, and delivery routes for epinephrine or other vasoactive drugs, including earlier use in very depressed newly born infants
- Indications for volume expansion, as well as optimal dosing, timing, and type of volume
- The management of pulseless electric activity

Specific Populations

- Management of the preterm newborn during and after resuscitation
- Management of congenital anomalies of the heart and lungs during and after resuscitation
- Resuscitation of newborns in the neonatal unit after the newly born period
- Resuscitation of newborns in other settings up to 28 days of age

Postresuscitation Care

- Optimal dose, route, and timing of surfactant in at-risk newborns, including less-invasive administration techniques
- Indications for therapeutic hypothermia in babies with mild HIE and in those born at less than 36 weeks' gestational age
- Adjunctive therapies to therapeutic hypothermia
- Optimal management of blood glucose
- Optimal rewarming strategy for newly born infants with unintentional hypothermia

For all these gaps, it is important that we have information on outcomes considered critical or important by both healthcare providers and families of newborn infants.

The research community needs to address the paucity of educational studies that provide outcomes with a high level of certainty. Internal validity might be better addressed by clearly defined primary outcomes, appropriate sample sizes, relevant and timed interventions and controls, and time series analyses in implementation studies. External validity might be improved by studying the relevant learner or provider populations and by measuring the impact on critical patient and system outcomes rather than limiting study to learner outcomes.

Researchers studying these gaps may need to consider innovations in clinical trial design; examples include pragmatic study designs and novel consent processes. As mortality and severe morbidities decline with biomedical advancements and improvements in healthcare delivery, there is decreased ability to have adequate power for some clinical questions using traditional individual patient randomized trials. Another barrier is the difficulty in obtaining antenatal consent for clinical trials in the delivery room. Adaptive trials, comparative effectiveness designs, and those using cluster randomization may be suitable for some questions, such as the best approach for MSAF in nonvigorous infants. High-quality observational studies of large populations may also add to the evidence. When feasible, well-designed multicenter randomized clinical trials are still optimal to generate the highest-quality evidence.

Finally, we wish to reinforce the importance of addressing the values and preferences of our key stakeholders, the families and teams who are involved in the process of resuscitation. Gaps in this domain, whether perceived or real, should be addressed at every stage in our research, educational, and clinical activities.

ARTICLE INFORMATION

The American Heart Association requests that this document be cited as follows: Aziz K, Lee HC, Escobedo MB, Hoover AV, Kamath-Rayne BD, Kapadia VS, Magid DJ, Niermeyer S, Schmölzer GM, Szyld E, Weiner GM, Wyckoff MH, Yamada NK, Zaichkin J. Part 5: neonatal resuscitation: 2020 American Heart Association Guidelines for Cardiopulmonary Resuscitation and Emergency Cardiovascular Care. *Circulation*. 2020;142(suppl 2):S524–S550. doi: 10.1161/CIR.0000000000000902

This article has been copublished in *Pediatrics*.

Acknowledgment

We thank Dr Abhrajit Ganguly for assistance in manuscript preparation.

Disclosures

Appendix 1. Writing Group Disclosures

Writing Group Member	Employment	Research Grant	Other Research Support	Speakers' Bureau/ Honoraria	Expert Witness	Ownership Interest	Consultant/ Advisory Board	Other
Khalid Aziz	University of Alberta Pediatrics	None	None	None	None	None	None	Salary: University of Alberta†
Henry C. Lee	Stanford University	NICHD (PI of R01 grant examining intensive care for infants born at extremely early gestational age)*	None	None	None	None	None	None
Marilyn B Escobedo	University of Oklahoma Medical School Pediatrics	None	None	None	None	None	None	None
Amber V. Hoover	American Heart Association	None	None	None	None	None	None	None
Beena D. Kamath-Rayne	American Academy of Pediatrics	None	None	None	None	None	None	None
Vishal S. Kapadia	UT Southwestern Pediatrics	NIH, NICHD†	None	None	None	None	None	None
David J. Magid	University of Colorado	NIH†; NHLBI†; CMS†; AHA†	None	None	None	None	None	American Heart Association (Senior Science Editor)†

(*Continued*)

Appendix 1. Continued

Writing Group Member	Employment	Research Grant	Other Research Support	Speakers' Bureau/ Honoraria	Expert Witness	Ownership Interest	Consultant/ Advisory Board	Other
Susan Niermeyer	University of Colorado Pediatrics	None	None	None	None	None	None	None
Georg M. Schmölzer	University of Alberta Pediatrics	Heart and Stroke Foundation Canada*; Canadian Institute of Health Research*; THRASHER Foundation*; Canadian Institute of Health Research*	None	None	None	Owner of RETAIN LABS Medical Inc*	None	None
Edgardo Szyld	University of Oklahoma	None	None	None	None	None	None	None
Gary M. Weiner	University of Michigan Pediatrics-Neonatology	None	None	None	None	None	None	None
Myra H. Wyckoff	UT Southwestern Pediatrics	None	None	None	None	None	None	None
Nicole K. Yamada	Stanford University	AHRQ†	None	None	None	None	None	None
Jeanette Zaichkin	Self used	None	None	None	None	None	American Academy of Pediatrics Neonatal Resuscitation Program†	None

This table represents the relationships of writing group members that may be perceived as actual or reasonably perceived conflicts of interest as reported on the Disclosure Questionnaire, which all members of the writing group are required to complete and submit. A relationship is considered to be "significant" if (a) the person receives $10 000 or more during any 12-month period, or 5% or more of the person's gross income; or (b) the person owns 5% or more of the voting stock or share of the entity, or owns $10 000 or more of the fair market value of the entity. A relationship is considered to be "modest" if it is less than "significant" under the preceding definition.

*Modest.

†Significant.

Appendix 2. Reviewer Disclosures

Reviewer	Employment	Research Grant	Other Research Support	Speakers' Bureau/ Honoraria	Expert Witness	Ownership Interest	Consultant/ Advisory Board	Other
Christoph Bührer	Charité University Medical Center (Germany)	None	None	University of Tübingen*	None	None	None	None
Praveen Chandrasekharan	SUNY Buffalo	None	None	None	None	None	None	None
Krithika Lingappan	Baylor College of Medicine	None	None	None	None	None	None	None
Ju-Lee Oei	Royal Hospital for Women (Australia)	None	None	None	None	None	None	None
Birju A. Shah	The University of Oklahoma	None	None	None	None	None	None	None

This table represents the relationships of reviewers that may be perceived as actual or reasonably perceived conflicts of interest as reported on the Disclosure Questionnaire, which all reviewers are required to complete and submit. A relationship is considered to be "significant" if (a) the person receives $10000 or more during any 12-month period, or 5% or more of the person's gross income; or (b) the person owns 5% or more of the voting stock or share of the entity, or owns $10000 or more of the fair market value of the entity. A relationship is considered to be "modest" if it is less than "significant" under the preceding definition.

*Modest.

Circulation

Part 6: Resuscitation Education Science

2020 American Heart Association Guidelines for Cardiopulmonary Resuscitation and Emergency Cardiovascular Care

Adam Cheng, MD, Chair
David J. Magid, MD, MPH
Marc Auerbach, MD, MSCE
Farhan Bhanji, MD, MEd
Blair L. Bigham, MD, MSc
Audrey L. Blewer, PhD, MPH
Katie N. Dainty, MSc, PhD
Emily Diederich, MD, MS
Yiqun Lin, MD, MHSc, PhD
Marion Leary, RN, MSN, MPH
Melissa Mahgoub, PhD
Mary E. Mancini, RN, PhD
Kenneth Navarro, PhD(c)
Aaron Donoghue, MD, MSCE, Vice Chair

TOP 10 TAKE-HOME MESSAGES

1. Effective education is an essential contributor to improved survival outcomes from cardiac arrest.
2. Use of a deliberate practice and mastery learning model during resuscitation training improves skill acquisition and retention for many critical tasks.
3. The addition of booster training to resuscitation courses is associated with improved cardiopulmonary resuscitation (CPR) skill retention over time and improved neonatal outcomes.
4. Implementation of a spaced learning approach for resuscitation training improves clinical performance and technical skills compared with massed learning.
5. The use of CPR feedback devices during resuscitation training promotes CPR skill acquisition and retention.
6. Teamwork and leadership training, high-fidelity manikins, in situ training, gamified learning, and virtual reality represent opportunities to enhance resuscitation training that may improve learning outcomes.
7. Self-directed CPR training represents a reasonable alternative to instructor-led CPR training for lay rescuers.
8. Middle school– and high school–age children should be taught how to perform high-quality CPR because this helps build the future cadre of trained community-based lay rescuers.
9. To increase bystander CPR rates, CPR training should be tailored to low–socioeconomic status neighborhoods and specific racial and ethnic communities, where there is currently a paucity of training opportunities.
10. Future resuscitation education research should include outcomes of clinical relevance, establish links between performance outcomes in training and patient outcomes, describe cost-effectiveness of interventions, and explore how instructional design can be tailored to specific skills.

PREAMBLE

Each year, millions of providers receive basic and advanced life support training with the aim of improving patient outcomes from cardiac arrest.[1] Resuscitation training programs incorporate evidence-based content while providing opportunities for learners to practice lifesaving skills in individual and team-based clinical environments. While resuscitation training is widespread, learners frequently fall short of achieving the desired performance outcomes, resulting in skills that do not consistently translate to clinical care with real patients.[1,2]

The International Liaison Committee on Resuscitation Formula for Survival (Figure) emphasizes 3 essential components influencing survival outcomes from

Key Words: AHA Scientific Statements ■ cardiopulmonary resuscitation ■ education ■ resuscitation ■ training

https://www.ahajournals.org/journal/circ

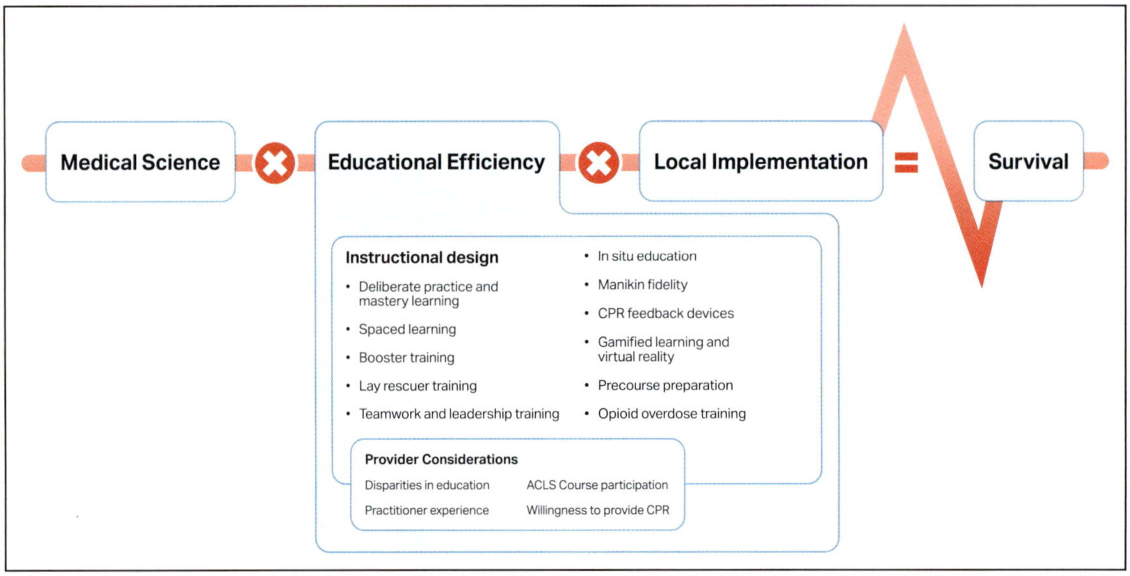

Figure. Formula for Survival in Resuscitation: Key Elements Contributing to Educational Efficiency.
ACLS indicates advanced cardiovascular life support; and CPR, cardiopulmonary resuscitation.

cardiac arrest: guidelines based on current resuscitation science, effective education of resuscitation providers, and local implementation of guidelines during patient care.[3] Greater emphasis on effective education will improve provider performance, enhance local implementation of guidelines, and potentially increase survival rates from cardiac arrest.

These guidelines contain recommendations for the design and delivery of resuscitation training for lay rescuers and healthcare providers. The provision of effective education is highly dependent on the instructional design of educational programs because this determines how content is delivered to the learner. In this Part, we explore the evidence informing different instructional design features and discuss how social determinants of health (eg, socioeconomic status [SES], race) and individual factors (eg, practitioner experience) may influence clinical performance and patient outcomes.

REFERENCES

1. Cheng A, Nadkarni VM, Mancini MB, Hunt EA, Sinz EH, Merchant RM, Donoghue A, Duff JP, Eppich W, Auerbach M, Bigham BL, Blewer AL, Chan PS, Bhanji F; American Heart Association Education Science Investigators; and on behalf of the American Heart Association Education Science and Programs Committee, Council on Cardiopulmonary, Critical Care, Perioperative and Resuscitation; Council on Cardiovascular and Stroke Nursing; and Council on Quality of Care and Outcomes Research. Resuscitation education science: educational strategies to improve outcomes from cardiac arrest: a scientific statement from the American Heart Association. *Circulation*. 2018;138:e82–e122. doi: 10.1161/CIR.0000000000000583
2. Bhanji F, Donoghue AJ, Wolff MS, Flores GE, Halamek LP, Berman JM, Sinz EH, Cheng A. Part 14: education: 2015 American Heart Association Guidelines Update for Cardiopulmonary Resuscitation and Emergency Cardiovascular Care. *Circulation*. 2015;132(suppl 2):S561–e573. doi: 10.1161/CIR.0000000000000268
3. Søreide E, Morrison L, Hillman K, Monsieurs K, Sunde K, Zideman D, Eisenberg M, Sterz F, Nadkarni VM, Soar J, Nolan JP; Utstein Formula for Survival Collaborators. The formula for survival in resuscitation. *Resuscitation*. 2013;84:1487–1493. doi: 10.1016/j.resuscitation.2013.07.020

INTRODUCTION

Scope of Guideline

Cardiac arrest remains a major public health problem, with more than 600 000 cardiac arrests per year in the United States.[1,2] Survival rates of patients with cardiac arrest remain low despite advancements in resuscitation science.[3] Each year, millions of people receive basic and advanced life support training in an effort to improve the quality of care delivered to cardiac arrest patients.[4] Resuscitation training programs are designed to convey evidence-based content and provide opportunities for learners (ie, those enrolled in resuscitation training programs) to apply knowledge and practice critical skills. These programs, however, frequently fall short of achieving the desired learning outcomes (eg, knowledge and skill acquisition), with performance that does not consistently translate over to the real-world clinical environment.[4,5] For example, cardiopulmonary resuscitation (CPR) skills that are acquired immediately after basic life support (BLS) training often show decay by as early as 3 months, resulting in many BLS-trained healthcare providers—such as physicians, nurses, respiratory therapists, and other healthcare professionals—struggling to perform guideline-compliant CPR during simulated and real cardiac arrests.[6–14] Additionally, current research on lay rescuer CPR training is lacking evidence describing the optimal methods to train bystanders to recognize cardiac arrest, initiate CPR, and use automated external defibrillators appropriately.[15–17] A dedicated focus on instructional design is essential to ensure that knowledge and skills acquired during training are applied when caring for patients in cardiac arrest.[4]

Improving survival from cardiac arrest is highly dependent on the quality of resuscitative care. Many key determinants of survival, such as immediate recognition of cardiac arrest, early initiation of CPR, early defibrillation, and high-quality chest compressions, are variables that can be targeted by resuscitation training programs to improve patient outcomes. Instructional design features are the key elements, or "active ingredients," of resuscitation training programs that determine how content is delivered to the learner.[18] A better understanding of the impact of instructional design features on learning outcomes will enable educators to design training programs that translate into outstanding clinical performance during cardiac arrests. Furthermore, appreciating how social determinants of health (eg, SES, race) and individual factors (eg, practitioner experience) influence the downstream impact of resuscitation education will help inform future policy and implementation strategies. In this Part, we describe the evidence supporting key elements of resuscitation education and provide recommendations aimed at improving learner outcomes and patient outcomes from cardiac arrest.

The following sections briefly describe the process of evidence review and guideline development. See "Part 2: Evidence Evaluation and Guidelines Development" in the 2020 ECC Guidelines for more details on this process.[19]

Organization of the Resuscitation Education Science Writing Group

The Resuscitation Education Science Writing Group comprised a diverse team of experts with backgrounds in resuscitation education, clinical medicine (ie, pediatrics, intensive care, emergency medicine), nursing, prehospital care, health services, and education research. Writing group members are American Heart Association (AHA) volunteers with an interest and recognized expertise in resuscitation and are selected by the AHA Emergency Cardiovascular Care (ECC) Committee. The AHA has rigorous conflict-of-interest policies and procedures to minimize the risk of bias and improper influence during development of the guidelines.[20] Before appointment, writing group members and peer reviewers disclosed all commercial relationships and other potential (including intellectual) conflicts. Disclosure information for writing group members is listed in Appendix 1.

Methodology and Evidence Review

This Part of the *2020 AHA Guidelines for CPR and ECC* is based on the extensive evidence evaluation performed in conjunction with the International Liaison Committee on Resuscitation and affiliated International Liaison Committee on Resuscitation member councils. Three different types of evidence reviews (systematic reviews, scoping reviews, and evidence updates) were used in the 2020 process. Each of these resulted in a description of the literature that facilitated guideline development.[21–25] Reviews were limited to the resuscitation education science literature, but many of the concepts reviewed have origins within other fields (eg, medical education, psychology).

Class of Recommendation and Level of Evidence

The AHA Resuscitation Education Science Writing Group reviewed all relevant and current *AHA Guidelines for CPR and ECC*[5,26–37] and the relevant *2020 International Consensus on CPR and ECC Science With Treatment Recommendations*[27] to determine if current guidelines should be reaffirmed, revised, or retired and whether new recommendations were needed. The writing group then drafted, reviewed, and approved recommendations (by majority vote among members), assigning to each a Level of Evidence (LOE; ie, quality) and Class of Recommendation (COR; ie, strength; see Table 1, Applying COR and LOE to Clinical Strategies, Interventions, Treatments, or Diagnostic Testing in Patient Care).

Importantly, applying Grading of Recommendations, Assessment, Development, and Evaluation (GRADE)[38] to educational studies yields greater challenges than its application to clinical studies. Specific considerations for studies involving educational outcomes (eg, improved "outcomes" in simulated patient settings or improved performance on summative assessment tools) are not provided in GRADE methodology; the writing group frequently assigned LOE to these studies according to a combination of a typical review of study quality, perceived importance of underlying constructs in the context of educational science, and (where possible) extrapolation of findings to analogous clinical phenomena (eg, outcomes in real patients as opposed to simulated ones).

Guideline Structure

The 2020 guidelines are organized into knowledge chunks, grouped into discrete modules of information on specific topics or management issues.[39] Each modular knowledge chunk includes a table of recommendations using standard AHA nomenclature of COR and LOE. A brief introduction or short synopsis puts the recommendations into context with important background information and overarching management or treatment concepts. Recommendation-specific supportive text clarifies the rationale and key study data supporting the recommendations. Hyperlinked references are provided to facilitate quick access and review.

Document Review and Approval

These guidelines were submitted for blinded peer review to subject matter experts nominated by the AHA.

Peer reviewer feedback was provided for guidelines in draft format and again in final format. The guidelines were reviewed and approved for publication by the AHA Science Advisory and Coordinating Committee and the AHA Executive Committee. Disclosure information for peer reviewers is listed in Appendix 2.

Abbreviations

Abbreviation	Meaning/Phrase
ACLS	advanced cardiovascular life support
AHA	American Heart Association
B-CPR	bystander cardiopulmonary resuscitation
BLS	basic life support
COR	Class of Recommendation
CPR	cardiopulmonary resuscitation
ECC	emergency cardiovascular care
EMS	emergency medical services
EO	expert opinion
LD	limited data
LOE	Level of Evidence
NR	nonrandomized
OHCA	out-of-hospital cardiac arrest
PALS	pediatric advanced life support
RCT	randomized controlled trial
ROSC	return of spontaneous circulation
SES	socioeconomic status
VR	virtual reality

REFERENCES

1. Andersen LW, Holmberg MJ, Berg KM, Donnino MW, Granfeldt A. In-hospital cardiac arrest: a review. *JAMA.* 2019;321:1200–1210. doi: 10.1001/jama.2019.1696
2. Benjamin EJ, Muntner P, Alonso A, Bittencourt MS, Callaway CW, Carson AP, Chamberlain AM, Chang AR, Cheng S, Das SR, et al; on behalf of the American Heart Association Council on Epidemiology and Prevention Statistics Committee and Stroke Statistics Subcommittee. Heart disease and stroke statistics–2019 update: a report from the American Heart Association. *Circulation.* 2019;139:e56–e528. doi: 10.1161/CIR.0000000000000659
3. Meaney PA, Bobrow BJ, Mancini ME, Christenson J, de Caen AR, Bhanji F, Abella BS, Kleinman ME, Edelson DP, Berg RA, et al; CPR Quality Summit Investigators, the American Heart Association Emergency Cardiovascular Care Committee, and the Council on Cardiopulmonary, Critical Care, Perioperative and Resuscitation. Cardiopulmonary resuscitation quality: [corrected] improving cardiac resuscitation outcomes both inside and outside the hospital: a consensus statement from the American Heart Association. *Circulation.* 2013;128:417–435. doi: 10.1161/CIR.0b013e31829d8654
4. Cheng A, Nadkarni VM, Mancini MB, Hunt EA, Sinz EH, Merchant RM, Donoghue A, Duff JP, Eppich W, Auerbach M, et al; American Heart Association Education Science Investigators; on behalf of the American Heart Association Education Science and Programs Committee, Council on Cardiopulmonary, Critical Care, Perioperative and Resuscitation; Council on Cardiovascular and Stroke Nursing; and Council on Quality of Care and Outcomes Research. Resuscitation education science: educational strategies to improve outcomes from cardiac arrest: a scientific statement from the American Heart Association. *Circulation.* 2018;138:e82–e122. doi: 10.1161/CIR.0000000000000583
5. Bhanji F, Donoghue AJ, Wolff MS, Flores GE, Halamek LP, Berman JM, Sinz EH, Cheng A. Part 14: education: 2015 American Heart Association Guidelines Update for Cardiopulmonary Resuscitation and Emergency Cardiovascular Care. *Circulation.* 2015;132(suppl 2):S561–573. doi: 10.1161/CIR.0000000000000268
6. Lin Y, Cheng A, Grant VJ, Currie GR, Hecker KG. Improving CPR quality with distributed practice and real-time feedback in pediatric healthcare providers - a randomized controlled trial. *Resuscitation.* 2018;130:6–12. doi: 10.1016/j.resuscitation.2018.06.025
7. Anderson R, Sebaldt A, Lin Y, Cheng A. Optimal training frequency for acquisition and retention of high-quality CPR skills: a randomized trial. *Resuscitation.*2019;135:153–161. doi: 10.1016/j.resuscitation.2018.10.033
8. Sutton RM, Case E, Brown SP, Atkins DL, Nadkarni VM, Kaltman J, Callaway C, Idris A, Nichol G, Hutchison J, et al; ROC Investigators. A quantitative analysis of out-of-hospital pediatric and adolescent resuscitation quality–a report from the ROC epistry-cardiac arrest. *Resuscitation.* 2015;93:150–157. doi: 10.1016/j.resuscitation.2015.04.010
9. Sutton RM, Niles D, French B, Maltese MR, Leffelman J, Eilevstjonn J, Wolfe H, Nishisaki A, Meaney PA, Berg RA, et al. First quantitative analysis of cardiopulmonary resuscitation quality during in-hospital cardiac arrests of young children. *Resuscitation.* 2014;85:70–74. doi: 10.1016/j.resuscitation.2013.08.014
10. Sutton RM, Niles D, Nysaether J, Abella BS, Arbogast KB, Nishisaki A, Maltese MR, Donoghue A, Bishnoi R, Helfaer MA, et al. Quantitative analysis of CPR quality during in-hospital resuscitation of older children and adolescents. *Pediatrics.* 2009;124:494–499. doi: 10.1542/peds.2008-1930
11. Stiell IG, Brown SP, Christenson J, Cheskes S, Nichol G, Powell J, Bigham B, Morrison LJ, Larsen J, Hess E, et al; Resuscitation Outcomes Consortium (ROC) Investigators. What is the role of chest compression depth during out-of-hospital cardiac arrest resuscitation? *Crit Care Med.* 2012;40:1192–1198. doi: 10.1097/CCM.0b013e31823bc8bb
12. Wik L, Steen PA, Bircher NG. Quality of bystander cardiopulmonary resuscitation influences outcome after prehospital cardiac arrest. *Resuscitation.* 1994;28:195–203. doi: 10.1016/0300-9572(94)90064-7
13. Idris AH, Guffey D, Aufderheide TP, Brown S, Morrison LJ, Nichols P, Powell J, Daya M, Bigham BL, Atkins DL, et al; Resuscitation Outcomes Consortium (ROC) Investigators. Relationship between chest compression rates and outcomes from cardiac arrest. *Circulation.* 2012;125:3004–3012. doi: 10.1161/CIRCULATIONAHA.111.059535
14. Cheng A, Hunt EA, Grant D, Lin Y, Grant V, Duff JP, White ML, Peterson DT, Zhong J, Gottesman R, et al; International Network for Simulation-based Pediatric Innovation, Research, and Education CPR Investigators. Variability in quality of chest compressions provided during simulated cardiac arrest across nine pediatric institutions. *Resuscitation.* 2015;97:13–19. doi: 10.1016/j.resuscitation.2015.08.024
15. Plant N, Taylor K. How best to teach CPR to schoolchildren: a systematic review. *Resuscitation.* 2013;84:415–421. doi: 10.1016/j.resuscitation.2012.12.008
16. Todd KH, Heron SL, Thompson M, Dennis R, O'Connor J, Kellermann AL. Simple CPR: a randomized, controlled trial of video self-instructional cardiopulmonary resuscitation training in an African American church congregation. *Ann Emerg Med.* 1999;34:730–737. doi: 10.1016/s0196-0644(99)70098-3
17. Castrén M, Nurmi J, Laakso JP, Kinnunen A, Backman R, Niemi-Murola L. Teaching public access defibrillation to lay volunteers–a professional health care provider is not a more effective instructor than a trained lay person. *Resuscitation.* 2004;63:305–310. doi: 10.1016/j.resuscitation.2004.06.011
18. Cook DA, Hamstra SJ, Brydges R, Zendejas B, Szostek JH, Wang AT, Erwin PJ, Hatala R. Comparative effectiveness of instructional design features in simulation-based education: systematic review and meta-analysis. *Med Teach.* 2013;35:e867–898. doi: 10.3109/0142159X.2012.714886
19. Magid DJ, Aziz K, Cheng A, Hazinski MF, Hoover AV, Mahgoub M, Panchal AR, Sasson C, Topjian AA, Rodriguez AJ, et al. Part 2: evidence evaluation and guidelines development: 2020 American Heart Association Guidelines for Cardiopulmonary Resuscitation and Emergency Cardiovascular Care. *Circulation.* 2020;142:(suppl 2):S358–S365. doi: 10.1161/CIR.0000000000000903
20. American Heart Association. Conflict of interest policy. https://www.heart.org/en/about-us/statements-and-policies/conflict-of-interest-policy. Accessed December 31, 2019.
21. Tricco AC, Lillie E, Zarin W, O'Brien KK, Colquhoun H, Levac D, Moher D, Peters MDJ, Horsley T, Weeks L, et al. PRISMA Extension for

Table 1. Applying Class of Recommendation and Level of Evidence to Clinical Strategies, Interventions, Treatments, or Diagnostic Testing in Patient Care (Updated May 2019)*

CLASS (STRENGTH) OF RECOMMENDATION	LEVEL (QUALITY) OF EVIDENCE‡
CLASS 1 (STRONG) — **Benefit >>> Risk**	**LEVEL A**
Suggested phrases for writing recommendations: • Is recommended • Is indicated/useful/effective/beneficial • Should be performed/administered/other • Comparative-Effectiveness Phrases†: – Treatment/strategy A is recommended/indicated in preference to treatment B – Treatment A should be chosen over treatment B	• High-quality evidence‡ from more than 1 RCT • Meta-analyses of high-quality RCTs • One or more RCTs corroborated by high-quality registry studies
	LEVEL B-R — **(Randomized)**
	• Moderate-quality evidence‡ from 1 or more RCTs • Meta-analyses of moderate-quality RCTs
CLASS 2a (MODERATE) — **Benefit >> Risk**	**LEVEL B-NR** — **(Nonrandomized)**
Suggested phrases for writing recommendations: • Is reasonable • Can be useful/effective/beneficial • Comparative-Effectiveness Phrases†: – Treatment/strategy A is probably recommended/indicated in preference to treatment B – It is reasonable to choose treatment A over treatment B	• Moderate-quality evidence‡ from 1 or more well-designed, well-executed nonrandomized studies, observational studies, or registry studies • Meta-analyses of such studies
	LEVEL C-LD — **(Limited Data)**
CLASS 2b (WEAK) — **Benefit ≥ Risk**	• Randomized or nonrandomized observational or registry studies with limitations of design or execution • Meta-analyses of such studies • Physiological or mechanistic studies in human subjects
Suggested phrases for writing recommendations: • May/might be reasonable • May/might be considered • Usefulness/effectiveness is unknown/unclear/uncertain or not well-established	**LEVEL C-EO** — **(Expert Opinion)** • Consensus of expert opinion based on clinical experience
CLASS 3: No Benefit (MODERATE) — **Benefit = Risk** **(Generally, LOE A or B use only)**	
Suggested phrases for writing recommendations: • Is not recommended • Is not indicated/useful/effective/beneficial • Should not be performed/administered/other	
Class 3: Harm (STRONG) — **Risk > Benefit**	
Suggested phrases for writing recommendations: • Potentially harmful • Causes harm • Associated with excess morbidity/mortality • Should not be performed/administered/other	

COR and LOE are determined independently (any COR may be paired with any LOE).

A recommendation with LOE C does not imply that the recommendation is weak. Many important clinical questions addressed in guidelines do not lend themselves to clinical trials. Although RCTs are unavailable, there may be a very clear clinical consensus that a particular test or therapy is useful or effective.

* The outcome or result of the intervention should be specified (an improved clinical outcome or increased diagnostic accuracy or incremental prognostic information).

† For comparative-effectiveness recommendations (COR 1 and 2a; LOE A and B only), studies that support the use of comparator verbs should involve direct comparisons of the treatments or strategies being evaluated.

‡ The method of assessing quality is evolving, including the application of standardized, widely-used, and preferably validated evidence grading tools; and for systematic reviews, the incorporation of an Evidence Review Committee.

COR indicates Class of Recommendation; EO, expert opinion; LD, limited data; LOE, Level of Evidence; NR, nonrandomized; R, randomized; and RCT, randomized controlled trial.

Scoping Reviews (PRISMAScR): checklist and explanation. *Ann Intern Med.* 2018;169:467–473. doi: 10.7326/M18-0850

22. International Liaison Committee on Resuscitation. Continuous evidence evaluation guidance and templates. https://www.ilcor.org/documents/continuous-evidence-evaluation-guidance-and-templates. Accessed December 31, 2019.
23. Institute of Medicine (US) Committee of Standards for Systematic Reviews of Comparative Effectiveness Research. *Finding What Works in Health Care: Standards for Systematic Reviews.* Eden J, Levit L, Berg A, Morton S, eds. Washington, DC: The National Academies Press; 2011.
24. PRISMA. PRISMA for scoping reviews. http://www.prisma-statement.org/Extensions/ScopingReviews. Accessed December 31, 2019.
25. International Liaison Committee on Resuscitation (ILCOR). Continuous evidence evaluation guidance and templates: 2020 evidence update process final. https://www.ilcor.org/documents/continuous-evidence-evaluationguidance-and-templates. Accessed December 31, 2019.
26. Bhanji F, Mancini ME, Sinz E, Rodgers DL, McNeil MA, Hoadley TA, Meeks RA, Hamilton MF, Meaney PA, Hunt EA, et al. Part 16: education, implementation, and teams: 2010 American Heart Association Guidelines for Cardiopulmonary Resuscitation and Emergency Cardiovascular Care. *Circulation.* 2010;122(suppl 3):S920–S933. doi: 10.1161/CIRCULATIONAHA.110.971135
27. Greif R, Bhanji F, Bigham BL, Bray J, Breckwoldt J, Cheng A, Duff JP, Gilfoyle E, Hsieh M-J, Iwami T, et al; on behalf of the Education, Implementation, and Teams Collaborators. Education, implementation, and teams: 2020 International Consensus on Cardiopulmonary Resuscitation and Emergency Cardiovascular Care Science With Treatment Recommendations. *Circulation.* 2020;142(suppl 1):S222–S283. doi: 10.1161/CIR.0000000000000896
28. Atkins DL, de Caen AR, Berger S, Samson RA, Schexnayder SM, Joyner BL Jr, Bigham BL, Niles DE, Duff JP, Hunt EA, et al. 2017 American Heart Association focused update on pediatric basic life support and cardiopulmonary resuscitation quality: an update to the American Heart Association Guidelines for Cardiopulmonary Resuscitation and Emergency Cardiovascular Care. *Circulation.* 2018;137:e1–e6. doi: 10.1161/CIR.0000000000000540
29. Kleinman ME, Goldberger ZD, Rea T, Swor RA, Bobrow BJ, Brennan EE, Terry M, Hemphill R, Gazmuri RJ, Hazinski MF, et al. 2017 American Heart Association focused update on adult basic life support and cardiopulmonary resuscitation quality: an update to the American Heart

Association Guidelines for Cardiopulmonary Resuscitation and Emergency Cardiovascular Care. *Circulation.* 2018;137:e7–e13. doi: 10.1161/CIR.0000000000000539
30. Panchal AR, Berg KM, Hirsch KG, Kudenchuk PJ, Del Rios M, Cabañas JG, Link MS, Kurz MC, Chan PS, Morley PT, et al. 2019 American Heart Association focused update on advanced cardiovascular life support: use of advanced airways, vasopressors, and extracorporeal cardiopulmonary resuscitation during cardiac arrest: an update to the American Heart Association Guidelines for Cardiopulmonary Resuscitation and Emergency Cardiovascular Care. *Circulation.* 2019;140:e881–e894. doi: 10.1161/CIR.0000000000000732
31. Panchal AR, Berg KM, Cabañas JG, Kurz MC, Link MS, Del Rios M, Hirsch KG, Chan PS, Hazinski MF, Morley PT, et al. 2019 American Heart Association focused update on systems of care: dispatcher-assisted cardiopulmonary resuscitation and cardiac arrest centers: an update to the American Heart Association Guidelines for Cardiopulmonary Resuscitation and Emergency Cardiovascular Care. *Circulation.* 2019;140:e895–e903. doi: 10.1161/CIR.0000000000000733
32. Panchal AR, Berg KM, Kudenchuk PJ, Del Rios M, Hirsch KG, Link MS, Kurz MC, Chan PS, Cabañas JG, Morley PT, et al. 2018 American Heart Association focused update on advanced cardiovascular life support use of antiarrhythmic drugs during and immediately after cardiac arrest: an update to the American Heart Association Guidelines for Cardiopulmonary Resuscitation and Emergency Cardiovascular Care. *Circulation.* 2018;138:e740–e749. doi: 10.1161/CIR.0000000000000613
33. Duff JP, Topjian A, Berg MD, Chan M, Haskell SE, Joyner BL Jr, Lasa JJ, Ley SJ, Raymond TT, Sutton RM, et al. 2018 American Heart Association focused update on pediatric advanced life support: an update to the American Heart Association Guidelines for Cardiopulmonary Resuscitation and Emergency Cardiovascular Care. *Circulation.* 2018;138:e731–e739. doi: 10.1161/CIR.0000000000000612
34. Escobedo MB, Aziz K, Kapadia VS, Lee HC, Niermeyer S, Schmölzer GM, Szyld E, Weiner GM, Wyckoff MH, Yamada NK, et al. 2019 American Heart Association focused update on neonatal resuscitation: an update to the American Heart Association Guidelines for Cardiopulmonary Resuscitation and Emergency Cardiovascular Care. *Circulation.* 2019;140:e922–e930. doi: 10.1161/CIR.0000000000000729
35. Charlton NP, Pellegrino JL, Kule A, Slater TM, Epstein JL, Flores GE, Goolsby CA, Orkin AM, Singletary EM, Swain JM. 2019 American Heart Association and American Red Cross focused update for first aid: presyncope: an update to the American Heart Association and American Red Cross Guidelines for First Aid. *Circulation.* 2019;140:e931–e938. doi: 10.1161/CIR.0000000000000730
36. Duff JP, Topjian AA, Berg MD, Chan M, Haskell SE, Joyner BL Jr, Lasa JJ, Ley SJ, Raymond TT, Sutton RM, et al. 2019 American Heart Association focused update on pediatric advanced life support: an update to the American Heart Association Guidelines for Cardiopulmonary Resuscitation and Emergency Cardiovascular Care. *Circulation.* 2019;140:e904–e914. doi: 10.1161/CIR.0000000000000731
37. Duff JP, Topjian AA, Berg MD, Chan M, Haskell SE, Joyner BL Jr, Lasa JJ, Ley SJ, Raymond TT, Sutton RM, et al. 2019 American Heart Association focused update on pediatric basic life support: an update to the American Heart Association guidelines for cardiopulmonary resuscitation and emergency cardiovascular care. *Circulation.* 2019;140:e915–e921. doi: 10.1161/CIR.0000000000000736
38. GRADE Working Group. 5.2.1. Study limitations (risk of bias). In: Schünemann HJ, Brożek J, Guyatt G, Oxman A, eds. *GRADE Handbook.* 2013. https://gdt.gradepro.org/app/handbook/handbook.html. Updated October 2013. Accessed December 31, 2019.
39. Levine GN, O'Gara PT, Beckman JA, Al-Khatib SM, Birtcher KK, Cigarroa JE, de Las Fuentes L, Deswal A, Fleisher LA, Gentile F, et al. Recent innovations, modifications, and evolution of ACC/AHA clinical practice guidelines: an update for our constituencies: a report of the American College of Cardiology/American Heart Association Task Force on Clinical Practice Guidelines. *Circulation.* 2019;139:e879–e886. doi: 10.1161/CIR.0000000000000651

MAJOR CONCEPTS

In 2018, the AHA published a scientific statement, titled "Resuscitation Education Science: Educational Strategies to Improve Outcomes From Cardiac Arrest,"[1] providing a comprehensive synthesis of the evidence supporting best educational practices for resuscitation. The topics explored in the statement were framed by the Formula for Survival in Resuscitation (Figure),[2] which describes the contributions of medical science (ie, guideline quality), educational efficiency (ie, quality and impact of education), and local implementation (ie, uptake and adoption of guidelines) toward improving survival outcomes from cardiac arrest. These guidelines complement the scientific statement by providing an updated review of the science and highlighting specific recommendations to support evidence-informed change in resuscitation education.

These guidelines comprise 3 main sections: instructional design, provider considerations, and knowledge gaps and future research. Resuscitation training programs may incorporate 1 key instructional design feature, or they may be blended in an effort to optimize learning outcomes. The best instructional designs are tailored to specific learning objectives, learner type, and context of learning. Here, we offer recommendations related to the use of deliberate practice and mastery learning, booster training and spaced learning, lay rescuer training, teamwork and leadership training, in situ education, manikin fidelity, CPR feedback devices in training, gamified learning and virtual reality (VR), precourse preparation for advanced courses, and special considerations for training in the management of opioid overdose. As highlighted in the Figure, instructional design features contribute to educational efficiency in the Formula for Survival.

In the second section, we describe how certain provider considerations may influence the overall impact of education. For example, disparities in access to resuscitation education (eg, SES, race) or prior provider experience may contribute positively or negatively to learning outcomes. Some providers may decide to take the AHA Advanced Cardiovascular Life Support (ACLS) Course, whereas others may not. How does this influence patient outcomes? All of these considerations feed into the potential impact of instructional design and ultimately influence the educational efficiency component of the Formula for Survival (Figure).

In reviewing content for these guidelines, the writing group identified and discussed many important topics relevant to resuscitation education, such as the role of cognitive load in learning, the use of augmented reality, blogs and podcasts as educational tools, learner assessment, training in low-resource settings, and the role of faculty development for training resuscitation educators. While these and other topics represent areas of interest, there was insufficient evidence examining the impact of these concepts on resuscitation education to support the development of recommendations. We refer interested readers to the AHA scientific statement "Resuscitation Education

Science: Educational Strategies to Improve Outcomes From Cardiac Arrest" for a discussion of these concepts.[1] More literature is required before these issues can be incorporated into future iterations of the AHA Guidelines. We conclude this Part of the 2020 Guidelines with a summary of current knowledge gaps in resuscitation education science and a discussion of future directions for optimizing the impact of resuscitation training programs.

REFERENCES

1. Cheng A, Nadkarni VM, Mancini MB, Hunt EA, Sinz EH, Merchant RM, Donoghue A, Duff JP, Eppich W, Auerbach M, Bigham BL, Blewer AL, Chan PS, Bhanji F; American Heart Association Education Science Investigators; and on behalf of the American Heart Association Education Science and Programs Committee, Council on Cardiopulmonary, Critical Care, Perioperative and Resuscitation; Council on Cardiovascular and Stroke Nursing; and Council on Quality of Care and Outcomes Research. Resuscitation Education Science: Educational Strategies to Improve Outcomes From Cardiac Arrest: A Scientific Statement From the American Heart Association. *Circulation.* 2018;138:e82–e122. doi: 10.1161/CIR.0000000000000583
2. Søreide E, Morrison L, Hillman K, Monsieurs K, Sunde K, Zideman D, Eisenberg M, Sterz F, Nadkarni VM, Soar J, Nolan JP; Utstein Formula for Survival Collaborators. The formula for survival in resuscitation. *Resuscitation.* 2013;84:1487–1493. doi: 10.1016/j.resuscitation.2013.07.020

INSTRUCTIONAL DESIGN FEATURES

Deliberate Practice and Mastery Learning

Recommendation for Deliberate Practice and Mastery Learning		
COR	**LOE**	**Recommendation**
2b	B-NR	1. Incorporating a deliberate practice and mastery learning model into basic or advanced life support courses may be considered for improving skill acquisition and performance.[1–12]

Synopsis

Deliberate practice is a training approach where learners are given (1) a discrete goal to achieve, (2) immediate feedback on their performance, and (3) ample time for repetition to improve performance.[13,14] *Mastery learning* is defined as the use of deliberate practice training along with testing that uses a set of criteria to define a specific passing standard that implies mastery of the tasks being learned.[15] A better understanding of how deliberate practice and mastery learning can be implemented in resuscitation training would help enhance training and patient outcomes. Twelve studies have examined the impact of deliberate practice and/or mastery learning in resuscitation training.[1–12] Eight studies demonstrated improved learner performance with deliberate practice and mastery learning (eg, scores on clinical assessments, time to interventions)[1,2,5–10] whereas other studies found no difference in learner outcomes.[3,4,11,12] Because the majority of studies report positive results, we recommend that deliberate practice and mastery learning be incorporated into basic and advanced life support training. Specifically, we recommend pairing repetition with customized feedback that is based on assessments, assigning specific exercises to address weaknesses, and providing learners sufficient time to attain the minimum passing standard for a specific skill. Future research should use consistent definitions for deliberate practice and mastery learning and seek to isolate the effect of deliberate practice and mastery learning through the use of appropriate and clearly defined comparator groups.

Recommendation-Specific Supportive Text

1. Two of 4 randomized controlled trials (RCTs) found that learners exposed to deliberate practice demonstrated improved clinical performance and decreased time to perform critical interventions (eg, time to ventilation, time to epinephrine) on simulated patients.[1,2] Two of 4 RCTs found no significant difference in learner outcomes with deliberate practice compared with traditional training.[3,4]

   Six of the 8 observational studies found an association between deliberate practice and mastery learning and improved performance measures in simulated patients (eg, time to compression, time to defibrillation, checklist scores).[5–10] Two studies involving lay rescuers (1 RCT and 1 observational) showed no improved performance associated with deliberate practice and mastery learning.[4,11]

   Skill decay was measured in 5 studies.[5,9–12] Four studies found no significant decay after deliberate practice and mastery learning for up to 6 months,[9–12] and 1 study found a significant linear decline ($P=0.039$) in performance at 6 months after training.[5] In one study, one-time costs associated with incorporating a deliberate practice and mastery learning model into resuscitation training were higher than for traditional training, whereas recurring costs were lower because of decreased instructor involvement.[12] Future studies should explore if deliberate practice and mastery learning are less costly over time for training larger groups of learners.

REFERENCES

1. Magee MJ, Farkouh-Karoleski C, Rosen TS. Improvement of Immediate Performance in Neonatal Resuscitation Through Rapid Cycle Deliberate Practice Training. *J Grad Med Educ.* 2018;10:192–197. doi: 10.4300/JGME-D-17-00467.1
2. Diederich E, Lineberry M, Blomquist M, Schott V, Reilly C, Murray M, Nazaran P, Rourk M, Werner R, Broski J. Balancing Deliberate Practice and Reflection: A Randomized Comparison Trial of Instructional Designs for Simulation-Based Training in Cardiopulmonary Resuscitation Skills. *Simul Healthc.* 2019;14:175–181. doi: 10.1097/SIH.0000000000000375
3. Lemke DS, Fielder EK, Hsu DC, Doughty CB. Improved Team Performance During Pediatric Resuscitations After Rapid Cycle Deliberate Practice Compared With Traditional Debriefing: A Pilot Study. *Pediatr Emerg Care.* 2019;35:480–486. doi: 10.1097/PEC.0000000000000940

4. Madou T, Iserbyt P. Mastery versus self-directed blended learning in basic life support: a randomised controlled trial. *Acta Cardiol.* 2019:1–7. doi: 10.1080/00015385.2019.1677374
5. Braun L, Sawyer T, Smith K, Hsu A, Behrens M, Chan D, Hutchinson J, Lu D, Singh R, Reyes J, Lopreiato J. Retention of pediatric resuscitation performance after a simulation-based mastery learning session: a multicenter randomized trial. *Pediatr Crit Care Med.* 2015;16:131–138. doi: 10.1097/PCC.0000000000000315
6. Cordero L, Hart BJ, Hardin R, Mahan JD, Nankervis CA. Deliberate practice improves pediatric residents' skills and team behaviors during simulated neonatal resuscitation. *Clin Pediatr (Phila).* 2013;52:747–752. doi: 10.1177/0009922813488646
7. Hunt EA, Duval-Arnould JM, Chime NO, Jones K, Rosen M, Hollingsworth M, Aksamit D, Twilley M, Camacho C, Nogee DP, Jung J, Nelson-McMillan K, Shilkofski N, Perretta JS. Integration of in-hospital cardiac arrest contextual curriculum into a basic life support course: a randomized, controlled simulation study. *Resuscitation.* 2017;114:127–132. doi: 10.1016/j.resuscitation.2017.03.014
8. Hunt EA, Duval-Arnould JM, Nelson-McMillan KL, Bradshaw JH, Diener-West M, Perretta JS, Shilkofski NA. Pediatric resident resuscitation skills improve after "rapid cycle deliberate practice" training. *Resuscitation.* 2014;85:945–951. doi: 10.1016/j.resuscitation.2014.02.025
9. Jeffers J, Eppich W, Trainor J, Mobley B, Adler M. Development and Evaluation of a Learning Intervention Targeting First-Year Resident Defibrillation Skills. *Pediatr Emerg Care.* 2016;32:210–216. doi: 10.1097/PEC.0000000000000765
10. Reed T, Pirotte M, McHugh M, Oh L, Lovett S, Hoyt AE, Quinones D, Adams W, Gruener G, McGaghie WC. Simulation-Based Mastery Learning Improves Medical Student Performance and Retention of Core Clinical Skills. *Simul Healthc.* 2016;11:173–180. doi: 10.1097/SIH.0000000000000154
11. Boet S, Bould MD, Pigford AA, Rössler B, Nambyiah P, Li Q, Bunting A, Schebesta K. Retention of Basic Life Support in Laypeople: Mastery Learning vs. Time-based Education. *Prehosp Emerg Care.* 2017;21:362–377. doi: 10.1080/10903127.2016.1258096
12. Devine LA, Donkers J, Brydges R, Perelman V, Cavalcanti RB, Issenberg SB. An Equivalence Trial Comparing Instructor-Regulated With Directed Self-Regulated Mastery Learning of Advanced Cardiac Life Support Skills. *Simul Healthc.* 2015;10:202–209. doi: 10.1097/SIH.0000000000000095
13. Ericsson KA. Deliberate practice and the acquisition and maintenance of expert performance in medicine and related domains. *Acad Med.* 2004;79(suppl):S70–81. doi: 10.1097/00001888-200410001-00022
14. Ericsson KA, Krampe RT, Tesch-Romer. The role of deliberate practice in the acquisition of expert performance. *Psychol Rev.* 1993;100:363–406. doi: 10.1037/0033-295X.100.3.363
15. McGaghie WC. When I say … mastery learning. *Med Educ.* 2015;49:558–559. doi: 10.1111/medu.12679

Booster Training and Spaced Learning

Most current resuscitation courses use a massed learning approach: a single training event lasting hours or days, with retraining every 1 to 2 years.[1] Other resuscitation courses use a spaced learning approach, involving the separation of training into multiple sessions, each lasting minutes to hours, with intervals of weeks to months between sessions.[2–5] Each spaced session involves the presentation of new content and/or the repetition of content from prior sessions. Booster training is another instructional design feature, involving brief weekly or monthly sessions focused on repetition of content presented in an initial massed learning course.[6–18]

Frequent booster trainings (at intervals of 1–6 months) were associated with improved CPR skills.[6–9,14,16,18] Reduced mortality was noted after implementation of weekly boosters for neonatal training.[13] One study reported that learners were less likely to attend all sessions with increased frequency of boosters, with the highest learner attrition in the group practicing every month.[6] No studies evaluated booster training for pediatric advanced life support (PALS) or ACLS courses. Spaced learning courses are of equal or greater effectiveness than massed learning courses for pediatric resuscitation training.[3–5] No studies compared spaced learning with massed learning for BLS, neonatal (eg, Neonatal Resuscitation Program), or ACLS courses. We recommend that resuscitation training programs implement boosters when a massed learning approach is used and consider implementing spaced learning courses in place of massed learning. Future research is needed to determine optimal training intervals while concurrently minimizing costs and ensuring learner engagement over time.

Recommendation for Booster Training

COR	LOE	Recommendation
1	B-R	1. It is recommended to implement booster sessions when utilizing a massed learning approach for resuscitation training.[6–18]

Recommendation-Specific Supportive Text

1. Seven RCTs compared booster CPR training, at intervals of 1 to 6 months, with no booster training and found improvements in CPR performance.[6–9,14,16,18] In 1 RCT, nurses randomized to more frequent CPR booster training demonstrated dose-dependent improvement in CPR skills at 1 year (proportion with overall excellent CPR at 12 months: 58% every 1 month boosters, 26% every 3 months, 21% every 6 months, 15% every 12 months).[6] The monthly group, however, was least likely to complete all sessions. In a second RCT, emergency department providers randomized to monthly CPR booster training demonstrated a higher percentage of providers who could perform excellent CPR at 12 months compared with those who received no boosters (excellent CPR on adult manikin: 54.3% versus 14.6%; $P<0.001$; infant manikin: 71.7% versus 19.5%; $P<0.001$).[14] Additional RCTs demonstrated improvements in knowledge and CPR skills after 30-minute boosters at 1, 3, and 6 months[7]; enhanced ventilations and compressions after 6-minute monthly boosters[8,16]; and shorter time to start compression and defibrillation after 15-minute boosters every 2, 3, or 6 months.[18]

   Three RCTs reported that more frequent Neonatal Resuscitation Program boosters (ie, weekly to every 9 months) were associated with improved skill performance over time,[10–12] and 1 observational study described improved clinical performance and reduced infant mortality (pre: 11.1/1000 versus post: 7.2/1000; $P=0.04$) after 3- to 5-minute weekly boosters.[13]

Recommendation for Spaced Learning		
COR	LOE	Recommendation
2a	B-R	1. It is reasonable to use a spaced learning approach in place of a massed learning approach for resuscitation training.[3–5]

Recommendation-Specific Supportive Text

1. Two RCTs and 1 observational study compared spaced learning with massed learning for pediatric resuscitation training.[3–5] In 1 RCT, emergency medical services (EMS) providers were randomized to either spaced learning (four 3.5-hour weekly sessions) or massed learning (2 sequential 7-hour days).[3] Compared with the massed learning group, the spaced learning group had superior retention of infant bag-mask ventilation and infant intraosseous insertion skills at 3 months but no difference in chest compression skills. Knowledge decay was noted in the massed learning group but not in the spaced learning group.[3]

   In another RCT, pediatric nurses and respiratory therapists were randomized to either spaced learning (six 30-minute sessions over 6 months) or massed learning (one 7.5-hour day) for PALS recertification.[5] Clinical performance scores improved in the spaced learning group. Both groups demonstrated similar improvements in teamwork measured at course completion.

   In an observational study, medical students completed either spaced learning (four 1.25-hour weekly sessions) or massed learning (one 5-hour session) for pediatric resuscitation skills. No difference was noted in knowledge or global ratings of skills (ie, bag-mask ventilation, intraosseous insertion, or chest compression) measured at 4 weeks after course completion between the groups.[4]

REFERENCES

1. Cheng A, Nadkarni VM, Mancini MB, Hunt EA, Sinz EH, Merchant RM, Donoghue A, Duff JP, Eppich W, Auerbach M, Bigham BL, Blewer AL, Chan PS, Bhanji F; American Heart Association Education Science Investigators; and on behalf of the American Heart Association Education Science and Programs Committee, Council on Cardiopulmonary, Critical Care, Perioperative and Resuscitation; Council on Cardiovascular and Stroke Nursing; and Council on Quality of Care and Outcomes Research. Resuscitation Education Science: Educational Strategies to Improve Outcomes From Cardiac Arrest: A Scientific Statement From the American Heart Association. *Circulation.* 2018;138:e82–e122. doi: 10.1161/CIR.0000000000000583
2. Greif R, Bhanji F, Bigham BL, Bray J, Breckwoldt J, Cheng A, Duff JP, Gilfoyle E, Hsieh M-J, Iwami T, et al; on behalf of the Education, Implementation, and Teams Collaborators. Education, implementation, and teams: 2020 International Consensus on Cardiopulmonary Resuscitation and Emergency Cardiovascular Care Science With Treatment Recommendations. *Circulation.* 2020;142(suppl 1):S222–S283. doi: 10.1161/CIR.0000000000000896
3. Patocka C, Cheng A, Sibbald M, Duff JP, Lai A, Lee-Nobbee P, Levin H, Varshney T, Weber B, Bhanji F. A randomized education trial of spaced versus massed instruction to improve acquisition and retention of paediatric resuscitation skills in emergency medical service (EMS) providers. *Resuscitation.* 2019;141:73–80. doi: 10.1016/j.resuscitation.2019.06.010
4. Patocka C, Khan F, Dubrovsky AS, Brody D, Bank I, Bhanji F. Pediatric resuscitation training-instruction all at once or spaced over time? *Resuscitation.* 2015;88:6–11. doi: 10.1016/j.resuscitation.2014.12.003
5. Kurosawa H, Ikeyama T, Achuff P, Perkel M, Watson C, Monachino A, Remy D, Deutsch E, Buchanan N, Anderson J, Berg RA, Nadkarni VM, Nishisaki A. A randomized, controlled trial of in situ pediatric advanced life support recertification ("pediatric advanced life support reconstructed") compared with standard pediatric advanced life support recertification for ICU frontline providers*. *Crit Care Med.* 2014;42:610–618. doi: 10.1097/CCM.0000000000000024
6. Anderson R, Sebaldt A, Lin Y, Cheng A. Optimal training frequency for acquisition and retention of high-quality CPR skills: A randomized trial. *Resuscitation.* 2019;135:153–161. doi: 10.1016/j.resuscitation.2018.10.033
7. O'Donnell CM, Skinner AC. An evaluation of a short course in resuscitation training in a district general hospital. *Resuscitation.* 1993;26:193–201. doi: 10.1016/0300-9572(93)90179-t
8. Oermann MH, Kardong-Edgren SE, Odom-Maryon T. Effects of monthly practice on nursing students' CPR psychomotor skill performance. *Resuscitation.* 2011;82:447–453. doi: 10.1016/j.resuscitation.2010.11.022
9. Nishiyama C, Iwami T, Murakami Y, Kitamura T, Okamoto Y, Marukawa S, Sakamoto T, Kawamura T. Effectiveness of simplified 15-min refresher BLS training program: a randomized controlled trial. *Resuscitation.* 2015;90:56–60. doi: 10.1016/j.resuscitation.2015.02.015
10. Tabangin ME, Josyula S, Taylor KK, Vasquez JC, Kamath-Rayne BD. Resuscitation skills after Helping Babies Breathe training: a comparison of varying practice frequency and impact on retention of skills in different types of providers. *Int Health.* 2018;10:163–171. doi: 10.1093/inthealth/ihy017
11. Bender J, Kennally K, Shields R, Overly F. Does simulation booster impact retention of resuscitation procedural skills and teamwork? *J Perinatol.* 2014;34:664–668. doi: 10.1038/jp.2014.72
12. Ernst KD, Cline WL, Dannaway DC, Davis EM, Anderson MP, Atchley CB, Thompson BM. Weekly and consecutive day neonatal intubation training: comparable on a pediatrics clerkship. *Acad Med.* 2014;89:505–510. doi: 10.1097/ACM.0000000000000150
13. Mduma E, Ersdal H, Svensen E, Kidanto H, Auestad B, Perlman J. Frequent brief on-site simulation training and reduction in 24-h neonatal mortality–an educational intervention study. *Resuscitation.* 2015;93:1–7. doi: 10.1016/j.resuscitation.2015.04.019
14. Lin Y, Cheng A, Grant VJ, Currie GR, Hecker KG. Improving CPR quality with distributed practice and real-time feedback in pediatric healthcare providers - A randomized controlled trial. *Resuscitation.* 2018;130:6–12. doi: 10.1016/j.resuscitation.2018.06.025
15. Montgomery C, Kardong-Edgren SE, Oermann MH, Odom-Maryon T. Student satisfaction and self report of CPR competency: HeartCode BLS courses, instructor-led CPR courses, and monthly voice advisory manikin practice for CPR skill maintenance. *Int J Nurs Educ Scholarsh.* 2012;9. doi: 10.1515/1548-923X.2361
16. Kardong-Edgren S, Oermann MH, Odom-Maryon T. Findings from a nursing student CPR study: implications for staff development educators. *J Nurses Staff Dev.* 2012;28:9–15. doi: 10.1097/NND.0b013e318240a6ad
17. Cepeda Brito JR, Hughes PG, Firestone KS, Ortiz Figueroa F, Johnson K, Ruthenburg T, McKinney R, Gothard MD, Ahmed R. Neonatal Resuscitation Program Rolling Refresher: Maintaining Chest Compression Proficiency Through the Use of Simulation-Based Education. *Adv Neonatal Care.* 2017;17:354–361. doi: 10.1097/ANC.0000000000000384
18. Sullivan NJ, Duval-Arnould J, Twilley M, Smith SP, Aksamit D, Boone-Guercio P, Jeffries PR, Hunt EA. Simulation exercise to improve retention of cardiopulmonary resuscitation priorities for in-hospital cardiac arrests: A randomized controlled trial. *Resuscitation.* 2015;86:6–13. doi: 10.1016/j.resuscitation.2014.10.021

Lay Rescuer Training

Recommendations for Lay Rescuer Training		
COR	LOE	Recommendations
1	C-LD	1. A combination of self-instruction and instructor-led teaching with hands-on training is recommended as an alternative to instructor-led courses for lay rescuers. If instructor-led training is not available, self-directed training is recommended for lay rescuers.[1–9]
1	C-LD	2. It is recommended to train middle school– and high school–age children in how to perform high-quality CPR.[10–18]
2a	C-LD	3. It is reasonable for communities to train bystanders in compression-only CPR for adult out-of-hospital cardiac arrest (OHCA) as an alternative to training in conventional CPR.[19–25]
2a	C-LD	4. It is reasonable to provide CPR training for primary caregivers and/or family members of high-risk patients.[26–39]
2a	A	5. Use of feedback devices can be effective in improving CPR performance during lay rescuer training.[40–47]
2b	B-R	6. If feedback devices are not available, auditory guidance (eg, metronome, music) may be considered to improve adherence to recommendations for chest compression rate only.[48–52]
2b	C-LD	7. It may be reasonable for CPR retraining to be completed more often than every 2 y by lay rescuers who are likely to encounter cardiac arrest.[4,53–57]

Synopsis

Immediate CPR can double or triple survival rates after cardiac arrest.[58,59] The primary goal of resuscitation training for lay rescuers (ie, non–healthcare professionals) is to increase immediate bystander CPR (B-CPR) rates, automated external defibrillator use, and timely emergency response system activation during an OHCA. Enhancing willingness to perform CPR in this population may have a direct impact on survival rates for OHCA.[60] This modular knowledge chunk looks at the question, *Among lay rescuers, what features of CPR training and/or the context of training affect willingness to perform CPR in actual resuscitations, skill-performance quality, and patient outcomes?*

The evidence reviewed suggests that lay rescuers should attend an instructor-led and/or self-directed CPR training session with real-time or delayed feedback to improve CPR skills.[1–4] Training sessions should use combinations of skill-specific training strategies designed to enhance CPR skill retention.[54–57] Refresher training, which focuses on skills and self-confidence rather than on knowledge, should be undertaken regularly, although the optimal time frame requires further study.[4,53–57] It is reasonable for communities to train lay rescuers in compression-only CPR rather than in traditional ventilation-and-compression CPR.[19,20] High-quality CPR is associated with improved survival; however, there are no studies to date that directly correlate CPR performance assessed on a manikin with real patient outcomes.

Recommendation-Specific Supportive Text

1. Four studies examined self-instruction without instructor involvement versus an instructor-led course and showed no significant difference.[1–4] Brief video instruction has shown improved compression rates compared with no training[5,6]; however, instructor-led training is slightly superior in improving compression depth and hand placement and minimizing interruptions.[6–9]
2. Multiple studies have found that middle school– and high school–age children are capable of learning and recalling high-quality CPR skills.[10–18] Early training in middle school and high school may instill confidence and a positive attitude toward responding in a real-life situation.
3. Studies have found that, compared with conventional CPR programs, compression-only CPR programs result in a greater number of appropriate chest compressions by lay rescuer learners.[19,20] When surveyed, lay rescuers report a greater willingness to provide compression-only CPR than they do for conventional CPR with assisted ventilations.[21–23] Two studies published after a statewide educational campaign for lay rescuers showed that the prevalence of both overall B-CPR and compression-only CPR increased over time, but no effect on patient survival was demonstrated.[24,25]
4. Many studies have looked at the effectiveness of BLS training in family members and/or caregivers of high-risk cardiac patients. Outcomes included frequency at which CPR is performed by family members; knowledge, skills, and adequacy of performance; and the survival rates of cardiac arrest victims receiving CPR from family members. The majority of trained lay rescuers were able to competently perform BLS skills, reported a willingness to use these skills, and experienced lower anxiety.[26–39] More research is required to demonstrate a clear benefit because many studies reported low numbers of OHCA and high loss of follow-up.
5. Lay rescuers who used devices that provided corrective feedback during CPR training had improved compression rate, depth, and recoil compared with learners performing CPR without feedback devices.[40–44] Evidence of the effect of feedback devices on CPR skill retention is limited, with 1 of 4 studies demonstrating improved retention.[41,45–47]

Circulation. 2020;142(suppl 2):S551–S579. DOI: 10.1161/CIR.0000000000000903

6. Three randomized trials examined the use of auditory guidance (ie, use of a metronome or music) to guide CPR performance during lay rescuer training.[48–50] All found that chest compression rate was improved when auditory guidance was used, although 1 study reported a negative impact on chest compression depth. Training with guidance from a popular song has been shown to prevent deterioration of chest compression rate over time.[48,51,52]
7. Studies have demonstrated the deterioration of CPR skills of lay rescuers in as little as 3 months after initial training.[4,53] Shorter and more frequent training sessions have demonstrated slight improvement in knowledge and chest compression performance and shorter time to defibrillation.[54–57]

REFERENCES

1. Reder S, Cummings P, Quan L. Comparison of three instructional methods for teaching cardiopulmonary resuscitation and use of an automatic external defibrillator to high school students. *Resuscitation.* 2006;69:443–453. doi: 10.1016/j.resuscitation.2005.08.020
2. Roppolo LP, Pepe PE, Campbell L, Ohman K, Kulkarni H, Miller R, Idris A, Bean L, Bettes TN, Idris AH. Prospective, randomized trial of the effectiveness and retention of 30-min layperson training for cardiopulmonary resuscitation and automated external defibrillators: The American Airlines Study. *Resuscitation.* 2007;74:276–285. doi: 10.1016/j.resuscitation.2006.12.017
3. de Vries W, Turner NM, Monsieurs KG, Bierens JJ, Koster RW. Comparison of instructor-led automated external defibrillation training and three alternative DVD-based training methods. *Resuscitation.* 2010;81:1004–1009. doi: 10.1016/j.resuscitation.2010.04.006
4. Saraç L, Ok A. The effects of different instructional methods on students' acquisition and retention of cardiopulmonary resuscitation skills. *Resuscitation.* 2010;81:555–561. doi: 10.1016/j.resuscitation.2009.08.030
5. Bobrow BJ, Vadeboncoeur TF, Spaite DW, Potts J, Denninghoff K, Chikani V, Brazil PR, Ramsey B, Abella BS. The effectiveness of ultrabrief and brief educational videos for training lay responders in hands-only cardiopulmonary resuscitation: implications for the future of citizen cardiopulmonary resuscitation training. *Circ Cardiovasc Qual Outcomes.* 2011;4:220–226. doi: 10.1161/CIRCOUTCOMES.110.959353
6. Panchal AR, Meziab O, Stolz U, Anderson W, Bartlett M, Spaite DW, Bobrow BJ, Kern KB. The impact of ultra-brief chest compression-only CPR video training on responsiveness, compression rate, and hands-off time interval among bystanders in a shopping mall. *Resuscitation.* 2014;85:1287–1290. doi: 10.1016/j.resuscitation.2014.06.013
7. Chung CH, Siu AY, Po LL, Lam CY, Wong PC. Comparing the effectiveness of video self-instruction versus traditional classroom instruction targeted at cardiopulmonary resuscitation skills for laypersons: a prospective randomised controlled trial. *Hong Kong Med J.* 2010;16:165–170.
8. Jones I, Handley AJ, Whitfield R, Newcombe R, Chamberlain D. A preliminary feasibility study of a short DVD-based distance-learning package for basic life support. *Resuscitation.* 2007;75:350–356. doi: 10.1016/j.resuscitation.2007.04.030
9. Beskind DL, Stolz U, Thiede R, Hoyer R, Robertson W, Brown J, Ludgate M, Tiutan T, Shane R, McMorrow D, Pleasants M, Kern KB, Panchal AR. Viewing an ultra-brief chest compression only video improves some measures of bystander CPR performance and responsiveness at a mass gathering event. *Resuscitation.* 2017;118:96–100. doi: 10.1016/j.resuscitation.2017.07.011
10. Zeleke BG, Biswas ES, Biswas M. Teaching Cardiopulmonary Resuscitation to Young Children (<12 Years Old). *Am J Cardiol.* 2019;123:1626–1627. doi: 10.1016/j.amjcard.2019.02.011
11. Schmid KM, García RQ, Fernandez MM, Mould-Millman NK, Lowenstein SR. Teaching Hands-Only CPR in Schools: A Program Evaluation in San José, Costa Rica. *Ann Glob Health.* 2018;84:612–617. doi: 10.9204/aogh.2367
12. Li H, Shen X, Xu X, Wang Y, Chu L, Zhao J, Wang Y, Wang H, Xie G, Cheng B, et al. Bystander cardiopulmonary resuscitation training in primary and secondary school children in China and the impact of neighborhood socioeconomic status: A prospective controlled trial. *Medicine (Baltimore).* 2018;97:e12673. doi: 10.1097/MD.0000000000012673
13. Paglino M, Contri E, Baggiani M, Tonani M, Costantini G, Bonomo MC, Baldi E. A video-based training to effectively teach CPR with long-term retention: the ScuolaSalvaVita.it ("SchoolSavesLives.it") project. *Intern Emerg Med.* 2019;14:275–279. doi: 10.1007/s11739-018-1946-3
14. Magid KH, Heard D, Sasson C. Addressing Gaps in Cardiopulmonary Resuscitation Education: Training Middle School Students in Hands-Only Cardiopulmonary Resuscitation. *J Sch Health.* 2018;88:524–530. doi: 10.1111/josh.12634
15. Andrews T, Price L, Mills B, Holmes L. Young adults' perception of mandatory CPR training in Australian high schools: a qualitative investigation. *Austr J Paramedicine.* 2018;15. doi: 10.33151/ajp.15.2.577
16. Aloush S, Tubaishat A, ALBashtawy M, Suliman M, Alrimawi I, Al Sabah A, Banikhaled Y. Effectiveness of Basic Life Support Training for Middle School Students. *J Sch Nurs.* 2019;35:262–267. doi: 10.1177/1059840517753879
17. Gabriel IO, Aluko JO. Theoretical knowledge and psychomotor skill acquisition of basic life support training programme among secondary school students. *World J Emerg Med.* 2019;10:81–87. doi: 10.5847/wjem.j.1920-8642.2019.02.003
18. Brown LE, Carroll T, Lynes C, Tripathi A, Halperin H, Dillon WC. CPR skill retention in 795 high school students following a 45-minute course with psychomotor practice. *Am J Emerg Med.* 2018;36:1110–1112. doi: 10.1016/j.ajem.2017.10.026
19. Nishiyama C, Iwami T, Kawamura T, Ando M, Yonemoto N, Hiraide A, Nonogi H. Effectiveness of simplified chest compression-only CPR training for the general public: a randomized controlled trial. *Resuscitation.* 2008;79:90–96. doi: 10.1016/j.resuscitation.2008.05.009
20. Heidenreich JW, Sanders AB, Higdon TA, Kern KB, Berg RA, Ewy GA. Uninterrupted chest compression CPR is easier to perform and remember than standard CPR. *Resuscitation.* 2004;63:123–130. doi: 10.1016/j.resuscitation.2004.04.011
21. Hawkes CA, Brown TP, Booth S, Fothergill RT, Siriwardena N, Zakaria S, Askew S, Williams J, Rees N, Ji C, et al. Attitudes to cardiopulmonary resuscitation and defibrillator use: a survey of UK adults in 2017. *J Am Heart Assoc.* 2019;8:e008267. doi: 10.1161/JAHA.117.008267
22. Cheskes L, Morrison LJ, Beaton D, Parsons J, Dainty KN. Are Canadians more willing to provide chest-compression-only cardiopulmonary resuscitation (CPR)?-a nation-wide public survey. *CJEM.* 2016;18:253–263. doi: 10.1017/cem.2015.113
23. Cho GC, Sohn YD, Kang KH, Lee WW, Lim KS, Kim W, Oh BJ, Choi DH, Yeom SR, Lim H. The effect of basic life support education on laypersons' willingness in performing bystander hands only cardiopulmonary resuscitation. *Resuscitation.* 2010;81:691–694. doi: 10.1016/j.resuscitation.2010.02.021
24. Bobrow BJ, Spaite DW, Berg RA, Stolz U, Sanders AB, Kern KB, Vadeboncoeur TF, Clark LL, Gallagher JV, Stapczynski JS, LoVecchio F, Mullins TJ, Humble WO, Ewy GA. Chest compression-only CPR by lay rescuers and survival from out-of-hospital cardiac arrest. *JAMA.* 2010;304:1447–1454. doi: 10.1001/jama.2010.1392
25. Panchal AR, Bobrow BJ, Spaite DW, Berg RA, Stolz U, Vadeboncoeur TF, Sanders AB, Kern KB, Ewy GA. Chest compression-only cardiopulmonary resuscitation performed by lay rescuers for adult out-of-hospital cardiac arrest due to non-cardiac aetiologies. *Resuscitation.* 2013;84:435–439. doi: 10.1016/j.resuscitation.2012.07.038
26. González-Salvado V, Abelairas-Gómez C, Gude F, Peña-Gil C, Neiro-Rey C, González-Juanatey JR, Rodriguez-Núñez A. Targeting relatives: Impact of a cardiac rehabilitation programme including basic life support training on their skills and attitudes. *Eur J Prev Cardiol.* 2019;26:795–805. doi: 10.1177/2047487319830190
27. Blewer AL, Leary M, Esposito EC, Gonzalez M, Riegel B, Bobrow BJ, Abella BS. Continuous chest compression cardiopulmonary resuscitation training promotes rescuer self-confidence and increased secondary training: a hospital-based randomized controlled trial*. *Crit Care Med.* 2012;40:787–792. doi: 10.1097/CCM.0b013e318236f2ca
28. Dracup K, Guzy PM, Taylor SE, Barry J. Cardiopulmonary resuscitation (CPR) training. Consequences for family members of high-risk cardiac patients. *Arch Intern Med.* 1986;146:1757–1761. doi: 10.1001/archinte.146.9.1757
29. Dracup K, Moser DK, Doering LV, Guzy PM, Juarbe T. A controlled trial of cardiopulmonary resuscitation training for ethnically diverse parents of infants at high risk for cardiopulmonary arrest. *Crit Care Med.* 2000;28:3289–3295. doi: 10.1097/00003246-200009000-00029

30. Moser DK, Dracup K, Doering LV. Effect of cardiopulmonary resuscitation training for parents of high-risk neonates on perceived anxiety, control, and burden. *Heart Lung.* 1999;28:326–333. doi: 10.1053/hl.1999.v28.a101053
31. Haugk M, Robak O, Sterz F, Uray T, Kliegel A, Losert H, Holzer M, Herkner H, Laggner AN, Domanovits H. High acceptance of a home AED programme by survivors of sudden cardiac arrest and their families. *Resuscitation.* 2006;70:263–274. doi: 10.1016/j.resuscitation.2006.03.010
32. Kliegel A, Scheinecker W, Sterz F, Eisenburger P, Holzer M, Laggner AN. The attitudes of cardiac arrest survivors and their family members towards CPR courses. *Resuscitation.* 2000;47:147–154. doi: 10.1016/s0300-9572(00)00214-8
33. Knight LJ, Wintch S, Nichols A, Arnolde V, Schroeder AR. Saving a life after discharge: CPR training for parents of high-risk children. *J Healthc Qual.* 2013;35:9–16; quiz17. doi: 10.1111/j.1945-1474.2012.00221.x
34. Tomatis Souverbielle C, González-Martínez F, González-Sánchez MI, CarrónM, GuerraMiguezL, ButragueñoL, GonzaloH, VillalbaT, PerezMorenoJ, Toledo B, Rodríguez-Fernández R. Strengthening the Chain of Survival: Cardiopulmonary Resuscitation Workshop for Caregivers of Children at Risk. *Pediatr Qual Saf.* 2019;4:e141. doi: 10.1097/pq9.0000000000000141
35. Dracup K, Moser DK, Doering LV, Guzy PM. Comparison of cardiopulmonary resuscitation training methods for parents of infants at high risk for cardiopulmonary arrest. *Ann Emerg Med.* 1998;32:170–177. doi: 10.1016/s0196-0644(98)70133-7
36. Dracup K, Moser DK, Guzy PM, Taylor SE, Marsden C. Is cardiopulmonary resuscitation training deleterious for family members of cardiac patients? *Am J Public Health.* 1994;84:116–118. doi: 10.2105/ajph.84.1.116
37. Higgins SS, Hardy CE, Higashino SM. Should parents of children with congenital heart disease and life-threatening dysrhythmias be taught cardiopulmonary resuscitation? *Pediatrics.* 1989;84:1102–1104.
38. McLauchlan CA, Ward A, Murphy NM, Griffith MJ, Skinner DV, Camm AJ. Resuscitation training for cardiac patients and their relatives–its effect on anxiety. *Resuscitation.* 1992;24:7–11. doi: 10.1016/0300-9572(92)90168-c
39. Pierick TA, Van Waning N, Patel SS, Atkins DL. Self-instructional CPR training for parents of high risk infants. *Resuscitation.* 2012;83:1140–1144. doi: 10.1016/j.resuscitation.2012.02.007
40. Renshaw AA, Mena-Allauca M, Gould EW, Sirintrapun SJ. Synoptic Reporting: Evidence-Based Review and Future Directions. *JCO Clin Cancer Inform.* 2018;2:1–9. doi: 10.1200/CCI.17.00088
41. Baldi E, Cornara S, Contri E, Epis F, Fina D, Zelaschi B, Dossena C, Fichtner F, Tonani M, Di Maggio M, Zambaiti E, Somaschini A. Real-time visual feedback during training improves laypersons' CPR quality: a randomized controlled manikin study. *CJEM.* 2017;19:480–487. doi: 10.1017/cem.2016.410
42. Saraç L. Effects of augmented feedback on cardiopulmonary resuscitation skill acquisition: concurrent versus terminal. *Eurasian J Educ Res.* 2017;72:83–106.
43. Yeung J, Davies R, Gao F, Perkins GD. A randomised control trial of prompt and feedback devices and their impact on quality of chest compressions—a simulation study. *Resuscitation.* 2014;85:553–559. doi: 10.1016/j.resuscitation.2014.01.015
44. Mpotos N, Yde L, Calle P, Deschepper E, Valcke M, Peersman W, Herregods L, Monsieurs K. Retraining basic life support skills using video, voice feedback or both: a randomised controlled trial. *Resuscitation.* 2013;84:72–77. doi: 10.1016/j.resuscitation.2012.08.320
45. Zhou XL, Wang J, Jin XQ, Zhao Y, Liu RL, Jiang C. Quality retention of chest compression after repetitive practices with or without feedback devices: A randomized manikin study. *Am J Emerg Med.* 2020;38:73–78. doi: 10.1016/j.ajem.2019.04.025
46. Wik L, Myklebust H, Auestad BH, Steen PA. Retention of basic life support skills 6 months after training with an automated voice advisory manikin system without instructor involvement. *Resuscitation.* 2002;52:273–279. doi: 10.1016/s0300-9572(01)00476-2
47. Williamson LJ, Larsen PD, Tzeng YC, Galletly DC. Effect of automatic external defibrillator audio prompts on cardiopulmonary resuscitation performance. *Emerg Med J.* 2005;22:140–143. doi: 10.1136/emj.2004.016444
48. Rawlins L, Woollard M, Williams J, Hallam P. Effect of listening to Nellie the Elephant during CPR training on performance of chest compressions by lay people: randomised crossover trial. *BMJ.* 2009;339:b4707. doi: 10.1136/bmj.b4707
49. Woollard M, Poposki J, McWhinnie B, Rawlins L, Munro G, O'Meara P. Achy breaky makey wakey heart? A randomised crossover trial of musical prompts. *Emerg Med J.* 2012;29:290–294. doi: 10.1136/emermed-2011-200187
50. Oh JH, Lee SJ, Kim SE, Lee KJ, Choe JW, Kim CW. Effects of audio tone guidance on performance of CPR in simulated cardiac arrest with an advanced airway. *Resuscitation.* 2008;79:273–277. doi: 10.1016/j.resuscitation.2008.06.022
51. Hafner JW, Jou AC, Wang H, Bleess BB, Tham SK. Death before disco: the effectiveness of a musical metronome in layperson cardiopulmonary resuscitation training. *J Emerg Med.* 2015;48:43–52. doi: 10.1016/j.jemermed.2014.07.048
52. Hong CK, Hwang SY, Lee KY, Kim YS, Ha YR, Park SO. Metronome vs. popular song: a comparison of long-term retention of chest compression skills after layperson training for cardiopulmonary resuscitation. *Hong Kong J Emerg Med.* 2016;32:145–152.
53. Papadimitriou L, Xanthos T, Bassiakou E, Stroumpoulis K, Barouxis D, Iacovidou N. Distribution of pre-course BLS/AED manuals does not influence skill acquisition and retention in lay rescuers: a randomised study. *Resuscitation.* 2010;81:348–352. doi: 10.1016/j.resuscitation.2009.11.020
54. Hsieh MJ, Chiang WC, Jan CF, Lin HY, Yang CW, Ma MH. The effect of different retraining intervals on the skill performance of cardiopulmonary resuscitation in laypeople-A three-armed randomized control study. *Resuscitation.* 2018;128:151–157. doi: 10.1016/j.resuscitation.2018.05.010
55. Niles D, Sutton RM, Donoghue A, Kalsi MS, Roberts K, Boyle L, Nishisaki A, Arbogast KB, Helfaer M, Nadkarni V. "Rolling Refreshers": a novel approach to maintain CPR psychomotor skill competence. *Resuscitation.* 2009;80:909–912. doi: 10.1016/j.resuscitation.2009.04.021
56. Woollard M, Whitfield R, Newcombe RG, Colquhoun M, Vetter N, Chamberlain D. Optimal refresher training intervals for AED and CPR skills: a randomised controlled trial. *Resuscitation.* 2006;71:237–247. doi: 10.1016/j.resuscitation.2006.04.005
57. Chamberlain D, Smith A, Woollard M, Colquhoun M, Handley AJ, Leaves S, Kern KB. Trials of teaching methods in basic life support (3): comparison of simulated CPR performance after first training and at 6 months, with a note on the value of re-training. *Resuscitation.* 2002;53:179–187. doi: 10.1016/s0300-9572(02)00025-4
58. Naim MY, Burke RV, McNally BF, Song L, Griffis HM, Berg RA, Vellano K, Markenson D, Bradley RN, Rossano JW. Association of Bystander Cardiopulmonary Resuscitation With Overall and Neurologically Favorable Survival After Pediatric Out-of-Hospital Cardiac Arrest in the United States: A Report From the Cardiac Arrest Registry to Enhance Survival Surveillance Registry. *JAMA Pediatr.* 2017;171:133–141. doi: 10.1001/jamapediatrics.2016.3643
59. Swor RA, Jackson RE, Cynar M, Sadler E, Basse E, Boji B, Rivera-Rivera EJ, Maher A, Grubb W, Jacobson R. Bystander CPR, ventricular fibrillation, and survival in witnessed, unmonitored out-of-hospital cardiac arrest. *Ann Emerg Med.* 1995;25:780–784. doi: 10.1016/s0196-0644(95)70207-5
60. McCarthy JJ, Carr B, Sasson C, Bobrow BJ, Callaway CW, Neumar RW, Ferrer JME, Garvey JL, Ornato JP, Gonzales L, Granger CB, Kleinman ME, Bjerke C, Nichol G; American Heart Association Emergency Cardiovascular Care Committee; Council on Cardiopulmonary, Critical Care, Perioperative and Resuscitation; and the Mission: Lifeline Resuscitation Subcommittee. Out-of-Hospital Cardiac Arrest Resuscitation Systems of Care: A Scientific Statement From the American Heart Association. *Circulation.* 2018;137:e645–e660. doi: 10.1161/CIR.0000000000000557

Teamwork and Leadership Training

Recommendation for Teamwork and Leadership Training		
COR	**LOE**	**Recommendation**
2a	B-NR	1. It is reasonable to include specific team and leadership training as part of advanced life support training for healthcare providers.[1–15]

Synopsis

Resuscitation of cardiac arrest patients relies on multiple providers working together to coordinate delivery of time-sensitive therapies, making teamwork and leadership indispensable components of providing optimal care.[16–18] Training that focuses on the communication and interpersonal skills required for teams to work as a coordinated unit can have a potential impact on patient outcomes.[19–21] Studies evaluating the effect of team and leadership training when included as part of advanced life support training for healthcare providers have found a positive impact on provider skills during simulated and real cardiac arrests.[1–15,22] These studies included a broad range of educational strategies (eg, video modules, simulation) and outcome measures (eg, quality of communication, adherence to recommended advanced life support practices). Despite the low-moderate quality of evidence, we recommend including team and leadership training as part of advanced life support training for healthcare providers. This recommendation is justified because the potential benefit from team and leadership training significantly outweighs the potential risks. Further studies are needed to define the optimal educational strategies for team and leadership training as well as to understand the interplay and relative benefit among team, leadership, and skills training on provider skill and patient outcomes.

Recommendation-Specific Supportive Text

1. Several studies examined the impact of team or leadership training on patient outcomes or provider skills in actual cardiac arrests. One prospective observational study reported an increase in survival from pediatric cardiac arrests from 33% to approximately 50% (P=0.00) within 1 year of implementing a formal hospital-wide mock code team training program.[1] One RCT of simulation-based leadership training found no effect on CPR quality during resuscitation of patients.[6] Four observational studies found an association between interventions to improve teamwork and CPR quality, communication, and deployment times for mechanical devices.[2–5]

   Seven RCTs and 1 multicenter prospective interventional study explored the impact of team and leadership training on performance of clinical tasks in simulated resuscitations, both at course completion and at follow-up from 3 to 15 months later.[7–14] Each of the studies showed improvement in 1 or more aspects of performance, although improvements were not universal across all measures. Improvements were seen in both specific aspects of clinical care, such as time to initiation of CPR and time to defibrillation,[7–13] and compliance with ACLS guidelines.[12–14] Ten RCTs reported that team or leadership training was associated with improvement in measures of teamwork and leadership during simulated resuscitations, such as frequency of leader vocalizations,[8,10,14] frequency of specific team skills,[7,11,13,23] and scores on various teamwork rating scales.[9,11,12,15]

REFERENCES

1. Andreatta P, Saxton E, Thompson M, Annich G. Simulation-based mock codes significantly correlate with improved pediatric patient cardiopulmonary arrest survival rates. *Pediatr Crit Care Med.* 2011;12:33–38. doi: 10.1097/PCC.0b013e3181e89270
2. Nadler I, Sanderson PM, Van Dyken CR, Davis PG, Liley HG. Presenting video recordings of newborn resuscitations in debriefings for teamwork training. *BMJ Qual Saf.* 2011;20:163–169. doi: 10.1136/bmjqs.2010.043547
3. Ong ME, Quah JL, Annathurai A, Noor NM, Koh ZX, Tan KB, Pothiawala S, Poh AH, Loy CK, Fook-Chong S. Improving the quality of cardiopulmonary resuscitation by training dedicated cardiac arrest teams incorporating a mechanical load-distributing device at the emergency department. *Resuscitation.* 2013;84:508–514. doi: 10.1016/j.resuscitation.2012.07.033
4. Su L, Spaeder MC, Jones MB, Sinha P, Nath DS, Jain PN, Berger JT, Williams L, Shankar V. Implementation of an extracorporeal cardiopulmonary resuscitation simulation program reduces extracorporeal cardiopulmonary resuscitation times in real patients. *Pediatr Crit Care Med.* 2014;15:856–860. doi: 10.1097/PCC.0000000000000234
5. Spitzer CR, Evans K, Buehler J, Ali NA, Besecker BY. Code blue pit crew model: A novel approach to in-hospital cardiac arrest resuscitation. *Resuscitation.* 2019;143:158–164. doi: 10.1016/j.resuscitation.2019.06.290
6. Weidman EK, Bell G, Walsh D, Small S, Edelson DP. Assessing the impact of immersive simulation on clinical performance during actual in-hospital cardiac arrest with CPR-sensing technology: A randomized feasibility study. *Resuscitation.* 2010;81:1556–1561. doi: 10.1016/j.resuscitation.2010.05.021
7. Thomas EJ, Williams AL, Reichman EF, Lasky RE, Crandell S, Taggart WR. Team training in the neonatal resuscitation program for interns: teamwork and quality of resuscitations. *Pediatrics.* 2010;125:539–546. doi: 10.1542/peds.2009-1635
8. Hunziker S, Bühlmann C, Tschan F, Balestra G, Legeret C, Schumacher C, Semmer NK, Hunziker P, Marsch S. Brief leadership instructions improve cardiopulmonary resuscitation in a high-fidelity simulation: a randomized controlled trial. *Crit Care Med.* 2010;38:1086–1091. doi: 10.1097/CCM.0b013e3181cf7383
9. Blackwood J, Duff JP, Nettel-Aguirre A, Djogovic D, Joynt C. Does teaching crisis resource management skills improve resuscitation performance in pediatric residents?*. *Pediatr Crit Care Med.* 2014;15:e168–e174. doi: 10.1097/PCC.0000000000000100
10. Fernandez Castelao E, Russo SG, Cremer S, Strack M, Kaminski L, Eich C, Timmermann A, Boos M. Positive impact of crisis resource management training on no-flow time and team member verbalisations during simulated cardiopulmonary resuscitation: a randomised controlled trial. *Resuscitation.* 2011;82:1338–1343. doi: 10.1016/j.resuscitation.2011.05.009
11. Haffner L, Mahling M, Muench A, Castan C, Schubert P, Naumann A, Reddersen S, Herrmann-Werner A, Reutershan J, Riessen R, Celebi N. Improved recognition of ineffective chest compressions after a brief Crew Resource Management (CRM) training: a prospective, randomised simulation study. *BMC Emerg Med.* 2017;17:7. doi: 10.1186/s12873-017-0117-6
12. Gilfoyle E, Koot DA, Annear JC, Bhanji F, Cheng A, Duff JP, Grant VJ, St George-Hyslop CE, Delaloye NJ, Kotsakis A, McCoy CD, Ramsay CE, Weiss MJ, Gottesman RD; Teams4Kids Investigators and the Canadian Critical Care Trials Group. Improved Clinical Performance and Teamwork of Pediatric Interprofessional Resuscitation Teams With a Simulation-Based Educational Intervention. *Pediatr Crit Care Med.* 2017;18:e62–e69. doi: 10.1097/PCC.0000000000001025
13. Jankouskas TS, Haidet KK, Hupcey JE, Kolanowski A, Murray WB. Targeted crisis resource management training improves performance among randomized nursing and medical students. *Simul Healthc.* 2011;6:316–326. doi: 10.1097/SIH.0b013e31822bc676
14. Fernandez Castelao E, Boos M, Ringer C, Eich C, Russo SG. Effect of CRM team leader training on team performance and leadership behavior in simulated cardiac arrest scenarios: a prospective, randomized, controlled study. *BMC Med Educ.* 2015;15:116. doi: 10.1186/s12909-015-0389-z
15. Cooper S. Developing leaders for advanced life support: evaluation of a training programme. *Resuscitation.* 2001;49:33–38. doi: 10.1016/s0300-9572(00)00345-2
16. Bhanji F, Finn JC, Lockey A, Monsieurs K, Frengley R, Iwami T, Lang E, Ma MH, Mancini ME, McNeil MA, et al; on behalf of the Education, Implementation, and Teams Chapter Collaborators. Part 8: education, implementation, and teams: 2015 International Consensus on Cardiopulmonary Resuscitation and Emergency Cardiovascular Care Science With Treatment Recommendations. *Circulation.* 2015;132(suppl 1):S242–S268. doi: 10.1161/CIR.0000000000000277
17. Bhanji F, Donoghue AJ, Wolff MS, Flores GE, Halamek LP, Berman JM, Sinz EH, Cheng A. Part 14: education: 2015 American Heart Association Guidelines Update for Cardiopulmonary Resuscitation and Emergency

Cardiovascular Care. *Circulation*. 2015;132(suppl 2):S561–573. doi: 10.1161/CIR.0000000000000268
18. Cheng A, Donoghue A, Gilfoyle E, Eppich W. Simulation-based crisis resource management training for pediatric critical care medicine: a review for instructors. *Pediatr Crit Care Med*. 2012;13:197–203. doi: 10.1097/PCC.0b013e3182192832
19. Rosen MA, DiazGranados D, Dietz AS, Benishek LE, Thompson D, Pronovost PJ, Weaver SJ. Teamwork in healthcare: Key discoveries enabling safer, high-quality care. *Am Psychol*. 2018;73:433–450. doi: 10.1037/amp0000298
20. Salas E, DiazGranados D, Weaver SJ, King H. Does team training work? Principles for health care. *Acad Emerg Med*. 2008;15:1002–1009. doi: 10.1111/j.1553-2712.2008.00254.x
21. Marlow SL, Hughes AM, Sonesh SC, Gregory ME, Lacerenza CN, Benishek LE, Woods AL, Hernandez C, Salas E. A Systematic Review of Team Training in Health Care: Ten Questions. *Jt Comm J Qual Patient Saf*. 2017;43:197–204. doi: 10.1016/j.jcjq.2016.12.004
22. Greif R, Bhanji F, Bigham BL, Bray J, Breckwoldt J, Cheng A, Duff JP, Gilfoyle E, Hsieh M-J, Iwami T, et al; on behalf of the Education, Implementation, and Teams Collaborators. Education, implementation, and teams: 2020 International Consensus on Cardiopulmonary Resuscitation and Emergency Cardiovascular Care Science With Treatment Recommendations. *Circulation*. 2020;142(suppl 1):S222–S283. doi: 10.1161/CIR.0000000000000896
23. Thomas EJ, Taggart B, Crandell S, Lasky RE, Williams AL, Love LJ, Sexton JB, Tyson JE, Helmreich RL. Teaching teamwork during the Neonatal Resuscitation Program: a randomized trial. *J Perinatol*. 2007;27:409–414. doi: 10.1038/sj.jp.7211771

In Situ Education

Recommendations for In Situ Education		
COR	**LOE**	**Recommendations**
2a	C-LD	1. It is reasonable to conduct in situ simulation-based resuscitation training in addition to traditional training.[1–12]
2b	B-R	2. It may be reasonable to conduct in situ simulation-based resuscitation training in place of traditional training.[13–15]

Synopsis

In situ simulation refers to a subset of simulation activities occurring in actual patient care areas (ie, real clinical environment).[16] In situ simulation can be used as a strategy to train individuals and/or healthcare teams.[17,18] The objectives for in situ training can be individual provider technical skills or team-based skills, including communication, leadership, role allocation, and situational awareness.[17,18] One distinct advantage of in situ training is that it provides learners with a more realistic training environment. In this review, we explored if in situ, simulation-based resuscitation training for healthcare providers leads to improved learning, performance, and/or patient outcomes.

Studies comparing in situ training to traditional training (ie, classroom or laboratory-based training) have not demonstrated significant differences in learning outcomes.[13–15] Compared with no intervention, in situ training added to other educational strategies has a positive impact on learning outcomes (eg, improved team performance, improved time to critical tasks),[2,7–12] performance change in the real clinical environment (eg, improved team performance, recognition of deteriorating patients),[2–4] and patient outcomes (eg, improved survival, neurological outcomes).[1,4–6] The advantages of in situ training should be weighed against the potential risks, including logistical challenges of conducting training in clinical spaces and risks of mixing training resources with real clinical resources (eg, simulated versus real medications or fluids).[19,20]

Recommendation-Specific Supportive Text

1. Three observational studies demonstrated that regular in situ simulation training, in combination with other educational strategies (ie, refresher of BLS/PALS training, introduction of code teams, distributed practice), is effective at improving team performance and time to recognize deteriorating patients.[2–4] Four additional observational studies assessing bundled interventions including in situ training demonstrated significant improvements in cardiac arrest survival.[1,4–6] Because in situ training was tested as part of a bundled intervention in these studies, the individual contribution of in situ training cannot be clearly elucidated.

   Two RCTs demonstrated that in situ cardiac arrest training coupled with spaced learning yields better learning outcomes (ie, improved clinical performance, decreased time to initiate compression and defibrillation) compared with training conducted in a massed-delivery format in the classroom.[8,9] One RCT and 4 prospective observational studies demonstrated that in situ simulation training results in improved clinical performance in simulated environments.[2,7,10–12] Most observational studies are limited by a lack of parallel control groups, a lack of performance measures with supportive validity evidence, and potential confounding factors.
2. Two RCTs and 1 observational study compared learning outcomes (ie, team performance, technical skills) of in situ simulation training with standard classroom or laboratory-based training settings and demonstrated no significant differences between the 2 settings.[13–15]

REFERENCES

1. Andreatta P, Saxton E, Thompson M, Annich G. Simulation-based mock codes significantly correlate with improved pediatric patient cardiopulmonary arrest survival rates. *Pediatr Crit Care Med*. 2011;12:33–38. doi: 10.1097/PCC.0b013e3181e89270
2. Steinemann S, Berg B, Skinner A, DiTulio A, Anzelon K, Terada K, Oliver C, Ho HC, Speck C. In situ, multidisciplinary, simulation-based teamwork training improves early trauma care. *J Surg Educ*. 2011;68:472–477. doi: 10.1016/j.jsurg.2011.05.009
3. Theilen U, Leonard P, Jones P, Ardill R, Weitz J, Agrawal D, Simpson D. Regular in situ simulation training of paediatric medical emergency team improves hospital response to deteriorating patients. *Resuscitation*. 2013;84:218–222. doi: 10.1016/j.resuscitation.2012.06.027

4. Knight LJ, Gabhart JM, Earnest KS, Leong KM, Anglemyer A, Franzon D. Improving code team performance and survival outcomes: implementation of pediatric resuscitation team training. *Crit Care Med.* 2014;42:243–251. doi: 10.1097/CCM.0b013e3182a6439d
5. Sodhi K, Singla MK, Shrivastava A. Institutional resuscitation protocols: do they affect cardiopulmonary resuscitation outcomes? A 6-year study in a single tertiary-care centre. *J Anesth.* 2015;29:87–95. doi: 10.1007/s00540-014-1873-z
6. Josey K, Smith ML, Kayani AS, Young G, Kasperski MD, Farrer P, Gerkin R, Theodorou A, Raschke RA. Hospitals with more-active participation in conducting standardized in-situ mock codes have improved survival after in-hospital cardiopulmonary arrest. *Resuscitation.* 2018;133:47–52. doi: 10.1016/j.resuscitation.2018.09.020
7. Clarke SO, Julie IM, Yao AP, Bang H, Barton JD, Alsomali SM, Kiefer MV, Al Khulaif AH, Aljahany M, Venugopal S, Bair AE. Longitudinal exploration of in situ mock code events and the performance of cardiac arrest skills. *BMJ Simul Technol Enhanc Learn.* 2019;5:29–33. doi: 10.1136/bmjstel-2017-000255
8. Kurosawa H, Ikeyama T, Achuff P, Perkel M, Watson C, Monachino A, Remy D, Deutsch E, Buchanan N, Anderson J, Berg RA, Nadkarni VM, Nishisaki A. A randomized, controlled trial of in situ pediatric advanced life support recertification ("pediatric advanced life support reconstructed") compared with standard pediatric advanced life support recertification for ICU frontline providers*. *Crit Care Med.* 2014;42:610–618. doi: 10.1097/CCM.0000000000000024
9. Sullivan NJ, Duval-Arnould J, Twilley M, Smith SP, Aksamit D, Boone-Guercio P, Jeffries PR, Hunt EA. Simulation exercise to improve retention of cardiopulmonary resuscitation priorities for in-hospital cardiac arrests: A randomized controlled trial. *Resuscitation.* 2015;86:6–13. doi: 10.1016/j.resuscitation.2014.10.021
10. Rubio-Gurung S, Putet G, Touzet S, Gauthier-Moulinier H, Jordan I, Beissel A, Labaune JM, Blanc S, Amamra N, Balandras C, Rudigoz RC, Colin C, Picaud JC. In situ simulation training for neonatal resuscitation: an RCT. *Pediatrics.* 2014;134:e790–e797. doi: 10.1542/peds.2013-3988
11. Saqe-Rockoff A, Ciardiello AV, Schubert FD. Low-Fidelity, In-Situ Pediatric Resuscitation Simulation Improves RN Competence and Self-Efficacy. *J Emerg Nurs.* 2019;45:538–544.e1. doi: 10.1016/j.jen.2019.02.003
12. Katznelson JH, Wang J, Stevens MW, Mills WA. Improving Pediatric Preparedness in Critical Access Hospital Emergency Departments: Impact of a Longitudinal In Situ Simulation Program. *Pediatr Emerg Care.* 2018;34:17–20. doi: 10.1097/PEC.0000000000001366
13. Crofts JF, Ellis D, Draycott TJ, Winter C, Hunt LP, Akande VA. Change in knowledge of midwives and obstetricians following obstetric emergency training: a randomised controlled trial of local hospital, simulation centre and teamwork training. *BJOG.* 2007;114:1534–1541. doi: 10.1111/j.1471-0528.2007.01493.x
14. Ellis D, Crofts JF, Hunt LP, Read M, Fox R, James M. Hospital, simulation center, and teamwork training for eclampsia management: a randomized controlled trial. *Obstet Gynecol.* 2008;111:723–731. doi: 10.1097/AOG.0b013e3181637a82
15. Couto TB, Kerrey BT, Taylor RG, FitzGerald M, Geis GL. Teamwork skills in actual, in situ, and in-center pediatric emergencies: performance levels across settings and perceptions of comparative educational impact. *Simul Healthc.* 2015;10:76–84. doi: 10.1097/SIH.0000000000000081
16. Kurup V, Matei V, Ray J. Role of in-situ simulation for training in healthcare: opportunities and challenges. *Curr Opin Anaesthesiol.* 2017;30:755–760. doi: 10.1097/ACO.0000000000000514
17. Goldshtein D, Krensky C, Doshi S, Perelman VS. In situ simulation and its effects on patient outcomes: a systematic review. *BMJ Simulation and Technology Enhanced Learning.* 2020;6:3–9. doi: 10.1136/bmjstel-2018-000387
18. Rosen MA, Hunt EA, Pronovost PJ, Federowicz MA, Weaver SJ. In situ simulation in continuing education for the health care professions: a systematic review. *J Contin Educ Health Prof.* 2012;32:243–254. doi: 10.1002/chp.21152
19. U.S. Food and Drug Administration. Simulated IV solutions from Wallcur: CDER statement—FDA's investigation into patients being injected. 2015. https://www.fdanews.com/ext/resources/files/01-15/01-15-2015-Saline-Safety-Warning.pdf?152088501. Accessed February 11, 2020.
20. Petrosoniak A, Auerbach M, Wong AH, Hicks CM. In situ simulation in emergency medicine: Moving beyond the simulation lab. *Emerg Med Australas.* 2017;29:83–88. doi: 10.1111/1742-6723.12705

Manikin Fidelity

Recommendations for Manikin Fidelity

COR	LOE	Recommendations
2a	B-R	1. The use of higher-fidelity manikins for advanced life support training can be beneficial for learners at training centers with available infrastructure and personnel.[1–4]
2b	C-LD	2. The use of lower-fidelity manikins during advanced life support training may be considered for training centers where cost, personnel, availability, or other considerations do not allow the use of higher-fidelity manikins.[1,3]
2b	C-EO	3. It may be reasonable for instructors to use manikins and manikin features in a manner that allows for alignment of learning objectives to the needs of individual learner groups.[1,5,6]

Synopsis

Learner engagement during resuscitation education is enhanced by optimizing the reality of the training experience.[1] Three different categories of fidelity (or realism) have been described: (a) conceptual fidelity (ie, the concepts and relationships presented in the simulation); (b) emotional fidelity (ie, the holistic experience of the simulation); and (c) physical fidelity (ie, the properties of the manikin and the environment).[7] Manikins are a full or partial body representation of a patient.[8] The term *manikin fidelity* has been used to refer to the presence of simulated physical features that can be used to more closely mimic a resuscitation patient.[2] Higher-fidelity manikins with advanced physical features allow simulation of patients across age groups (eg, newborn, infant, child, adult) and physiological states (eg, traumatic injury, pregnancy, cardiac arrest). Use of higher-fidelity manikins could theoretically improve learner immersion and engagement in scenario-based learning. Disadvantages of higher-fidelity manikins include increased costs to purchase, the need for trained personnel to operate them, and the need for ongoing maintenance.[1]

Studies examining the impact of higher-fidelity manikins during resuscitation education have yielded varied results. A recent systematic review found that using higher-fidelity manikins in resuscitation training led to improved skill acquisition at course completion but no impact on long-term skills or knowledge.[2] For the current update, we identified 2 RCTs examining the impact of manikin fidelity on trainee knowledge and psychomotor skill, with mixed results.[3,4] No studies assess the impact of manikin fidelity on patient outcomes. Using higher-fidelity manikins can be beneficial when availability and supportive infrastructure permit their use. This recommendation must be balanced against the cost and training requirements for manikin operators as well as the need for accurate alignment of manikin features with learning objectives.

Recommendation-Specific Supportive Text

1. A meta-analysis of studies assessing the impact of higher-fidelity manikins during resuscitation education found a moderate benefit on skill performance at course conclusion but no impact on long-term skills or knowledge.[2] The review acknowledged the increased cost and the need for trained personnel to operate higher-fidelity manikins. One nonrandomized trial of PALS training compared knowledge (examination score) and skill (task performance time) for intervention group trainees who used a higher-fidelity infant manikin with control group trainees who used a standard manikin. No differences were found in knowledge or skill at course completion, though knowledge at 6 months after course completion was higher in the higher-fidelity group.[4]
2. An RCT of a neonatal resuscitation program training medical students compared knowledge (ie, examination score) and skill (ie, Megacode score) for intervention trainees who used a higher-fidelity manikin (ie, with observable vital signs, cyanosis, limb movements, and breath sounds) with control trainees who used a basic manikin without these features. No significant differences were found in skill or knowledge at course completion or at 3 months between the intervention and control groups.[3]
3. Tailoring manikin selection (ie, physical features) to the needs of the scenario and the scope of trainees' practice ensures that required physical features are present to maximize learner engagement.[6]

REFERENCES

1. Cheng A, Nadkarni VM, Mancini MB, Hunt EA, Sinz EH, Merchant RM, Donoghue A, Duff JP, Eppich W, Auerbach M, Bigham BL, Blewer AL, Chan PS, Bhanji F; American Heart Association Education Science Investigators; and on behalf of the American Heart Association Education Science and Programs Committee, Council on Cardiopulmonary, Critical Care, Perioperative and Resuscitation; Council on Cardiovascular and Stroke Nursing; and Council on Quality of Care and Outcomes Research. Resuscitation Education Science: Educational Strategies to Improve Outcomes From Cardiac Arrest: A Scientific Statement From the American Heart Association. *Circulation*. 2018;138:e82–e122. doi: 10.1161/CIR.0000000000000583
2. Cheng A, Lockey A, Bhanji F, Lin Y, Hunt EA, Lang E. The use of high-fidelity manikins for advanced life support training–A systematic review and meta-analysis. *Resuscitation*. 2015;93:142–149. doi: 10.1016/j.resuscitation.2015.04.004
3. Nimbalkar A, Patel D, Kungwani A, Phatak A, Vasa R, Nimbalkar S. Randomized control trial of high fidelity vs low fidelity simulation for training undergraduate students in neonatal resuscitation. *BMC Res Notes*. 2015;8:636. doi: 10.1186/s13104-015-1623-9
4. Stellflug SM, Lowe NK. The Effect of High Fidelity Simulators on Knowledge Retention and Skill Self Efficacy in Pediatric Advanced Life Support Courses in a Rural State. *J Pediatr Nurs*. 2018;39:21–26. doi: 10.1016/j.pedn.2017.12.006
5. Donoghue AJ, Durbin DR, Nadel FM, Stryjewski GR, Kost SI, Nadkarni VM. Perception of realism during mock resuscitations by pediatric housestaff: the impact of simulated physical features. *Simul Healthc*. 2010;5:16–20. doi: 10.1097/SIH.0b013e3181a46aa1
6. Hamstra SJ, Brydges R, Hatala R, Zendejas B, Cook DA. Reconsidering fidelity in simulation-based training. *Acad Med*. 2014;89:387–392. doi: 10.1097/ACM.0000000000000130
7. Rudolph JW, Simon R, Raemer DB. Which reality matters? Questions on the path to high engagement in healthcare simulation. *Simul Healthc*. 2007;2:161–163. doi: 10.1097/SIH.0b013e31813d1035
8. Lopreiato JO. *Heatlhcare Simulation Dictionary*. Rockville, MD: Agency for Healthcare Research and Quality; 2016. https://www.ahrq.gov/sites/default/files/publications/files/sim-dictionary.pdf. Accessed April 27, 2020.

CPR Feedback Devices in Training

Recommendation for CPR Feedback Devices in Training		
COR	**LOE**	**Recommendation**
2a	B-R	1. Use of feedback devices during training can be effective in improving CPR performance.[1–10]

Synopsis

Accurate assessment of CPR skills is critical to helping learners improve performance.[11] Prior studies demonstrate that visual assessment of CPR quality is neither reliable nor accurate, making it challenging for instructors to provide consistently meaningful feedback during CPR training.[12–15] Feedback devices address this problem by providing objective feedback to learners and instructors during practice. CPR feedback devices can be grouped into 2 categories: corrective feedback devices (eg, visual display of depth) and prompt devices that provide an auditory tone for the provider to follow (eg, metronome). In this review, we assessed if the use of CPR feedback devices during training, compared with no use of feedback devices during training, improves CPR skills, clinical performance, and patient outcomes.[16]

Studies examining the use of CPR feedback devices during training showed mixed results, with 6 of 8 studies demonstrating improved CPR skill performance at the conclusion of training.[1–6,17,18] The use of corrective feedback devices during training resulted in improved skill retention at 7 days to 3 months after initial training compared with learners trained without a feedback device.[2,6–10,19] No studies have reported the cost-effectiveness of feedback device use during training or the impact on healthcare providers' performance in clinical settings and patient outcomes. The benefit of feedback use during training should be balanced with the cost of such devices as well as the potential increased cognitive processing for learners during CPR training.

Recommendation-Specific Supportive Text

1. Seven RCTs and 1 observational study examined the use of feedback devices during training relative to no use of feedback devices during training or instructor-led training.[1–6,17,18] Six studies demonstrated significant improvement in CPR skills at course completion when feedback devices were used during training,[1–6] whereas 2 studies failed to demonstrate benefit with CPR feedback device

use.[17,18] Five RCTs and 2 observational studies demonstrated that feedback device use during training was associated with significantly improved CPR skill retention at 7 days to 3 months.[2,6–10,19]

Some studies used lay rescuers, junior trainees, or medical students as the study population, limiting the generalizability of the findings to practicing healthcare providers.[2,3,5,9,10,17–19] Other studies combined real-time feedback with other educational strategies,[6,19] making it difficult to isolate the true impact of feedback device use. Future research should consider linking CPR feedback device use during training with actual patient outcomes or clinical performance of healthcare providers and reporting the cost-effectiveness of feedback device use during training.

REFERENCES

1. Cheng A, Brown LL, Duff JP, Davidson J, Overly F, Tofil NM, Peterson DT, White ML, Bhanji F, Bank I, et al; on behalf of the International Network for Simulation-Based Pediatric Innovation, Research, & Education (INSPIRE) CPR Investigators. Improving cardiopulmonary resuscitation with a CPR feedback device and refresher simulations (CPR CARES Study): a randomized clinical trial. *JAMA Pediatr.* 2015;169:137–144. doi: 10.1001/jamapediatrics.2014.2616
2. Katipoglu B, Madziala MA, Evrin T, Gawlowski P, Szarpak A, Dabrowska A, Bialka S, Ladny JR, Szarpak L, Konert A, et al. How should we teach cardiopulmonary resuscitation? Randomized multi-center study. *Cardiol J.* 2019:Epub ahead of print. doi: 10.5603/CJ.a2019.0092
3. McCoy CE, Rahman A, Rendon JC, Anderson CL, Langdorf MI, Lotfipour S, Chakravarthy B. Randomized controlled trial of simulation vs. standard training for teaching medical students high-quality cardiopulmonary resuscitation. *West J Emerg Med.* 2019;20:15–22. doi: 10.5811/westjem.2018.11.39040
4. Navarro-Patón R, Freire-Tellado M, Basanta-Camiño S, Barcala-Furelos R, Arufe-Giraldez V, Rodriguez-Fernández JE. Effect of 3basic life support training programs in future primary school teachers. A quasi-experimental design. *Med Intensiva.* 2018;42:207–215. doi: 10.1016/j.medin.2017.06.005
5. Wagner M, Bibl K, Hrdliczka E, Steinbauer P, Stiller M, Gröpel P, Goeral K, Salzer-Muhar U, Berger A, Schmölzer GM, et al. Effects of feedback on chest compression quality: a randomized simulation study. *Pediatrics.* 2019;143:e20182441. doi: 10.1542/peds.2018-2441
6. Lin Y, Cheng A, Grant VJ, Currie GR, Hecker KG. Improving CPR quality with distributed practice and real-time feedback in pediatric healthcare providers - A randomized controlled trial. *Resuscitation.* 2018;130:6–12. doi: 10.1016/j.resuscitation.2018.06.025
7. Niles DE, Nishisaki A, Sutton RM, Elci OU, Meaney PA, O'Connor KA, Leffelman J, Kramer-Johansen J, Berg RA, Nadkarni V. Improved Retention of Chest Compression Psychomotor Skills With Brief "Rolling Refresher" Training. *Simul Healthc.* 2017;12:213–219. doi: 10.1097/SIH.0000000000000228
8. Smart JR, Kranz K, Carmona F, Lindner TW, Newton A. Does real-time objective feedback and competition improve performance and quality in manikin CPR training–a prospective observational study from several European EMS. *Scand J Trauma Resusc Emerg Med.* 2015;23:79. doi: 10.1186/s13049-015-0160-9
9. Smereka J, Szarpak L, Czekajlo M, Abelson A, Zwolinski P, Plusa T, Dunder D, Dabrowski M, Wiesniewska Z, Robak O, et al. The TrueCPR device in the process of teaching cardiopulmonary resuscitation: a randomized simulation trial. *Medicine (Baltimore).* 2019;98:e15995. doi: 10.1097/MD.0000000000015995
10. Zhou XL, Wang J, Jin XQ, Zhao Y, Liu RL, Jiang C. Quality retention of chest compression after repetitive practices with or without feedback devices: A randomized manikin study. *Am J Emerg Med.* 2020;38:73–78. doi: 10.1016/j.ajem.2019.04.025
11. Ende J. Feedback in clinical medical education. *JAMA.* 1983;250:777–781.
12. Jones A, Lin Y, Nettel-Aguirre A, Gilfoyle E, Cheng A. Visual assessment of CPR quality during pediatric cardiac arrest: does point of view matter? *Resuscitation.* 2015;90:50–55. doi: 10.1016/j.resuscitation.2015.01.036
13. Cheng A, Overly F, Kessler D, Nadkarni VM, Lin Y, Doan Q, Duff JP, Tofil NM, Bhanji F, Adler M, Charnovich A, Hunt EA, Brown LL; International Network for Simulation-based Pediatric Innovation, Research, Education (INSPIRE) CPR Investigators. Perception of CPR quality: Influence of CPR feedback, Just-in-Time CPR training and provider role. *Resuscitation.* 2015;87:44–50. doi: 10.1016/j.resuscitation.2014.11.015
14. Hansen C, Bang C, Stærk M, Krogh K, Løfgren B. Certified Basic Life Support Instructors Identify Improper Cardiopulmonary Resuscitation Skills Poorly: Instructor Assessments Versus Resuscitation Manikin Data. *Simul Healthc.* 2019;14:281–286. doi: 10.1097/SIH.0000000000000386
15. Cheng A, Kessler D, Lin Y, Tofil NM, Hunt EA, Davidson J, Chatfield J, Duff JP; International Network for Simulation-based Pediatric Innovation, Research and Education (INSPIRE) CPR Investigators. Influence of Cardiopulmonary Resuscitation Coaching and Provider Role on Perception of Cardiopulmonary Resuscitation Quality During Simulated Pediatric Cardiac Arrest. *Pediatr Crit Care Med.* 2019;20:e191–e198. doi: 10.1097/PCC.0000000000001871
16. Greif R, Bhanji F, Bigham BL, Bray J, Breckwoldt J, Cheng A, Duff JP, Gilfoyle E, Hsieh M-J, Iwami T, et al; on behalf of the Education, Implementation, and Teams Collaborators. Education, implementation, and teams: 2020 International Consensus on Cardiopulmonary Resuscitation and Emergency Cardiovascular Care Science With Treatment Recommendations. *Circulation.* 2020;142(suppl 1):S222–S283. doi: 10.1161/CIR.0000000000000896
17. Min MK, Yeom SR, Ryu JH, Kim YI, Park MR, Han SK, Lee SH, Park SW, Park SC. Comparison between an instructor-led course and training using a voice advisory manikin in initial cardiopulmonary resuscitation skill acquisition. *Clin Exp Emerg Med.* 2016;3:158–164. doi: 10.15441/ceem.15.114
18. Pavo N, Goliasch G, Nierscher FJ, Stumpf D, Haugk M, Breckwoldt J, Ruetzler K, Greif R, Fischer H. Short structured feedback training is equivalent to a mechanical feedback device in two-rescuer BLS: a randomised simulation study. *Scand J Trauma Resusc Emerg Med.* 2016;24:70. doi: 10.1186/s13049-016-0265-9
19. Cortegiani A, Russotto V, Montalto F, Iozzo P, Meschis R, Pugliesi M, Mariano D, Benenati V, Raineri SM, Gregoretti C, Giarratano A. Use of a Real-Time Training Software (Laerdal QCPR®) Compared to Instructor-Based Feedback for High-Quality Chest Compressions Acquisition in Secondary School Students: A Randomized Trial. *PLoS One.* 2017;12:e0169591. doi: 10.1371/journal.pone.0169591

Gamified Learning and VR

Recommendations for Gamified Learning and VR

COR	LOE	Recommendations
2b	B-R	1. The use of gamified learning may be considered for basic or advanced life support training for lay rescuers and/or healthcare providers.[1–6]
2b	B-NR	2. The use of VR may be considered for basic or advanced life support training for lay rescuers and/or healthcare providers.[7–10]

Synopsis

Increasingly, the use of gamified learning and VR is being considered for training lay rescuers and healthcare providers.[11,12] Gamified learning includes leaderboards and serious games. *Leaderboards* are used for the purpose of increasing the frequency of practice by incorporating competition among trainees, whereas *serious games* are designed specifically for use of play (ie, board games, computer-based games) around a "serious" topic, such as resuscitation.[6,13] VR is a computer-generated interface with which a user can interact in a three-dimensional world in which objects have a sense of spatial presence.[14,15]

Review of the gamified learning and VR literature demonstrated mixed results, with some studies showing improved knowledge acquisition, knowledge retention, and CPR skills with these learning modalities,[1–5,7,16] whereas other studies showed no benefit.[6,8–10,17,18] No studies demonstrated a negative impact on learning. The effect of gamified learning and VR on performance during real cardiac arrests or on patient outcomes is unknown. Incorporation of gamified learning and VR into resuscitation programs should consider start-up costs associated with purchasing equipment and relevant software. *Augmented reality,* which incorporates a computer-generated holographic image overlaid into the real environment, was not included in this review because of a lack of relevant research.

Recommendation-Specific Supportive Text

1. Several studies evaluating the effect of gamified learning demonstrated an improvement in knowledge acquisition, knowledge retention, and CPR skills.[2–5] No studies demonstrated a negative impact on learning or notable adverse effects. The use of leaderboards demonstrated similarly mixed results, with 1 study showing improved CPR performance[1] and others demonstrating no significant improvement in frequency of CPR practice of CPR skill.[6]
2. Of the studies that evaluated VR for CPR training, 1 randomized and 1 observational cross-sectional study showed that VR improves knowledge and skills performance in both lay rescuers and healthcare providers.[7,8] One randomized study showed no difference compared with ACLS training with feedback in healthcare providers,[9] and 1 randomized study found that VR improved bystander response metrics (eg, requesting automated external defibrillator) but decreased chest compression depth, though neither cohort performed chest compression depth within guidelines.[10]

REFERENCES

1. MacKinnon RJ, Stoeter R, Doherty C, Fullwood C, Cheng A, Nadkarni V, Stenfors-Hayes T, Chang TP. Self-motivated learning with gamification improves infant CPR performance, a randomised controlled trial. *BMJ Stel* 2015;1:71–76.
2. Boada I, Rodriguez-Benitez A, Garcia-Gonzalez JM, Olivet J, Carreras V, Sbert M. Using a serious game to complement CPR instruction in a nurse faculty. *Comput Methods Programs Biomed.* 2015;122:282–291. doi: 10.1016/j.cmpb.2015.08.006
3. Desailly V, Hajage D, Pasquier P, Brun P, Iglesias P, Huet J, Masseran C, Claudon A, Ebeyer C, Truong T, et al. The use of the serious game Stayingalive® at school improves basic life support performed by secondary pupils: a randomized controlled study: proceedings of Réanimation 2017, the French Intensive Care Society International Congress. *Ann Intensive Care.* 2017;7:P49.
4. Otero-Agra M, Barcala-Furelos R, Besada-Saavedra I, Peixoto-Pino L, Martínez-Isasi S, Rodríguez-Núñez A. Let the kids play: gamification as a CPR training methodology in secondary school students. A quasi-experimental manikin simulation study. *Emerg Med J.* 2019;36:653–659. doi: 10.1136/emermed-2018-208108
5. Semeraro F, Frisoli A, Loconsole C, Mastronicola N, Stroppa F, Ristagno G, Scapigliati A, Marchetti L, Cerchiari E. Kids (learn how to) save lives in the school with the serious game Relive. *Resuscitation.* 2017;116:27–32. doi: 10.1016/j.resuscitation.2017.04.038
6. Chang TP, Raymond T, Dewan M, MacKinnon R, Whitfill T, Harwayne-Gidansky I, Doughty C, Frisell K, Kessler D, Wolfe H, Auerbach M, Rutledge C, Mitchell D, Jani P, Walsh CM; INSPIRE In-Hospital QCPR Leaderboard Investigators. The effect of an International competitive leaderboard on self-motivated simulation-based CPR practice among healthcare professionals: A randomized control trial. *Resuscitation.* 2019;138:273–281. doi: 10.1016/j.resuscitation.2019.02.050
7. Semeraro F, Frisoli A, Loconsole C, Bannò F, Tammaro G, Imbriaco G, Marchetti L, Cerchiari EL. Motion detection technology as a tool for cardiopulmonary resuscitation (CPR) quality training: a randomised crossover mannequin pilot study. *Resuscitation.* 2013;84:501–507. doi: 10.1016/j.resuscitation.2012.12.006
8. Espinoza ED. Virtual reality in cardiopulmonary resuscitation training: a randomized trial [in Spanish]. *Emergencias.* 2019:43.
9. Khanal P, Vankipuram A, Ashby A, Vankipuram M, Gupta A, Drumm-Gurnee D, Josey K, Tinker L, Smith M. Collaborative virtual reality based advanced cardiac life support training simulator using virtual reality principles. *J Biomed Inform.* 2014;51:49–59. doi: 10.1016/j.jbi.2014.04.005
10. Leary M, McGovern SK, Chaudhary Z, Patel J, Abella BS, Blewer AL. Comparing bystander response to a sudden cardiac arrest using a virtual reality CPR training mobile app versus a standard CPR training mobile app. *Resuscitation.* 2019;139:167–173. doi: 10.1016/j.resuscitation.2019.04.017
11. Cheng A, Nadkarni VM, Mancini MB, Hunt EA, Sinz EH, Merchant RM, Donoghue A, Duff JP, Eppich W, Auerbach M, Bigham BL, Blewer AL, Chan PS, Bhanji F; American Heart Association Education Science Investigators; and on behalf of the American Heart Association Education Science and Programs Committee, Council on Cardiopulmonary, Critical Care, Perioperative and Resuscitation; Council on Cardiovascular and Stroke Nursing; and Council on Quality of Care and Outcomes Research. Resuscitation Education Science: Educational Strategies to Improve Outcomes From Cardiac Arrest: A Scientific Statement From the American Heart Association. *Circulation.* 2018;138:e82–e122. doi: 10.1161/CIR.0000000000000583
12. Rumsfeld JS, Brooks SC, Aufderheide TP, Leary M, Bradley SM, Nkonde-Price C, Schwamm LH, Jessup M, Ferrer JM, Merchant RM; American Heart Association Emergency Cardiovascular Care Committee; Council on Cardiopulmonary, Critical Care, Perioperative and Resuscitation; Council on Quality of Care and Outcomes Research; Council on Cardiovascular and Stroke Nursing; and Council on Epidemiology and Prevention. Use of Mobile Devices, Social Media, and Crowdsourcing as Digital Strategies to Improve Emergency Cardiovascular Care: A Scientific Statement From the American Heart Association. *Circulation.* 2016;134:e87–e108. doi: 10.1161/CIR.0000000000000428
13. Graafland M, Schraagen JM, Schijven MP. Systematic review of serious games for medical education and surgical skills training. *Br J Surg.* 2012;99:1322–1330. doi: 10.1002/bjs.8819
14. Lopreiato JO. *Heatlhcare Simulation Dictionary.* Rockville, MD: Agency for Healthcare Research and Quality; 2016. https://www.ahrq.gov/sites/default/files/publications/files/sim-dictionary.pdf. Accessed April 27, 2020.
15. Giraldi G, Silva R, de Oliveira JC. Introduction to virtual reality. https://www.lncc.br/~jauvane/papers/RelatorioTecnicoLNCC-0603.pdf. Accessed February 14, 2020.
16. Ghoman SK, Patel SD, Cutumisu M, von Hauff P, Jeffery T, Brown MRG, Schmölzer GM. Serious games, a game changer in teaching neonatal resuscitation? A review. *Arch Dis Child Fetal Neonatal Ed.* 2020;105:98–107. doi: 10.1136/archdischild-2019-317011
17. Drummond D, Delval P, Abdenouri S, Truchot J, Ceccaldi PF, Plaisance P, Hadchouel A, Tesnière A. Serious game versus online course for pretraining medical students before a simulation-based mastery learning course on cardiopulmonary resuscitation: A randomised controlled study. *Eur J Anaesthesiol.* 2017;34:836–844. doi: 10.1097/EJA.0000000000000675
18. Yeung J, Kovic I, Vidacic M, Skilton E, Higgins D, Melody T, Lockey A. The school Lifesavers study-A randomised controlled trial comparing the impact of Lifesaver only, face-to-face training only, and Lifesaver with face-to-face training on CPR knowledge, skills and attitudes in UK school children. *Resuscitation.* 2017;120:138–145. doi: 10.1016/j.resuscitation.2017.08.010

Precourse Preparation for Advanced Courses

Recommendation for Precourse Preparation for Advanced Courses		
COR	LOE	Recommendation
2b	C-LD	1. It may be reasonable to incorporate precourse eLearning into existing advanced courses.[1,2]

Synopsis

Learners can maximize their learning opportunities during advanced life support courses by being well prepared before arriving in the classroom.[3] Learners can accomplish this by completing precourse learning assignments or reviewing course materials before attending class. Courses providing precourse preparation, such as screen-based simulation,[1,2] allow the instructor to focus classroom time on blending newly acquired knowledge with technical skill and teamwork practice necessary to improve learning outcomes. We reviewed the literature to determine if precourse preparation was effective as a supplement to traditional advanced life support training conducted with an instructor.[4] Two RCTs addressed the research question; 1 study demonstrated improved performance on some individual CPR performance variables, but neither demonstrated improved overall pass rates.[1,2] The literature search identified 3 additional studies in which precourse preparation replaced the first day of a traditional 2-day advanced life support course; these studies were excluded from the current review. Given the unclear benefit and low risk, it may be reasonable to incorporate precourse learning when possible. Future studies should examine the comparative effectiveness of different modes of content delivery in precourse learning.

Recommendation-Specific Supportive Text

1. A systematic review identified 2 RCTs relevant to the research question.[1,2] In both studies, learners were given access to a computer-based simulation program from 2 to 4 weeks before the start of the course. In 1 RCT, precourse preparation was associated with improved time to defibrillate ventricular fibrillation (112 seconds versus 149.9 seconds; $P<0.05$) and improved time to pacing of symptomatic bradycardia (95.1 seconds versus 154.9 seconds; $P<0.05$) but no improvement in course pass rates.[1] A second RCT demonstrated no improvement in clinical performance and knowledge with the addition of precourse preparation via screen-based learning.[2] It is difficult to fully understand the impact of precourse preparation because both studies provided precourse access for all learners but only 1 trial subjectively monitored whether the learner actually participated in the simulation exercises.[2] In that trial, one third of the learners came to class without accessing the precourse simulations. Those learners who did access the simulations spent about 2 hours on average.

REFERENCES

1. Nacca N, Holliday J, Ko PY. Randomized trial of a novel ACLS teaching tool: does it improve student performance? *West J Emerg Med.* 2014;15:913–918. doi: 10.5811/westjem.2014.9.20149
2. Perkins GD, Fullerton JN, Davis-Gomez N, Davies RP, Baldock C, Stevens H, Bullock I, Lockey AS. The effect of pre-course e-learning prior to advanced life support training: a randomised controlled trial. *Resuscitation.* 2010;81:877–881. doi: 10.1016/j.resuscitation.2010.03.019
3. Bhanji F, Donoghue AJ, Wolff MS, Flores GE, Halamek LP, Berman JM, Sinz EH, Cheng A. Part 14: education: 2015 American Heart Association Guidelines Update for Cardiopulmonary Resuscitation and Emergency Cardiovascular Care. *Circulation.* 2015;132(suppl 2):S561–573. doi: 10.1161/CIR.0000000000000268
4. Greif R, Bhanji F, Bigham BL, Bray J, Breckwoldt J, Cheng A, Duff JP, Gilfoyle E, Hsieh M-J, Iwami T, et al; on behalf of the Education, Implementation, and Teams Collaborators. Education, implementation, and teams: 2020 International Consensus on Cardiopulmonary Resuscitation and Emergency Cardiovascular Care Science With Treatment Recommendations. *Circulation.* 2020;142(suppl 1):S222–S283. doi: 10.1161/CIR.0000000000000896

Opioid Overdose Training for Lay Rescuers

Recommendation for Opioid Overdose Training for Lay Rescuers		
COR	LOE	Recommendation
2a	C-LD	1. It is reasonable for lay rescuers to receive training in responding to opioid overdose, including provision of naloxone.[1–8]

Synopsis

According to the Centers for Disease Control and Prevention, opioid overdose deaths in the United States have more than doubled in the past decade, from 18 515 in 2007 to 47 600 in 2017.[9] Improving recognition of opioid overdose and increasing lay rescuers' willingness and ability to administer naloxone has the potential to improve outcomes. A scoping review was conducted to determine the impact of targeted resuscitation and naloxone training on opioid users and lay rescuers likely to encounter an opioid overdose.[10] Educational interventions included training programs for family members of opioid users (including naloxone distribution), computer-based training of opioid users, peer-to-peer training (ie, opioid users teaching other opioid users), and brief counseling by emergency department staff.[1–8]

Educating opioid users[5,7] and their friends, families,[1] and close contacts[5] improves willingness and ability to administer naloxone, risk awareness, overdose knowledge recognition, and attitudes toward calling EMS.[3,10] We suggest that people who use opioids or those who may witness an opioid overdose receive training in responding to opioid overdose, including the administration of naloxone. The data reviewed are limited by the inability to link population-level interventions to individual patient outcomes. More research is required to determine which educational interventions provide the greatest benefit by measuring both learner and patient outcomes.

Recommendation-Specific Supportive Text

1. Eight studies (1 RCT and 7 observational studies)[1–8] assessed the impact of opioid training using a comparator group. These studies evaluated the impact of short educational courses, with opioid users, friends, and family members as participants. Outcomes were heterogenous and included knowledge of risk, identifying overdose, knowledge and skill to respond to overdose, and willingness to aid or phone for help.[1,3–8]

   One RCT found that 60% of witnessed overdoses involving an individual who had been trained within the prior 3 months received first aid and/or naloxone compared with zero in the comparator group.[1] In an observational study, 40% of participants who witnessed an overdose in the 12 months after education administered naloxone.[5] Another study found that the rate of naloxone administration was higher in those who had received opioid training compared with those who did not (32% versus 0%).[4] They found no difference in the rates of calling 9-1-1 or delivering rescue breaths between the 2 groups.[4] Another study found no difference in the provision of aid between trained and untrained responders.[2] Interventions that included skills practice (ie, naloxone administration) were more likely to lead to improved clinical performance compared with interventions without skills practice.[1,11–22]

REFERENCES

1. Williams AV, Marsden J, Strang J. Training family members to manage heroin overdose and administer naloxone: randomized trial of effects on knowledge and attitudes. *Addiction.* 2014;109:250–259. doi: 10.1111/add.12360
2. Doe-Simkins M, Quinn E, Xuan Z, Sorensen-Alawad A, Hackman H, Ozonoff A, Walley AY. Overdose rescues by trained and untrained participants and change in opioid use among substance-using participants in overdose education and naloxone distribution programs: a retrospective cohort study. *BMC Public Health.* 2014;14:297. doi: 10.1186/1471-2458-14-297
3. Dunn KE, Yepez-Laubach C, Nuzzo PA, Fingerhood M, Kelly A, Berman S, Bigelow GE. Randomized controlled trial of a computerized opioid overdose education intervention. *Drug Alcohol Depend.* 2017;173 Suppl 1:S39–S47. doi: 10.1016/j.drugalcdep.2016.12.003
4. Dwyer K, Walley AY, Langlois BK, Mitchell PM, Nelson KP, Cromwell J, Bernstein E. Opioid education and nasal naloxone rescue kits in the emergency department. *West J Emerg Med.* 2015;16:381–384. doi: 10.5811/westjem.2015.2.24909
5. Espelt A, Bosque-Prous M, Folch C, Sarasa-Renedo A, Majó X, Casabona J, Brugal MT; REDAN Group. Is systematic training in opioid overdose prevention effective? *PLoS One.* 2017;12:e0186833. doi: 10.1371/journal.pone.0186833
6. Franko TS II, Distefano D, Lewis L. A novel naloxone training compared with current recommended training in an overdose simulation. *J Am Pharm Assoc (2003).* 2019;59:375–378. doi: 10.1016/j.japh.2018.12.022
7. Jones JD, Roux P, Stancliff S, Matthews W, Comer SD. Brief overdose education can significantly increase accurate recognition of opioid overdose among heroin users. *Int J Drug Policy.* 2014;25:166–170. doi: 10.1016/j.drugpo.2013.05.006
8. Lott DC, Rhodes J. Opioid overdose and naloxone education in a substance use disorder treatment program. *Am J Addict.* 2016;25:221–226. doi: 10.1111/ajad.12364
9. National Institute on Drug Abuse. Overdose death rates. 2020. https://www.drugabuse.gov/related-topics/trends-statistics/overdose-death-rates. Updated March 2020. Accessed March 18, 2020.
10. Greif R, Bhanji F, Bigham BL, Bray J, Breckwoldt J, Cheng A, Duff JP, Gilfoyle E, Hsieh M-J, Iwami T, et al; on behalf of the Education, Implementation, and Teams Collaborators. Education, implementation, and teams: 2020 International Consensus on Cardiopulmonary Resuscitation and Emergency Cardiovascular Care Science With Treatment Recommendations. *Circulation.* 2020;142(suppl 1):S222–S283. DOI: 10.1161/CIR.0000000000000896
11. Pietrusza LM, Puskar KR, Ren D, Mitchell AM. Evaluation of an Opiate Overdose Educational Intervention and Naloxone Prescribing Program in Homeless Adults Who Use Opiates. *J Addict Nurs.* 2018;29:188–195. doi: 10.1097/JAN.0000000000000235
12. Katzman JG, Greenberg NH, Takeda MY, Moya Balasch M. Characteristics of Patients With Opioid Use Disorder Associated With Performing Overdose Reversals in the Community: An Opioid Treatment Program Analysis. *J Addict Med.* 2019;13:131–138. doi: 10.1097/ADM.0000000000000461
13. Piper TM, Stancliff S, Rudenstine S, Sherman S, Nandi V, Clear A, Galea S. Evaluation of a naloxone distribution and administration program in New York City. *Subst Use Misuse.* 2008;43:858–870. doi: 10.1080/10826080701801261
14. Walley AY, Doe-Simkins M, Quinn E, Pierce C, Xuan Z, Ozonoff A. Opioid overdose prevention with intranasal naloxone among people who take methadone. *J Subst Abuse Treat.* 2013;44:241–247. doi: 10.1016/j.jsat.2012.07.004
15. Walley AY, Xuan Z, Hackman HH, Quinn E, Doe-Simkins M, Sorensen-Alawad A, Ruiz S, Ozonoff A. Opioid overdose rates and implementation of overdose education and nasal naloxone distribution in Massachusetts: interrupted time series analysis. *BMJ.* 2013;346:f174. doi: 10.1136/bmj.f174
16. Wagner KD, Bovet LJ, Haynes B, Joshua A, Davidson PJ. Training law enforcement to respond to opioid overdose with naloxone: Impact on knowledge, attitudes, and interactions with community members. *Drug Alcohol Depend.* 2016;165:22–28. doi: 10.1016/j.drugalcdep.2016.05.008
17. Dahlem CHG, King L, Anderson G, Marr A, Waddell JE, Scalera M. Beyond rescue: Implementation and evaluation of revised naloxone training for law enforcement officers. *Public Health Nurs.* 2017;34:516–521. doi: 10.1111/phn.12365
18. Panther SG, Bray BS, White JR. The implementation of a naloxone rescue program in university students. *J Am Pharm Assoc (2003).* 2017;57:S107–S112 e102. doi: 10.1016/j.japh.2016.11.002
19. Mcauley A, Lindsay G, Woods M, Louttit D. Responsible management and use of a personal take-home naloxone supply: a pilot project. *Drugs: Education, Prevention and Policy.* 2010;17:388–399.
20. Seal KH, Thawley R, Gee L, Bamberger J, Kral AH, CiccaroneD, DowningM, EdlinBR. Naloxonedistributionandcardiopulmonary resuscitation training for injection drug users to prevent heroin overdose death: a pilot intervention study. *J Urban Health.* 2005;82:303–311. doi: 10.1093/jurban/jti053
21. Tobin KE, Sherman SG, Beilenson P, Welsh C, Latkin CA. Evaluation of the Staying Alive programme: training injection drug users to properly administer naloxone and save lives. *Int J Drug Policy.* 2009;20:131–136. doi: 10.1016/j.drugpo.2008.03.002
22. Lankenau SE, Wagner KD, Silva K, Kecojevic A, Iverson E, McNeely M, Kral AH. Injection drug users trained by overdose prevention programs: responses to witnessed overdoses. *J Community Health.* 2013;38:133–141. doi: 10.1007/s10900-012-9591-7

PROVIDER CONSIDERATIONS

Disparities in Education

Recommendations for Disparities in Education		
COR	LOE	Recommendations
1	B-NR	1. It is recommended to target and tailor layperson CPR training to specific racial and ethnic populations and neighborhoods in the United States.[1–10]
1	B-NR	2. It is recommended to target low-SES populations and neighborhoods for layperson CPR training and awareness efforts.[11–20]
2a	C-LD	3. It is reasonable to address barriers to B-CPR for female victims through educational training and public awareness efforts.[21–24]

Synopsis

Health disparities adversely affect groups that have systematically experienced greater obstacles to health based on social determinants such as race, ethnicity, SES, and gender.[25] We defined racial and ethnic populations as individuals and neighborhoods that have historically experienced inequity or prejudice, such as black or Hispanic people and linguistically isolated communities with limited English proficiency. SES was characterized by self-identified income and education by individual or neighborhood. Gender was defined on the individual level as self-identified or clinician-identified male or female gender. We examined whether race, ethnicity, SES, and gender are associated with lower rates of B-CPR or CPR training to understand if targeted training for these populations is warranted.[1–24] Predominantly black, Hispanic, and low-SES neighborhoods have lower rates of B-CPR and CPR training.[3–5,16] Language barriers are associated with lower rates of CPR training.[9,10] Women are less likely to receive B-CPR, which may be because bystanders fear injuring female victims or accusations of inappropriate touching.[22,23] The targeting of specific racial, ethnic, and low-SES populations for CPR education and modification of education to address gender differences could eliminate disparities in CPR training and B-CPR and potentially enhance outcomes from cardiac arrest in these populations. Future work examining the racial, socioeconomic, and gender barriers to B-CPR and CPR education is critical to advance our understanding of these important issues.

Recommendation-Specific Supportive Text

1. Four retrospective cohort studies and 1 cross-sectional study found that residents of black and Hispanic neighborhoods were less likely to receive B-CPR and that black residents were less likely to be CPR trained.[1–5] A descriptive investigation found few high-quality CPR educational resources for Spanish-speaking populations.[6] Mixed qualitative studies suggest that language barriers, financial considerations, and lack of information are associated with low rates of B-CPR in linguistically isolated communities.[6–10]
2. Several retrospective cohort studies have demonstrated that low SES is associated with a lower likelihood of receiving B-CPR.[11–16] In addition, recent cross-sectional studies found that low SES is associated with a lower likelihood of CPR training.[17,18] To address this, retrospective studies have demonstrated the feasibility of using neighborhood mapping to identify low-SES neighborhoods for targeted training.[19,20]
3. A recent study examining gender differences in the delivery of B-CPR found that men were more likely than women to receive B-CPR in public locations.[21] Cross-sectional survey studies suggest that layperson responders are fearful of being accused of inappropriate touching, sexual assault, and causing injury to female victims in need of B-CPR.[22,23] A randomized simulation study found that subjects were less likely to remove the clothing of a female manikin than a male manikin.[24]

REFERENCES

1. Brookoff D, Kellermann AL, Hackman BB, Somes G, Dobyns P. Do blacks get bystander cardiopulmonary resuscitation as often as whites? *Ann Emerg Med.* 1994;24:1147–1150. doi: 10.1016/s0196-0644(94)70246-2
2. Vadeboncoeur TF, Richman PB, Darkoh M, Chikani V, Clark L, Bobrow BJ. Bystander cardiopulmonary resuscitation for out-of-hospital cardiac arrest in the Hispanic vs the non-Hispanic populations. *Am J Emerg Med.* 2008;26:655–660. doi: 10.1016/j.ajem.2007.10.002
3. Anderson ML, Cox M, Al-Khatib SM, Nichol G, Thomas KL, Chan PS, Saha-Chaudhuri P, Fosbol EL, Eigel B, Clendenen B, Peterson ED. Rates of cardiopulmonary resuscitation training in the United States. *JAMA Intern Med.* 2014;174:194–201. doi: 10.1001/jamainternmed.2013.11320
4. Fosbøl EL, Dupre ME, Strauss B, Swanson DR, Myers B, McNally BF, Anderson ML, Bagai A, Monk L, Garvey JL, Bitner M, Jollis JG, Granger CB. Association of neighborhood characteristics with incidence of out-of-hospital cardiac arrest and rates of bystander-initiated CPR: implications for community-based education intervention. *Resuscitation.* 2014;85:1512–1517. doi: 10.1016/j.resuscitation.2014.08.013
5. Blewer AL, Schmicker RH, Morrison LJ, Aufderheide TP, Daya M, Starks MA, May S, Idris AH, Callaway CW, Kudenchuk PJ, Vilke GM, Abella BS; Resuscitation Outcomes Consortium Investigators. Variation in Bystander Cardiopulmonary Resuscitation Delivery and Subsequent Survival From Out-of-Hospital Cardiac Arrest Based on Neighborhood-Level Ethnic Characteristics. *Circulation.* 2020;141:34–41. doi: 10.1161/CIRCULATIONAHA.119.041541
6. Liu KY, Haukoos JS, Sasson C. Availability and quality of cardiopulmonary resuscitation information for Spanish-speaking population on the Internet. *Resuscitation.* 2014;85:131–137. doi: 10.1016/j.resuscitation.2013.08.274
7. Yip MP, Ong B, Tu SP, Chavez D, Ike B, Painter I, Lam I, Bradley SM, Coronado GD, Meischke HW. Diffusion of cardiopulmonary resuscitation training to Chinese immigrants with limited English proficiency. *Emerg Med Int.* 2011;2011:685249. doi: 10.1155/2011/685249
8. Meischke H, Taylor V, Calhoun R, Liu Q, Sos C, Tu SP, Yip MP, Eisenberg D. Preparedness for cardiac emergencies among Cambodians with limited English proficiency. *J Community Health.* 2012;37:176–180. doi: 10.1007/s10900-011-9433-z
9. Sasson C, Haukoos JS, Bond C, Rabe M, Colbert SH, King R, Sayre M, Heisler M. Barriers and facilitators to learning and performing cardiopulmonary resuscitation in neighborhoods with low bystander cardiopulmonary resuscitation prevalence and high rates of cardiac arrest in Columbus, OH. *Circ Cardiovasc Qual Outcomes.* 2013;6:550–558. doi: 10.1161/CIRCOUTCOMES.111.000097

10. Sasson C, Haukoos JS, Ben-Youssef L, Ramirez L, Bull S, Eigel B, Magid DJ, Padilla R. Barriers to calling 911 and learning and performing cardiopulmonary resuscitation for residents of primarily Latino, high-risk neighborhoods in Denver, Colorado. *Ann Emerg Med.* 2015;65:545–552.e2. doi: 10.1016/j.annemergmed.2014.10.028
11. Mitchell MJ, Stubbs BA, Eisenberg MS. Socioeconomic status is associated with provision of bystander cardiopulmonary resuscitation. *Prehosp Emerg Care.* 2009;13:478–486. doi: 10.1080/10903120903144833
12. Vaillancourt C, Lui A, De Maio VJ, Wells GA, Stiell IG. Socioeconomic status influences bystander CPR and survival rates for out-of-hospital cardiac arrest victims. *Resuscitation.* 2008;79:417–423. doi: 10.1016/j.resuscitation.2008.07.012
13. Chiang WC, Ko PC, Chang AM, Chen WT, Liu SS, Huang YS, Chen SY, Lin CH, Cheng MT, Chong KM, Wang HC, Yang CW, Liao MW, Wang CH, Chien YC, Lin CH, Liu YP, Lee BC, Chien KL, Lai MS, Ma MH. Bystander-initiated CPR in an Asian metropolitan: does the socioeconomic status matter? *Resuscitation.* 2014;85:53–58. doi: 10.1016/j.resuscitation.2013.07.033
14. Moncur L, Ainsborough N, Ghose R, Kendal SP, Salvatori M, Wright J. Does the level of socioeconomic deprivation at the location of cardiac arrest in an English region influence the likelihood of receiving bystander-initiated cardiopulmonary resuscitation? *Emerg Med J.* 2016;33:105–108. doi: 10.1136/emermed-2015-204643
15. Dahan B, Jabre P, Karam N, Misslin R, Tafflet M, Bougouin W, Jost D, Beganton F, Marijon E, Jouven X. Impact of neighbourhood socio-economic status on bystander cardiopulmonary resuscitation in Paris. *Resuscitation.* 2017;110:107–113. doi: 10.1016/j.resuscitation.2016.10.028
16. Brown TP, Booth S, Hawkes CA, Soar J, Mark J, Mapstone J, Fothergill RT, Black S, Pocock H, Bichmann A, Gunson I, Perkins GD. Characteristics of neighbourhoods with high incidence of out-of-hospital cardiac arrest and low bystander cardiopulmonary resuscitation rates in England. *Eur Heart J Qual Care Clin Outcomes.* 2019;5:51–62. doi: 10.1093/ehjqcco/qcy026
17. Blewer AL, Ibrahim SA, Leary M, Dutwin D, McNally B, Anderson ML, Morrison LJ, Aufderheide TP, Daya M, Idris AH, et al. Cardiopulmonary resuscitation training disparities in the United States *J Am Heart Assoc.* 2017;6:e006124. doi: 10.1161/JAHA.117.006124
18. Abdulhay NM, Totolos K, McGovern S, Hewitt N, Bhardwaj A, Buckler DG, Leary M, Abella BS. Socioeconomic disparities in layperson CPR training within a large U.S. city. *Resuscitation.* 2019;141:13–18. doi: 10.1016/j.resuscitation.2019.05.038
19. Sasson C, Keirns CC, Smith DM, Sayre MR, Macy ML, Meurer WJ, McNally BF, Kellermann AL, Iwashyna TJ. Examining the contextual effects of neighborhood on out-of-hospital cardiac arrest and the provision of bystander cardiopulmonary resuscitation. *Resuscitation.* 2011;82:674–679. doi: 10.1016/j.resuscitation.2011.02.002
20. Root ED, Gonzales L, Persse DE, Hinchey PR, McNally B, Sasson C. A tale of two cities: the role of neighborhood socioeconomic status in spatial clustering of bystander CPR in Austin and Houston. *Resuscitation.* 2013;84:752–759. doi: 10.1016/j.resuscitation.2013.01.007
21. Blewer AL, McGovern SK, Schmicker RH, May S, Morrison LJ, Aufderheide TP, Daya M, Idris AH, Callaway CW, Kudenchuk PJ, Vilke GM, Abella BS; Resuscitation Outcomes Consortium (ROC) Investigators. Gender Disparities Among Adult Recipients of Bystander Cardiopulmonary Resuscitation in the Public. *Circ Cardiovasc Qual Outcomes.* 2018;11:e004710. doi: 10.1161/CIRCOUTCOMES.118.004710
22. Becker TK, Gul SS, Cohen SA, Maciel CB, Baron-Lee J, Murphy TW, Youn TS, Tyndall JA, Gibbons C, Hart L, Alviar CL; Florida Cardiac Arrest Resource Team. Public perception towards bystander cardiopulmonary resuscitation. *Emerg Med J.* 2019;36:660–665. doi: 10.1136/emermed-2018-208234
23. Perman SM, Shelton SK, Knoepke C, Rappaport K, Matlock DD, Adelgais K, Havranek EP, Daugherty SL. Public Perceptions on Why Women Receive Less Bystander Cardiopulmonary Resuscitation Than Men in Out-of-Hospital Cardiac Arrest. *Circulation.* 2019;139:1060–1068. doi: 10.1161/CIRCULATIONAHA.118.037692
24. Kramer CE, Wilkins MS, Davies JM, Caird JK, Hallihan GM. Does the sex of a simulated patient affect CPR? *Resuscitation.* 2015;86:82–87. doi: 10.1016/j.resuscitation.2014.10.016
25. LaVeist TA. *Race, Ethnicity, and Health: A Public Health Reader.* Hoboken, NJ: John Wiley & Sons, Inc; 2002.

EMS Practitioner Experience and Exposure to OHCA

Recommendation for EMS Practitioner Experience and Exposure to OHCA		
COR	**LOE**	**Recommendation**
2a	C-LD	1. It is reasonable for EMS systems to monitor clinical personnel's exposure to resuscitation to ensure treating teams have members competent in the management of cardiac arrest cases. Competence of teams may be supported through staffing or training strategies.[1–6]

Synopsis

Appropriate provision of prehospital resuscitative care is an important element in determining outcomes from OHCA.[7] Understanding the impact of ongoing exposure (ie, caring for actual patients in cardiac arrest) or general experience (ie, time on the job) on patient outcomes from OHCA may inform staffing and training strategies. A systematic review suggests that EMS provider exposure—both the number of cardiac arrest cases managed over time and the most recent exposure to cardiac arrest (less than 6 months)—is associated with improved return of spontaneous circulation (ROSC)[2,3] and survival to hospital discharge.[1,8] Results of the individual studies were inconsistent, but those of higher quality that adjusted for known predictors of survival demonstrated improved survival outcomes with higher EMS provider exposure.[1] EMS provider experience (years on the job) was not associated with improved survival to discharge.[1]

It is reasonable for EMS systems to monitor provider exposure to resuscitation to implement strategies to address issues of low exposure or to ensure that treating teams have members with recent exposure to cardiac arrest cases. The benefits of adjusting staffing or supplementing exposure through simulation-based training need to be weighed against the practicality of scheduling and the additional costs of training because they may come at the expense of other potentially beneficial quality improvement activities. We are unable to make any recommendations on the exposure required to care for pediatric cardiac arrest victims.

Recommendation-Specific Supportive Text

1. Results of a systematic review identified 2 observational studies that evaluated an impact of provider exposure.[1,3] The larger study reporting adjusted outcomes found improved survival to discharge with higher team exposure (number of cardiac arrests in the preceding 3 years). Compared with teams with 6 or fewer exposures, the likelihood of survival was higher in groups with more than 6 to 11 exposures (adjusted odds ratio, 1.26; 95% CI, 1.04–1.54), 11 to 17 exposures (adjusted odds ratio, 1.29; 95% CI, 1.04–1.59), and more than 17 exposures (adjusted odds ratio, 1.50; 95% CI, 1.22–1.86), suggesting

a "dose-response" relationship with exposure.[1] The remaining observational study reporting unadjusted outcomes found no association between exposure and survival to hospital discharge.

One observational study found lower survival to discharge in patients treated by teams with no exposure in the preceding 6 months compared with those with recent (less than 1 month) exposure (adjusted odds ratio, 0.70; 95% CI, 0.54–0.91).[1] Additional studies found no association between team leader cardiac arrest exposure and event survival[3] and no association between years of clinical experience of the EMS provider or EMS team and survival to hospital discharge.[1,4,9] Two studies reported improved ROSC with higher primary treating paramedic exposure.[2,3]

REFERENCES

1. Dyson K, Bray JE, Smith K, Bernard S, Straney L, Finn J. Paramedic Exposure to Out-of-Hospital Cardiac Arrest Resuscitation Is Associated With Patient Survival. *Circ Cardiovasc Qual Outcomes.* 2016;9:154–160. doi: 10.1161/CIRCOUTCOMES.115.002317
2. Tuttle JE, Hubble MW. Paramedic out-of-hospital cardiac arrest case volume is a predictor of return of spontaneous circulation *West J Emerg Med.* 2018;19:654–659. doi: 10.5811/westjem.2018.3.37051
3. Weiss N, Ross E, Cooley C, Polk J, Velasquez C, Harper S, Walrath B, Redman T, Mapp J, Wampler D. Does Experience Matter? Paramedic Cardiac Resuscitation Experience Effect on Out-of-Hospital Cardiac Arrest Outcomes. *Prehosp Emerg Care.* 2018;22:332–337. doi: 10.1080/10903127.2017.1392665
4. Gold LS, Eisenberg MS. The effect of paramedic experience on survival from cardiac arrest. *Prehosp Emerg Care.* 2009;13:341–344. doi: 10.1080/10903120902935389
5. Soo LH, Gray D, Young T, Skene A, Hampton JR. Influence of ambulance crew's length of experience on the outcome of out-of-hospital cardiac arrest. *Eur Heart J.* 1999;20:535–540.
6. Bjornsson HM, Marelsson S, Magnusson V, Sigurdsson G, Thorgeirsson G. Physician experience in addition to ACLS training does not significantly affect the outcome of prehospital cardiac arrest. *Eur J Emerg Med.* 2011;18:64–67. doi: 10.1097/MEJ.0b013e32833c6642
7. Perkins GD, Jacobs IG, Nadkarni VM, Berg RA, Bhanji F, Biarent D, Bossaert LL, Brett SJ, Chamberlain D, de Caen AR, Deakin CD, Finn JC, Gräsner JT, Hazinski MF, Iwami T, Koster RW, Lim SH, Huei-Ming Ma M, McNally BF, Morley PT, Morrison LJ, Monsieurs KG, Montgomery W, Nichol G, Okada K, Eng Hock Ong M, Travers AH, Nolan JP; Utstein Collaborators. Cardiac arrest and cardiopulmonary resuscitation outcome reports: update of the Utstein Resuscitation Registry Templates for Out-of-Hospital Cardiac Arrest: a statement for healthcare professionals from a task force of the International Liaison Committee on Resuscitation (American Heart Association, European Resuscitation Council, Australian and New Zealand Council on Resuscitation, Heart and Stroke Foundation of Canada, InterAmerican Heart Foundation, Resuscitation Council of Southern Africa, Resuscitation Council of Asia); and the American Heart Association Emergency Cardiovascular Care Committee and the Council on Cardiopulmonary, Critical Care, Perioperative and Resuscitation. *Circulation.* 2015;132:1286–1300. doi: 10.1161/CIR.0000000000000144
8. Greif R, Bhanji F, Bigham BL, Bray J, Breckwoldt J, Cheng A, Duff JP, Gilfoyle E, Hsieh M-J, Iwami T, et al; on behalf of the Education, Implementation, and Teams Collaborators. Education, implementation, and teams: 2020 International Consensus on Cardiopulmonary Resuscitation and Emergency Cardiovascular Care Science With Treatment Recommendations. *Circulation.* 2020;142(suppl 1):S222–S283. doi: 10.1161/CIR.0000000000000896
9. Lukić A, Lulić I, Lulić D, Ognjanović Z, Cerovečki D, Telebar S, Mašić I. Analysis of out-of-hospital cardiac arrest in Croatia—survival, bystander cardiopulmonary resuscitation, and impact of physician's experience on cardiac arrest management: a single center observational study. *Croat Med J.* 2016;57:591–600. doi: 10.3325/cmj.2016.57.591

ACLS Course Participation

Recommendation for ACLS Course Participation		
COR	**LOE**	**Recommendation**
2a	C-LD	1. It is reasonable for healthcare professionals to take an adult ACLS course or equivalent training.[1–9]

Synopsis

Resuscitation councils have offered adult advanced life support courses (eg, ACLS offered by the AHA, Advanced Life Support course offered by the European Resuscitation Council) for more than 3 decades, providing the knowledge and skills required to recognize and treat critically ill adult patients.[10] The course is intended for healthcare professionals likely to manage adult patients with cardiac arrest. ACLS course content and instructional design is updated every 5 years to reflect the most current resuscitation guidelines, and recent versions have focused on interprofessional, team-based care via simulation-based training.[10–12] A meta-analysis of relevant studies found that resuscitation teams with 1 or more team members having previous participation in an ACLS course results in improved patient outcomes, including ROSC, survival to hospital discharge, and survival to 30 days.[9,13] For this reason, we recommend that all healthcare professionals likely to participate in the care of adult cardiac arrest patients take the ACLS course or equivalent training.

The benefits of course participation should be weighed against the costs of taking the course, particularly in low-resource settings where taking ACLS may come at the expense of other beneficial interventions. We are unable to make a recommendation for neonatal and pediatric healthcare providers, given the lack of evidence evaluating patient outcomes from PALS and Neonatal Resuscitation Program courses.

Recommendation-Specific Supportive Text

1. A recent systematic review found evidence from 6 observational studies[3–8] enrolling 1461 patients with higher rates of ROSC for adult in-hospital cardiac arrest cared for by a resuscitation team with at least 1 member completing an accredited ACLS course compared with patients cared for by a team without members with prior ACLS training (odds ratio, 1.64; 95% CI, 1.12–2.41).[9] The systematic review found evidence from 7 observational studies[1–3,5–8] enrolling 1507 adult in-hospital cardiac arrest patients for improved survival to hospital discharge or survival to 30 days for patients cared for by a team with at least 1 member completing an accredited ACLS course (odds ratio, 2.43; 95% CI, 1.04–5.70).[9] Pooled data from 2 observational studies[5,6] enrolling 455 patients showed no significant association between 1-year survival and ACLS training.[9]

Additional benefits of ACLS training include faster time to ROSC,[5] decreased treatment errors (eg, incorrect rhythm assessment),[4] and an association between the number of team members trained and higher ROSC.[5]

No studies report the impact of ACLS training on intact neurological survival or the impact of course components on patient outcomes. Among the studies reviewed, there was a high risk of selection bias due to differences between study populations. Most studies were conducted before 2010 and may not accurately reflect current standards of care and current ACLS course design, which has a greater focus on team-based care and simulation-based learning.

REFERENCES

1. Camp BN, Parish DC, Andrews RH. Effect of advanced cardiac life support training on resuscitation efforts and survival in a rural hospital. *Ann Emerg Med.* 1997;29:529–533. doi: 10.1016/s0196-0644(97)70228-2
2. Dane FC, Russell-Lindgren KS, Parish DC, Durham MD, Brown TD. In-hospital resuscitation: association between ACLS training and survival to discharge. *Resuscitation.* 2000;47:83–87. doi: 10.1016/s0300-9572(00)00210-0
3. Lowenstein SR, Sabyan EM, Lassen CF, Kern DC. Benefits of training physicians in advanced cardiac life support. *Chest.* 1986;89:512–516. doi: 10.1378/chest.89.4.512
4. Makker R, Gray-Siracusa K, Evers M. Evaluation of advanced cardiac life support in a community teaching hospital by use of actual cardiac arrests. *Heart Lung.* 1995;24:116–120. doi: 10.1016/s0147-9563(05)80005-6
5. Moretti MA, Cesar LA, Nusbacher A, Kern KB, Timerman S, Ramires JA. Advanced cardiac life support training improves long-term survival from in-hospital cardiac arrest. *Resuscitation.* 2007;72:458–465. doi: 10.1016/j.resuscitation.2006.06.039
6. Pottle A, Brant S. Does resuscitation training affect outcome from cardiac arrest? *Accid Emerg Nurs.* 2000;8:46–51. doi: 10.1054/aaen.1999.0089
7. Sanders AB, Berg RA, Burress M, Genova RT, Kern KB, Ewy GA. The efficacy of an ACLS training program for resuscitation from cardiac arrest in a rural community. *Ann Emerg Med.* 1994;23:56–59. doi: 10.1016/s0196-0644(94)70009-5
8. Sodhi K, Singla MK, Shrivastava A. Impact of advanced cardiac life support training program on the outcome of cardiopulmonary resuscitation in a tertiary care hospital. *Indian J Crit Care Med.* 2011;15:209–212. doi: 10.4103/0972-5229.92070
9. Lockey A, Lin Y, Cheng A. Impact of adult advanced cardiac life support course participation on patient outcomes-A systematic review and meta-analysis. *Resuscitation.* 2018;129:48–54. doi: 10.1016/j.resuscitation.2018.05.034
10. Bhanji F, Donoghue AJ, Wolff MS, Flores GE, Halamek LP, Berman JM, Sinz EH, Cheng A. Part 14: education: 2015 American Heart Association Guidelines Update for Cardiopulmonary Resuscitation and Emergency Cardiovascular Care. *Circulation.* 2015;132(suppl 2):S561–573. doi: 10.1161/CIR.0000000000000268
11. Cheng A, Lockey A, Bhanji F, Lin Y, Hunt EA, Lang E. The use of high-fidelity manikins for advanced life support training–A systematic review and meta-analysis. *Resuscitation.* 2015;93:142–149. doi: 10.1016/j.resuscitation.2015.04.004
12. Cheng A, Nadkarni VM, Mancini MB, Hunt EA, Sinz EH, Merchant RM, Donoghue A, Duff JP, Eppich W, Auerbach M, Bigham BL, Blewer AL, Chan PS, Bhanji F; American Heart Association Education Science Investigators; and on behalf of the American Heart Association Education Science and Programs Committee, Council on Cardiopulmonary, Critical Care, Perioperative and Resuscitation; Council on Cardiovascular and Stroke Nursing; and Council on Quality of Care and Outcomes Research. Resuscitation Education Science: Educational Strategies to Improve Outcomes From Cardiac Arrest: A Scientific Statement From the American Heart Association. *Circulation.* 2018;138:e82–e122. doi: 10.1161/CIR.0000000000000583
13. Greif R, Bhanji F, Bigham BL, Bray J, Breckwoldt J, Cheng A, Duff JP, Gilfoyle E, Hsieh M-J, Iwami T, et al; on behalf of the Education, Implementation, and Teams Collaborators. Education, implementation, and teams: 2020 International Consensus on Cardiopulmonary Resuscitation and Emergency Cardiovascular Care Science With Treatment Recommendations. *Circulation.* 2020;142(suppl1):S222–S283. doi: 10.1161/CIR.0000000000000896

Willingness to Perform B-CPR

Recommendations for Willingness to Perform B-CPR

COR	LOE	Recommendations
2a	C-LD	1. It is reasonable to increase bystander willingness to perform CPR through CPR training, mass CPR training, CPR awareness initiatives, and promotion of Hands-Only CPR.[1-4]
2b	C-LD	2. It may be reasonable for lay rescuer CPR training programs to raise awareness of physical barriers that may affect bystanders' willingness to perform CPR.[2,5-11]
2b	C-LD	3. It may be reasonable for lay rescuer CPR training programs to address emotional barriers that may impact bystanders' willingness to perform CPR.[3,6,12]

Synopsis

Prompt delivery of B-CPR doubles a victim's chance of survival from sudden cardiac arrest, yet fewer than 40% of victims receive B-CPR in many communities.[13,14] Given the relatively low B-CPR rate, assessment of the facilitators and barriers to the performance of B-CPR is warranted. Individual-level facilitators that increase willingness to perform B-CPR include previous CPR training, younger age, and family relationship to the cardiac arrest patient.[2,12,15,16] Community-level facilitators include Hands-Only CPR training, mass CPR training (ie, training large numbers), and CPR awareness initiatives to increase bystander performance.[1-4] Barriers to bystanders' initiating CPR include individual-level emotional barriers (eg, fear, panic, lack of confidence, concern of injuring the victim),[3,8,12] perception of the victim's physical characteristics (eg, vomit, blood, female gender, perceived futility of the situation, positioning of the patient),[2,5,7-11] and community-level low SES and racial composition.[16-21] We suggest that bystander willingness to perform CPR be enhanced through mass CPR training, CPR awareness initiatives, and promotion of Hands-Only CPR. We also suggest that layperson CPR training programs address physical and emotional barriers to bystander willingness to perform CPR. These efforts may improve bystanders' initiation of CPR and provide avenues for future initiatives tailored to address these known barriers.

Recommendation-Specific Supportive Text

1. A cohort study demonstrated that bystanders with previous CPR training were 3 times more likely to perform CPR.[2] A 40-minute mass, Hands-Only CPR training of more than 5 500 university students

was found to promote B-CPR.[3] Community-level promotion of Hands-Only CPR training was associated with increased B-CPR and an increased incidence of survival with favorable neurological outcome.[1] Communities with a higher proportion of residents identifying as having CPR awareness, prior CPR training, and higher self-efficacy were associated with an increased likelihood of B-CPR.[4] Some studies were limited by prior CPR training and ecological community-level measurements.

2. Several survey-based studies of bystanders described vomit, alcohol on the victim's breath, and visible blood as physical barriers to initiating CPR.[5,6] Analyses of dispatch-assisted CPR tapes found that inability to move patients to a hard, flat surface was associated with reduced rates of CPR.[7,8] Four retrospective cohort studies found that women are less likely to receive B-CPR compared with men.[2,9–11]
3. Observational studies found that panic, lack of confidence, perceptions of futility, and fear of injury were emotional barriers to initiating CPR.[6,12] A survey of university students cited burden of responsibility and difficulty in judging a cardiac arrest as additional barriers.[3] These studies suggest that tailored CPR training to address these emotional barriers and providing general awareness of these barriers may improve bystander willingness to perform CPR.

REFERENCES

1. Iwami T, Kitamura T, Kiyohara K, Kawamura T. Dissemination of Chest Compression-Only Cardiopulmonary Resuscitation and Survival After Out-of-Hospital Cardiac Arrest. *Circulation*. 2015;132:415–422. doi: 10.1161/CIRCULATIONAHA.114.014905
2. Tanigawa K, Iwami T, Nishiyama C, Nonogi H, Kawamura T. Are trained individuals more likely to perform bystander CPR? An observational study. *Resuscitation*. 2011;82:523–528. doi: 10.1016/j.resuscitation.2011.01.027
3. Nishiyama C, Sato R, Baba M, Kuroki H, Kawamura T, Kiguchi T, Kobayashi D, Shimamoto T, Koike K, Tanaka S, Naito C, Iwami T. Actual resuscitation actions after the training of chest compression-only CPR and AED use among new university students. *Resuscitation*. 2019;141:63–68. doi: 10.1016/j.resuscitation.2019.05.040
4. Ro YS, Shin SD, Song KJ, Hong SO, Kim YT, Lee DW, Cho SI. Public awareness and self-efficacy of cardiopulmonary resuscitation in communities and outcomes of out-of-hospital cardiac arrest: A multi-level analysis. *Resuscitation*. 2016;102:17–24. doi: 10.1016/j.resuscitation.2016.02.004
5. McCormack AP, Damon SK, Eisenberg MS. Disagreeable physical characteristics affecting bystander CPR. *Ann Emerg Med*. 1989;18:283–285. doi: 10.1016/s0196-0644(89)80415-9
6. Axelsson A, Herlitz J, Ekström L, Holmberg S. Bystander-initiated cardiopulmonary resuscitation out-of-hospital. A first description of the bystanders and their experiences. *Resuscitation*. 1996;33:3–11. doi: 10.1016/s0300-9572(96)00993-8
7. Langlais BT, Panczyk M, Sutter J, Fukushima H, Wu Z, Iwami T, Spaite D, Bobrow B. Barriers to patient positioning for telephone cardiopulmonary resuscitation in out-of-hospital cardiac arrest. *Resuscitation*. 2017;115:163–168. doi: 10.1016/j.resuscitation.2017.03.034
8. Case R, Cartledge S, Siedenburg J, Smith K, Straney L, Barger B, Finn J, Bray JE. Identifying barriers to the provision of bystander cardiopulmonary resuscitation (CPR) in high-risk regions: A qualitative review of emergency calls. *Resuscitation*. 2018;129:43–47. doi: 10.1016/j.resuscitation.2018.06.001
9. Blewer AL, McGovern SK, Schmicker RH, May S, Morrison LJ, Aufderheide TP, Daya M, Idris AH, Callaway CW, Kudenchuk PJ, Vilke GM, Abella BS; Resuscitation Outcomes Consortium (ROC) Investigators. Gender Disparities Among Adult Recipients of Bystander Cardiopulmonary Resuscitation in the Public. *Circ Cardiovasc Qual Outcomes*. 2018;11:e004710. doi: 10.1161/CIRCOUTCOMES.118.004710
10. Matsuyama T, Okubo M, Kiyohara K, Kiguchi T, Kobayashi D, Nishiyama C, Okabayashi S, Shimamoto T, Izawa J, Komukai S, Gibo K, Ohta B, Kitamura T, Kawamura T, Iwami T. Sex-Based Disparities in Receiving Bystander Cardiopulmonary Resuscitation by Location of Cardiac Arrest in Japan. *Mayo Clin Proc*. 2019;94:577–587. doi: 10.1016/j.mayocp.2018.12.028
11. Matsui S, Kitamura T, Kiyohara K, Sado J, Ayusawa M, Nitta M, Iwami T, Nakata K, Kitamura Y, Sobue T; SPIRITS Investigators. Sex Disparities in Receipt of Bystander Interventions for Students Who Experienced Cardiac Arrest in Japan. *JAMA Netw Open*. 2019;2:e195111. doi: 10.1001/jamanetworkopen.2019.5111
12. Swor R, Khan I, Domeier R, Honeycutt L, Chu K, Compton S. CPR training and CPR performance: do CPR-trained bystanders perform CPR? *Acad Emerg Med*. 2006;13:596–601. doi: 10.1197/j.aem.2005.12.021
13. Girotra S, van Diepen S, Nallamothu BK, Carrel M, Vellano K, Anderson ML, McNally B, Abella BS, Sasson C, Chan PS; CARES Surveillance Group and the HeartRescue Project. Regional Variation in Out-of-Hospital Cardiac Arrest Survival in the United States. *Circulation*. 2016;133:2159–2168. doi: 10.1161/CIRCULATIONAHA.115.018175
14. Iwami T, Nichol G, Hiraide A, Hayashi Y, Nishiuchi T, Kajino K, Morita H, Yukioka H, Ikeuchi H, Sugimoto H, Nonogi H, Kawamura T. Continuous improvements in "chain of survival" increased survival after out-of-hospital cardiac arrests: a large-scale population-based study. *Circulation*. 2009;119:728–734. doi: 10.1161/CIRCULATIONAHA.108.802058
15. Greif R, Bhanji F, Bigham BL, Bray J, Breckwoldt J, Cheng A, Duff JP, Gilfoyle E, Hsieh M-J, Iwami T, et al; on behalf of the Education, Implementation, and Teams Collaborators. Education, implementation, and teams: 2020 International Consensus on Cardiopulmonary Resuscitation and Emergency Cardiovascular Care Science With Treatment Recommendations. *Circulation*. 2020;142(suppl 1):S222–S283. doi: 10.1161/CIR.0000000000000896
16. Chang I, Kwak YH, Shin SD, Ro YS, Kim DK. Characteristics of bystander cardiopulmonary resuscitation for paediatric out-of-hospital cardiac arrests: A national observational study from 2012 to 2014. *Resuscitation*. 2017;111:26–33. doi: 10.1016/j.resuscitation.2016.11.007
17. Chiang WC, Ko PC, Chang AM, Chen WT, Liu SS, Huang YS, Chen SY, Lin CH, Cheng MT, Chong KM, Wang HC, Yang CW, Liao MW, Wang CH, Chien YC, Lin CH, Liu YP, Lee BC, Chien KL, Lai MS, Ma MH. Bystander-initiated CPR in an Asian metropolitan: does the socioeconomic status matter? *Resuscitation*. 2014;85:53–58. doi: 10.1016/j.resuscitation.2013.07.033
18. Dahan B, Jabre P, Karam N, Misslin R, Tafflet M, Bougouin W, Jost D, Beganton F, Marijon E, Jouven X. Impact of neighbourhood socio-economic status on bystander cardiopulmonary resuscitation in Paris. *Resuscitation*. 2017;110:107–113. doi: 10.1016/j.resuscitation.2016.10.028
19. Moncur L, Ainsborough N, Ghose R, Kendal SP, Salvatori M, Wright J. Does the level of socioeconomic deprivation at the location of cardiac arrest in an English region influence the likelihood of receiving bystander-initiated cardiopulmonary resuscitation? *Emerg Med J*. 2016;33:105–108. doi: 10.1136/emermed-2015-204643
20. Vaillancourt C, Lui A, De Maio VJ, Wells GA, Stiell IG. Socioeconomic status influences bystander CPR and survival rates for out-of-hospital cardiac arrest victims. *Resuscitation*. 2008;79:417–423. doi: 10.1016/j.resuscitation.2008.07.012
21. Sasson C, Magid DJ, Chan P, Root ED, McNally BF, Kellermann AL, Haukoos JS; CARES Surveillance Group. Association of neighborhood characteristics with bystander-initiated CPR. *N Engl J Med*. 2012;367:1607–1615. doi: 10.1056/NEJMoa1110700

KNOWLEDGE GAPS AND FUTURE RESEARCH

Defining the optimal means of delivering resuscitation education requires robustly designed studies that address important knowledge gaps. Resuscitation education research has been hampered by unique limitations compared with clinical resuscitation research. This can be readily appreciated with the predominance of

Table 2. Overarching Knowledge Gaps in Resuscitation Education

Topic Area	Sample Research Question
Relevance of outcomes	Is there an association between educational outcomes in training (ie, knowledge and skill), clinical performance, and patient outcomes?
Patient outcomes	What is the impact of educational interventions and/or specific instructional design elements on patient outcomes?
Standardized reporting	How can outcomes from resuscitation education research be standardized to reduce heterogeneity among studies?
Cost-effectiveness	What is the cost-effectiveness of different educational interventions?
Optimizing instructional design	How can instructional design features be combined to best optimize learning and patient outcomes?
Tailoring instructional design	Which resuscitation skills/competencies are best suited for each instructional design feature?
Learning curves and skill retention	What are the learning curves for key resuscitation skills, and how can training be structured to optimize long-term retention of skills?

recommendations in this chapter that are classified as weak and are based on levels of evidence classified as low, according to GRADE criteria.[1] We believe that this, in part, reflects inherent limitations associated with the use of GRADE for the evaluation of educational research. Many of the studies we reviewed were insufficiently powered, single-center studies, making it difficult to determine the true impact of the intervention of interest. Collaboration in the form of multicenter research studies would help to address this problem.[2] Education research networks provide the infrastructure necessary to support mentorship, grant applications, study design and implementation, and knowledge dissemination.[2,3] Another overarching issue prevalent among resuscitation education research is outcome selection.[4,5] In a manner relatively different from other scientific areas, direct linkage of provider performance in simulated environments to performance during actual patient care (or patient outcomes) remains relatively elusive. Over the past several years, a handful of studies have successfully linked educational interventions to clinical outcomes after actual patient events,[6–10] but most educational studies examine the surrogate outcomes of learner knowledge and skill performance in the simulated setting. Resuscitation researchers should aspire to report clinical outcomes from educational interventions (Table 2). When the selection of patient outcomes is not feasible, we encourage educational researchers to select quantitative measures that have a known association with improved clinical outcomes from cardiac arrest (eg, chest compression depth). Doing so will allow researchers to establish causal links among outcomes that are similarly reported in simulation-based and clinical studies.[11]

Our review of the literature identified significant heterogeneity in intervention type and outcome measure type, making it difficult to conduct meta-analyses for many of the key topics. Even for outcomes common across many studies (eg, CPR depth), there was variability in the outcome measure type (eg, mean CPR depth versus percentage compliance with CPR depth per 30-second epoch versus percentage compliance with CPR depth per event). The establishment of standardized reporting guidelines for outcomes from resuscitation education research would address this issue and enable meta-analysis of key questions in the future (Table 2). Acknowledging these shortcomings, it remains true that educational research, like other areas of resuscitation science, has gaps in essential knowledge that require further investigation.

Several general questions bear mentioning as essential considerations for future research in resuscitation education. Because very few studies link educational interventions to patient outcomes, additional research is needed to examine the connections between educational outcomes and survival from cardiac arrest, as well as from other intermediate clinical outcomes known to be contributors to survival (eg, high-quality CPR, time to defibrillation, time to initiation of CPR). Among the studies examining knowledge and skill as outcomes, a disproportionate number examine these outcomes only at a single time point immediately after course conclusion. Future studies should focus on retention of knowledge and skill over longer periods of time rather than exclusively at the end of course delivery, particularly in light of the fact that some teaching strategies may show good short-term improvements but poor long-term learning outcomes. Many of the studies we identified examined certain instructional design features in isolation, or they executed a study design that failed to appropriately isolate the variable of interest. Future studies should be designed to control for potential confounding variables (eg, concurrent educational opportunities, prior experiences, rater blinding) and/or include statistical analyses that adjust for variables of interest. Furthermore, a greater understanding of the combined effect of instructional design features, when applied to specific resuscitation skills, will facilitate improved learning outcomes in the future.

Significant knowledge gaps exist with respect to the economic evaluation of resuscitation education. Economic evaluation is a type of research that examines both the cost and the consequences of at least 2 alternatives (eg, BLS training with and without CPR feedback devices).[12] Although current literature has provided evidence supporting the effectiveness of certain instructional design features, educational programs still must balance the potential benefits with costs when deciding whether to adopt a certain method of training. A properly conducted cost-effectiveness analysis can inform these decisions. Future educational research should explore both the effectiveness and the associated costs of training (Table 2). This helps not only to promote the implementation of certain instructional designs but also to establish evidence on how to maximize learning outcomes with limited resources.

Table 3. Specific Knowledge Gaps in Resuscitation Education by Topic

Topic Area	Sample Research Question
Mastery learning	What are the minimal passing standards for different resuscitation skills, and does incorporation of these standards into a mastery learning model of training improve skill acquisition and retention?
Booster training	What are the ideal booster training intervals for key resuscitation skills to prevent skill decay over time?
Layperson training	How do we optimize layperson training to improve bystander CPR rates, quality of CPR, and patient outcomes?
Teamwork and leadership training	How can resuscitation team structure be modified (eg, inclusion of a CPR coach) to enhance performance, and can training in these new structures improve outcomes?
Feedback and debriefing	How does the source, frequency, structure, content, and timing of feedback and debriefing during resuscitation training influence outcomes?
Technology in training	How can new and emerging technologies (eg, VR, augmented reality, eye tracking, artificial intelligence) be used to improve resuscitation performance and patient outcomes?
Disparities in education	What are the optimal methods to address racial, ethnic, socioeconomic, and gender disparities in resuscitation education?
Faculty development	What is the best method of training resuscitation instructors that is both scalable and effective?
Assessment of learners	What is the most effective assessment strategy during resuscitation training?
Cognitive aids in training	How can cognitive aids be effectively incorporated into resuscitation training programs to support learning?

CPR indicates cardiopulmonary resuscitation; and VR, virtual reality.

The writing group identified several key content areas with glaring knowledge gaps. Assessment that drives learning is among the AHA's core educational concepts, yet there is a relative paucity of research informing the practice of assessment in resuscitation education.[5] Research exploring the source (ie, instructor, manikin, device), timing, and structure of feedback is necessary to inform future course design. A growing number of instruments for formative and summative assessment of learners in resuscitation courses exist in published literature.[4] Assessment of healthcare providers spans the domains of clinical knowledge, technical skills, and teamwork. Selecting the appropriate instrument for specific domains should be part of the assessment strategy for training programs. Instruments designed for these purposes should be rigorously tested for reliability and generalizability. Future research would benefit from a description of rater training strategies and greater standardization of use of these instruments across different learner groups and settings (Table 3).

Faculty development opportunities for resuscitation educators ensures that resuscitation training programs are delivered effectively. Although existing literature describes key features of effective faculty development in medical education,[13] there is a lack of research as it applies to the training of resuscitation educators. Finally, topics such as the use of cognitive aids during training, hybrid course design (eg, with eLearning and/or other features), artificial intelligence, and augmented reality are of interest but require a greater body of evidence before recommendations to inform future practice can be made (Table 3).

While these guidelines covered some newer educational strategies, such as VR and gamified learning, we also continue to focus on basic constructs, such as spaced learning, booster training, deliberate practice, and feedback. In all of these areas, important knowledge gaps—and thereby opportunities for future study—remain (Table 3). We challenge funding agencies to recognize the critical role of resuscitation education in improving cardiac arrest outcomes by providing focused funding opportunities for research in resuscitation education. With appropriate funding, researchers will be able to explore newer or novel phenomena and also continue to evaluate long-standing paradigms of resuscitation education. With this approach, we will continue to push for enhanced educational efficiency and improved outcomes from cardiac arrest.

REFERENCES

1. Magid DJ, Aziz K, Cheng A, Hazinski MF, Hoover AV, Mahgoub M, Panchal AR, Sasson C, Topjian AA, Rodriguez AJ, et al. Part 2: evidence evaluation and guidelines development: 2020 American Heart Association Guidelines for Cardiopulmonary Resuscitation and Emergency Cardiovascular Care. *Circulation*. 2020;142(suppl 2):S358–S365. doi: 10.1161/CIR.0000000000000898
2. Schwartz A, Young R, Hicks PJ, Appd L. Medical education practice-based research networks: Facilitating collaborative research. *Med Teach*. 2016;38:64–74. doi: 10.3109/0142159X.2014.970991
3. Cheng A, Auerbach M, Calhoun A, Mackinnon R, Chang TP, Nadkarni V, Hunt EA, Duval-Arnould J, Peiris N, Kessler DatII. Building a community of practice for researchers: the international network for simulation-based pediatric innovation, research and education. *Simul Healthc*. 2018;13(suppl 1):S28–S34. doi: 10.1097/SIH.0000000000000269
4. Cheng A, Nadkarni VM, Mancini MB, Hunt EA, Sinz EH, Merchant RM, Donoghue A, Duff JP, Eppich W, Auerbach M, Bigham BL, Blewer AL, Chan PS, Bhanji F; American Heart Association Education Science Investigators; and on behalf of the American Heart Association Education Science and Programs Committee, Council on Cardiopulmonary, Critical Care, Perioperative and Resuscitation; Council on Cardiovascular and Stroke Nursing; and Council on Quality of Care and Outcomes Research. Resuscitation Education Science: Educational Strategies to Improve Outcomes From Cardiac Arrest: A Scientific Statement From the American Heart Association. *Circulation*. 2018;138:e82–e122. doi: 10.1161/CIR.0000000000000583
5. Bhanji F, Donoghue AJ, Wolff MS, Flores GE, Halamek LP, Berman JM, Sinz EH, Cheng A. Part 14: education: 2015 American Heart Association Guidelines Update for Cardiopulmonary Resuscitation and Emergency Cardiovascular Care. *Circulation*. 2015;132(suppl 2):S561–573. doi: 10.1161/CIR.0000000000000268
6. Wayne DB, Didwania A, Feinglass J, Fudala MJ, Barsuk JH, McGaghie WC. Simulation-based education improves quality of care during cardiac arrest team responses at an academic teaching hospital: a case-control study. *Chest*. 2008;133:56–61. doi: 10.1378/chest.07-0131
7. Edelson DP, Litzinger B, Arora V, Walsh D, Kim S, Lauderdale DS, Vanden Hoek TL, Becker LB, Abella BS. Improving in-hospital cardiac arrest process and outcomes with performance debriefing. *Arch Intern Med*. 2008;168:1063–1069. doi: 10.1001/archinte.168.10.1063
8. Wolfe H, Zebuhr C, Topjian AA, Nishisaki A, Niles DE, Meaney PA, Boyle L, Giordano RT, Davis D, Priestley M, Apkon M, Berg RA, Nadkarni VM, Sutton RM. Interdisciplinary ICU cardiac arrest debriefing improves survival outcomes*. *Crit Care Med*. 2014;42:1688–1695. doi: 10.1097/CCM.0000000000000327

9. Bobrow BJ, Spaite DW, Vadeboncoeur TF, Hu C, Mullins T, Tormala W, Dameff C, Gallagher J, Smith G, Panczyk M. Implementation of a Regional Telephone Cardiopulmonary Resuscitation Program and Outcomes After Out-of-Hospital Cardiac Arrest. *JAMA Cardiol.* 2016;1:294–302. doi: 10.1001/jamacardio.2016.0251
10. Morrison LJ, Brooks SC, Dainty KN, Dorian P, Needham DM, Ferguson ND, Rubenfeld GD, Slutsky AS, Wax RS, Zwarenstein M, Thorpe K, Zhan C, Scales DC; Strategies for Post-Arrest Care Network. Improving use of targeted temperature management after out-of-hospital cardiac arrest: a stepped wedge cluster randomized controlled trial. *Crit Care Med.* 2015;43:954–964. doi: 10.1097/CCM.0000000000000864
11. Cook DA, West CP. Perspective: reconsidering the focus on "outcomes research" in medical education: a cautionary note. *Acad Med.* 2013;88:162–167. doi: 10.1097/ACM.0b013e31827c3d78
12. Lin Y, Cheng A, Hecker K, Grant V, Currie GR. Implementing economic evaluation in simulation-based medical education: challenges and opportunities. *Med Educ.* 2018;52:150–160. doi: 10.1111/medu.13411
13. Steinert Y, Mann K, Anderson B, Barnett BM, Centeno A, Naismith L, Prideaux D, Spencer J, Tullo E, Viggiano T, Ward H, Dolmans D. A systematic review of faculty development initiatives designed to enhance teaching effectiveness: A 10-year update: BEME Guide No. 40. *Med Teach.* 2016;38:769–786. doi: 10.1080/0142159X.2016.1181851

ARTICLE INFORMATION

The American Heart Association requests that this document be cited as follows: Cheng A, Magid DJ, Auerbach M, Bhanji F, Bigham BL, Blewer AL, Dainty KN, Diederich E, Lin Y, Leary M, Mahgoub M, Mancini ME, Navarro K, Donoghue A. Part 6: resuscitation education science: 2020 American Heart Association Guidelines for Cardiopulmonary Resuscitation and Emergency Cardiovascular Care. *Circulation*. 2020;142(suppl 2):S551–S579. doi: 10.1161/CIR.0000000000000903

Disclosures

Appendix 1. Writing Group Disclosures

Writing Group Member	Employment	Research Grant	Other Research Support	Speakers' Bureau/ Honoraria	Expert Witness	Ownership Interest	Consultant/ Advisory Board	Other
Adam Cheng	University of Calgary	None	None	None	None	None	None	None
Aaron Donoghue	The Children's Hospital of Philadelphia, University of Pennsylvania School of Medicine	None	None	None	Atkinson, Haskins, Nellis, Brittingham, Gladd & Fiasco*	None	None	None
Marc Auerbach	Yale University	None	None	None	None	None	None	None
Farhan Bhanji	McGill University	None	None	None	None	None	None	None
Blair L. Bigham	McMaster University Emergency Medicine	None	None	None	None	None	None	None
Audrey L. Blewer	Duke University	None	None	None	None	None	None	None
Katie N. Dainty	North York General Hospital Research and Innovation	None	None	None	None	None	None	None
Emily Diederich	University of Kansas Medical Center Internal Medicine	None	None	None	None	None	None	None
Marion Leary	Center for Resuscitation Science	None	None	None	None	None	None	None
Yiqun Lin	Alberta Children's Hospital KidSIM Simulation Research Program	None	None	None	None	None	None	None
David J. Magid	University of Colorado	NIH†; NHLBI†; CMS†; AHA†	None	None	None	None	None	American Heart Association (Senior Science Editor)†
Melissa Mahgoub	American Heart Association	None	None	None	None	None	None	None
Mary E. Mancini	The University of Texas at Arlington College of Nursing and Health Innovation	None	None	Stryker*	None	None	None	None
Kenneth Navarro	The University of Texas Southwestern Medical Center at Dallas Emergency Medicine	None	None	None	None	None	None	None

This table represents the relationships of writing group members that may be perceived as actual or reasonably perceived conflicts of interest as reported on the Disclosure Questionnaire, which all members of the writing group are required to complete and submit. A relationship is considered to be "significant" if (a) the person receives $10 000 or more during any 12-month period, or 5% or more of the person's gross income; or (b) the person owns 5% or more of the voting stock or share of the entity, or owns $10 000 or more of the fair market value of the entity. A relationship is considered to be "modest" if it is less than "significant" under the preceding definition.

*Modest.

†Significant.

Appendix 2. Reviewer Disclosures

Reviewer	Employment	Research Grant	Other Research Support	Speakers' Bureau/ Honoraria	Expert Witness	Ownership Interest	Consultant/ Advisory Board	Other
Jeffrey M. Berman	UNC Hospitals	None	None	None	None	None	None	None
Aaron W. Calhoun	University of Louisville	None	None	None	None	None	None	None
Maia Dorsett	University of Rochester Medical Center	None	None	None	None	None	None	None
Joyce Foresman-Capuzzi	Lankenau Medical Center	None	None	None	None	None	None	None
Louis P. Halamek	Stanford University	None	None	None	None	None	None	None
Mary Ann McNeil	University of Minnesota	None	None	None	None	None	None	None
Catherine Patocka	University of Calgary (Canada)	None	None	None	None	None	None	None
David L. Rodgers	Penn State	None	None	None	None	None	None	None

This table represents the relationships of reviewers that may be perceived as actual or reasonably perceived conflicts of interest as reported on the Disclosure Questionnaire, which all reviewers are required to complete and submit. A relationship is considered to be "significant" if (a) the person receives $10 000 or more during any 12-month period, or 5% or more of the person's gross income; or (b) the person owns 5% or more of the voting stock or share of the entity, or owns $10 000 or more of the fair market value of the entity. A relationship is considered to be "modest" if it is less than "significant" under the preceding definition.

Circulation

Part 7: Systems of Care

2020 American Heart Association Guidelines for Cardiopulmonary Resuscitation and Emergency Cardiovascular Care

ABSTRACT: Survival after cardiac arrest requires an integrated system of people, training, equipment, and organizations working together to achieve a common goal. Part 7 of the *2020 American Heart Association Guidelines for Cardiopulmonary Resuscitation and Emergency Cardiovascular Care* focuses on systems of care, with an emphasis on elements that are relevant to a broad range of resuscitation situations. Previous systems of care guidelines have identified a Chain of Survival, beginning with prevention and early identification of cardiac arrest and proceeding through resuscitation to post–cardiac arrest care. This concept is reinforced by the addition of recovery as an important stage in cardiac arrest survival. Debriefing and other quality improvement strategies were previously mentioned and are now emphasized. Specific to out-of-hospital cardiac arrest, this Part contains recommendations about community initiatives to promote cardiac arrest recognition, cardiopulmonary resuscitation, public access defibrillation, mobile phone technologies to summon first responders, and an enhanced role for emergency telecommunicators. Germane to in-hospital cardiac arrest are recommendations about the recognition and stabilization of hospital patients at risk for developing cardiac arrest. This Part also includes recommendations about clinical debriefing, transport to specialized cardiac arrest centers, organ donation, and performance measurement across the continuum of resuscitation situations.

Katherine M. Berg, MD, Chair
Adam Cheng, MD
Ashish R. Panchal, MD, PhD
Alexis A. Topjian, MD, MSCE
Khalid Aziz, MBBS, MA, MEd(IT)
Farhan Bhanji, MD, MSc (Ed)
Blair L. Bigham, MD, MSc
Karen G. Hirsch, MD
Amber V. Hoover, RN, MSN
Michael C. Kurz, MD, MS
Arielle Levy, MD, MEd
Yiqun Lin, MD, MHSc, PhD
David J. Magid, MD, MPH
Melissa Mahgoub, PhD
Mary Ann Peberdy, MD
Amber J. Rodriguez, PhD
Comilla Sasson, MD, PhD
Eric J. Lavonas, MD, MS
On behalf of the Adult Basic and Advanced Life Support, Pediatric Basic and Advanced Life Support, Neonatal Life Support, and Resuscitation Education Science Writing Groups

Key Words: AHA Scientific Statements ■ cardiopulmonary resuscitation ■ delivery of health care ■ emergency medical dispatcher ■ hospital rapid response team ■ organ transplantation ■ patient care team ■ quality improvement

https://www.ahajournals.org/journal/circ

TOP 10 TAKE-HOME MESSAGES: SYSTEMS OF CARE

1. Recovery is a critical component of the resuscitation Chain of Survival.
2. Efforts to support the ability and willingness of members of the general public to perform cardiopulmonary resuscitation (CPR), and to use an automated external defibrillator, improve resuscitation outcomes in communities.
3. Novel methods to use mobile phone technology to alert trained lay rescuers of events requiring CPR have shown promise in some urban communities and deserve more study.
4. Emergency system telecommunicators can instruct bystanders to perform hands-only CPR for adults. The No-No-Go framework is effective.
5. Early warning scoring systems and rapid response teams can prevent cardiac arrest in both pediatric and adult hospitals, but the literature is too varied to understand what components of these systems are associated with benefit.
6. Cognitive aids may improve resuscitation performance by untrained laypersons, but their use results in a delay to starting CPR. More development and study are needed before these systems can be fully endorsed.
7. Surprisingly little is known about the effect of cognitive aids on the performance of emergency medical services or hospital-based resuscitation teams.
8. Although specialized cardiac arrest centers offer protocols and technology not available at all hospitals, the available literature about their impact on resuscitation outcomes is mixed.
9. Team feedback matters. Structured debriefing protocols improve the performance of resuscitation teams in subsequent resuscitation events.
10. System-wide feedback matters. Implementing structured data collection and review leads to improved resuscitation processes and survival in both in-hospital and out-of-hospital settings.

PREAMBLE

Successful resuscitation requires swift and coordinated action by trained providers, each performing an important role within an organizational framework. Willing bystanders, property owners who maintain automated external defibrillators (AEDs), emergency service telecommunicators (also known as *dispatchers* or *call-takers*), and basic life support (BLS) and advanced life support (ALS) providers working within emergency medical services (EMS) systems all contribute to successful resuscitation from out-of-hospital cardiac arrest (OHCA). Within the hospital, the work of physicians, nurses, respiratory therapists, pharmacists, and many other professionals supports resuscitation outcomes. Successful resuscitation also depends on the contributions of equipment manufacturers, pharmaceutical companies, resuscitation instructors and instructor trainers, guidelines developers, and many others. Long-term recovery after cardiac arrest requires support from family and professional caregivers, including, in many cases, experts in cognitive, physical, and psychological rehabilitation and recovery. A systems-wide approach to learning and advancing at every level of care, from prevention to recognition to treatment, is essential to achieving successful outcomes after cardiac arrest.

These systems of care guidelines focus on aspects of resuscitation that are broadly applicable to persons of all ages. The guidelines emphasize strategies at every step in the continuum of care to improve cardiac arrest survival: to increase the proportion of patients with OHCA who receive prompt cardiopulmonary resuscitation (CPR) and early defibrillation; to prevent in-hospital cardiac arrest (IHCA); and to examine the use of cognitive aids to improve resuscitation team performance, the role of specialized cardiac arrest centers, organ donation, and measures to improve resuscitation team performance and resuscitation outcomes.

INTRODUCTION

Scope of the Guidelines

These guidelines are designed primarily for North American healthcare providers who are looking for an up-to-date summary for clinical care and the design and operation of resuscitation systems, as well as for those who are seeking more in-depth information on resuscitation science and gaps in current knowledge. The emphasis in this Part of the *2020 American Heart Association* (AHA) *Guidelines for CPR and Emergency Cardiovascular Care* (ECC) is on elements of care involving coordination between different contributors to the Chain of Survival (eg, emergency telecommunicators and untrained lay rescuers), those elements common to the resuscitation of different populations (eg, community CPR training and public access to defibrillation, early interventions to prevent IHCA), and means to improve the performance of resuscitation teams and systems.

Some recommendations are directly relevant to lay rescuers who may or may not have received CPR training and who have little or no access to resuscitation equipment. Other recommendations are relevant to persons with more advanced resuscitation training, functioning either with or without access to resuscitation drugs and devices, working either within or outside of a hospital. Recommendations for actions by emergency telecommunicators who provide instructions before the arrival of EMS are provided. Some treatment recommendations

Table 1. Applying Class of Recommendation and Level of Evidence to Clinical Strategies, Interventions, Treatments, or Diagnostic Testing in Patient Care (Updated May 2019)*

CLASS (STRENGTH) OF RECOMMENDATION	
CLASS 1 (STRONG)	**Benefit >>> Risk**
Suggested phrases for writing recommendations: • Is recommended • Is indicated/useful/effective/beneficial • Should be performed/administered/other • Comparative-Effectiveness Phrases†: – Treatment/strategy A is recommended/indicated in preference to treatment B – Treatment A should be chosen over treatment B	
CLASS 2a (MODERATE)	**Benefit >> Risk**
Suggested phrases for writing recommendations: • Is reasonable • Can be useful/effective/beneficial • Comparative-Effectiveness Phrases†: – Treatment/strategy A is probably recommended/indicated in preference to treatment B – It is reasonable to choose treatment A over treatment B	
CLASS 2b (WEAK)	**Benefit ≥ Risk**
Suggested phrases for writing recommendations: • May/might be reasonable • May/might be considered • Usefulness/effectiveness is unknown/unclear/uncertain or not well-established	
CLASS 3: No Benefit (MODERATE) **(Generally, LOE A or B use only)**	**Benefit = Risk**
Suggested phrases for writing recommendations: • Is not recommended • Is not indicated/useful/effective/beneficial • Should not be performed/administered/other	
Class 3: Harm (STRONG)	**Risk > Benefit**
Suggested phrases for writing recommendations: • Potentially harmful • Causes harm • Associated with excess morbidity/mortality • Should not be performed/administered/other	

LEVEL (QUALITY) OF EVIDENCE‡	
LEVEL A	
• High-quality evidence‡ from more than 1 RCT • Meta-analyses of high-quality RCTs • One or more RCTs corroborated by high-quality registry studies	
LEVEL B-R	**(Randomized)**
• Moderate-quality evidence‡ from 1 or more RCTs • Meta-analyses of moderate-quality RCTs	
LEVEL B-NR	**(Nonrandomized)**
• Moderate-quality evidence‡ from 1 or more well-designed, well-executed nonrandomized studies, observational studies, or registry studies • Meta-analyses of such studies	
LEVEL C-LD	**(Limited Data)**
• Randomized or nonrandomized observational or registry studies with limitations of design or execution • Meta-analyses of such studies • Physiological or mechanistic studies in human subjects	
LEVEL C-EO	**(Expert Opinion)**
• Consensus of expert opinion based on clinical experience	

COR and LOE are determined independently (any COR may be paired with any LOE).

A recommendation with LOE C does not imply that the recommendation is weak. Many important clinical questions addressed in guidelines do not lend themselves to clinical trials. Although RCTs are unavailable, there may be a very clear clinical consensus that a particular test or therapy is useful or effective.

* The outcome or result of the intervention should be specified (an improved clinical outcome or increased diagnostic accuracy or incremental prognostic information).

† For comparative-effectiveness recommendations (COR 1 and 2a; LOE A and B only), studies that support the use of comparator verbs should involve direct comparisons of the treatments or strategies being evaluated.

‡ The method of assessing quality is evolving, including the application of standardized, widely-used, and preferably validated evidence grading tools; and for systematic reviews, the incorporation of an Evidence Review Committee.

COR indicates Class of Recommendation; EO, expert opinion; LD, limited data; LOE, Level of Evidence; NR, nonrandomized; R, randomized; and RCT, randomized controlled trial.

involve medical care and decision-making after return of spontaneous circulation (ROSC) or after resuscitation has been unsuccessful. Importantly, recommendations are provided related to team debriefing and systematic feedback to increase future resuscitation success.

Coronavirus Disease 2019 (COVID-19) Guidance

Together with other professional societies, the AHA has provided interim guidance for basic and advanced life support in adults, children, and neonates with suspected or confirmed COVID-19 infection. Because evidence and guidance are evolving with the COVID-19 situation, this interim guidance is maintained separately from the ECC guidelines. Readers are directed to the AHA CPR and ECC website (cpr.heart.org) for the most recent guidance.[1]

Organization of the Systems of Care Writing Group

The Systems of Care Writing Group included a diverse group of experts with backgrounds in clinical medicine, education, research, and public health. Because the systems of care guidelines draw material from each of the main writing groups, the Chairs of each writing group collaborated to develop the systems of care guidelines along with content experts, AHA staff, and the AHA Senior Science Editors. Each recommendation was developed and formally approved by the writing group from which it originated.

The AHA has rigorous conflict of interest policies and procedures to minimize the risk of bias or improper influence during the development of guidelines. Prior to appointment, writing group members disclosed all commercial relationships and other potential (including intellectual) conflicts. These procedures are described more fully in "Part 2: Evidence Evaluation and Guidelines Development."[2] Disclosure information for writing group members is listed in Appendix 1.

METHODOLOGY AND EVIDENCE REVIEW

These systems of care guidelines are based on the extensive evidence evaluation performed in conjunction with the International Liaison Committee on Resuscitation (ILCOR) and affiliated ILCOR member councils. Three different types of evidence reviews (systematic reviews, scoping reviews, and evidence updates) were used in the 2020 process. Each of these resulted in a description of the literature that facilitated guideline development. A more comprehensive description of these methods is provided in "Part 2: Evidence Evaluation and Guidelines Development."[2]

Class of Recommendation and Level of Evidence

As with all AHA guidelines, each 2020 recommendation is assigned a Class of Recommendation (COR) based on the strength and consistency of the evidence, alternative treatment options, and the impact on patients and society. The Level of Evidence (LOE) is based on the quality, quantity, relevance, and consistency of the available evidence (Table 1).

For each recommendation in "Part 7: Systems of Care," the originating writing group discussed and approved specific recommendation wording and the COR and LOE assignments. In determining the COR, the writing group considered the LOE and other factors, including systems issues, economic factors, and ethical factors such as equity, acceptability, and feasibility. These evidence-review methods, including specific criteria used to determine COR and LOE, are described more fully in "Part 2: Evidence Evaluation and Guidelines Development."[2] The Systems of Care Writing Group members had final authority over and formally approved these recommendations.

Guideline Structure

The 2020 guidelines are organized into "knowledge chunks," grouped into discrete modules of information on specific topics or management issues.[3] Each modular knowledge chunk includes a table of recommendations that uses standard AHA nomenclature of COR and LOE. A brief introduction or short synopsis is provided to put the recommendations into context with important background information and overarching management or treatment concepts. Recommendation-specific text clarifies the rationale and key study data supporting the recommendations. When appropriate, flow diagrams or additional tables are included. Hyperlinked references are provided to facilitate quick access and review.

Document Review and Approval

Each *2020 AHA Guidelines for CPR and ECC* document was submitted for blinded peer review to 5 subject matter experts nominated by the AHA. Before appointment, all peer reviewers were required to disclose relationships with industry and any other potential conflicts of interest, and all disclosures were reviewed by AHA staff. Peer reviewer feedback was provided for guidelines in draft format and again in final format. All guidelines were reviewed and approved for publication by the AHA Science Advisory and Coordinating Committee and AHA Executive Committee. Disclosure information for peer reviewers is listed in Appendix 2.

Abbreviations

Abbreviation	Meaning/Phrase
ALS	advanced life support
AED	automated external defibrillator
AHA	American Heart Association
BLS	basic life support
CAC	cardiac arrest center
COR	Class of Recommendation
CPR	cardiopulmonary resuscitation
EMS	emergency medical services
IHCA	in-hospital cardiac arrest
ILCOR	International Liaison Committee on Resuscitation
LOE	Level of Evidence
MET	medical emergency team
OHCA	out-of-hospital cardiac arrest
OR	odds ratio
PAD	public access defibrillation
RCT	randomized controlled trial
ROSC	return of spontaneous circulation
RR, aRR	relative risk, adjusted relative risk
RRT	rapid response team
T-CPR	telecommunicator CPR instructions

REFERENCES

1. American Heart Association. CPR & ECC. https://cpr.heart.org/. Accessed June 19, 2020.
2. Magid DJ, Aziz K, Cheng A, Hazinski MF, Hoover AV, Mahgoub M, Panchal AR, Sasson C, Topjian AA, Rodriguez AJ, et al. Part 2: evidence evaluation and guidelines development: 2020 American Heart Association Guidelines for Cardiopulmonary Resuscitation and Emergency Cardiovascular Care. *Circulation*. 2020;142(suppl 2):S358–S365. doi: 10.1161/CIR.0000000000000898

3. Levine GN, O'Gara PT, Beckman JA, Al-Khatib SM, Birtcher KK, Cigarroa JE, de Las Fuentes L, Deswal A, Fleisher LA, Gentile F, Goldberger ZD, Hlatky MA, Joglar JA, Piano MR, Wijeysundera DN. Recent innovations, modifications, and evolution of ACC/AHA clinical practice guidelines: an update for our constituencies: a report of the American College of Cardiology/American Heart Association Task Force on Clinical Practice Guidelines. *Circulation*. 2019;139:e879–e886. doi: 10.1161/CIR.0000000000000651

MAJOR CONCEPTS

The Utstein Formula for Survival

The development and implementation of resuscitation systems of care is founded on the Utstein Formula for Survival.[1] The Utstein Formula holds that resuscitation survival is based on synergy achieved by the development and dissemination of medical science (ie, resuscitation guidelines based on the best available evidence); educational efficiency, which includes the effective training of resuscitation providers and members of the general public; and local implementation, which includes seamless collaboration between caregivers involved in all stages of resuscitation and post–cardiac arrest care (Figure 1). Parts 3 through 5 of the 2020 Guidelines represent the AHA's creation of guidelines based on the best available resuscitation science. In "Part 6: Resuscitation Education Science," the AHA critically evaluates the science of training medical professionals and the general public to assist a person in cardiac arrest. In "Part 7: Systems of Care," we explore resuscitation topics that are common to the resuscitation of infants, children, and adults.

The AHA Chain of Survival

Since 1991, the AHA has emphasized the concept of a *chain of survival*, the coordinated effort used to implement resuscitation science and training.[2] With minor variations for the BLS, ALS, and pediatric ALS care settings, the AHA's Chain of Survival emphasized early recognition of cardiac arrest, activation of the emergency response system, early defibrillation, high quality CPR, advanced resuscitation techniques, and post–cardiac arrest care.

Several improvements have been made to the Chain of Survival concept in these guidelines. Because the causes and treatment of cardiac arrest differ between adults and infants/children as well as between IHCA and OHCA, specific Chains of Survival have been created for different age groups and situations (Figure 2). Each chain has also been lengthened by adding a link for recovery. The neonatal Chain of Survival concept (not supported by a graphic) differs somewhat, because there are far greater opportunities for community and facility preparation before birth, and neonatal resuscitation teams can anticipate and prepare with advance warning and parental involvement. However, the principles of the Chain of Survival and the formula for survival may be universally applied. This Part focuses on recommendations for broad interventions along the entire Chain of Survival that can improve outcomes for all rather than for merely one patient.

Although there are intentional differences in content and sequence due to populations and context, each Chain of Survival includes elements of the following:

- **Prevention and preparedness**, including responder training, early recognition of cardiac arrest, and rapid response
- **Activation of the emergency response system**, either outside of or within the hospital
- **High-quality CPR**, including **early defibrillation** of ventricular fibrillation and pulseless ventricular tachycardia
- **Advanced resuscitation interventions**, including medications, advanced airway interventions, and extracorporeal CPR
- **Post–cardiac arrest care**, including critical care interventions and targeted temperature management
- **Recovery**, including effective support for physical, cognitive, emotional, and family needs

Prevention of cardiac arrest in the out-of-hospital setting includes measures to improve the health of communities and individuals as well as public awareness campaigns to help people recognize the signs and symptoms of acute coronary syndromes and cardiac arrest. In the hospital setting, **preparedness** includes early recognition of and response to the patient who may need resuscitation (including preparation for high-risk deliveries), rapid response teams (see Prevention of IHCA), and training of individuals and resuscitation teams. Extensive information about individual and team training is also provided in "Part 6: Resuscitation Education Science."[3] Emergency response system development, layperson and dispatcher training in the recognition of cardiac arrest, community CPR training, widespread AED availability, and telecommunicator

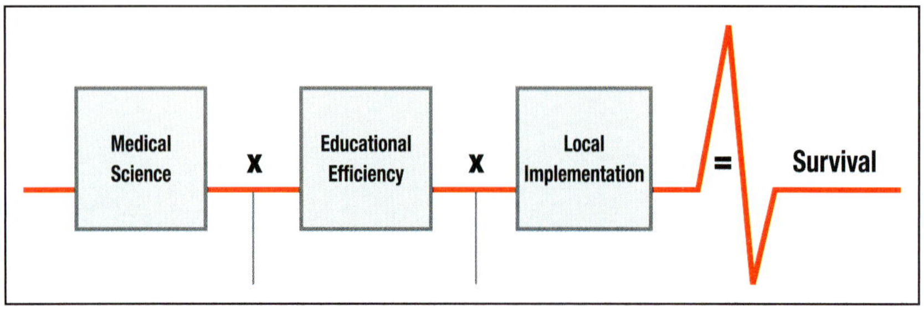

Figure 1. **The Utstein Formula for Survival.**[1]

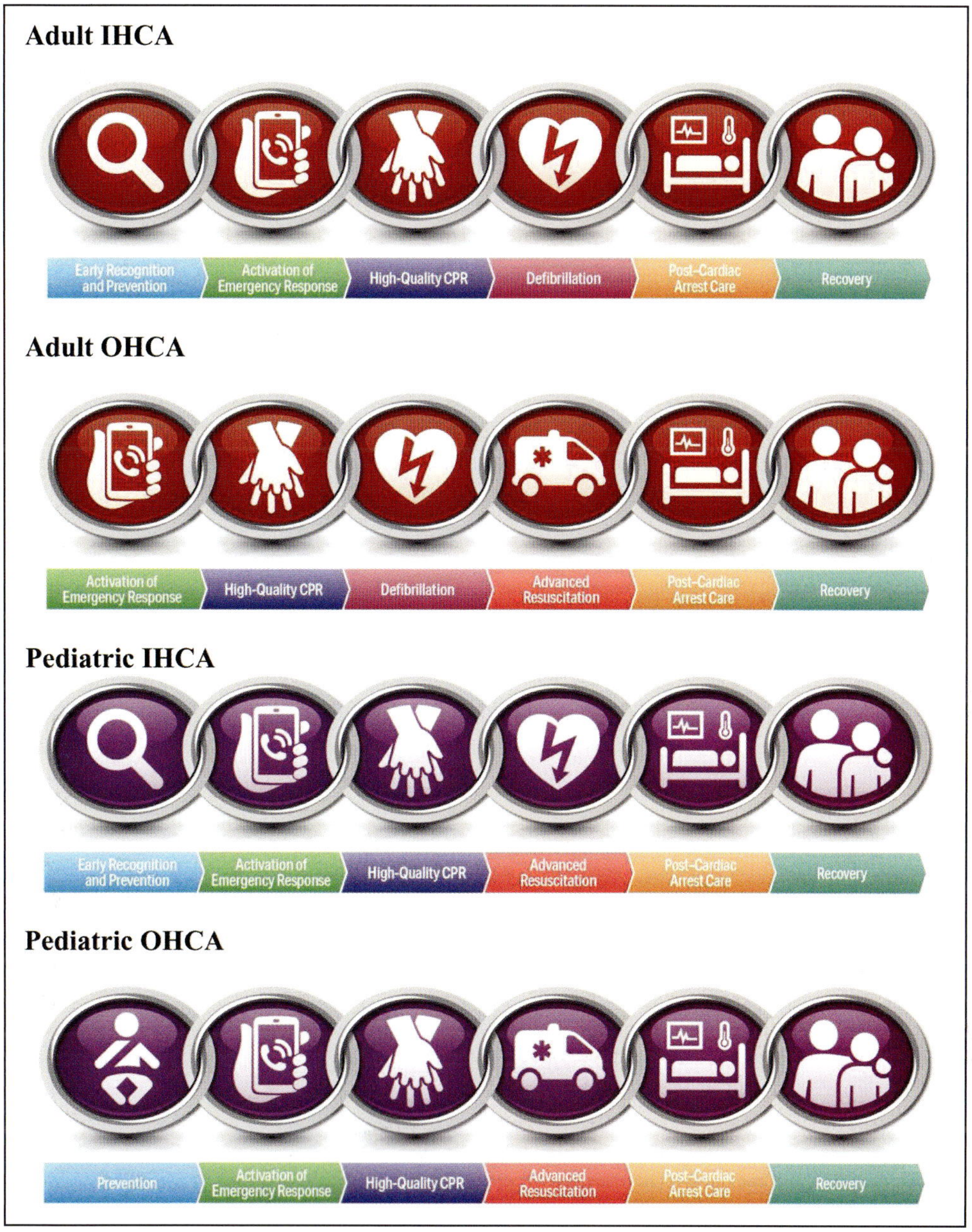

Figure 2. The Updated AHA Chains of Survival.
AHA indicates American Heart Association; CPR, cardiopulmonary resuscitation; IHCA, in-hospital cardiac arrest; and OHCA, out-of-hospital cardiac arrest.

instructions that enable members of the general public to initiate high-quality CPR and perform early defibrillation are all important components of this step in the out-of-hospital setting. Recent innovations include using mobile phone technology to summon members of the public who are trained in CPR (see Mobile Phone Technologies to Alert Bystanders of Events Requiring CPR). As described in "Part 5: Neonatal Resuscitation," predelivery preparedness is an essential component of successful neonatal resuscitation.[4]

Activation of the emergency response system typically begins with shouting for nearby help. Outside the hospital, immediate next steps include phoning the universal emergency response number (eg, 9-1-1) and sending someone to get the nearest AED. For IHCA, parallel steps include summoning the hospital's resuscitation team.

High-quality CPR, with minimal interruptions and continuous monitoring of CPR quality, and **early defibrillation** of ventricular fibrillation and pulseless ventricular tachycardia together form the cornerstone of modern resuscitation and are the interventions most closely related to good resuscitation outcomes. Importantly, these time-sensitive interventions can be provided by members of the public as well as by healthcare professionals. Similarly, in cases of opioid-associated respiratory arrest, early administration of naloxone by bystanders or trained rescuers can be lifesaving.

Advanced resuscitation interventions, including pharmacotherapy, advanced airway interventions (endotracheal intubation or supraglottic airway placement), and extracorporeal CPR may also improve outcomes in specific resuscitation situations.

Post–cardiac arrest care includes routine critical care support (eg, mechanical ventilation, intravenous vasopressors) and also specific, evidence-based interventions that improve outcomes in patients who achieve ROSC after successful resuscitation, such as targeted temperature management. Specific recommendations for targeted temperature management are found in Parts 3, 4, and 5, which provide the 2020 AHA adult,[5] pediatric,[6] and neonatal guidelines,[4] respectively. Because there is no earlier method to reliably identify patients in whom a poor neurological outcome is inevitable, current guidelines for adults recommend against withdrawal of life support for at least 72 hours after resuscitation and rewarming from any induced hypothermia, and perhaps longer.[5,8,9] A great deal of active research is underway to develop additional neuroprotective strategies and biomarkers to indicate a good, or poor, prognosis after ROSC.

Recovery from cardiac arrest continues long after hospital discharge. Depending on the outcome achieved, important elements of recovery may include measures to address the underlying cause of cardiac arrest, secondary-prevention cardiac rehabilitation, neurologically focused rehabilitative care, and psychological support for the patient and family. A growing and important body of research examines interventions to benefit the cardiac arrest survivor.[10]

Use of Data for Continuous Improvement

Although the Chain of Survival emphasizes key elements in the care of an individual patient, it does not sufficiently emphasize steps that are necessary for improving future performance. Examples include conducting a structured team debriefing after a resuscitation event, responding to data on IHCAs collected through the AHA's Get With The Guidelines initiative, and reviewing data collected for OHCA by using the Utstein framework (Table 2). Several formal process-improvement frameworks, including Lean, Six Sigma, the High Reliability Organization framework, and the Deming Model for Improvement, exist to facilitate continuous improvement. The AHA and other organizations have recommended structures for specific performance-improvement initiatives in resuscitation. The goal is to become a "learning healthcare system"[11] that uses data to continually improve preparedness and resuscitation outcomes. Application of this concept to resuscitation systems of care has been previously supported, and is ongoing in many resuscitation organizations.[12,13]

For OHCA, major contributors to resuscitation success are early and effective CPR and early defibrillation.

Table 2. Examples of the Use of Data for Systems Improvement

After reading about the role of AEDs in the workplace, the manager of a busy office building installed an AED and obtained hands-only CPR training for all of her staff.
In response to data that showed a large number of opioid overdoses at the main branch of the public library, an EMS agency provided library staff with naloxone kits and training.
During resuscitation, the Team Leader identified that the rescuer who was providing bag-mask ventilation via endotracheal tube was hyperventilating the patient. The Team Leader coached the rescuer to compress the bag only enough to achieve chest rise.
In response to data showing low bystander CPR rates in some neighborhoods, free CPR classes were provided in community centers in those neighborhoods.
During the team debriefing after a difficult but successful pediatric resuscitation, an error in epinephrine dosing was discovered. The root cause was traced to the need to calculate drug volume under pressure. A reference book was created, listing standard resuscitation medication volumes in milliliters for children of different weights.
In response to research showing that women who are victims of cardiac arrest are less likely than men to receive bystander CPR, focus groups were held to identify the root causes for this reluctance, and training was adjusted to target these barriers.
In response to data showing that many newly born infants became hypothermic during resuscitation, a predelivery checklist was introduced to ensure that steps were carried out to prevent this complication.

AED indicates automated external defibrillator; CPR, cardiopulmonary resuscitation; and EMS, emergency medical services.

Measures to reduce delays to CPR, improve the effectiveness of that CPR, and ensure early defibrillation for patients with shockable rhythms are therefore a major component of these guidelines.

For IHCA, the major contributors to resuscitation success are similar, but the presence of healthcare professionals affords the opportunity to prevent cardiac arrest. The median time from hospital admission to IHCA in adult patients is 2 days.[13] Early identification of the decompensating patient may allow for stabilization that prevents cardiac arrest. This intervention includes 2 steps: identifying the patient at risk, and providing early intervention, either by the patient's current caregivers or by members of a dedicated team, to prevent deterioration. Because there are separate adult and pediatric evidence bases for these questions, the Adult Basic and Advanced Life Support Writing Group and the Pediatric Basic and Advanced Life Support Writing Group performed parallel evaluations of the evidence about early warning scoring systems as well as about rapid response teams (RRTs) and medical emergency teams (METs).

REFERENCES

1. Søreide E, Morrison L, Hillman K, Monsieurs K, Sunde K, Zideman D, Eisenberg M, Sterz F, Nadkarni VM, Soar J, Nolan JP; Utstein Formula for Survival Collaborators. The formula for survival in resuscitation. *Resuscitation*. 2013;84:1487–1493. doi: 10.1016/j.resuscitation.2013.07.020

2. Cummins RO, Ornato JP, Thies WH, Pepe PE. Improving survival from sudden cardiac arrest: the "chain of survival" concept. A statement for health professionals from the Advanced Cardiac Life Support Subcommittee and the Emergency Cardiac Care Committee, American Heart Association. *Circulation*. 1991;83:1832–1847. doi: 10.1161/01.cir.83.5.1832
3. Cheng A, Magid DJ, Auerbach M, Bhanji F, Bigham BL, Blewer AL, Dainty KN, Diederich E, Lin Y, Leary M, et al. Part 6: resuscitation education science: 2020 American Heart Association Guidelines for Cardiopulmonary Resuscitation and Emergency Cardiovascular Care. *Circulation*. 2020;142(suppl 2):S551–S579. doi: 10.1161/CIR.0000000000000903
4. Aziz K, Lee HC, Escobedo MB, Hoover AV, Kamath-Rayne BD, Kapadia VS, Magid DJ, Niermeyer S, Schmölzer GM, Szyld E, et al. Part 5: neonatal resuscitation: 2020 American Heart Association Guidelines for Cardiopulmonary Resuscitation and Emergency Cardiovascular Care. *Circulation*. 2020;142(suppl 2):S524–S550. doi: 10.1161/CIR.0000000000000902
5. Panchal AR, Bartos JA, Cabañas JG, Donnino MW, Drennan IR, Hirsch KG, Kudenchuk PJ, Kurz MC, Lavonas EJ, Morley PT, et al; on behalf of the Adult Basic and Advanced Life Support Writing Group. Part 3: adult basic and advanced life support: 2020 American Heart Association Guidelines for Cardiopulmonary Resuscitation and Emergency Cardiovascular Care. *Circulation*. 2020;142(suppl 2):S366–S468. doi: 10.1161/CIR.0000000000000916
6. Topjian AA, Raymond TT, Atkins D, Chan M, Duff JP, Joyner BL Jr, Lasa JJ, Lavonas EJ, Levy A, Mahgoub M, et al; on behalf of the Pediatric Basic and Advanced Life Support Collaborators. Part 4: pediatric basic and advanced life support: 2020 American Heart Association Guidelines for Cardiopulmonary Resuscitation and Emergency Cardiovascular Care. *Circulation*. 2020;142(suppl 2):S469–S523. doi: 10.1161/CIR.0000000000000901
7. Deleted in proof.
8. Callaway CW, Donnino MW, Fink EL, Geocadin RG, Golan E, Kern KB, Leary M, Meurer WJ, Peberdy MA, Thompson TM, et al. Part 8: post–cardiac arrest care: 2015 American Heart Association Guidelines Update for Cardiopulmonary Resuscitation and Emergency Cardiovascular Care. *Circulation*. 2015;132(suppl 2):S465–482. doi: 10.1161/cir.0000000000000262
9. Geocadin RG, Callaway CW, Fink EL, Golan E, Greer DM, Ko NU, Lang E, Licht DJ, Marino BS, McNair ND, Peberdy MA, Perman SM, Sims DB, Soar J, Sandroni C; American Heart Association Emergency Cardiovascular Care Committee. Standards for Studies of Neurological Prognostication in Comatose Survivors of Cardiac Arrest: A Scientific Statement From the American Heart Association. *Circulation*. 2019;140:e517–e542. doi: 10.1161/CIR.0000000000000702
10. Sawyer KN, Camp-Rogers TR, Kotini-Shah P, Del Rios M, Gossip MR, Moitra VK, Haywood KL, Dougherty CM, Lubitz SA, Rabinstein AA, Rittenberger JC, Callaway CW, Abella BS, Geocadin RG, Kurz MC; American Heart Association Emergency Cardiovascular Care Committee; Council on Cardiovascular and Stroke Nursing; Council on Genomic and Precision Medicine; Council on Quality of Care and Outcomes Research; and Stroke Council. Sudden Cardiac Arrest Survivorship: A Scientific Statement From the American Heart Association. *Circulation*. 2020;141:e654–e685. doi: 10.1161/CIR.0000000000000747
11. *Institute of Medicine (US) Roundtable on Evidence-Based Medicine*. Olsen LA, Aisner D, McGinnis JM, eds. Washington DC: National Academies Press; 2007.
12. Committee on the Treatment of Cardiac Arrest: Current Status and Future Directions; Board on Health Sciences Policy; Institute of Medicine. *Strategies to Improve Cardiac Arrest Survival: A Time to Act*. Graham R, McCoy MA, Schultz AM, eds. Washington DC; 2015. https://www.ncbi.nlm.nih.gov/pubmed/26225413. Accessed February 14, 2020.
13. Neumar RW, Eigel B, Callaway CW, Estes NA 3rd, Jollis JG, Kleinman ME, Morrison LJ, Peberdy MA, Rabinstein A, Rea TD, et al; on behalf of the American Heart Association. American Heart Association response to the 2015 Institute of Medicine report on strategies to improve cardiac arrest survival. *Circulation*. 2015;132:1049–1070. doi: 10.1161/CIR.0000000000000233
14. Deleted in proof.
15. Nolan JP, Soar J, Smith GB, Gwinnutt C, Parrott F, Power S, Harrison DA, Nixon E, Rowan K; National Cardiac Arrest Audit. Incidence and outcome of in-hospital cardiac arrest in the United Kingdom National Cardiac Arrest Audit. *Resuscitation*. 2014;85:987–992. doi: 10.1016/j.resuscitation.2014.04.002

PREHOSPITAL SYSTEMS OF CARE

Community Initiatives to Promote CPR Implementation

Recommendation for Community Initiatives to Promote CPR Implementation		
COR	LOE	Recommendation
2b	C-LD	1. It may be reasonable for communities to implement strategies for increasing awareness and delivery of bystander CPR.[1–12]

Synopsis

CPR and AED use are lifesaving interventions, but rates of bystander action are low.[13] Mass media campaigns (eg, advertisements, mass distribution of educational materials), instructor-led training (ie, instructor-facilitated CPR training in small or large groups), and various types of bundled interventions have all been studied to improve rates of bystander CPR in communities.[1–12] Bundled interventions include multipronged approaches to enhancing several links in the Chain of Survival, involving targeted (based on postal code or risk assessment) or untargeted (mass) instruction incorporating instructors, peers, digital media (ie, video), or self-instruction. Depending on the context, *community* could refer to a group of neighborhoods; 1 or more cities, towns, or regions; or a whole nation.[14]

Recommendation-Specific Supportive Text

1. A 2020 ILCOR systematic review[14] identified 1 randomized controlled trial (RCT)[15] and 16 observational studies[1–12,16–19] reporting bystander CPR rates and/or survival outcomes. Bystander CPR rates improved in 12 of these studies.[1–12]

Instructor-Led Training: Six observational studies assessed the impact of instructor-led training.[1–4,17–19] Two of 4 studies found improvement in survival with good neurological outcomes after implementation of instructor-led training.[1,2,17,18] Two of 3 studies reported improvements in survival to hospital discharge,[1,3,18] and 1 study demonstrated an improvement in ROSC after instructor-led training.[3] Instructor-led training improved bystander CPR rates by 10% to 19% in 4 studies.[1–4]

Mass Media Campaigns: One observational study reported a 12% absolute increase in bystander CPR rates after a campaign of television advertisements promoting bystander CPR.[6] However, mass distribution (via mail) of a 10-minute CPR instructional video to 8659 households resulted in no significant improvement in bystander CPR rates when compared with a community with households that did not receive a video (47% in intervention households, 53% in controls).[15]

Bundled Interventions: Nine observational studies evaluated the impact of bundled interventions on bystander

CPR rates and survival outcomes.[5,7–12,16,19] Bystander CPR rates were improved in 7 of these studies.[4,5,7–12,16]

These recommendations were created by the AHA Resuscitation Education Science Writing Group and are supported by a 2020 ILCOR systematic review.[14]

REFERENCES

1. Fordyce CB, Hansen CM, Kragholm K, Dupre ME, Jollis JG, Roettig ML, Becker LB, Hansen SM, Hinohara TT, Corbett CC, Monk L, Nelson RD, Pearson DA, Tyson C, van Diepen S, Anderson ML, McNally B, Granger CB. Association of public health initiatives with outcomes for out-of-hospital cardiac arrest at home and in public locations. *JAMA Cardiol.* 2017;2:1226–1235. doi: 10.1001/jamacardio.2017.3471
2. Malta Hansen C, Kragholm K, Pearson DA, Tyson C, Monk L, Myers B, Nelson D, Dupre ME, Fosbol EL, Jollis JG, et al. Association of bystander and first-responder intervention with survival after out-of-hospital cardiac arrest in North Carolina, 2010-2013. *JAMA.* 2015;314:255–264. doi: 10.1001/jama.2015.7938
3. Tay PJM, Pek PP, Fan Q, Ng YY, Leong BS, Gan HN, Mao DR, Chia MYC, Cheah SO, Doctor N, Tham LP, Ong MEH. Effectiveness of a community based out-of-hospital cardiac arrest (OHCA) interventional bundle: Results of a pilot study. *Resuscitation.* 2020;146:220–228. doi: 10.1016/j.resuscitation.2019.10.015
4. Boland LL, Formanek MB, Harkins KK, Frazee CL, Kamrud JW, Stevens AC, Lick CJ, Yannopoulos D. Minnesota Heart Safe Communities: Are community-based initiatives increasing pre-ambulance CPR and AED use? *Resuscitation.* 2017;119:33–36. doi: 10.1016/j.resuscitation.2017.07.031
5. Bergamo C, Bui QM, Gonzales L, Hinchey P, Sasson C, Cabanas JG. TAKE10: A community approach to teaching compression-only CPR to high-risk zip codes. *Resuscitation.* 2016;102:75–79. doi: 10.1016/j.resuscitation.2016.02.019
6. Becker L, Vath J, Eisenberg M, Meischke H. The impact of television public service announcements on the rate of bystander CPR. *Prehosp Emerg Care.* 1999;3:353–356. doi: 10.1080/10903129908958968
7. Hwang WS, Park JS, Kim SJ, Hong YS, Moon SW, Lee SW. A system-wide approach from the community to the hospital for improving neurologic outcomes in out-of-hospital cardiac arrest patients. *Eur J Emerg Med.* 2017;24:87–95. doi: 10.1097/MEJ.0000000000000313
8. Ro YS, Shin SD, Song KJ, Hong SO, Kim YT, Lee DW, Cho SI. Public awareness and self-efficacy of cardiopulmonary resuscitation in communities and outcomes of out-of-hospital cardiac arrest: A multi-level analysis. *Resuscitation.* 2016;102:17–24. doi: 10.1016/j.resuscitation.2016.02.004
9. Nielsen AM, Isbye DL, Lippert FK, Rasmussen LS. Persisting effect of community approaches to resuscitation. *Resuscitation.* 2014;85:1450–1454. doi: 10.1016/j.resuscitation.2014.08.019
10. Møller Nielsen A, Lou Isbye D, Knudsen Lippert F, Rasmussen LS. Engaging a whole community in resuscitation. *Resuscitation.* 2012;83:1067–1071. doi: 10.1016/j.resuscitation.2012.04.012
11. Wissenberg M, Lippert FK, Folke F, Weeke P, Hansen CM, Christensen EF, Jans H, Hansen PA, Lang-Jensen T, Olesen JB, Lindhardsen J, Fosbol EL, Nielsen SL, Gislason GH, Kober L, Torp-Pedersen C. Association of national initiatives to improve cardiac arrest management with rates of bystander intervention and patient survival after out-of-hospital cardiac arrest. *JAMA.* 2013;310:1377–1384. doi: 10.1001/jama.2013.278483
12. Ro YS, Song KJ, Shin SD, Hong KJ, Park JH, Kong SY, Cho SI. Association between county-level cardiopulmonary resuscitation training and changes in Survival Outcomes after out-of-hospital cardiac arrest over 5years: A multilevel analysis. *Resuscitation.* 2019;139:291–298. doi: 10.1016/j.resuscitation.2019.01.012
13. Girotra S, van Diepen S, Nallamothu BK, Carrel M, Vellano K, Anderson ML, McNally B, Abella BS, Sasson C, Chan PS; CARES Surveillance Group and the HeartRescue Project. Regional Variation in Out-of-Hospital Cardiac Arrest Survival in the United States. *Circulation.* 2016;133:2159–2168. doi: 10.1161/CIRCULATIONAHA.115.018175
14. Olasveengen TM, Mancini ME, Perkins GD, Avis S, Brooks S, Castrén M, Chung SP, Considine J, Couper K, Escalante R, et al; on behalf of the Adult Basic Life Support Collaborators. Adult basic life support: 2020 International Consensus on Cardiopulmonary Resuscitation and Emergency Cardiovascular Care Science With Treatment Recommendations. *Circulation.* 2020;142(suppl 1):S41–S91. doi: 10.1161/CIR.0000000000000892
15. Eisenberg M, Damon S, Mandel L, Tewodros A, Meischke H, Beaupied E, Bennett J, Guildner C, Ewell C, Gordon M. CPR instruction by videotape: results of a community project. *Ann Emerg Med.* 1995;25:198–202. doi: 10.1016/s0196-0644(95)70324-1
16. Del Rios M, Han J, Cano A, Ramirez V, Morales G, Campbell TL, Vanden Hoek T. Pay it forward: high school video-based instruction can disseminate CPR knowledge in priority neighborhoods. *West J Emerg Med.* 2018;19:423–429. doi: 10.5811/westjem.2017.10.35108
17. Nishiyama C, Kitamura T, Sakai T, Murakami Y, Shimamoto T, Kawamura T, Yonezawa T, Nakai S, Marukawa S, Sakamoto T, Iwami T. Community-wide dissemination of bystander cardiopulmonary resuscitation and automated external defibrillator use using a 45-minute chest compression-only cardiopulmonary resuscitation training. *J Am Heart Assoc.* 2019;8:e009436. doi: 10.1161/JAHA.118.009436
18. Uber A, Sadler RC, Chassee T, Reynolds JC. Does non-targeted community CPR training increase bystander CPR frequency? *Prehosp Emerg Care.* 2018;22:753–761. doi: 10.1080/10903127.2018.1459978
19. Isbye DL, Rasmussen LS, Ringsted C, Lippert FK. Disseminating cardiopulmonary resuscitation training by distributing 35,000 personal manikins among school children. *Circulation.* 2007;116:1380–1385. doi: 10.1161/CIRCULATIONAHA.107.710616

Public Access Defibrillation

Recommendation for Public Access Defibrillation		
COR	**LOE**	**Recommendation**
1	B-NR	1. We recommend that public access defibrillation programs for patients with OHCA be implemented in communities at risk for cardiac arrest.[1–33]

Synopsis

Early defibrillation significantly increases survival rates from OHCA.[34–37] Public access defibrillation (PAD) programs are designed to reduce the time to defibrillation by placing AEDs in public places and training members of the public to use them. Compared with traditional EMS systems without a PAD program, persons who experience an OHCA in EMS systems with a PAD program have higher rates of ROSC; higher rates of survival to hospital discharge and at 30 days after OHCA; and higher rates of survival with favorable neurological outcome at hospital discharge, at 30 days, and at 1 year after OHCA.[9,10,33] On the basis of this evidence, we recommend that PAD be implemented in communities with individuals at risk for cardiac arrest (eg, office buildings, casinos, apartment buildings, public gatherings). Although the existing evidence supports the effectiveness of PAD programs, the use of public access defibrillators by lay rescuers remains low.[38,39] Additional research is needed on strategies to improve public access defibrillation by lay rescuers, including the role of the emergency medical dispatcher in identifying the nearest AED and alerting callers to its location, the optimal placement of AEDs, and the use of technology to enhance rescuers' ability to deliver timely defibrillation.[33,40]

Recommendation-Specific Supportive Text

1. Of 31 studies that assessed the impact of PAD programs, 27 (1 RCT[20] and 26 observational studies[1–3,5,7,8,11–19,21–23,25–28,30–32,41] found improved outcomes while 4 observational studies[4,6,24,29] found no difference in outcomes.

A 2020 ILCOR systematic review[33] found low-quality evidence of improved survival with favorable neurological outcome for systems with a PAD program compared with those without a program, at 1 year from 1 observational study[4] enrolling 62 patients (43% versus 0%, P=0.02), at 30 days from 7 observational studies[3,22,25,26,29,30,41] enrolling 43 116 patients (odds ratio [OR], 6.60; 95% CI 3.54–12.28), and at hospital discharge from 8 observational studies[1,2,4,7,11–13,24] enrolling 11 837 patients (OR, 2.89; 95% CI, 1.79–4.66).

This same review found low- to moderate-quality evidence of improved survival for systems with a PAD program compared with those without a program, at 30 days from 8 observational studies[3,5,15,17,22,28–30] enrolling 85 589 patients (OR, 3.66; 95% CI, 2.63–5.11) and at hospital discharge from 1 RCT[20] enrolling 235 patients (RR, 2.0; 95% CI, 1.07–3.77) and 16 observational studies[1,2,6–8,11,13,14,16,18,19,21,24,27,31,32] enrolling 40 243 patients (OR, 3.24; 95% CI, 2.13–4.92).

Low-quality evidence from 13 observational studies[3–7,11,17,19,22,28–31] enrolling 95 354 patients found improved ROSC in EMS systems with a PAD program compared with systems without a PAD program (OR, 2.45; 95% CI, 1.88–3.18).

These recommendations were created by the AHA Adult Basic and Advanced Life Support Writing Group and are supported by a 2020 ILCOR systematic review.[33]

REFERENCES

1. Berdowski J, Blom MT, Bardai A, Tan HL, Tijssen JG, Koster RW. Impact of onsite or dispatched automated external defibrillator use on survival after out-of-hospital cardiac arrest. *Circulation*. 2011;124:2225–2232. doi: 10.1161/CIRCULATIONAHA.110.015545
2. Fordyce CB, Hansen CM, Kragholm K, Dupre ME, Jollis JG, Roettig ML, Becker LB, Hansen SM, Hinohara TT, Corbett CC, Monk L, Nelson RD, Pearson DA, Tyson C, van Diepen S, Anderson ML, McNally B, Granger CB. Association of public health initiatives with outcomes for out-of-hospital cardiac arrest at home and in public locations. *JAMA Cardiol*. 2017;2:1226–1235. doi: 10.1001/jamacardio.2017.3471
3. Fukuda T, Ohashi-Fukuda N, Kobayashi H, Gunshin M, Sera T, Kondo Y, Yahagi N. Public access defibrillation and outcomes after pediatric out-of-hospital cardiac arrest. *Resuscitation*. 2017;111:1–7. doi: 10.1016/j.resuscitation.2016.11.010
4. Gianotto-Oliveira R, Gonzalez MM, Vianna CB, Monteiro Alves M, Timerman S, Kalil Filho R, Kern KB. Survival after ventricular fibrillation cardiac arrest in the Sao Paulo Metropolitan subway system: first successful targeted automated external defibrillator (AED) program in Latin America. *J Am Heart Assoc*. 2015;4:e002185. doi: 10.1161/JAHA.115.002185
5. Hansen SM, Hansen CM, Folke F, Rajan S, Kragholm K, Ejlskov L, Gislason G, Køber L, Gerds TA, Hjortshøj S, Lippert F, Torp-Pedersen C, Wissenberg M. Bystander defibrillation for out-of-hospital cardiac arrest in public vs residential locations. *JAMA Cardiol*. 2017;2:507–514. doi: 10.1001/jamacardio.2017.0008
6. Nas J, Thannhauser J, Herrmann JJ, van der Wulp K, van Grunsven PM, van Royen N, de Boer MJ, Bonnes JL, Brouwer MA. Changes in automated external defibrillator use and survival after out-of-hospital cardiac arrest in the Nijmegen area. *Neth Heart J*. 2018;26:600–605. doi: 10.1007/s12471-018-1162-9
7. Pollack RA, Brown SP, Rea T, Aufderheide T, Barbic D, Buick JE, Christenson J, Idris AH, Jasti J, Kampp M, Kudenchuk P, May S, Muhr M, Nichol G, Ornato JP, Sopko G, Vaillancourt C, Morrison L, Weisfeldt M; ROC Investigators. Impact of bystander automated external defibrillator use on survival and functional outcomes in shockable observed public cardiac arrests. *Circulation*. 2018;137:2104–2113. doi: 10.1161/CIRCULATIONAHA.117.030700
8. Weisfeldt ML, Sitlani CM, Ornato JP, Rea T, Aufderheide TP, Davis D, Dreyer J, Hess EP, Jui J, Maloney J, Sopko G, Powell J, Nichol G, Morrison LJ; ROC Investigators. Survival after application of automatic external defibrillators before arrival of the emergency medical system: evaluation in the resuscitation outcomes consortium population of 21 million. *J Am Coll Cardiol*. 2010;55:1713–1720. doi: 10.1016/j.jacc.2009.11.077
9. Bækgaard JS, Viereck S, Møller TP, Ersbøll AK, Lippert F, Folke F. The effects of public access defibrillation on survival after out-of-hospital cardiac arrest: a systematic review of observational studies. *Circulation*. 2017;136:954–965. doi: 10.1161/CIRCULATIONAHA.117.029067
10. Holmberg MJ, Vognsen M, Andersen MS, Donnino MW, Andersen LW. Bystander automated external defibrillator use and clinical outcomes after out-of-hospital cardiac arrest: A systematic review and meta-analysis. *Resuscitation*. 2017;120:77–87. doi: 10.1016/j.resuscitation.2017.09.003
11. Andersen LW, Holmberg MJ, Granfeldt A, Løfgren B, Vellano K, McNally BF, Siegerink B, Kurth T, Donnino MW; CARES Surveillance Group. Neighborhood characteristics, bystander automated external defibrillator use, and patient outcomes in public out-of-hospital cardiac arrest. *Resuscitation*. 2018;126:72–79. doi: 10.1016/j.resuscitation.2018.02.021
12. Aschieri D, Penela D, Pelizzoni V, Guerra F, Vermi AC, Rossi L, Torretta L, Losi G, Villani GQ, Capucci A. Outcomes after sudden cardiac arrest in sports centres with and without on-site external defibrillators. *Heart*. 2018;104:1344–1349. doi: 10.1136/heartjnl-2017-312441
13. Capucci A, Aschieri D, Piepoli MF, Bardy GH, Iconomu E, Arvedi M. Tripling survival from sudden cardiac arrest via early defibrillation without traditional education in cardiopulmonary resuscitation. *Circulation*. 2002;106:1065–1070. doi: 10.1161/01.cir.0000028148.62305.69
14. Capucci A, Aschieri D, Guerra F, Pelizzoni V, Nani S, Villani GQ, Bardy GH. Community-based automated external defibrillator only resuscitation for out-of-hospital cardiac arrest patients. *Am Heart J*. 2016;172:192–200. doi: 10.1016/j.ahj.2015.10.018
15. Claesson A, Herlitz J, Svensson L, Ottosson L, Bergfeldt L, Engdahl J, Ericson C, Sandén P, Axelsson C, Bremer A. Defibrillation before EMS arrival in western Sweden. *Am J Emerg Med*. 2017;35:1043–1048. doi: 10.1016/j.ajem.2017.02.030
16. Culley LL, Rea TD, Murray JA, Welles B, Fahrenbruch CE, Olsufka M, Eisenberg MS, Copass MK. Public access defibrillation in out-of-hospital cardiac arrest: a community-based study. *Circulation*. 2004;109:1859–1863. doi: 10.1161/01.CIR.0000124721.83385.B2
17. Dicker B, Davey P, Smith T, Beck B. Incidence and outcomes of out-of-hospital cardiac arrest: A New Zealand perspective. *Emerg Med Australas*. 2018;30:662–671. doi: 10.1111/1742-6723.12966
18. Edwards MJ, Fothergill RT. Exercise-related sudden cardiac arrest in London: incidence, survival and bystander response. *Open Heart*. 2015;2:e000281. doi: 10.1136/openhrt-2015-000281
19. Garcia EL, Caffrey-Villari S, Ramirez D, Caron JL, Mannhart P, Reuter PG, Lapostolle F, Adnet F. [Impact of onsite or dispatched automated external defibrillator use on early survival after sudden cardiac arrest occurring in international airports]. *Presse Med*. 2017;46:e63–e68. doi: 10.1016/j.lpm.2016.09.027
20. Hallstrom AP, Ornato JP, Weisfeldt M, Travers A, Christenson J, McBurnie MA, Zalenski R, Becker LB, Schron EB, Proschan M; Public Access Defibrillation Trial Investigators. Public-access defibrillation and survival after out-of-hospital cardiac arrest. *N Engl J Med*. 2004;351:637–646. doi: 10.1056/NEJMoa040566
21. Karam N, Marijon E, Dumas F, Offredo L, Beganton F, Bougouin W, Jost D, Lamhaut L, Empana JP, Cariou A, Spaulding C, Jouven X; Paris Sudden Death Expertise Center. Characteristics and outcomes of out-of-hospital sudden cardiac arrest according to the time of occurrence. *Resuscitation*. 2017;116:16–21. doi: 10.1016/j.resuscitation.2017.04.024
22. Kiguchi T, Kiyohara K, Kitamura T, Nishiyama C, Kobayashi D, Okabayashi S, Shimamoto T, Matsuyama T, Kawamura T, Iwami T. Public-access defibrillation and survival of out-of-hospital cardiac arrest in public vs. residential locations in Japan. *Circ J*. 2019;83:1682–1688. doi: 10.1253/circj.CJ-19-0065
23. Kim JH, Uhm TH. Survival to admission after out-of-hospital cardiac arrest in Seoul, South Korea. *Open Access Emerg Med*. 2014;6:63–68. doi: 10.2147/OAEM.S68758
24. Kuisma M, Castrén M, Nurminen K. Public access defibrillation in Helsinki–costs and potential benefits from a community-based pilot study. *Resuscitation*. 2003;56:149–152. doi: 10.1016/s0300-9572(02)00344-1
25. Matsui S, Kitamura T, Sado J, Kiyohara K, Kobayashi D, Kiguchi T, Nishiyama C, Okabayashi S, Shimamoto T, Matsuyama T, Kawamura T, Iwami T, Tanaka R, Kurosawa H, Nitta M, Sobue T. Location of arrest and survival from out-of-hospital cardiac arrest among children in the public-access defibrillation era in Japan. *Resuscitation*. 2019;140:150–158. doi: 10.1016/j.resuscitation.2019.04.045

26. Nakahara S, Tomio J, Ichikawa M, Nakamura F, Nishida M, Takahashi H, Morimura N, Sakamoto T. Association of bystander interventions with neurologically intact survival among patients with bystander-witnessed out-of-hospital cardiac arrest in Japan. *JAMA.* 2015;314:247–254. doi: 10.1001/jama.2015.8068
27. Nehme Z, Andrew E, Bernard S, Haskins B, Smith K. Trends in survival from out-of-hospital cardiac arrests defibrillated by paramedics, first responders and bystanders. *Resuscitation.* 2019;143:85–91. doi: 10.1016/j.resuscitation.2019.08.018
28. Ringh M, Jonsson M, Nordberg P, Fredman D, Hasselqvist-Ax I, Håkansson F, Claesson A, Riva G, Hollenberg J. Survival after public access defibrillation in Stockholm, Sweden–a striking success. *Resuscitation.* 2015;91:1–7. doi: 10.1016/j.resuscitation.2015.02.032
29. Tay PJM, Pek PP, Fan Q, Ng YY, Leong BS, Gan HN, Mao DR, Chia MYC, Cheah SO, Doctor N, Tham LP, Ong MEH. Effectiveness of a community based out-of-hospital cardiac arrest (OHCA) interventional bundle: Results of a pilot study. *Resuscitation.* 2020;146:220–228. doi: 10.1016/j.resuscitation.2019.10.015
30. Kitamura T, Kiyohara K, Sakai T, Matsuyama T, Hatakeyama T, Shimamoto T, Izawa J, Fujii T, Nishiyama C, Kawamura T, Iwami T. Public-access defibrillation and out-of-hospital cardiac arrest in Japan. *N Engl J Med.* 2016;375:1649–1659. doi: 10.1056/NEJMsa1600011
31. Colquhoun MC, Chamberlain DA, Newcombe RG, Harris R, Harris S, Peel K, Davies CS, Boyle R. A national scheme for public access defibrillation in England and Wales: early results. *Resuscitation.* 2008;78:275–280. doi: 10.1016/j.resuscitation.2008.03.226
32. Fleischhackl R, Roessler B, Domanovits H, Singer F, Fleischhackl S, Foitik G, Czech G, Mittlboeck M, Malzer R, Eisenburger P, Hoerauf K. Results from Austria's nationwide public access defibrillation (ANPAD) programme collected over 2 years. *Resuscitation.* 2008;77:195–200. doi: 10.1016/j.resuscitation.2007.11.019
33. Olasveengen TM, Mancini ME, Perkins GD, Avis S, Brooks S, Castrén M, Chung SP, Considine J, Couper K, Escalante R, et al; on behalf of the Adult Basic Life Support Collaborators. Adult basic life support: 2020 International Consensus on Cardiopulmonary Resuscitation and Emergency Cardiovascular Care Science With Treatment Recommendations. *Circulation.* 2020;142(suppl 1):S41–S91. doi: 10.1161/CIR.0000000000000892
34. Sasson C, Rogers MA, Dahl J, Kellermann AL. Predictors of survival from out-of-hospital cardiac arrest: a systematic review and meta-analysis. *Circ Cardiovasc Qual Outcomes.* 2010;3:63–81. doi: 10.1161/CIRCOUTCOMES.109.889576
35. Wissenberg M, Lippert FK, Folke F, Weeke P, Hansen CM, Christensen EF, Jans H, Hansen PA, Lang-Jensen T, Olesen JB, Lindhardsen J, Fosbol EL, Nielsen SL, Gislason GH, Kober L, Torp-Pedersen C. Association of national initiatives to improve cardiac arrest management with rates of bystander intervention and patient survival after out-of-hospital cardiac arrest. *JAMA.* 2013;310:1377–1384. doi: 10.1001/jama.2013.278483
36. Larsen MP, Eisenberg MS, Cummins RO, Hallstrom AP. Predicting survival from out-of-hospital cardiac arrest: a graphic model. *Ann Emerg Med.* 1993;22:1652–1658. doi: 10.1016/s0196-0644(05)81302-2
37. Perkins GD, Handley AJ, Koster RW, Castren M, Smyth MA, Olasveengen T, Monsieurs KG, Raffay V, Grasner JT, Wenzel V, et al; on behalf of the adult basic life support and automated external defibrillation section collaborators. European Resuscitation Council guidelines for resuscitation 2015: Section 2: adult basic life support and automated external defibrillation. *Resuscitation.* 2015;95:81–99. doi: 10.1016/j.resuscitation.2015.07.015
38. Ringh M, Hollenberg J, Palsgaard-Moeller T, Svensson L, Rosenqvist M, Lippert FK, Wissenberg M, Malta Hansen C, Claesson A, Viereck S, Zijlstra JA, Koster RW, Herlitz J, Blom MT, Kramer-Johansen J, Tan HL, Beesems SG, Hulleman M, Olasveengen TM, Folke F; COSTA study group (research collaboration between Copenhagen, Oslo, STockholm, and Amsterdam). The challenges and possibilities of public access defibrillation. *J Intern Med.* 2018;283:238–256. doi: 10.1111/joim.12730
39. Myat A, Baumbach A. Public-access defibrillation: a call to shock. *Lancet.* 2020;394:2204–2206. doi: 10.1016/S0140-6736(19)32560-7
40. Mao RD, Ong ME. Public access defibrillation: improving accessibility and outcomes. *Br Med Bull.* 2016;118:25–32. doi: 10.1093/bmb/ldw011
41. Takeuchi I, Nagasawa H, Jitsuiki K, Kondo A, Ohsaka H, Yanagawa Y. Impact of automated external defibrillator as a recent innovation for the resuscitation of cardiac arrest patients in an urban city of Japan. *J Emerg Trauma Shock.* 2018;11:217–220. doi: 10.4103/JETS.JETS_79_17

Mobile Phone Technologies to Alert Bystanders of Events Requiring CPR

Recommendation for Mobile Phone Technologies to Alert Bystanders of Events Requiring CPR

COR	LOE	Recommendation
2a	B-NR	1. The use of mobile phone technology by emergency dispatch systems to alert willing bystanders to nearby events that may require CPR or AED use is reasonable.[1–7]

Synopsis

Despite the recognized role of lay first responders in improving OHCA outcomes, most communities experience low rates of bystander CPR[8] and AED use.[1] Mobile phone technology, such as text messages and smartphone applications, is increasingly being used to summon bystander assistance to OHCA events. For example, some smartphone apps allow emergency dispatch telecommunicators to send out alerts to CPR-trained community members who are within close proximity to a cardiac arrest event and use mapping technology to guide citizens to nearby AEDs and cardiac arrest victims.[2]

An ILCOR systematic review[10] found that notification of lay rescuers via a smartphone app or text message alert is associated with shorter bystander response times,[2] higher bystander CPR rates,[5,6] shorter time to defibrillation,[1] and higher rates of survival to hospital discharge[3–5,7] for individuals who experience OHCA. Technology currently exists for emergency dispatch systems to use mobile phone technology to summon willing bystanders to nearby events where CPR and/or defibrillation may be required. As these technologies become more ubiquitous, they are likely to play an expanding role in the Chain of Survival. Randomized controlled trials, cost-effectiveness studies, and studies exploring this intervention for diverse patient, community, and geographical contexts are required. The psychological impact of engaging citizens to provide care to bystanders is unclear.

Recommendation-Specific Supportive Text

1. A systematic review[9] identified 1 RCT[6] and 6 observational studies[1–5,7] reporting uniformly positive data supportive of using mobile phone technology to summon bystanders. Meta-analysis of 4 observational studies enrolling 2905 OHCA events showed improvement in survival to hospital discharge when a citizen responder was notified of an OHCA by mobile phone technology (adjusted relative risk [aRR], 1.70; 95% CI 1.16–2.48) compared to no notification.[3–5,7] This evidence is of low certainty due to the biases inherent in observational work. One RCT[6] enrolling 667 patients

with OHCA found that bystander CPR rates were increased by 14% (aRR, 1.27; CI 1.10–1.46) when citizen responders were notified by mobile phone technology, although ROSC and survival were not increased. An observational study of 1696 OHCA events reported an increase of 16% in bystander CPR rate (aRR, 1.29; CI 1.20–1.37) when lay rescuers were notified via text message.[5] Four observational studies including 1833 OHCA episodes showed that lay rescuers notified by mobile phone technology arrived between 3 and 4 minutes faster than ambulances.[1–3,7] Time to defibrillation was reduced by 2 minutes and 39 seconds when citizens were notified via text message to bring an AED compared with ambulance response.[1] No study reported the occurrence of any adverse events related to citizen notification. To date, there have been no studies conducted in North America, and important cultural and geographic differences could alter the effect of these technologies between countries and regions. Further studies are required to establish efficacy.

These recommendations were created by the AHA Resuscitation Education Science Writing Group and are supported by a 2020 ILCOR systematic review.[10]

REFERENCES

1. Zijlstra JA, Stieglis R, Riedijk F, Smeekes M, van der Worp WE, Koster RW. Local lay rescuers with AEDs, alerted by text messages, contribute to early defibrillation in a Dutch out-of-hospital cardiac arrest dispatch system. *Resuscitation.* 2014;85:1444–1449. doi: 10.1016/j.resuscitation.2014.07.020
2. Berglund E, Claesson A, Nordberg P, Djärv T, Lundgren P, Folke F, Forsberg S, Riva G, Ringh M. A smartphone application for dispatch of lay responders to out-of-hospital cardiac arrests. *Resuscitation.* 2018;126:160–165. doi: 10.1016/j.resuscitation.2018.01.039
3. Caputo ML, Muschietti S, Burkart R, Benvenuti C, Conte G, Regoli F, Mauri R, Klersy C, Moccetti T, Auricchio A. Lay persons alerted by mobile application system initiate earlier cardio-pulmonary resuscitation: A comparison with SMS-based system notification. *Resuscitation.* 2017;114:73–78. doi: 10.1016/j.resuscitation.2017.03.003
4. Pijls RW, Nelemans PJ, Rahel BM, Gorgels AP. A text message alert system for trained volunteers improves out-of-hospital cardiac arrest survival. *Resuscitation.* 2016;105:182–187. doi: 10.1016/j.resuscitation.2016.06.006
5. Lee SY, Shin SD, Lee YJ, Song KJ, Hong KJ, Ro YS, Lee EJ, Kong SY. Text message alert system and resuscitation outcomes after out-of-hospital cardiac arrest: A before-and-after population-based study. *Resuscitation.* 2019;138:198–207. doi: 10.1016/j.resuscitation.2019.01.045
6. Ringh M, Rosenqvist M, Hollenberg J, Jonsson M, Fredman D, Nordberg P, Järnbert-Pettersson H, Hasselqvist-Ax I, Riva G, Svensson L. Mobile-phone dispatch of laypersons for CPR in out-of-hospital cardiac arrest. *N Engl J Med.* 2015;372:2316–2325. doi: 10.1056/NEJMoa1406038
7. Stroop R, Kerner T, Strickmann B, Hensel M. Mobile phone-based alerting of CPR-trained volunteers simultaneously with the ambulance can reduce the resuscitation-free interval and improve outcome after out-of-hospital cardiac arrest: A German, population-based cohort study. *Resuscitation.* 2020;147:57–64. doi: 10.1016/j.resuscitation.2019.12.012
8. Girotra S, van Diepen S, Nallamothu BK, Carrel M, Vellano K, Anderson ML, McNally B, Abella BS, Sasson C, Chan PS; CARES Surveillance Group and the HeartRescue Project. Regional Variation in Out-of-Hospital Cardiac Arrest Survival in the United States. *Circulation.* 2016;133:2159–2168. doi: 10.1161/CIRCULATIONAHA.115.018175
9. Semeraro F, Zace D, Bigham BL, Scapigliati A, Ristagno G, Bhanji F, Bray JE, Breckwoldt J, Cheng A, Duff JP, et al. First responder engaged by technology (EIT #878): systematic review: consensus on science with treatment recommendations. https://costr.ilcor.org/document/first-responder-engaged-by-technology-systematic-review. Accessed February 17, 2020.
10. Greif R, Bhanji F, Bigham BL, Bray J, Breckwoldt J, Cheng A, Duff JP, Gilfoyle E, Hsieh M-J, Iwami T, et al; on behalf of the Education, Implementation, and Teams Collaborators. Education, implementation, and teams: 2020 International Consensus on Cardiopulmonary Resuscitation and Emergency Cardiovascular Care Science With Treatment Recommendations. *Circulation.* 2020;142(suppl 1):S222–S283. doi: 10.1161/CIR.0000000000000896

Telecommunicator Roles in the Management of OHCA

Introduction

Early, effective bystander CPR is a critical component of the OHCA Chain of Survival. Unfortunately, rates of bystander CPR remain low for both adults and children. As the initial public safety interface with the lay public in a medical emergency, telecommunicators are a critical link in the OHCA Chain of Survival. In adults and children with OHCA, the provision of CPR instructions by emergency telecommunicators (commonly called *call takers* or *dispatchers*) is associated with increased rates of bystander CPR and improved patient outcomes. EMS systems that offer telecommunicator CPR instructions (T-CPR; sometimes referred to as *dispatcher-assisted CPR*, or DA-CPR) document higher bystander CPR rates in both adult and pediatric OHCA.[1–3] Unfortunately, bystander CPR rates for pediatric OHCA remain low, even when T-CPR is offered. The T-CPR process should be scripted to maximize the number of OHCA victims receiving bystander CPR, and quality improvement mechanisms should be used routinely.

Because the evidence base for this question is distinct for adult and pediatric patient populations, the AHA Adult Basic and Advanced Life Support Writing Group and the AHA Pediatric Basic and Advanced Life Support Writing Group performed separate reviews.

REFERENCES

1. Duff JP, Topjian AA, Berg MD, Chan M, Haskell SE, Joyner BL Jr, Lasa JJ, Ley SJ, Raymond TT, Sutton RM, et al. 2019 American Heart Association focused update on pediatric basic life support: an update to the American Heart Association guidelines for cardiopulmonary resuscitation and emergency cardiovascular care. *Circulation.* 2019;140:e915–e921. doi: 10.1161/CIR.0000000000000736
2. Panchal AR, Berg KM, Cabañas JG, Kurz MC, Link MS, Del Rios M, Hirsch KG, Chan PS, Hazinski MF, Morley PT, Donnino MW, Kudenchuk PJ. 2019 American Heart Association focused update on systems of care: dispatcher-assisted cardiopulmonary resuscitation and cardiac arrest centers: an update to the American Heart Association Guidelines for Cardiopulmonary Resuscitation and Emergency Cardiovascular Care. *Circulation.* 2019;140:e895–e903. doi: 10.1161/CIR.0000000000000733
3. Kurz MC BB, Buckingham J, Cabanas JG, Eisenberg M, Fromm P, Panczyk MJ, Rea T, Seaman K, Vaillancourt C. Telephone cardiopulmonary resuscitation: an advocacy statement from the American Heart Association. *Circulation.* 2020;141:e686–e700. doi: 10.1161/CIR.0000000000000744

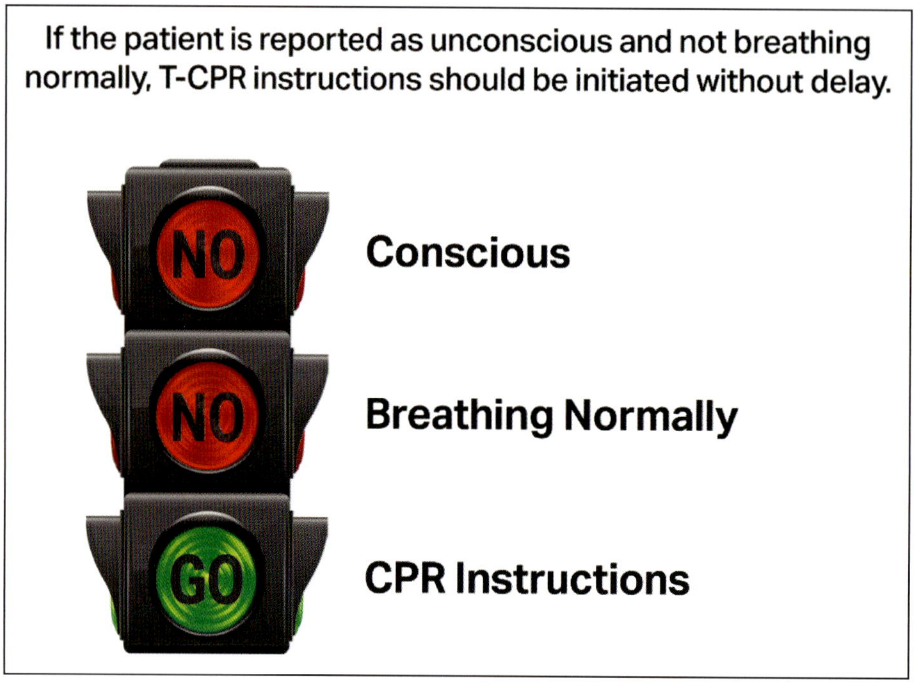

If the patient is reported as unconscious and not breathing normally, T-CPR instructions should be initiated without delay.
NO
Conscious
NO
Breathing Normally
GO
CPR Instructions

Figure 3. **The No-No-Go Mnemonic for Initiation of Bystander CPR.**
From The Road to Recognition and Resuscitation: The Role of Telecommunicators and Telephone CPR Quality Improvement in Cardiac Arrest Survival. With permission from The Resuscitation Academy, Seattle, WA. CPR indicates cardiopulmonary resuscitation; and T-CPR, telephone cardiopulmonary resuscitation.

Telecommunicator Roles in OHCA in Adults

Recommendations for Telecommunicator Recognition of Cardiac Arrest in Adults

COR	LOE	Recommendations
1	C-LD	1. Telecommunicators should acquire the requisite information to determine the location of the event before questions to identify OHCA, to allow for simultaneous dispatching of EMS response.[1,2]
2a	C-LD	2. If the patient is unresponsive with abnormal, agonal, or absent breathing, it is reasonable for the emergency dispatcher to assume that the patient is in cardiac arrest.[3,4]

Recommendation-Specific Supportive Text

1. A telecommunicator receiving an emergency call for service (ie, a 9-1-1 call) for an adult patient in suspected cardiac arrest first should acquire the location of the emergency so that appropriate emergency medical response can be dispatched simultaneous to OHCA identification.[1] Asking the 2 scripted questions from the No-No-Go process (Figure 3) to determine if a victim is unresponsive with abnormal breathing may positively identify up to 92% of people suffering OHCA.[2]
2. When a caller describes an adult victim as unresponsive, with absent or abnormal breathing, telecommunicators should conclude that the victim is experiencing OHCA and should immediately provide T-CPR instructions.[3,5] To address the variation in OHCA presentations, telecommunicators should be trained to identify OHCA across a broad range of circumstances, including agonal gasping and brief myoclonus.[4]

These recommendations were created by the AHA Adult Basic and Advanced Life Support Writing Group and are supported by the "2019 AHA Focused Update on Systems of Care: Dispatcher-Assisted CPR and Cardiac Arrest Centers: An Update to the AHA Guidelines for CPR and ECC," a 2018 ILCOR systematic review, and a 2020 AHA statement.[3,5,6]

Recommendations for T-CPR Instructions for Adults in Suspected Cardiac Arrest

COR	LOE	Recommendations
1	C-LD	1. We recommend that emergency dispatch centers offer CPR instructions and empower dispatchers to provide such instructions for adult patients in cardiac arrest.[7]
1	C-LD	2. Telecommunicators should instruct callers to initiate CPR for adults with suspected OHCA.[7]
1	C-LD	3. We recommend that dispatchers should provide chest compression–only CPR instructions to callers for adults with suspected OHCA.[7]

Recommendation-Specific Supportive Text

1. Early access to EMS via emergency dispatch centers (ie, 9-1-1) and early CPR are the first 2 links

Circulation. 2020;142(suppl 2):S580–S604. DOI: 10.1161/CIR.0000000000000899

in the Chain of Survival for adult OHCA. In 3 adjusted observational studies, T-CPR was associated with a greater than 5-fold likelihood of provision of bystander CPR,[8–10] and CPR was initiated 7 minutes sooner[9] compared with no T-CPR.

2. The delivery of bystander CPR before the arrival of professional responders is associated with survival and favorable neurological outcome in 6 observational studies.[8,9,11–14] In 2 studies, offering T-CPR was associated with increased survival with favorable neurological outcome at 1 month after discharge, even after adjustment for multiple variables.[9,12] Therefore, every emergency communications center should provide timely T-CPR instructions in all calls in which an OHCA victim is identified.[3]
3. Based on meta-analysis of the 2 largest randomized trials comparing dispatcher compression-only CPR with conventional CPR (total n=2496), dispatcher instruction in compression-only CPR was associated with long-term survival benefit compared with instruction in chest compressions and rescue breathing.[6,15]

Recommendation for T-CPR Quality Improvement

COR	LOE	Recommendation
1	B-NR	1. The delivery of T-CPR instructions should be reviewed and evaluated as part of an EMS system quality improvement process.[16,17]

Recommendation-Specific Supportive Text

1. Successful T-CPR programs should have a robust quality improvement process, including auditory review of OHCA calls, to ensure that T-CPR is being provided as broadly, rapidly, and appropriately as possible.[16,17]

These recommendations were created by the AHA Adult Basic and Advanced Life Support Writing Group and are supported by the "2019 AHA Focused Update on Systems of Care: Dispatcher-Assisted CPR and Cardiac Arrest Centers: An Update to the AHA Guidelines for CPR and ECC"; a 2018 ILCOR systematic review; and a 2020 AHA statement.[3,5,6]

REFERENCES

1. Lerner EB, Rea TD, Bobrow BJ, Acker JE III, Berg RA, Brooks SC, Cone DC, Gay M, Gent LM, Mears G, Nadkarni VM, O'Connor RE, Potts J, Sayre MR, Swor RA, Travers AH; American Heart Association Emergency Cardiovascular Care Committee; Council on Cardiopulmonary, Critical Care, Perioperative and Resuscitation. Emergency medical service dispatch cardiopulmonary resuscitation prearrival instructions to improve survival from out-of-hospital cardiac arrest: a scientific statement from the American Heart Association. *Circulation*. 2012;125:648–655. doi: 10.1161/CIR.0b013e31823ee5fc
2. Lewis M, Stubbs BA, Eisenberg MS. Dispatcher-assisted cardiopulmonary resuscitation: time to identify cardiac arrest and deliver chest compression instructions. *Circulation*. 2013;128:1522–1530. doi: 10.1161/CIRCULATIONAHA.113.002627
3. Kurz MC BB, Buckingham J, Cabanas JG, Eisenberg M, Fromm P, Panczyk MJ, Rea T, Seaman K, Vaillancourt C. Telephone cardiopulmonary resuscitation: an advocacy statement from the American Heart Association. *Circulation*. 2020;141:e686–e700. doi: 10.1161/CIR.0000000000000744
4. Bång A, Herlitz J, Martinell S. Interaction between emergency medical dispatcher and caller in suspected out-of-hospital cardiac arrest calls with focus on agonal breathing. A review of 100 tape recordings of true cardiac arrest cases. *Resuscitation*. 2003;56:25–34. doi: 10.1016/s0300-9572(02)00278-2
5. Panchal AR, Berg KM, Cabañas JG, Kurz MC, Link MS, Del Rios M, Hirsch KG, Chan PS, Hazinski MF, Morley PT, Donnino MW, Kudenchuk PJ. 2019 American Heart Association focused update on systems of care: dispatcher-assisted cardiopulmonary resuscitation and cardiac arrest centers: an update to the American Heart Association Guidelines for Cardiopulmonary Resuscitation and Emergency Cardiovascular Care. *Circulation*. 2019;140:e895–e903. doi: 10.1161/CIR.0000000000000733
6. Olasveengen TM, Mancini ME, Perkins GD, Avis S, Brooks S, Castrén M, Chung SP, Considine J, Couper K, Escalante R, et al; on behalf of the Adult Basic Life Support Collaborators. Adult basic life support: 2020 International Consensus on Cardiopulmonary Resuscitation and Emergency Cardiovascular Care Science With Treatment Recommendations. *Circulation*. 2020;142(suppl 1):S41–S91. doi: 10.1161/CIR.0000000000000892
7. Nikolaou N, Dainty KN, Couper K, Morley P, Tijssen J, Vaillancourt C; International Liaison Committee on Resuscitation's (ILCOR) Basic Life Support and Pediatric Task Forces. A systematic review and meta-analysis of the effect of dispatcher-assisted CPR on outcomes from sudden cardiac arrest in adults and children. *Resuscitation*. 2019;138:82–105. doi: 10.1016/j.resuscitation.2019.02.035
8. Song KJ, Shin SD, Park CB, Kim JY, Kim DK, Kim CH, Ha SY, Eng Hock Ong M, Bobrow BJ, McNally B. Dispatcher-assisted bystander cardiopulmonary resuscitation in a metropolitan city: a before-after population-based study. *Resuscitation*. 2014;85:34–41. doi: 10.1016/j.resuscitation.2013.06.004
9. Goto Y, Maeda T, Goto Y. Impact of dispatcher-assisted bystander cardiopulmonary resuscitation on neurological outcomes in children with out-of-hospital cardiac arrests: a prospective, nationwide, population-based cohort study. *J Am Heart Assoc*. 2014;3:e000499. doi: 10.1161/JAHA.113.000499
10. Fukushima H, Panczyk M, Hu C, Dameff C, Chikani V, Vadeboncoeur T, Spaite DW, Bobrow BJ. Description of abnormal breathing is associated with improved outcomes and delayed telephone cardiopulmonary resuscitation instructions. *J Am Heart Assoc*. 2017;6:e005058. doi: 10.1161/JAHA.116.005058
11. Besnier E, Damm C, Jardel B, Veber B, Compere V, Dureuil B. Dispatcher-assisted cardiopulmonary resuscitation protocol improves diagnosis and resuscitation recommendations for out-of-hospital cardiac arrest. *Emerg Med Australas*. 2015;27:590–596. doi: 10.1111/1742-6723.12493
12. Harjanto S, Na MX, Hao Y, Ng YY, Doctor N, Goh ES, Leong BS, Gan HN, Chia MY, Tham LP, Cheah SO, Shahidah N, Ong ME; PAROS study group. A before-after interventional trial of dispatcher-assisted cardio-pulmonary resuscitation for out-of-hospital cardiac arrests in Singapore. *Resuscitation*. 2016;102:85–93. doi: 10.1016/j.resuscitation.2016.02.014
13. Hiltunen PV, Silfvast TO, Jäntti TH, Kuisma MJ, Kurola JO; FINNRESUSCI Prehospital Study Group. Emergency dispatch process and patient outcome in bystander-witnessed out-of-hospital cardiac arrest with a shockable rhythm. *Eur J Emerg Med*. 2015;22:266–272. doi: 10.1097/MEJ.0000000000000151
14. Takahashi H, Sagisaka R, Natsume Y, Tanaka S, Takyu H, Tanaka H. Does dispatcher-assisted CPR generate the same outcomes as spontaneously delivered bystander CPR in Japan? *Am J Emerg Med*. 2018;36:384–391. doi: 10.1016/j.ajem.2017.08.034
15. Hüpfl M, Selig HF, Nagele P. Chest-compression-only versus standard cardiopulmonary resuscitation: a meta-analysis. *Lancet*. 2010;376:1552–1557. doi: 10.1016/S0140-6736(10)61454-7
16. Tanaka Y, Taniguchi J, Wato Y, Yoshida Y, Inaba H. The continuous quality improvement project for telephone-assisted instruction of cardiopulmonary resuscitation increased the incidence of bystander CPR and improved the outcomes of out-of-hospital cardiac arrests. *Resuscitation*. 2012;83:1235–1241. doi: 10.1016/j.resuscitation.2012.02.013
17. Bobrow BJ, Spaite DW, Vadeboncoeur TF, Hu C, Mullins T, Tormala W, Dameff C, Gallagher J, Smith G, Panczyk M. Implementation of a regional telephone cardiopulmonary resuscitation program and outcomes after out-of-hospital cardiac arrest. *JAMA Cardiol*. 2016;1:294–302. doi: 10.1001/jamacardio.2016.0251

Telecommunicator Roles in OHCA—Infants and Children

Recommendations for T-CPR—Infants and Children		
COR	LOE	Recommendations
1	C-LD	1. We recommend that emergency medical dispatch centers offer T-CPR instructions for presumed pediatric cardiac arrest.[1–5]
1	C-LD	2. We recommend that emergency dispatchers provide T-CPR instructions for pediatric cardiac arrest when no bystander CPR is in progress.[1–5]

Recommendation-Specific Supportive Text

1. A recent ILCOR systematic review provides evidence that T-CPR is associated with improved patient outcomes in children and adults compared to no T-CPR.[6] An observational study reported the association of T-CPR with increased survival at 1 month in children with OHCA.[1] An observational study of 5009 cardiac arrest patients showed that offered dispatcher-assisted CPR was associated with improved 1-month survival but not with 1-month favorable neurological outcome. The provision of bystander CPR, with or without dispatcher instruction, was associated with improved odds of survival and survival with favorable neurological outcomes compared with no bystander CPR.[2]
2. A cross-sectional registry study demonstrated that both T-CPR and unassisted bystander CPR were associated with increased likelihood of favorable neurological outcome at hospital discharge compared with no bystander CPR.[3] A more recent cross-sectional study of children with OHCA from the same database noted the association of bystander CPR with more than double the survival with favorable neurological function at hospital discharge, whether that bystander CPR was delivered with or without dispatcher assistance.[4]

These recommendations were created by the AHA Pediatric Basic and Advanced Life Support Writing Group and are supported by the "2019 AHA Focused Update on Pediatric Basic Life Support: An Update to the AHA Guidelines for CPR and ECC" and a 2019 ILCOR systematic review.[6]

REFERENCES

1. Akahane M, Ogawa T, Tanabe S, Koike S, Horiguchi H, Yasunaga H, Imamura T. Impact of telephone dispatcher assistance on the outcomes of pediatric out-of-hospital cardiac arrest. *Crit Care Med*. 2012;40:1410–1416. doi: 10.1097/CCM.0b013e31823e99ae
2. Goto Y, Maeda T, Goto Y. Impact of dispatcher-assisted bystander cardiopulmonary resuscitation on neurological outcomes in children with out-of-hospital cardiac arrests: a prospective, nationwide, population-based cohort study. *J Am Heart Assoc*. 2014;3:e000499. doi: 10.1161/JAHA.113.000499
3. Ro YS, Shin SD, Song KJ, Hong KJ, Ahn KO, Kim DK, Kwak YH. Effects of Dispatcher-assisted Cardiopulmonary Resuscitation on Survival Outcomes in Infants, Children, and Adolescents with Out-of-hospital Cardiac Arrests. *Resuscitation*. 2016;108:20–26. doi: 10.1016/j.resuscitation.2016.08.026
4. Chang I, Ro YS, Shin SD, Song KJ, Park JH, Kong SY. Association of dispatcher-assisted bystander cardiopulmonary resuscitation with survival outcomes after pediatric out-of-hospital cardiac arrest by community property value. *Resuscitation*. 2018;132:120–126. doi: 10.1016/j.resuscitation.2018.09.008
5. Nikolaou N, Dainty KN, Couper K, Morley P, Tijssen J, Vaillancourt C; International Liaison Committee on Resuscitation's (ILCOR) Basic Life Support and Pediatric Task Forces. A systematic review and meta-analysis of the effect of dispatcher-assisted CPR on outcomes from sudden cardiac arrest in adults and children. *Resuscitation*. 2019;138:82–105. doi: 10.1016/j.resuscitation.2019.02.035
6. Olasveengen TM, Mancini ME, Perkins GD, Avis S, Brooks S, Castrén M, Chung SP, Considine J, Couper K, Escalante R, et al; on behalf of the Adult Basic Life Support Collaborators. Adult basic life support: 2020 International Consensus on Cardiopulmonary Resuscitation and Emergency Cardiovascular Care Science With Treatment Recommendations. *Circulation*. 2020;142(suppl 1):S41–S91. doi: 10.1161/CIR.0000000000000892

PREVENTION OF IHCA

Introduction

Survival from IHCA remains variable, particularly for adults.[1] Patients who arrest in an unmonitored or unwitnessed setting, as is typical on most general wards, have the worst outcomes. Outcomes from pediatric IHCA have improved, and survival rates are as high as 38%,[2] and most pediatric IHCAs occur in ICUs.[3] In-hospital cardiac or respiratory arrest can potentially be prevented by systems that recognize and dedicate resources to the deteriorating patient. MET or RRT activation by the bedside care team or family members ideally occurs as a response to changes noted in a patient's condition. These teams respond to patients with acute physiological decline in an effort to prevent in-hospital cardiopulmonary arrest and death. Although rapid response systems have been widely adopted, outcome studies have shown inconsistent results. The composition of the responding teams, the consistency of team activation and response, as well as the elements comprising the early warning scoring systems vary widely between hospitals, thus making widespread scientific conclusions on the efficacy of such interventions difficult.

Because the evidence base for this question is distinct for adult and pediatric patient populations and pediatric patient populations, the AHA Adult Basic and Advanced Life Support Writing Group and the AHA Pediatric Basic and Advanced Life Support Writing Group performed separate reviews.

REFERENCES

1. Virani SS, Alonso A, Benjamin EJ, Bittencourt MS, Callaway CW, Carson AP, Chamberlain AM, Chang AR, Cheng S, Delling FN, et al: on behalf of the American Heart Association Council on Epidemiology and Prevention Statistics Committee and Stroke Statistics Subcommittee. Heart disease and stroke statistics—2020 update: a report from the American Heart Association. *Circulation*. 2020;141:e139–e596. doi: 10.1161/CIR.0000000000000757
2. Holmberg MJ, Wiberg S, Ross CE, Kleinman M, Hoeyer-Nielsen AK, Donnino MW, Andersen LW. Trends in survival after pediatric in-hospital cardiac arrest in the United States. *Circulation*. 2019;140:1398–1408. doi: 10.1161/CIRCULATIONAHA.119.041667
3. Berg RA, Sutton RM, Holubkov R, Nicholson CE, Dean JM, Harrison R, Heidemann S, Meert K, Newth C, Moler F, Pollack M, Dalton H, Doctor A, Wessel D, Berger J, Shanley T, Carcillo J, Nadkarni VM; Eunice Kennedy Shriver National Institute of Child Health and Human Development Collaborative Pediatric Critical Care Research Network and for

the American Heart Association's Get With the Guidelines-Resuscitation (formerly the National Registry of Cardiopulmonary Resuscitation) Investigators. Ratio of PICU versus ward cardiopulmonary resuscitation events is increasing. *Crit Care Med.* 2013;41:2292–2297. doi: 10.1097/CCM.0b013e31828cf0c0

Clinical Early Warning Systems and Rapid Response Teams to Prevent IHCA in Adults

Recommendations for Prevention of IHCA—Adult Patients		
COR	LOE	Recommendations
2a	C-LD	1. For hospitalized adults, response systems such as rapid response teams or medical emergency teams can be effective in reducing the incidence of cardiac arrest, particularly in general care wards.[1]
2b	C-LD	2. The use of early warning scoring systems may be considered for hospitalized adults.[1]

Recommendation-Specific Supportive Text

1. A recent ILCOR systematic review found inconsistency in the results of observational studies of RRT/MET system implementation, with 17 studies demonstrating a significant improvement in cardiac arrest rates and 7 studies finding no such improvement.[1] One large RCT demonstrated no benefit in cardiac arrest occurrence or mortality.[2] On the basis of this evidence, it appears that implementation of an RRT/MET system can be effective in decreasing non-ICU cardiac arrests, and possibly mortality, but further evaluations are necessary. Higher-intensity systems (eg, higher RRT/MET activation rates, senior medical staff on RRTs/METs) appear to be more effective. Heterogeneity in study design, context, patient populations, response team composition, team activation criteria, and outcomes studied prevent critical analysis of data across studies.
2. The systematic review focused primarily on the effect of RRT/MET systems, but the use of early warning systems was also included. No RCTs were identified on the use of early warning scoring systems with the specific goal of decreasing adult IHCA. One observational study was included, which found that the Modified Early Warning Score had an inconsistent ability to predict IHCA.[1,3] More recently, there is growing interest in machine learning and other approaches to aid in early detection of deterioration, and further study of these is warranted.[4]

These recommendations were created by the AHA Adult Basic and Advanced Life Support Writing Group and are based on a 2020 ILCOR systematic review that focused on RRT/MET implementation.[1]

REFERENCES

1. Greif R, Bhanji F, Bigham BL, Bray J, Breckwoldt J, Cheng A, Duff JP, Gilfoyle E, Hsieh M-J, Iwami T, et al; on behalf of the Education, Implementation, and Teams Collaborators. Education, implementation, and teams: 2020 International Consensus on Cardiopulmonary Resuscitation and Emergency Cardiovascular Care Science With Treatment Recommendations. *Circulation.* 2020;142(suppl 1):S222–S283. doi: 10.1161/CIR.0000000000000896
2. Hillman K, Chen J, Cretikos M, Bellomo R, Brown D, Doig G, Finfer S, Flabouris A; MERIT study investigators. Introduction of the medical emergency team (MET) system: a cluster-randomised controlled trial. *Lancet.* 2005;365:2091–2097. doi: 10.1016/S0140-6736(05)66733-5
3. Subbe CP, Davies RG, Williams E, Rutherford P, Gemmell L. Effect of introducing the Modified Early Warning score on clinical outcomes, cardio-pulmonary arrests and intensive care utilisation in acute medical admissions. *Anaesthesia.* 2003;58:797–802. doi: 10.1046/j.1365-2044.2003.03258.x
4. Kwon JM, Lee Y, Lee Y, Lee S, Park J. An algorithm based on deep learning for predicting in-hospital cardiac arrest. *J Am Heart Assoc.* 2018;7:e008678. doi: 10.1161/jaha.118.008678

Clinical Early Warning Systems and Rapid Response Teams to Prevent IHCA in Infants, Children, and Adolescents

Recommendations for Prevention of IHCA—Infants, Children, and Adolescents		
COR	LOE	Recommendations
2a	C-LD	1. Pediatric rapid response team/medical emergency team systems can be beneficial in facilities where children with high-risk illnesses are cared for on general inpatient units.[1–4]
2b	B-R	2. Pediatric early warning/trigger scores may be considered in addition to pediatric rapid response/medical emergency teams to detect high-risk infants and children for early transfer to a higher level of care.[1,5–9]

Recommendation-Specific Supportive Text

1. RRT/MET systems are associated with reductions in hospital mortality and cardiopulmonary arrest rates in both adult and pediatric populations.[1–3] One observational registry study of 38 pediatric hospitals found no difference in risk-adjusted mortality rates associated with RRT/MET implementation.[4] There is low-quantity and low-quality evidence evaluating the role of RRT/MET systems to prevent pediatric cardiac arrest. Major limitations are the low rate of pediatric cardiac arrests and mortality (especially outside the ICU setting) and the heterogeneity of the patient populations.
2. In a multicenter, international cluster randomized trial, implementation of the bedside pediatric early warning system was associated with a decrease in clinically important deteriorations on the wards of nontertiary care in community hospitals, but not with all-cause mortality.[5] Four recent systematic reviews and 1 recent scoping review found limited evidence that the use of the pediatric early warning system leads to reductions in deterioration.[1,6–9] One scoping review found evidence, though limited, suggesting that the pediatric early warning system is useful in low- or middle-income countries.[8]

These recommendations were created by the AHA Pediatric Basic and Advanced Life Support Writing Group and are based on a 2019 ILCOR scoping review and a 2020 evidence review.[10]

REFERENCES

1. Maharaj R, Raffaele I, Wendon J. Rapid response systems: a systematic review and meta-analysis. *Crit Care.* 2015;19:254. doi: 10.1186/s13054-015-0973-y
2. Bonafide CP, Localio AR, Roberts KE, Nadkarni VM, Weirich CM, Keren R. Impact of rapid response system implementation on critical deterioration events in children. *JAMA Pediatr.* 2014;168:25–33. doi: 10.1001/jamapediatrics.2013.3266
3. Kolovos NS, Gill J, Michelson PH, Doctor A, Hartman ME. Reduction in mortality following pediatric rapid response team implementation. *Pediatr Crit Care Med.* 2018;19:477–482. doi: 10.1097/PCC.0000000000001519
4. Kutty S, Jones PG, Karels Q, Joseph N, Spertus JA, Chan PS. Association of Pediatric Medical Emergency Teams With Hospital Mortality. *Circulation.* 2018;137:38–46. doi: 10.1161/CIRCULATIONAHA.117.029535
5. Parshuram CS, Dryden-Palmer K, Farrell C, Gottesman R, Gray M, Hutchison JS, Helfaer M, Hunt EA, Joffe AR, Lacroix J, Moga MA, Nadkarni V, Ninis N, Parkin PC, Wensley D, Willan AR, Tomlinson GA; Canadian Critical Care Trials Group and the EPOCH Investigators. Effect of a pediatric early warning system on all-cause mortality in hospitalized pediatric patients: the EPOCH randomized clinical trial. *JAMA.* 2018;319:1002–1012. doi: 10.1001/jama.2018.0948
6. Trubey R, Huang C, Lugg-Widger FV, Hood K, Allen D, Edwards D, Lacy D, Lloyd A, Mann M, Mason B, Oliver A, Roland D, Sefton G, Skone R, Thomas-Jones E, Tume LN, Powell C. Validity and effectiveness of paediatric early warning systems and track and trigger tools for identifying and reducing clinical deterioration in hospitalised children: a systematic review. *BMJ Open.* 2019;9:e022105. doi: 10.1136/bmjopen-2018-022105
7. Chapman SM, Wray J, Oulton K, Peters MJ. Systematic review of paediatric track and trigger systems for hospitalised children. *Resuscitation.* 2016;109:87–109. doi: 10.1016/j.resuscitation.2016.07.230
8. Brown SR, Martinez Garcia D, Agulnik A. Scoping review of pediatric early warning systems (PEWS) in resource-limited and humanitarian settings. *Front Pediatr.* 2018;6:410. doi: 10.3389/fped.2018.00410
9. Lambert V, Matthews A, MacDonell R, Fitzsimons J. Paediatric early warning systems for detecting and responding to clinical deterioration in children: a systematic review. *BMJ Open.* 2017;7:e014497. doi: 10.1136/bmjopen-2016-014497
10. Maconochie IK, Aickin R, Hazinski MF, Atkins DL, Bingham R, Couto TB, Guerguerian A-M, Nadkarni VM, Ng K-C, Nuthall GA, et al; on behalf of the Pediatric Life Support Collaborators. Pediatric life support: 2020 International Consensus on Cardiopulmonary Resuscitation and Emergency Cardiovascular Care Science With Treatment Recommendations. *Circulation.* 2020;142(suppl 1):S140–S184. doi: 10.1161/CIR.0000000000000894

PERFORMANCE OF RESUSCITATION

Cognitive Aids in Resuscitation

Recommendations for the Use of Cognitive Aids in Resuscitation

COR	LOE	Recommendations
2b	C-LD	1. The effectiveness of cognitive aids for lay rescuers responding to a cardiac arrest is unclear and requires additional study before broad implementation.[1–5]
2b	C-LD	2. It may be reasonable to use cognitive aids to improve team performance of healthcare providers during cardiopulmonary resuscitation.[6–9]

Synopsis

Cognitive aids improve patient care in nonacute settings,[10,11] yet little is known of their impact in critical situations. Understanding if, when, and how cognitive aids can be useful may help improve the resuscitation efforts of lay providers and healthcare professionals, thereby saving more lives. We considered cognitive aids as a "presentation of prompts aimed to encourage recall of information in order to increase the likelihood of desired behaviors, decisions, and outcomes."[12] Examples include checklists, alarms, mobile applications, and mnemonics.

An ILCOR systematic review suggests that the use of cognitive aids by lay rescuers results in a delay in initiating CPR during simulated cardiac arrest, which could potentially cause considerable harm in real patients.[14] The use of cognitive aids for lay providers during cardiac arrests requires additional study before broad implementation. No studies were identified evaluating the use of cognitive aids among healthcare teams during cardiac arrest. Evidence from trauma resuscitation suggests that the use of cognitive aids improves adherence to resuscitation guidelines, reduces errors, and improves survival of the most severely injured patients. It may be reasonable for healthcare providers to use cognitive aids during cardiac arrest. Extrapolation from a closely related field is appropriate but requires further study. Future research should explore whether cognitive aids support the actions of bystanders and healthcare providers during actual cardiac arrests.

Recommendation-Specific Supportive Text

1. Results from a systematic review[14] identified 4 randomized trials[1–4] demonstrating a statistically significant and clinically relevant delay in initiating CPR when lay rescuers used cognitive aids (30-second–70-second difference between groups in each study). Once CPR is initiated, rescuers who are using cognitive aids appear to have less hands-off time[1,2,4,5] and are more confident in their ability to act,[4] which may ultimately be important to support a lay provider in responding to a cardiac arrest.
2. The systematic review identified no studies analyzing survival to discharge using cognitive aids in cardiac arrest, but it did identify 3 studies related to trauma resuscitation, including 1 RCT[6] and 2 observational studies.[7,9] Survival to hospital discharge was higher in the observational studies for those with the most significant injury (Injury Severity Score 25 or greater) when a cognitive aid was used.[7,9] The RCT included patients with lower injury severity and did not demonstrate a difference in survival.[6] Measures of resuscitation performance (eg, fewer errors, completion of primary and secondary surveys, quicker performance of tasks), although inconsistently used as metrics in each study, generally favored the use of cognitive aids in trauma resuscitation.[6–9]

These recommendations were created by the AHA Resuscitation Education Science Writing Group and are supported by a 2020 ILCOR systematic review.[14]

REFERENCES

1. Hunt EA, Heine M, Shilkofski NS, Bradshaw JH, Nelson-McMillan K, Duval-Arnould J, Elfenbein R. Exploration of the impact of a voice activated decision support system (VADSS) with video on resuscitation performance by lay rescuers during simulated cardiopulmonary arrest. *Emerg Med J.* 2015;32:189–194. doi: 10.1136/emermed-2013-202867
2. Merchant RM, Abella BS, Abotsi EJ, Smith TM, Long JA, Trudeau ME, Leary M, Groeneveld PW, Becker LB, Asch DA. Cell phone cardiopulmonary resuscitation: audio instructions when needed by lay rescuers: a randomized, controlled trial. *Ann Emerg Med.* 2010;55:538–543.e1. doi: 10.1016/j.annemergmed.2010.01.020
3. Paal P, Pircher I, Baur T, Gruber E, Strasak AM, Herff H, Brugger H, Wenzel V, Mitterlechner T. Mobile phone-assisted basic life support augmented with a metronome. *J Emerg Med.* 2012;43:472–477. doi: 10.1016/j.jemermed.2011.09.011
4. Rössler B, Ziegler M, Hüpfl M, Fleischhackl R, Krychtiuk KA, Schebesta K. Can a flowchart improve the quality of bystander cardiopulmonary resuscitation? *Resuscitation.* 2013;84:982–986. doi: 10.1016/j.resuscitation.2013.01.001
5. Hawkes GA, Murphy G, Dempsey EM, Ryan AC. Randomised controlled trial of a mobile phone infant resuscitation guide. *J Paediatr Child Health.* 2015;51:1084–1088. doi: 10.1111/jpc.12968
6. Fitzgerald M, Cameron P, Mackenzie C, Farrow N, Scicluna P, Gocentas R, Bystrzycki A, Lee G, O'Reilly G, Andrianopoulos N, Dziukas L, Cooper DJ, Silvers A, Mori A, Murray A, Smith S, Xiao Y, Stub D, McDermott FT, Rosenfeld JV. Trauma resuscitation errors and computer-assisted decision support. *Arch Surg.* 2011;146:218–225. doi: 10.1001/archsurg.2010.333
7. Bernhard M, Becker TK, Nowe T, Mohorovicic M, Sikinger M, Brenner T, Richter GM, Radeleff B, Meeder PJ, Büchler MW, Böttiger BW, Martin E, Gries A. Introduction of a treatment algorithm can improve the early management of emergency patients in the resuscitation room. *Resuscitation.* 2007;73:362–373. doi: 10.1016/j.resuscitation.2006.09.014
8. Kelleher DC, Carter EA, Waterhouse LJ, Parsons SE, Fritzeen JL, Burd RS. Effect of a checklist on advanced trauma life support task performance during pediatric trauma resuscitation. *Acad Emerg Med.* 2014;21:1129–1134. doi: 10.1111/acem.12487
9. Lashoher A, Schneider EB, Juillard C, Stevens K, Colantuoni E, Berry WR, Bloem C, Chadbunchachai W, Dharap S, Dy SM, Dziekan G, Gruen RL, Henry JA, Huwer C, Joshipura M, Kelley E, Krug E, Kumar V, Kyamanywa P, Mefire AC, Musafir M, Nathens AB, Ngendahayo E, Nguyen TS, Roy N, Pronovost PJ, Khan IQ, Razzak JA, Rubiano AM, Turner JA, Varghese M, Zakirova R, Mock C. Implementation of the World Health Organization Trauma Care Checklist program in 11 centers across multiple economic strata: effect on care process measures. *World J Surg.* 2017;41:954–962. doi: 10.1007/s00268-016-3759-8
10. de Vries EN, Prins HA, Crolla RM, den Outer AJ, van Andel G, van Helden SH, Schlack WS, van Putten MA, Gouma DJ, Dijkgraaf MG, Smorenburg SM, Boermeester MA; SURPASS Collaborative Group. Effect of a comprehensive surgical safety system on patient outcomes. *N Engl J Med.* 2010;363:1928–1937. doi: 10.1056/NEJMsa0911535
11. Haynes AB, Weiser TG, Berry WR, Lipsitz SR, Breizat AH, Dellinger EP, Herbosa T, Joseph S, Kibatala PL, Lapitan MC, Merry AF, Moorthy K, Reznick RK, Taylor B, Gawande AA; Safe Surgery Saves Lives Study Group. A surgical safety checklist to reduce morbidity and mortality in a global population. *N Engl J Med.* 2009;360:491–499. doi: 10.1056/NEJMsa0810119
12. Fletcher KA, Bedwell WL. Cognitive aids: design suggestions for the medical field. *Proc Int Symp Human Factors Ergonomics Health Care.* 2014;3:148–152. doi: 10.1177/2327857914031024
13. Deleted in proof.
14. Greif R, Bhanji F, Bigham BL, Bray J, Breckwoldt J, Cheng A, Duff JP, Gilfoyle E, Hsieh M-J, Iwami T, et al; on behalf of the Education, Implementation, and Teams Collaborators. Education, implementation, and teams: 2020 International Consensus on Cardiopulmonary Resuscitation and Emergency Cardiovascular Care Science With Treatment Recommendations. *Circulation.* 2020;142(suppl 1):S222–S283. doi: 10.1161/CIR.0000000000000896

POST–CARDIAC ARREST CARE

Cardiac Arrest Centers

Recommendation for Cardiac Arrest Centers		
COR	**LOE**	**Recommendation**
2a	C-LD	1. A regionalized approach to post–cardiac arrest care that includes transport of acutely resuscitated patients directly to specialized cardiac arrest centers is reasonable when comprehensive postarrest care is not available at local facilities.[1–10]

Synopsis

Cardiac arrest centers (CACs), although still lacking official criteria for designation as has been established for other centers of expertise, are specialized facilities that provide comprehensive, evidence-based post–cardiac arrest care, including emergent cardiac catheterization, targeted temperature management, hemodynamic support, and neurological expertise. A CAC may also have protocols and quality improvement programs to ensure guideline-compliant care. A growing number of CACs also have the capability to provide extracorporeal membrane oxygenation and/or other forms of circulatory support. Patients may be transported directly to CACs by EMS either during resuscitation or after ROSC, or they may be transferred from another hospital to a CAC after ROSC. Important considerations in this decision-making process must include transport time, the stability of the patient, and the ability of the transporting service to provide needed care.

Although supportive evidence for comprehensive post–cardiac arrest interventions remains largely observational (particularly when they are administered together as bundled care at specialized centers) and the results of these studies are mixed, CACs may nonetheless represent a logical clinical link between successful resuscitation and ultimate survival. Taken together with experience from regionalized approaches to other emergencies such as trauma, stroke, and ST-segment elevation acute myocardial infarction, when a suitable complement of post–cardiac arrest services is not available locally, direct transport of the resuscitated patient to a regional center offering such support may be beneficial and is a reasonable approach when feasible.

Recommendation-Specific Supportive Text

1. Evidence-based, comprehensive post–cardiac arrest care is critically important for resuscitated patients. The adjusted analyses from 2 observational studies found that treatment at CACs was not associated with increased survival with favorable neurological outcome at 30 days,[2,3] whereas 2 other studies found that admission to a CAC was associated with improved survival to hospital discharge with good neurological outcome.[4,7] Treatment at CACs was associated with

increased 30-day survival[5,6] and survival to hospital discharge[4,7–10] compared with treatment at non-CACs. An interim feasibility report (n=40 patients) of a randomized trial evaluating expedited transport to a CAC demonstrated no difference in clinical outcomes, but it is preliminary and underpowered for this outcome.[11]

These recommendations were created by the AHA Adult Basic and Advanced Life Support Writing Group and are supported by a 2019 ILCOR systematic review.[12]

REFERENCES

1. Panchal AR, Berg KM, Cabañas JG, Kurz MC, Link MS, Del Rios M, Hirsch KG, Chan PS, Hazinski MF, Morley PT, Donnino MW, Kudenchuk PJ. 2019 American Heart Association focused update on systems of care: dispatcher-assisted cardiopulmonary resuscitation and cardiac arrest centers: an update to the American Heart Association Guidelines for Cardiopulmonary Resuscitation and Emergency Cardiovascular Care. *Circulation.* 2019;140:e895–e903. doi: 10.1161/CIR.0000000000000733
2. Matsuyama T, Kiyohara K, Kitamura T, Nishiyama C, Nishiuchi T, Hayashi Y, Kawamura T, Ohta B, Iwami T. Hospital characteristics and favourable neurological outcome among patients with out-of-hospital cardiac arrest in Osaka, Japan. *Resuscitation.* 2017;110:146–153. doi: 10.1016/j.resuscitation.2016.11.009
3. Tagami T, Hirata K, Takeshige T, Matsui J, Takinami M, Satake M, Satake S, Yui T, Itabashi K, Sakata T, Tosa R, Kushimoto S, Yokota H, Hirama H. Implementation of the fifth link of the chain of survival concept for out-of-hospital cardiac arrest. *Circulation.* 2012;126:589–597. doi: 10.1161/CIRCULATIONAHA.111.086173
4. Kragholm K, Malta Hansen C, Dupre ME, Xian Y, Strauss B, Tyson C, Monk L, Corbett C, Fordyce CB, Pearson DA, et al. Direct transport to a percutaneous cardiac intervention center and outcomes in patients with out-of-hospital cardiac arrest. *Circ Cardiovasc Qual Outcomes.* 2017;10:e003414. doi: 10.1161/CIRCOUTCOMES.116.003414
5. Harnod D, Ma MHM, Chang WH, Chang RE, Chang CH. Mortality factors in out-of-hospital cardiac arrest patients: a nationwide population-based study in Taiwan. *Int J Gerontology.* 2013;7:216–220.
6. Søholm H, Wachtell K, Nielsen SL, Bro-Jeppesen J, Pedersen F, Wanscher M, Boesgaard S, Møller JE, Hassager C, Kjaergaard J. Tertiary centres have improved survival compared to other hospitals in the Copenhagen area after out-of-hospital cardiac arrest. *Resuscitation.* 2013;84:162–167. doi: 10.1016/j.resuscitation.2012.06.029
7. Spaite DW, Bobrow BJ, Stolz U, Berg RA, Sanders AB, Kern KB, Chikani V, Humble W, Mullins T, Stapczynski JS, Ewy GA; Arizona Cardiac Receiving Center Consortium. Statewide regionalization of postarrest care for out-of-hospital cardiac arrest: association with survival and neurologic outcome. *Ann Emerg Med.* 2014;64:496–506.e1. doi: 10.1016/j.annemergmed.2014.05.028
8. Cournoyer A, Notebaert É, de Montigny L, Ross D, Cossette S, Londei-Leduc L, Iseppon M, Lamarche Y, Sokoloff C, Potter BJ, Vadeboncoeur A, Larose D, Morris J, Daoust R, Chauny JM, Piette É, Paquet J, Cavayas YA, de Champlain F, Segal E, Albert M, Guertin MC, Denault A. Impact of the direct transfer to percutaneous coronary intervention-capable hospitals on survival to hospital discharge for patients with out-of-hospital cardiac arrest. *Resuscitation.* 2018;125:28–33. doi: 10.1016/j.resuscitation.2018.01.048
9. Lick CJ, Aufderheide TP, Niskanen RA, Steinkamp JE, Davis SP, Nygaard SD, Bemenderfer KK, Gonzales L, Kalla JA, Wald SK, Gillquist DL, Sayre MR, Osaki Holm SY, Oski Holm SY, Oakes DA, Provo TA, Racht EM, Olsen JD, Yannopoulos D, Lurie KG. Take Heart America: A comprehensive, community-wide, systems-based approach to the treatment of cardiac arrest. *Crit Care Med.* 2011;39:26–33. doi: 10.1097/CCM.0b013e3181fa7ce4
10. Stub D, Smith K, Bray JE, Bernard S, Duffy SJ, Kaye DM. Hospital characteristics are associated with patient outcomes following out-of-hospital cardiac arrest. *Heart.* 2011;97:1489–1494. doi: 10.1136/hrt.2011.226431
11. Patterson T, Perkins GD, Joseph J, Wilson K, Van Dyck L, Robertson S, Nguyen H, McConkey H, Whitbread M, Fothergill R, Nevett J, Dalby M, Rakhit R, MacCarthy P, Perera D, Nolan JP, Redwood SR. A randomised trial of expedited transfer to a cardiac arrest centre for non-ST elevation ventricular fibrillation out-of-hospital cardiac arrest: The ARREST pilot randomised trial. *Resuscitation.* 2017;115:185–191. doi: 10.1016/j.resuscitation.2017.01.020
12. Yeung J, Matsuyama T, Bray J, Reynolds J, Skrifvars MB. Does care at a cardiac arrest centre improve outcome after out-of-hospital cardiac arrest? - A systematic review. *Resuscitation.* 2019;137:102–115. doi: 10.1016/j.resuscitation.2019.02.006

Organ Donation

Recommendations for Organ Donation

COR	LOE	Recommendations
1	B-NR	1. We recommend that all patients who are resuscitated from cardiac arrest but who subsequently progress to death be evaluated for organ donation.[1]
2b	B-NR	2. Patients who do not have ROSC after resuscitation efforts and who would otherwise have termination of resuscitative efforts may be considered candidates for donation in settings where such programs exist.[1]

Synopsis

Organ donation can occur after death by neurological criteria or after death by circulatory criteria. Donation after circulatory death may occur in controlled and uncontrolled settings. Controlled donation after circulatory death usually takes place in the hospital after withdrawal of life support. Uncontrolled donation usually takes place in an emergency department after exhaustive efforts at resuscitation have failed to achieve ROSC. Organ donation in any setting raises important ethical issues. Decisions for termination of resuscitative efforts or withdrawal of life-sustaining measures must be independent from processes of organ donation.

In 2015, the ILCOR Advanced Life Support Task Force reviewed the evidence for the impact that a donor having received CPR has on graft function. The 2 general comparisons were 1) controlled organ donation using organs from a donor who had previously received CPR and obtained ROSC compared with a donor who had not received CPR and 2) uncontrolled donation using organs from a donor receiving ongoing CPR, for whom ongoing resuscitation was deemed futile, compared with other types of donors,[1] on the question of whether an organ retrieved in the setting of controlled donation versus uncontrolled donation had an impact on survival and complications.

Recommendation-Specific Supportive Text

1 and 2. Studies comparing transplanted organ function between organs from donors who had received successful CPR before donation and organs from donors who had not received CPR before donation have found no difference in transplanted organ function.[2–6] Outcomes studied include immediate graft function, 1-year graft function, and 5-year graft function.

Studies have also shown no evidence of worse outcome in transplanted kidneys and livers from adult donors who have not had ROSC after CPR (uncontrolled donation) compared with those from other types of donors.[7–9] There is broad consensus that decisions for termination of resuscitative efforts and the pursuit of organ donation need to be carried out by independent parties.[10–13]

These recommendations were created by the AHA Adult Basic and Advanced Life Support Writing Group and are supported by a 2015 systematic evidence review.[1,14] A comprehensive ILCOR review is anticipated in 2020.

REFERENCES

1. Soar J, Callaway CW, Aibiki M, Böttiger BW, Brooks SC, Deakin CD, Donnino MW, Drajer S, Kloeck W, Morley PT, et al; on behalf of the Advanced Life Support Chapter Collaborators. Part 4: advanced life support: 2015 International Consensus on Cardiopulmonary Resuscitation and Emergency Cardiovascular Care Science with Treatment Recommendations. *Resuscitation*. 2015;95:e71–e120. doi: 10.1016/j.resuscitation.2015.07.042
2. Orioles A, Morrison WE, Rossano JW, Shore PM, Hasz RD, Martiner AC, Berg RA, Nadkarni VM. An under-recognized benefit of cardiopulmonary resuscitation: organ transplantation. *Crit Care Med*. 2013;41:2794–2799. doi: 10.1097/CCM.0b013e31829a7202
3. Adrie C, Haouache H, Saleh M, Memain N, Laurent I, Thuong M, Darques L, Guerrini P, Monchi M. An underrecognized source of organ donors: patients with brain death after successfully resuscitated cardiac arrest. *Intensive Care Med*. 2008;34:132–137. doi: 10.1007/s00134-007-0885-7
4. Quader MA, Wolfe LG, Kasirajan V. Heart transplantation outcomes from cardiac arrest-resuscitated donors. *J Heart Lung Transplant*. 2013;32:1090–1095. doi: 10.1016/j.healun.2013.08.002
5. Pilarczyk K, Osswald BR, Pizanis N, Tsagakis K, Massoudy P, Heckmann J, Jakob HG, Kamler M. Use of donors who have suffered cardiopulmonary arrest and resuscitation in lung transplantation. *Eur J Cardiothorac Surg*. 2011;39:342–347. doi: 10.1016/j.ejcts.2010.06.038
6. Southerland KW, Castleberry AW, Williams JB, Daneshmand MA, Ali AA, Milano CA. Impact of donor cardiac arrest on heart transplantation. *Surgery*. 2013;154:312–319. doi: 10.1016/j.surg.2013.04.028
7. Fondevila C, Hessheimer AJ, Flores E, Ruiz A, Mestres N, Calatayud D, Paredes D, Rodríguez C, Fuster J, Navasa M, Rimola A, Taurá P, García-Valdecasas JC. Applicability and results of Maastricht type 2 donation after cardiac death liver transplantation. *Am J Transplant*. 2012;12:162–170. doi: 10.1111/j.1600-6143.2011.03834.x
8. Alonso A, Fernández-Rivera C, Villaverde P, Oliver J, Cillero S, Lorenzo D, Valdés F. Renal transplantation from non-heart-beating donors: a single-center 10-year experience. *Transplant Proc*. 2005;37:3658–3660. doi: 10.1016/j.transproceed.2005.09.104
9. Morozumi J, Matsuno N, Sakurai E, Nakamura Y, Arai T, Ohta S. Application of an automated cardiopulmonary resuscitation device for kidney transplantation from uncontrolled donation after cardiac death donors in the emergency department. *Clin Transplant*. 2010;24:620–625. doi: 10.1111/j.1399-0012.2009.01140.x
10. Dalle Ave AL, Shaw DM, Gardiner D. Extracorporeal membrane oxygenation (ECMO) assisted cardiopulmonary resuscitation or uncontrolled donation after the circulatory determination of death following out-of-hospital refractory cardiac arrest-An ethical analysis of an unresolved clinical dilemma. *Resuscitation*. 2016;108:87–94. doi: 10.1016/j.resuscitation.2016.07.003
11. Steinbrook R. Organ donation after cardiac death. *N Engl J Med*. 2007;357:209–213. doi: 10.1056/NEJMp078066
12. Gallagher TK, Skaro AI, Abecassis MM. Emerging ethical considerations of donation after circulatory death: getting to the heart of the matter. *Ann Surg*. 2016;263:217–218. doi: 10.1097/SLA.0000000000001585
13. Truog RD, Miller FG, Halpern SD. The dead-donor rule and the future of organ donation. *N Engl J Med*. 2013;369:1287–1289. doi: 10.1056/NEJMp1307220
14. Mancini ME, Diekema DS, Hoadley TA, Kadlec KD, Leveille MH, McGowan JE, Munkwitz MM, Panchal AR, Sayre MR, Sinz EH. Part 3: ethical issues: 2015 American Heart Association Guidelines Update for Cardiopulmonary Resuscitation and Emergency Cardiovascular Care. *Circulation*. 2015;132(suppl 2):S383–S396. doi: 10.1161/CIR.0000000000000254

IMPROVING RESUSCITATION PERFORMANCE

Debriefing

Recommendations for Clinical Debriefing

COR	LOE	Recommendations
2a	B-NR	1. Performance-focused debriefing of rescuers after cardiac arrest can be effective for out-of-hospital systems of care.[1]
2a	B-NR	2. Performance-focused debriefing of rescuers after cardiac arrest can be effective for in-hospital systems of care.[1–3]
2a	B-NR	3. Review of objective and quantitative resuscitation data during postevent debriefing can be effective.[1–5]
2a	C-EO	4. It is reasonable for debriefings to be facilitated by healthcare professionals familiar with established debriefing processes.[1–5]

Synopsis

Post-event debriefing is defined as "a discussion between 2 or more individuals in which aspects of performance are analyzed,"[6] with the goal of improving future clinical practice.[7] During debriefing, resuscitation team members may discuss process and quality of care (eg, algorithm adherence), review quantitative data collected during the event (eg, CPR metrics), reflect on teamwork and leadership issues, and address emotional responses to the event.[8–13] A facilitator, typically a healthcare professional, leads a discussion focused on identifying opportunities and strategies for improving performance.[8,9,11,13,14] Debriefings may occur either immediately after a resuscitation event (*hot debriefing*) or at a later time (*cold debriefing*).[7,9,15] Some debriefings take the form of personalized reflective feedback conversations,[1,4] while others involve group discussion among a larger, multidisciplinary resuscitation team.[2,3] We examined the impact of postevent clinical debriefing on process measures (eg, CPR quality) and patient outcomes (eg, survival). Studies related to critical incident stress debriefing (ie, psychological debriefing), which is a process intended to prevent or limit post-traumatic stress symptoms, were excluded from the review but have been well reviewed elsewhere.[16] Data-informed debriefing of providers after cardiac arrest has potential benefit for both in-hospital and out-of-hospital systems of care; discussion should ideally be facilitated by healthcare professionals.[1–4]

Recommendation-Specific Supportive Text

1. One prospective, observational study of post-OHCA debriefing among prehospital personnel demonstrated improved quality of resuscitation (ie, increased chest compression fraction, reduced pause duration) but no improvement in survival to discharge.[1] Good and poor performance were highlighted during discussion.
2. Three prospective observational studies of post-IHCA debriefing among multidisciplinary resuscitation team members show mixed results.[2–4] Meta-analysis of these studies demonstrated improved ROSC and mean chest compression depth in the period after implementation of debriefing. Two studies demonstrating improvements in quality of resuscitation (ie, chest compression depth, chest compression fraction, pause duration, excellent CPR) and survival outcomes (ie, ROSC, survival with favorable neurological outcome),[2,3] and 1 study demonstrated no improvement in patient or process-focused outcomes.[4]
3. Because provider recall of events and self-assessment of performance are often poor,[9,17,18] debriefings should be supplemented by discussion of objective, quantitative data such as CPR quality performance data (chest compression rate, depth, and fraction; telemetry and defibrillator tracings; end-tidal CO_2 tracings; and resuscitation records.[1–4]
4. In all studies reviewed, debriefings were facilitated by healthcare professionals familiar with the recommended debriefing process or structure, which in some cases was supported by the use of a cognitive aid or checklist.[1–4] Discussions were tailored to participant type and group size and were individualized to the nature of performance during the event.

These recommendations were created by the AHA Resuscitation Education Science Writing Group and are supported by a 2019 ILCOR systematic review.[19]

REFERENCES

1. Bleijenberg E, Koster RW, de Vries H, Beesems SG. The impact of post-resuscitation feedback for paramedics on the quality of cardiopulmonary resuscitation. *Resuscitation.* 2017;110:1–5. doi: 10.1016/j.resuscitation.2016.08.034
2. Wolfe H, Zebuhr C, Topjian AA, Nishisaki A, Niles DE, Meaney PA, Boyle L, Giordano RT, Davis D, Priestley M, Apkon M, Berg RA, Nadkarni VM, Sutton RM. Interdisciplinary ICU cardiac arrest debriefing improves survival outcomes. *Crit Care Med.* 2014;42:1688–1695. doi: 10.1097/CCM.0000000000000327
3. Edelson DP, Litzinger B, Arora V, Walsh D, Kim S, Lauderdale DS, Vanden Hoek TL, Becker LB, Abella BS. Improving in-hospital cardiac arrest process and outcomes with performance debriefing. *Arch Intern Med.* 2008;168:1063–1069. doi: 10.1001/archinte.168.10.1063
4. Couper K, Kimani PK, Davies RP, Baker A, Davies M, Husselbee N, Melody T, Griffiths F, Perkins GD. An evaluation of three methods of in-hospital cardiac arrest educational debriefing: The cardiopulmonary resuscitation debriefing study. *Resuscitation.* 2016;105:130–137. doi: 10.1016/j.resuscitation.2016.05.005
5. Cheng A, Nadkarni VM, Mancini MB, Hunt EA, Sinz EH, Merchant RM, Donoghue A, Duff JP, Eppich W, Auerbach M, Bigham BL, Blewer AL, Chan PS, Bhanji F; American Heart Association Education Science Investigators; and on behalf of the American Heart Association Education Science and Programs Committee, Council on Cardiopulmonary, Critical Care, Perioperative and Resuscitation; Council on Cardiovascular and Stroke Nursing; and Council on Quality of Care and Outcomes Research. Resuscitation education science: educational strategies to improve outcomes from cardiac arrest: a scientific statement from the American Heart Association. *Circulation.* 2018;138:e82–e122. doi: 10.1161/CIR.0000000000000583
6. Cheng A, Eppich W, Grant V, Sherbino J, Zendejas B, Cook DA. Debriefing for technology-enhanced simulation: a systematic review and meta-analysis. *Med Educ.* 2014;48:657–666. doi: 10.1111/medu.12432
7. Kronick SL, Kurz MC, Lin S, Edelson DP, Berg RA, Billi JE, Cabanas JG, Cone DC, Diercks DB, Foster JJ, et al. Part 4: systems of care and continuous quality improvement: 2015 American Heart Association Guidelines Update for Cardiopulmonary Resuscitation and Emergency Cardiovascular Care. *Circulation.* 2015;132(suppl 2):S397–S413. doi: 10.1161/CIR.0000000000000258
8. Kessler DO, Cheng A, Mullan PC. Debriefing in the emergency department after clinical events: a practical guide. *Ann Emerg Med.* 2015;65:690–698. doi: 10.1016/j.annemergmed.2014.10.019
9. Mullan PC, Cochrane NH, Chamberlain JM, Burd RS, Brown FD, Zinns LE, Crandall KM, O'Connell KJ. Accuracy of postresuscitation team debriefings in a pediatric emergency department. *Ann Emerg Med.* 2017;70:311–319. doi: 10.1016/j.annemergmed.2017.01.034
10. Mullan PC, Kessler DO, Cheng A. Educational opportunities with postevent debriefing. *JAMA.* 2014;312:2333–2334. doi: 10.1001/jama.2014.15741
11. Zinns LE, O'Connell KJ, Mullan PC, Ryan LM, Wratney AT. National survey of pediatric emergency medicine fellows on debriefing after medical resuscitations. *Pediatr Emerg Care.* 2015;31:551–554. doi: 10.1097/PEC.0000000000000196
12. Eppich W, Cheng A. Promoting Excellence and Reflective Learning in Simulation (PEARLS): development and rationale for a blended approach to health care simulation debriefing. *Simul Healthc.* 2015;10:106–115. doi: 10.1097/SIH.0000000000000072
13. Couper K, Salman B, Soar J, Finn J, Perkins GD. Debriefing to improve outcomes from critical illness: a systematic review and meta-analysis. *Intensive Care Med.* 2013;39:1513–1523. doi: 10.1007/s00134-013-2951-7
14. Rose S, Cheng A. Charge nurse facilitated clinical debriefing in the emergency department. *CJEM.* 2018;20:781–785. doi: 10.1017/cem.2018.369
15. Sweberg T, Sen AI, Mullan PC, Cheng A, Knight L, Del Castillo J, Ikeyama T, Seshadri R, Hazinski MF, Raymond T, Niles DE, Nadkarni V, Wolfe H; pediatric resuscitation quality (pediRES-Q) collaborative investigators. Description of hot debriefings after in-hospital cardiac arrests in an international pediatric quality improvement collaborative. *Resuscitation.* 2018;128:181–187. doi: 10.1016/j.resuscitation.2018.05.015
16. Rose SC, Bisson J, Churchill R, Wessely S. Psychological debriefing for preventing post traumatic stress disorder (PTSD). *Cochrane Database Syst Rev.* 2002; doi: 10.1002/14651858.CD000560
17. Cheng A, Overly F, Kessler D, Nadkarni VM, Lin Y, Doan Q, Duff JP, Tofil NM, Bhanji F, Adler M, Charnovich A, Hunt EA, Brown LL; International Network for Simulation-based Pediatric Innovation, Research, Education (INSPIRE) CPR Investigators. Perception of CPR quality: Influence of CPR feedback, Just-in-Time CPR training and provider role. *Resuscitation.* 2015;87:44–50. doi: 10.1016/j.resuscitation.2014.11.015
18. Cheng A, Kessler D, Lin Y, Tofil NM, Hunt EA, Davidson J, Chatfield J, Duff JP; International Network for Simulation-based Pediatric Innovation, Research and Education (INSPIRE) CPR Investigators. Influence of cardiopulmonary resuscitation coaching and provider role on perception of cardiopulmonary resuscitation quality during simulated pediatric cardiac arrest. *Pediatr Crit Care Med.* 2019;20:e191–e198. doi: 10.1097/PCC.0000000000001871
19. Greif R, Bhanji F, Bigham BL, Bray J, Breckwoldt J, Cheng A, Duff JP, Gilfoyle E, Hsieh M-J, Iwami T, et al; on behalf of the Education, Implementation, and Teams Collaborators. Education, implementation, and teams: 2020 International Consensus on Cardiopulmonary Resuscitation and Emergency Cardiovascular Care Science With Treatment Recommendations. *Circulation.* 2020;142(suppl 1):S222–S283. doi: 10.1161/CIR.0000000000000896

Data Registries to Improve System Performance

Recommendation for Data Registries to Improve System Performance		
COR	LOE	Recommendation
2a	C-LD	1. It is reasonable for organizations that treat cardiac arrest patients to collect processes-of-care data and outcomes.[1–6]

Synopsis

Many industries, including healthcare, collect and assess performance data to measure quality and identify opportunities for improvement. This can be done at the local, regional, or national level through participation in data registries that collect information on processes of care (CPR performance data, defibrillation times, adherence to guidelines) and outcomes of care (ROSC, survival) associated with cardiac arrest. The AHA's Get With The Guidelines–Resuscitation registry is one such initiative to capture, analyze, and report processes and outcomes for IHCA.

A recent ILCOR systematic review[7] found that most studies assessing the impact of data registries, with or without public reporting, demonstrate improvement in cardiac arrest survival outcomes after the implementation of such systems.[1–6,8–21] Although hospitals act on recorded metrics in other situations, it is unclear what exact changes are made in response to these analytics. The collection and reporting of performance and survival data and the implementation of performance improvement plans, with or without public reporting of metrics, may lead to improved systems performance and, ultimately, benefit patients. Use of registries to target interventions for communities with particular need is of interest, and further study is needed to inform optimal implementation strategies of such systems in the future.

Recommendation-Specific Supportive Text

1. A recent ILCOR systematic review[7] found 6 observational studies demonstrating that the implementation of cardiac arrest registry was associated with improved survival and adherence to key performance indicators (CPR process measures, time to defibrillator application, adherence to guidelines) over time.[1–6]

In an observational study of a registry that included 104 732 patients with IHCA, for each additional year of hospital participation in the registry, survival from cardiac arrest increased over time (OR, 1.02 per year of participation; CI, 1.00–1.04; *P*=0.046).[1] Another observational study of a multistate registry included 64 988 OHCA and found that all-rhythm survival doubled (8.0% preregistry, 16.1% postregistry; *P*<0.001) after registry implementation.[6] A state OHCA registry enrolling 15 145 patients found improved survival to hospital discharge (8.6%–16%) over the 10-year study period.[5] In another study that included a state registry of 128 888 OHCAs that mandated public reporting of outcomes, survival increased over a decade from 1.2% to 4.1%.[4]

These recommendations were created by the AHA Resuscitation Education Science Writing Group and are supported by a 2020 ILCOR systematic review.[7]

REFERENCES

1. Bradley SM, Huszti E, Warren SA, Merchant RM, Sayre MR, Nichol G. Duration of hospital participation in Get With the Guidelines-Resuscitation and survival of in-hospital cardiac arrest. *Resuscitation.* 2012;83:1349–1357. doi: 10.1016/j.resuscitation.2012.03.014
2. Nehme Z, Bernard S, Cameron P, Bray JE, Meredith IT, Lijovic M, Smith K. Using a cardiac arrest registry to measure the quality of emergency medical service care: decade of findings from the Victorian Ambulance Cardiac Arrest Registry. *Circ Cardiovasc Qual Outcomes.* 2015;8:56–66. doi: 10.1161/CIRCOUTCOMES.114.001185
3. Stub D, Schmicker RH, Anderson ML, Callaway CW, Daya MR, Sayre MR, Elmer J, Grunau BE, Aufderheide TP, Lin S, Buick JE, Zive D, Peterson ED, Nichol G; ROC Investigators. Association between hospital post-resuscitative performance and clinical outcomes after out-of-hospital cardiac arrest. *Resuscitation.* 2015;92:45–52. doi: 10.1016/j.resuscitation.2015.04.015
4. Kim YT, Shin SD, Hong SO, Ahn KO, Ro YS, Song KJ, Hong KJ. Effect of national implementation of utstein recommendation from the global resuscitation alliance on ten steps to improve outcomes from Out-of-Hospital cardiac arrest: a ten-year observational study in Korea. *BMJ Open.* 2017;7:e016925. doi: 10.1136/bmjopen-2017-016925
5. Grunau B, Kawano T, Dick W, Straight R, Connolly H, Schlamp R, Scheuermeyer FX, Fordyce CB, Barbic D, Tallon J, et al. Trends in care processes and survival following prehospital resuscitation improvement initiatives for out-of-hospital cardiac arrest in British Columbia, 2006-2016. *Resuscitation.* 2018;125:118–125. doi: 10.1016/j.resuscitation.2018.01.049
6. van Diepen S, Girotra S, Abella BS, Becker LB, Bobrow BJ, Chan PS, Fahrenbruch C, Granger CB, Jollis JG, McNally B, et al. Multistate 5-year initiative to improve care for out-of-hospital cardiac arrest: primary results from the heartrescue project. *J Am Heart Assoc.* 2017;6:e005716. doi: 10.1161/JAHA.117.005716
7. Greif R, Bhanji F, Bigham BL, Bray J, Breckwoldt J, Cheng A, Duff JP, Gilfoyle E, Hsieh M-J, Iwami T, et al; on behalf of the Education, Implementation, and Teams Collaborators. Education, implementation, and teams: 2020 International Consensus on Cardiopulmonary Resuscitation and Emergency Cardiovascular Care Science With Treatment Recommendations. *Circulation.* 2020;142(suppl 1):S222–S283. doi: 10.1161/CIR.0000000000000896
8. Hostler D, Everson-Stewart S, Rea TD, Stiell IG, Callaway CW, Kudenchuk PJ, Sears GK, Emerson SS, Nichol G; Resuscitation Outcomes Consortium Investigators. Effect of real-time feedback during cardiopulmonary resuscitation outside hospital: prospective, cluster-randomised trial. *BMJ.* 2011;342:d512. doi: 10.1136/bmj.d512
9. Wolfe H, Zebuhr C, Topjian AA, Nishisaki A, Niles DE, Meaney PA, Boyle L, Giordano RT, Davis D, Priestley M, Apkon M, Berg RA, Nadkarni VM, Sutton RM. Interdisciplinary ICU cardiac arrest debriefing improves survival outcomes*. *Crit Care Med.* 2014;42:1688–1695. doi: 10.1097/CCM.0000000000000327
10. Couper K, Kimani PK, Abella BS, Chilwan M, Cooke MW, Davies RP, Field RA, Gao F, Quinton S, Stallard N, Woolley S, Perkins GD; Cardiopulmonary Resuscitation Quality Improvement Initiative Collaborators. The system-wide effect of real-time audiovisual feedback and postevent debriefing for in-hospital cardiac arrest: the cardiopulmonary resuscitation quality improvement initiative. *Crit Care Med.* 2015;43:2321–2331. doi: 10.1097/CCM.0000000000001202
11. Knight LJ, Gabhart JM, Earnest KS, Leong KM, Anglemyer A, Franzon D. Improving code team performance and survival outcomes: implementation of pediatric resuscitation team training. *Crit Care Med.* 2014;42:243–251. doi: 10.1097/CCM.0b013e3182a6439d

12. Davis DP, Graham PG, Husa RD, Lawrence B, Minokadeh A, Altieri K, Sell RE. A performance improvement-based resuscitation programme reduces arrest incidence and increases survival from in-hospital cardiac arrest. *Resuscitation.* 2015;92:63–69. doi: 10.1016/j.resuscitation.2015.04.008
13. Hwang WS, Park JS, Kim SJ, Hong YS, Moon SW, Lee SW. A system-wide approach from the community to the hospital for improving neurologic outcomes in out-of-hospital cardiac arrest patients. *Eur J Emerg Med.* 2017;24:87–95. doi: 10.1097/MEJ.0000000000000313
14. Pearson DA, Darrell Nelson R, Monk L, Tyson C, Jollis JG, Granger CB, Corbett C, Garvey L, Runyon MS. Comparison of team-focused CPR vs standard CPR in resuscitation from out-of-hospital cardiac arrest: Results from a statewide quality improvement initiative. *Resuscitation.* 2016;105:165–172. doi: 10.1016/j.resuscitation.2016.04.008
15. Sporer K, Jacobs M, Derevin L, Duval S, Pointer J. Continuous quality improvement efforts increase survival with favorable neurologic outcome after out-of-hospital cardiac arrest. *Prehosp Emerg Care.* 2017;21:1–6. doi: 10.1080/10903127.2016.1218980
16. Park JH, Shin SD, Ro YS, Song KJ, Hong KJ, Kim TH, Lee EJ, Kong SY. Implementation of a bundle of Utstein cardiopulmonary resuscitation programs to improve survival outcomes after out-of-hospital cardiac arrest in a metropolis: A before and after study. *Resuscitation.* 2018;130:124–132. doi: 10.1016/j.resuscitation.2018.07.019
17. Hubner P, Lobmeyr E, Wallmüller C, Poppe M, Datler P, Keferböck M, Zeiner S, Nürnberger A, Zajicek A, Laggner A, Sterz F, Sulzgruber P. Improvements in the quality of advanced life support and patient outcome after implementation of a standardized real-life post-resuscitation feedback system. *Resuscitation.* 2017;120:38–44. doi: 10.1016/j.resuscitation.2017.08.235
18. Anderson ML, Nichol G, Dai D, Chan PS, Thomas L, Al-Khatib SM, Berg RA, Bradley SM, Peterson ED; American Heart Association's Get With the Guidelines–Resuscitation Investigators. Association between hospital process composite performance and patient outcomes after in-hospital cardiac arrest care. *JAMA Cardiol.* 2016;1:37–45. doi: 10.1001/jamacardio.2015.0275
19. Del Rios M, Weber J, Pugach O, Nguyen H, Campbell T, Islam S, Stein Spencer L, Markul E, Bunney EB, Vanden Hoek T. Large urban center improves out-of-hospital cardiac arrest survival. *Resuscitation.* 2019;139:234–240. doi: 10.1016/j.resuscitation.2019.04.019
20. Ewy GA, Sanders AB. Alternative approach to improving survival of patients with out-of-hospital primary cardiac arrest. *J Am Coll Cardiol.* 2013;61:113–118. doi: 10.1016/j.jacc.2012.06.064
21. Hopkins CL, Burk C, Moser S, Meersman J, Baldwin C, Youngquist ST. Implementation of pit crew approach and cardiopulmonary resuscitation metrics for out-of-hospital cardiac arrest improves patient survival and neurological outcome. *J Am Heart Assoc.* 2016;5 doi: 10.1161/JAHA.115.002892

KNOWLEDGE GAPS AND PRIORITIES FOR RESEARCH

Resuscitation science, including understanding about integrated systems of care, continues to evolve. Among the many high-priority unresolved questions are the following:

- Although the clinical effectiveness of community CPR and AED programs is well established, the populations and settings in which these interventions are cost-effective requires further study.
- Preliminary studies of drone delivery of AEDs are promising.[1,2] Given the time-sensitive benefit to defibrillation, this concept and other means for just-in-time AED delivery deserve further study.
- The RRT/MET concept seems promising, but current data are too heterogeneous to support strong conclusions. Systematic data collection would greatly improve understanding of the types of interventions and characteristics of patients who benefit from RRT/MET interventions as well as the makeup and activities of successful teams.
- Along the same lines, validated clinical criteria, perhaps developed by machine-learning technology, may have value to identify and direct interventions toward patients at risk of IHCA.
- Although the concept is logical, cognitive aids (other than T-CPR) to assist bystanders in performing CPR have not yet proven effective. Given the ubiquity of smartphones and the innovation of smartphone app platforms, additional study is warranted.
- Low rates of bystander CPR persist for women, children, and members of minority communities. Efforts to improve bystander response in these populations should be implemented and evaluated for effectiveness.
- Creating a culture of action is an important part of bystander response. More research is needed to understand what key drivers would influence bystanders to perform CPR and/or use an AED.
- Additional research is needed on cognitive aids to assist healthcare providers and teams managing OHCA and IHCA to improve resuscitation team performance.
- Although the value of immediate feedback (eg, team debriefing) and data-driven systems feedback is well established, specific high-yield components of that feedback have yet to be identified.
- More research is needed to better understand how to use technology to drive data and quality improvement both inside and outside of the hospital for cardiac arrest patients.

REFERENCES

1. Boutilier JJ, Brooks SC, Janmohamed A, Byers A, Buick JE, Zhan C, Schoellig AP, Cheskes S, Morrison LJ, Chan TCY; Rescu Epistry Investigators. Optimizing a drone network to deliver automated external defibrillators. *Circulation.* 2017;135:2454–2465. doi: 10.1161/CIRCULATIONAHA.116.026318
2. Cheskes S, Snobelen P, McLeod S, Brooks S, Vaillancourt C, Chan T, Dainty KN, Nolan M. AED on the fly: a drone delivery feasibility study for rural and remote out-of-hospital cardiac arrest [abstract 147]. *Circulation.* 2019;140:A147. doi:10.1161/circ.140.suppl_2.147

ARTICLE INFORMATION

The American Heart Association requests that this document be cited as follows: Berg KM, Cheng A, Panchal AR, Topjian AA, Aziz K, Bhanji F, Bigham BL, Hirsch KG, Hoover AV, Kurz MC, Levy A, Lin Y, Magid DJ, Mahgoub M, Peberdy MA, Rodriguez AJ, Sasson C, Lavonas EJ; on behalf of the Adult Basic and Advanced Life Support, Pediatric Basic and Advanced Life Support, Neonatal Life Support, and Resuscitation Education Science Writing Groups. Part 7: systems of care: 2020 American Heart Association Guidelines for Cardiopulmonary Resuscitation and Emergency Cardiovascular Care. *Circulation.* 2020;142(suppl 2):S580–S604. doi: 10.1161/CIR.0000000000000899

Acknowledgments

The authors thank Dr Monica Kleinman for her contributions.

Disclosures

Appendix 1. Writing Group Disclosures

Writing Group Member	Employment	Research Grant	Other Research Support	Speakers' Bureau/ Honoraria	Expert Witness	Ownership Interest	Consultant/ Advisory Board	Other
Katherine M. Berg	Beth Israel Deaconess Medical Center	NHLBI Grant K23 HL128814†	None	None	None	None	None	None
Khalid Aziz	University of Alberta (Canada)	None	None	None	None	None	None	University of Alberta (Professor of Pediatrics)†
Farhan Bhanji	McGill University (Canada)	None	None	None	None	None	None	None
Blair L. Bigham	McMaster University (Canada)	None	None	None	None	None	None	None
Adam Cheng	Alberta Children's Hospital (Canada)	None	None	None	None	None	None	None
Karen G. Hirsch	Stanford University	American Heart Association (cardiac arrest research)*	None	None	Stroke and TBI cases (not cardiac arrest)*	None	None	None
Amber V. Hoover	American Heart Association	None	None	None	None	None	None	None
Michael C. Kurz	University of Alabama at Birmingham	DOD (DSMB for Pre-Hospital Airway Control Trial [PACT])*; NIH (Co-PI for R21 examining mast-cell degranulation in OHCA)*	None	Zoll Medical Corp*	None	None	Zoll Circulation, Inc†	Zoll Circulation, Inc†
Eric J. Lavonas	Denver Health Emergency Medicine	BTG Pharmaceuticals (Denver Health (Dr Lavonas' employer) has research, call center, consulting, and teaching agreements with BTG Pharmaceuticals. BTG manufactures the digoxin antidote, DigiFab. Dr Lavonas does not receive bonus or incentive compensation, and these agreements involve an unrelated product. When these guidelines were developed, Dr Lavonas recused from discussions related to digoxin poisoning.)†	None	None	None	None	None	American Heart Association (Senior Science Editor)†
Arielle Levy	University of Montreal (Canada)	None	None	None	None	None	None	None
Yiqun Lin	Alberta Children's Hospital (Canada)	None	None	None	None	None	None	None
David J. Magid	University of Colorado	NIH†; NHLBI†; CMS†; AHA†	None	None	None	None	None	American Heart Association (Senior Science Editor)†
Melissa Mahgoub	American Heart Association	None	None	None	None	None	None	None
Ashish R. Panchal	The Ohio State University	None	None	None	None	None	None	None

(Continued)

Appendix 1. Continued

Writing Group Member	Employment	Research Grant	Other Research Support	Speakers' Bureau/ Honoraria	Expert Witness	Ownership Interest	Consultant/ Advisory Board	Other
Mary Ann Peberdy	Virginia Commonwealth University	None	None	None	None	None	None	None
Amber J. Rodriguez	American Heart Association	None	None	None	None	None	None	None
Comilla Sasson	American Heart Association	None	None	None	None	None	None	None
Alexis A. Topjian	The Children's Hospital of Philadelphia	NIH (POCCA trial site PI)*	None	None	None	None	None	None

This table represents the relationships of writing group members that may be perceived as actual or reasonably perceived conflicts of interest as reported on the Disclosure Questionnaire, which all members of the writing group are required to complete and submit. A relationship is considered to be "significant" if (a) the person receives $10 000 or more during any 12-month period, or 5% or more of the person's gross income; or (b) the person owns 5% or more of the voting stock or share of the entity, or owns $10 000 or more of the fair market value of the entity. A relationship is considered to be "modest" if it is less than "significant" under the preceding definition.

*Modest.

†Significant.

Appendix 2. Reviewer Disclosures

Reviewer	Employment	Research Grant	Other Research Support	Speakers' Bureau/ Honoraria	Expert Witness	Ownership Interest	Consultant/ Advisory Board	Other
Alix Carter	Dalhousie University (Canada)	Maritime Heart*	None	None	None	None	None	None
Henry Halperin	Johns Hopkins University	Zoll Medical†; NIH†	None	None	None	None	None	None
Jonathan Jui	Oregon Health and Science University	NIH*	None	None	None	None	None	None
Fred Severyn	Denver Health and Hospital Authority and University of Colorado Anschutz Medical Campus; University of Arkansas	None	None	None	None	None	None	None
Robert A. Swor	William Beaumont Hospital	None	None	None	None	None	None	None
Andrew H. Travers	Emergency Health Services (Canada)	None	None	None	None	None	None	None

This table represents the relationships of reviewers that may be perceived as actual or reasonably perceived conflicts of interest as reported on the Disclosure Questionnaire, which all reviewers are required to complete and submit. A relationship is considered to be "significant" if (a) the person receives $10 000 or more during any 12-month period, or 5% or more of the person's gross income; or (b) the person owns 5% or more of the voting stock or share of the entity, or owns $10 000 or more of the fair market value of the entity. A relationship is considered to be "modest" if it is less than "significant" under the preceding definition.

*Modest.

†Significant.